HOME HEALTH NURSING PRACTICE
Concepts & Application

HOME HEALTH NURSING PRACTICE
Concepts & Application

Robyn Rice, RN, MSN

Clinical Associate Professor
Barnes College of Nursing
The University of Missouri–St. Louis
St. Louis, Missouri

Home Health Clinical Nurse Specialist
Saint Anthony's Health Center
Alton, Illinois

Second Edition

with 95 illustrations

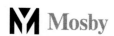 Mosby

St. Louis   Baltimore   Boston   Carlsbad   Chicago   Naples   New York   Philadelphia   Portland
London   Madrid   Mexico City   Singapore   Sydney   Tokyo   Toronto   Wiesbaden

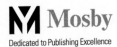

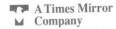

Vice President and Publisher: Nancy L. Coon
Executive Editor: N. Darlene Como
Senior Developmental Editor: Laurie Sparks
Project Manager: Deborah Vogel
Editing and Production: Carlisle Publishers Services
Designer: Pati Pye
Manufacturing Supervisor: Linda Ierardi

SECOND EDITION

Copyright © 1996 by Mosby-Year Book, Inc.

Previous edition copyrighted 1992

Printed in the United States of America
Composition by Carlisle Communications, Ltd.
Printing/binding by R. R. Donnelley & Sons Company

Mosby–Year Book, Inc.
11830 Westline Industrial Drive
St. Louis, Missouri 63146

Library of Congress Cataloging in Publication Data
Rice, Robyn.
    Home health nursing practice : concepts and application / Robyn
Rice -- 2nd ed.
      p. cm.
    Rev. ed. of: Home health nursing practice / [edited by] Robyn
Rice. c1992.
    Includes bibliographical references and index.
    ISBN 0-8151-7240-0 (pbk.)
    1. Home nursing. I. Title.
    [DNLM: 1. Home Care Services. WY 115 R495h 1995]
RT120.H65 1995
362.1'4--dc20
DNLM/DLC
for Library of Congress
                95-39774
                CIP

95 96 97 98 99 / 9 8 7 6 5 4 3 2 1

Contributors

Ellen Barker, RN, MSN, CNRN
President
Neuroscience Nursing Consultants
Newark, Delaware

Karen Balakas, RN, MSN
Clinical Associate Professor
Barnes College of Nursing
The University of Missouri–St. Louis
St. Louis, Missouri

Elizabeth A. Buck, RN, PhD
Professor
Jewish Hospital College of Nursing and Allied Health
St. Louis, Missouri

Jacquelyn M. Clement, RN, PhD
Associate Professor
School of Nursing
Southern Illinois University
Edwardsville, Illinois

Virginia Drake, RN, PhD
Associate Professor
Barnes College of Nursing
The University of Missouri–St. Louis
St. Louis, Missouri

Patricia Freed, RN, EdD
Instructor
Barnes College of Nursing
The University of Missouri–St. Louis
St. Louis, Missouri

Debra Haire-Joshu, RN, PhD
Research Associate Professor of Medicine
Diabetes Research and Training Center
Washington University School of Medicine
St. Louis, Missouri

Dorothy O. Hauk, RN, MSN
Psychiatric Clinical Nurse Specialist
The Visiting Nurse Association of Greater St. Louis
St. Louis, Missouri

Susan Heady, RN, PhD
Associate Professor
School of Nursing
Webster University
St. Louis, Missouri

Kathyrn A. Houston, RN, MSN
Geriatric Clinical Nurse Specialist
St. Louis University
St. Louis, Missouri

Diane Huntley, RNC, MS
Hospice Supervisor
HealthReach Hospice
Augustana, Maine

Irene Kalnins, RN, EdD
Associate Clinical Professor
School of Nursing
St. Louis University
St. Louis, Missouri

Carol A. Keene, PhD
Associate Professor and Chair of the Department
of Philosophical Studies
Southern Illinois University
Edwardsville, Illinois

Roberta Kordish, RN, MSN
Professional Nurse Associates, Inc.
Cleveland, Ohio

Annette M. Lynch, RN, MSN
Professional Nurse Associates, Inc.
Cleveland, Ohio

Troy McMullin, PharmD
Clinical Assistant Professor
St. Louis College of Pharmacy
St. Louis, Missouri

Laurie Rappl, PT
Embracing Concepts, Inc.
Rochester, New York

Robyn Rice, RN, MSN(R)
Clinical Associate Professor
Barnes College of Nursing
The University of Missouri–St. Louis
St. Louis, Missouri;
Home Health Clinical Nurse Specialist
Saint Anthony's Health Center
Alton, Illinois

David Ritchie, PharmD, BCPS
Assistant Professor of Pharmacy Practice
St. Louis College of Pharmacy
St. Louis, Missouri;
Clinical Pharmacist, Infectious Diseases
Barnes and Jewish Hospitals
St. Louis, Missouri

Jacalyn Wickline Ryberg, RN, MSN, CPN
Home Health Consultant
O'Fallon, Illinois

Anne Schappe, RN, MSN, MA
Clinical Associate Professor
Barnes College of Nursing
The University of Missouri–St. Louis
St. Louis, Missouri

Saundra J. Triplett, RN, MSN
Home Care Consultant
St. Louis, Missouri

Joanne P. Sheehan, RN, JD
Principal in Law Firm of
Friedman, Mellitz, and Newman
Fairfield, Connecticut

Dolores V. Smiley, RN, EdD
Associate Professor
School of Nursing
St. Louis University
St. Louis, Missouri

Gayle H. Sullivan, RN, JD
Medical Liability Consultant
Quality Assurance Associates, Inc.
Fairfield, Connecticut

Lori B. Watkins, RN, MSN
Intake Coordinator
Barnes Home IV Services
Barnes Hospital at Washington University
Medical Center
St. Louis, Missouri

Catherine A. White, RN, MSN
Neonatal Education Specialist
St. Louis Children's Hospital
St. Louis, Missouri

Laurel A. Wiersema, RN, MSN
Medical and Surgical Clinical Nurse Specialist
Barnes Hospital at Washington University
Medical Center
St. Louis, Missouri

Nancy Van Fleet Wilens, RN, MSN
Unit Leader
Johnston Bowman Health Center
Chicago, Illinois

Gail Wilkerson, RNCS, MSN
Geriatric Clinical Nurse Specialist
Barnes and Jewish Home Health Services
St. Louis, Missouri

Lenore R. Williams, RN, MSN
Professional Nurse Associates, Inc.
Cleveland, Ohio

Consultants

Arlene Bradford, RN, C, BA
Director of Mental Health Nursing
South Hills Health System
Home Health Agency
Homestead, Pennsylvania

Linda Boccialetti, RN
Pediatric Program Manager
VNA Health Care, Inc.
Waterbury, Connecticut

Bob Dehaemers, RN, MA
Clinical Operations Specialist
Nursefinders
Arlington, Texas

Loretta M. Chillemi, BS, MS, MSN
Clinical Nursing Supervisor
VNA Health Care, Inc.
Waterbury, Connecticut

Mary Lou Ende, RN, MNEd
Director of Pediatric/Maternal-Child Nursing
South Hills Health System
Home Health Agency
Homestead, Pennsylvania

Lisa A. Gorski, MS, RNC
Clinical Nurse Specialist
Franciscan Home Health, Inc.
Milwaukee, Wisconsin

Cheryl A. Grande, RN, BSN
Staff Nurse
VNA Health Care, Inc.
Waterbury, Connecticut

Suzanne Hatch, RN, BSN, MEd
Staff Development Coordinator
Lee Visiting Nurse Association, Inc.
Lee, Massachusetts

Maxine Reed Johnson, RN, BSN
Home Health Nurse
Barnes Home Health Department
Barnes Hospital at Washington University
Medical Center
St. Louis, Missouri

Irene Kalnins, RN, EdD
Associate Professor
School of Nursing
St. Louis University
St. Louis, Missouri

Marilee Kuhrik, RN, MSN
Assistant Professor
Jewish Hospital College of Nursing and Allied Health
St. Louis, Missouri

Lori Neave, RN
IV Coordinator
VNA Health Care, Inc.
Waterbury, Connecticut

Katherine Porpora, RN, MSN
Private Practice, Pediatric Home Care
Westchester, New York

Joan Quint Randall, RN, MS
VNA Home Health Systems
Orange, California

Kate Salvato, RNC, BSN
Provider Relations Coordinator
Visiting Nurse Association of Delaware
New Castle, Delaware

Carla Scheffert, RN
Home Health Consultant
Minneapolis, Minnesota

George F. Schuster, RN, DNSc
Associate Professor
College of Nursing
University of New Mexico
Albuquerque, New Mexico

Janet A. Sipple, RN, EdD
Associate Professor and Associate Dean
(Undergraduate)
Barnes College of Nursing
The University of Missouri–St. Louis
St. Louis, Missouri

Gale A. Spencer, PhD, RN
Director, Center for Nursing Research
Decker School of Nursing
Binghamton University
Binghamton, New York

Marie Sweeney, RN, MSN
Psychiatric Clinical Nurse Specialist
VNA Health Care, Inc.
Waterbury, Connecticut

Dennis Tureson, CRTT, RRT
Clinical Manager
Aequitron Medical, Inc.
Minneapolis, Minnesota

Pamela Becker Weilitz, RNCS, MSN(R)
Manager of Nursing Care Delivery
Barnes and Jewish Hospitals
St. Louis, Missouri

For Jack

About the Author

Robyn Rice, RN, MSN, is a clinician, educator, author, and nurse advocate. She has worked in home care for more than 10 years specializing in high-tech home health services. Ms. Rice has authored *Handbook of Home Health Nursing Procedures* and *Manual of Home Health Nursing Procedures*, as well as numerous chapters and articles. She serves on the editorial board for the *Journal of Home Health Care Nursing* and is an item writer for the ANCC Home Health Nursing Certification Examination.

Ms. Rice has presented numerous workshops and seminars at local, state, and national levels. She was the keynote speaker for the state of Alaska's first home care conference in 1993. She has also lectured on infection control in the home for the Missouri League of Nursing and on home health topics at a national level for Mosby and American Nursing Development.

At present, Ms. Rice is a clinical associate professor at Barnes College of Nursing at the University of Missouri–St. Louis, where she developed the working model for the senior home health student clinical practicum, and serves as a home health clinical nurse specialist for Saint Anthony's Health Center in Alton, Illinois. She is currently pursuing her doctorate in public policy at St. Louis University, St. Louis.

Preface

As a home health clinical nurse specialist for more than 10 years, I have been struck by the tremendous growth of home care. Unfortunately, this growth has not always been accompanied with adequate learning resources for home health nurses. Because there is so much change occurring in home care, the literature quickly falls behind the times.

The second edition of *Home Health Nursing Practice: Concepts & Application* was designed to meet current learning needs of practicing home health nurses. Student nurses and registered nurses considering entering home care will also benefit from the book. Nurses involved in administrative and educational aspects of agency operation will find it a useful resource for orientation and clinical support purposes.

The special challenges of the home care setting call for nurses to be self-directed professionals with a concern for quality patient care. This book was written to give guidance and vision of practice to those nurses choosing to work in home health. Material in the second edition has been completely updated with many new chapters added to meet the growing clinical practice needs of field staff.

The book is organized into four major parts. Part I, Concepts of Home Health Nursing, reviews concepts pertinent to general nursing practice within the home milieu. Discussions include role preparation and implementation, staff safety concerns, recommendations for working with student nurses, developing the plan of care, Medicare-based documentation guidelines, infection control measure, and quality care concerns.

In the second edition, several new chapters have been added to Part I. Nurses who can articulate their role drive clinical policy; therefore, Chapter 2, Understanding Home Health Care: Applying Theory to Clinical Practice, addresses the purpose of home health and the role of the home health nurse. Chapter 5, Patient Education in the Home, discusses issues of health teaching for patients across the lifespan. Chapter 7, Legal and Ethical

Issues in Home Care, provides sound clinical practice guidelines for nurses working in the sometimes unpredictable environment of the home milieu. Chapter 8, Case Management and Leadership Strategies for Home Health Nurses, discusses issues such as case load organization, collaborating with the multidisciplinary team, clinical leadership strategies such as committee work, and care path development.

Part II, Clinical Application, discusses patients typically visited in the home. Nursing interventions for patients with chronic obstructive pulmonary disease, congestive heart failure, diabetes, bowel and bladder dysfunction, and AIDS are discussed, as well as caregiving concerns related to wound care and home rehabilitation. High-technology care, such as home mechanical ventilation and home IV therapy, are also included. A new chapter, The Patient with Neurological Dysfunction, provides clinical guidelines for patients with Alzheimer's disease, cerebral vascular accident, and multiple sclerosis. Part II provides a detailed discussion of the role of the home medical equipment vendor and the equipment and products available for home use. Descriptions of commonly used home care products and equipment will assist the reader to use them appropriately and effectively. (The description of a particular product or piece of equipment is not intended to be an endorsement on the part of the author or publisher.) To reinforce the importance of patient teaching, I have highlighted patient education guidelines throughout the clinical chapters.

Part III, Special Clinical Issues, addresses special patient populations the home health nurse is likely to encounter. Individual chapters deal with pediatric, geriatric, mental health, and hospice patients. Topics include family role theory and parent support guidelines, clinical recommendations for patients experiencing schizophrenia or acute depression, physiological changes associated with aging and associated nursing interventions, in addition to spiritual as well as palliative care issues. A new chapter on the postpartum patient provides excellent assessment and care guidelines for the newborn.

Part IV, Future Trends, considers the health care needs of the patients of tomorrow; societal responsibility in the allocation of health care resources; the ethical, legal, and economic issues likely to influence home health nursing practice; and the need for the home health nurse to deal effectively with changes in health care delivery.

Two points should be noted. First, the term *caregiver* is used throughout the book to denote the patient's family, friend, or significant other who may assist the patient and the nurse in carrying out the plan of care. Although most patients live at home with their families, some patients receive care and support from other sources. For this reason, I chose to use the term *caregiver* to encompass the services of all who provide assistance. Second, as a primary component of patient education, clean technique is commonly taught in the home setting today. As a standard of practice, home health nurses should perform procedures using aseptic technique whenever possible. Infection control precautions should

provide safety for the patient, caregiver, and home care team. The Centers for Disease Control and Prevention is set to revise Universal Precautions in 1996. I advise nurses to implement these changes when they are published.

The information in this book will assist home health nurses in caring for patients with different educational, social, economic, and cultural backgrounds. In addition, my intent is that the book be used to increase the nurse's understanding of clinical issues and high technology related to patient care, the importance of working with caregivers or family members, the purpose and use of a multidisciplinary approach, the impact of patient education in fostering self-care management, and the basics of Medicare regulations governing reimbursement for services rendered. I wrote the book to inspire autonomy of nursing practice and creative, new ways of thinking. I sincerely hope that the information and recommendations in this book be integrated with a sensitivity to the special concerns and special privileges that home health nursing practice provides.

Robyn Rice

Acknowledgments

Acknowledgments present opportunities to be self-indulgent with thank yous. *My thank yous are many and heart felt.*

First, I wish to thank my husband, Jack, for his support of this project. Jack, I just really could not have done it without you!

Second, I wish to thank my mother, Tommie Sue Thorpe, and the rest of my family—including the Rices—for understanding that my work takes up a lot of my time. I love them all.

I think a librarian is the noblest profession. I wish to thank Beth Carlin, our librarian at Barnes, for helping me with the numerous literature searches required for this project.

Writing is a lonely process. There is some risk taking that goes along with stepping away from the crowd and being different. I truly believe, however, that if we do not take the time to write down our vision and record our history, it will be lost; therefore, it was very important to me to do the *best second edition* possible. I realized very quickly that the work involved would be tremendous and time consuming. I wish to thank Dean Shirley Martin and Dr. Janet Sipple for granting me an academic leave of absence from the university so that I could devote my complete attention to this project. Their support was greatly appreciated.

I was allowed permission to reproduce numerous forms and pictures from educational centers and home health agencies. I would like to thank and acknowledge them in alphabetical order:

American Nursing Development of Maryville, Maryville, Illinois;

Barnes College of Nursing at the University of Missouri-St. Louis, St. Louis, Missouri;

Barnes Home Health Department, St. Louis, Missouri;

Ruth Constant and Associates, Beaumont, Texas;

DePaul Hospital Home Health Department, St. Louis, Missouri;

Lincoln-Lancaster Public Health Department, Omaha, Nebraska;

Methodist Hospital Home Health Department, Omaha, Nebraska;

The Home Health Department at Gila Regional Medical Center, Silver City, New Mexico;

The Home Health Department at Saint Anthony's Health Center, Alton, Ilinois;

The Family Services and Visiting Nurse Association, Alton, Illinois;

The Visiting Nurse Association of Greater St. Louis, St. Louis, Missouri.

I wish to thank the consultants who lent their special expertise to this project. Their comments and suggestions were very helpful in fine-tuning the manuscript.

I wish to thank my Editor, Darlene Como, and Senior Developmental Editor, Laurie Sparks, at Mosby for their assistance in the development of this manuscript. On behalf of myself and the chapter contributors, I especially wish to thank Darlene and Laurie for allowing us the freedom to write from our hearts.

Last, but not least, I wish to thank the chapter contributors. They all worked very hard to make this second edition a wonderful book. It was my honor to work with each of them in bringing this project to fruition. On a professional level, I found the chapter contributors to be visionaries and leaders in health care. On a personal level, I found them to be warm and supportive people. *They are the caring kind. . .*

Contents

PART

I Concepts of Home Health Nursing

1 Historical Perspectives

Robyn Rice and *Dolores V. Smiley*

The advent and growth of the home care industry has resulted from public demand for quality health care and societal pressure for cost containment of medical services. Diagnostic-related groups (DRGs) were legislated in the 1980s to control cost inflation in the health care system.[2] As a result, many patients are now discharged from the hospital into the home "sicker and quicker." Home health nursing continues to evolve within this setting, providing care for patients with complex and diverse health care needs.

Home health nursing consists of principles of nursing practice that are both old and new. Although intricately bound to government policy regulating reimbursement of services, home health nursing blends concepts of community health nursing with high-technology, disease-focused care. The evolution and continued development of home health nursing is best understood by exploring historical, societal, and governmental regulatory events that have shaped this special kind of nursing practice.

HISTORICAL PERSPECTIVES

The following chronology outlines significant events in understanding the history of home care. Home care services have their roots in visits made to the sick poor by religious orders during the late 1700s.[13] In 1796 the Boston Dispensary was one of the first to provide home care in the United States.[12] A founding principle of the Boston Dispensary reveals its home health care philosophy:[7] "The sick, without being pained by separation from their families, may be attended and relieved at home."

The first visiting nurses in America were called *district nurses,* a British term credited to Florence Nightingale (1820-1910) for nurses who cared for the sick at home (Figure 1-1). In the late 1800s home nursing services were organized and administered by laypersons. These agencies provided unlicensed, skilled nursing care and taught cleanliness and home care techniques to the ill and their families. In 1877 the Women's Branch of the New York City Mission was the first group to employ a graduate nurse to care for the sick at home.

A voluntary agency was established in 1885 in Buffalo, New York, to provide home nursing care. In 1886 other voluntary agencies providing patients with similar home health care services emerged in Boston and Philadelphia.[13] These would later become Visiting Nurse Associations (VNAs).

In 1893 the Henry Street Settlement House in New York City was established by Lillian Wald and Mary Brewster to provide care for the sick and poor.[10] Home health care nurses were employed to tend the health needs of tenement residents (Figure 1-2).

In 1898 graduate nurses were hired by the Los Angeles County Health Department to make visits to the sick poor.[13] This was the first governmental health department to set up such services. The term *public health nurse* was subsequently coined.

By 1890 there were 21 VNAs in the United States, most of them employing only one nurse. Late in the nineteenth century, VNAs increased in number. The growing social consciousness and the increasing wealth of the United States to fund such services were contributing factors.[13] In 1909 some

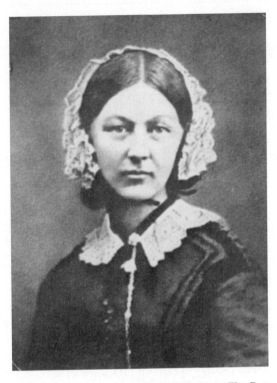

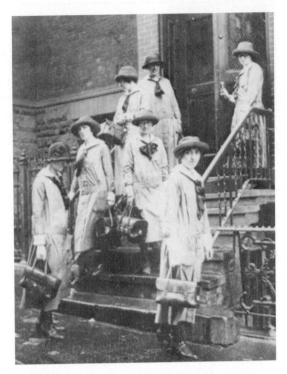

Figure 1-1 Florence Nightingale. (Courtesy The Bettman Archive.)

Figure 1-2 Nurses at the Henry Street Settlement House, early 1900s. (Courtesy The Bettman Archive.)

home care services were covered for policyholders of Metropolitan Life Insurance in New York City.[10]

With the dawn of the 1900s the Frontier Nursing Services were established in rural Kentucky by Mary Breckinridge. Their purpose was to provide home care to rural mountain people (Figure 1-3). Home health nursing continued to serve urban needs as well (Figure 1-4).

The number of home care agencies grew during World War II as home visits by physicians began to decline.[9] After World War II, home care services developed at an ever-increasing rate, with tremendous growth experienced by nonprofit or"voluntary" home health agencies such as the VNAs as well as public health departments.[9] Today the home care industry continues to grow as the delivery of patient care and scope of services reflect societal demands for cost-effective, quality health care available to all Americans.

SOCIAL PERSPECTIVES

The following chronology describes social factors that influenced home care. Before the 1960s home care was viewed as a community service. While the focus of community and public health nursing was one of health promotion, home health nursing focused on health restoration and caring for the sick. Agencies such as the VNAs established the fundamentals of bringing health care services into homes. The essential mission of these agencies was to provide quality home care to all patients without regard for their ability to pay for services. Government intervention, private foundations and endowments, and other organizations such as the United Way made agency operation possible.

In the mid-1960s a growing elderly population, advances in medical technology, and public demand for universal access to the health care system had tremendous influence on the home care

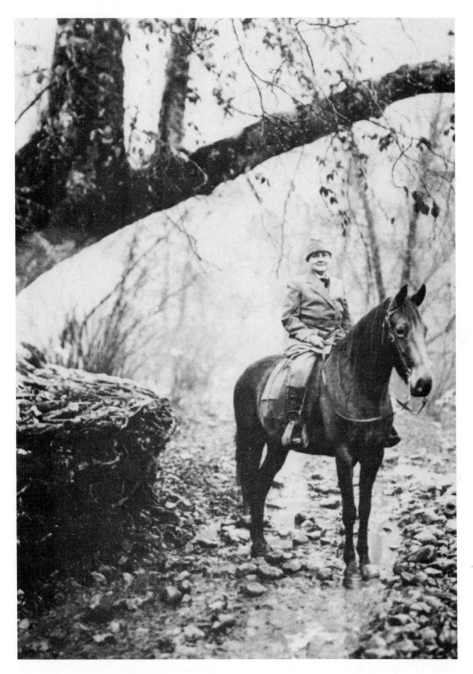

Figure 1-3 Mary Breckinridge, founder of Frontier Nursing Services. (Courtesy Frontier Nursing Services, Wendover, Ky.)

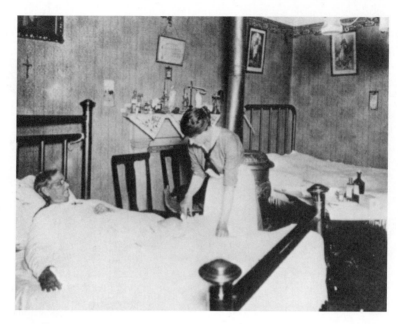

Figure 1-4 The visiting nurse in the patient's home. (Courtesy Visiting Nurse Association of Greater St Louis.)

industry. There were more patients to be seen and fewer resources to cover the cost of visits.

Medicare and Medicaid, public managed care systems, were legislated in 1965 in response to societal pressures that demanded easily accessible health care for the elderly, poor, and mentally ill. Medicare is a federal program and Medicaid is a state program.

Under Medicare, home health care programs were established in 1966. Since the enactment of Medicare, Medicare-certified home health agencies have generated a significant portion of their income from care provided to Medicare beneficiaries. Medicare home health agency benefit payments have grown from $4.8 billion in fiscal year 1992 to $7.1 billion in 1993, an increase of nearly 48%.[5] Of note, medicare remains the largest single payer of home care services.[11]

Medicare is Title XVIII of the Social Security Act. Although eligibility requirements continue to broaden, it ensures federally financed health insurance for those over age 65 as covered by Social Security or the Railroad System. Administered initially by the Bureau of Insurance in the Department of Health, Education, and Welfare (DHEW), Medicare has been managed by the Health Care Financing Administration (HCFA) in the Department of Health and Human Services (DHHS) since 1978.

Medicare has two parts: A and B. Part A reimburses hospital or posthospital costs (including home health care) and is funded by Social Security revenues. Part B is primarily funded by the insured's monthly premiums and covers physician services, laboratory services, medical equipment and supplies, speech and physical therapy, and a variety of other health services and supplies.[6]

Currently, to receive Medicare coverage for home health services, patients must have (1) homebound status, (2) a need for part-time or intermittent skilled care (services may not be duplicated; e.g., SN and therapists cannot perform the same services), and (3) a medically reasonable and necessary need for treatment with (4) a plan of care authorized by a physician. Medicare eligibility criteria for coverage are reviewed in Chapter 4.

Most home health services under Medicare are subject to claims reviews by intermediaries, private insurance companies approved by Medicare as claims processors. Intermediaries, located in certain geographical regions across the country, are under contract to the government. Their purpose is to ensure appropriate disbursement of Medicare monies to home health agencies operating within their geographical region. Intermediaries accomplish this purpose by reviewing the delivery of home care services using government guidelines outlined in the Home Health Insurance Manual, Publication Number 11 (HIM-11). Periodic on-site home health agency inspection to examine patient care, documentation, and operation is also a part of the review. A major intermediary is Blue Cross.

Carriers such as Blue Shield process claims for services covered under Medicare Part B. Under Medicare Part B, payments are made to the providers or beneficiaries. Carriers determine reimbursement using "customary and prevailing charges," whereas intermediaries determine reimbursement based on "reasonable cost," both defined by the HIM-11.[7] Cited as "the bible of home health," the HIM-11 and the HCFA Federal Register provide stringent Medicare guidelines and updates for reimbursement, as well as delineating the scope of home health services. The boxes on the following pages provide excerpts from these publications.[6]

Medicaid and other government sources along with third-party payers provide additional coverage for home health services. Medicaid was legislated by Title XIX of the Social Security Act providing health care to low-income populations. Medicare provides coverage for elderly adults, while Medicaid frequently subsidizes health care of needy children.[13]

Administered by the states, Medicaid monies are subsidized by state and federal governments. Medicaid covers skilled and unskilled home health services as directed by a physician. Medicaid limits some of the home health services normally provided under Medicare. It becomes the primary payment source when the patient is no longer eligible for Medicare. Medicaid coverage of home health services varies from state to state.

Title III of the Older American Act (OAA) and Title XX (Grant-In-Aid), legislated in the 1960s and 1970s, also subsidize home health services but to a more limited degree than Medicare/Medicaid. Title III of the OAA and Title XX are designed to subsidize home health services for the elderly and for low-income populations. Both of these programs are directed toward health restoration and self-care management at home.[3]

HIM-11—COVERAGE OF SERVICES

Home health agency

A home health agency is a public agency or private organization, or a subdivision of such an agency or organization, which meets the following requirements:

A. It is primarily engaged in providing skilled nursing services and other therapeutic services, such as physical, speech, or occupational therapy, medical social services, and home health aide services. A public or voluntary nonprofit health agency may qualify by:
   1. Furnishing both skilled nursing and at least one other therapeutic service directly to patients, or
   2. Furnishing directly either skilled nursing services or at least one other therapeutic service and having arrangements with another public or voluntary nonprofit agency to furnish the services which it does not provide directly.

A proprietary agency can qualify only by providing directly both skilled nursing services and at least one other therapeutic service.

B. It has policies established by a professional group associated with the agency or organization (including at least one physician and at least one registered professional nurse) to govern the services, and provides for supervision of such services by a physician or a registered professional nurse.
C. It maintains clinical records on all patients.
D. It is licensed in accordance with State or local law or is approved by the State or local licensing agency as meeting the licensing standards (where State or local law provides for the licensing of such agencies or organizations).
E. It meets other conditions found by the Secretary of Health, Education, and Welfare to be necessary for health and safety.

From Health Care Financing Administration: *Home Health Insurance Manual,* Pub No 11 -Thru T273, Rev 3/95, Washington DC, 1995, US Department of Health and Human Services.

Home health services are viewed as financially advantageous when compared with institutional (hospital) care. For example, according to a report published by The National Association for Home Care (NAHC), monthly costs of health care for a

---

HCFA: FEDERAL REGISTER DEFINITIONS PERTINENT TO HOME CARE

Branch office means a location or site from which a home health agency provides services within a portion of the total geographic area served by the parent agency. The branch office is part of the home health agency and is located sufficiently close to share administration, supervision, and services in a manner that renders it unnecessary for the branch independently to meet the conditions of participation as a home health agency.

Clinical note means a notation of a contact with a patient that is written and dated by a member of the health team, and that describes signs and symptoms, treatment and drugs administered and the patient's reaction, and any changes in physical or emotional condition.

HHA stands for home health agency.

Nonprofit agency means an agency exempt from Federal income taxation under section 501 of the Internal Revenue Code of 1954.

Parent home health agency means the agency that develops and maintains administrative controls of subunits and/or branch offices.

Primary home health agency means the agency that is responsible for the services furnished to patients and for implementation of the plan of care.

Progress note means a written notation, dated and signed by a member of the health team, that summarizes facts about care furnished and the patient's response during a given period of time.

Proprietary agency means a private profit-making agency licensed by the State.

Public agency means an agency operated by a State or local government.

Subdivision means a component of a multi-function health agency, such as the home care department of a hospital or the nursing division of a health department, which independently meets the conditions of participation for HHAs. A subdivision that has subunits or branch offices is considered a parent agency.

Subunit means a semi-autonomous organization that:

1. Serves patients in a geographic area different from that of the parent agency; and
2. Must independently meet the conditions of participation for HHAs because it is too far from the parent agency to share administration, supervision, and services on a daily basis.

Summary report means the compilation of the pertinent factors of a patient's clinical notes and progress notes that is submitted to the patient's physician.

Supervision means authoritative procedural guidance by a qualified person for the accomplishment of a function or activity.

From Health Care Financing Administration: *Home Health Insurance Manual,* Pub No 11 -Thru T273, Rev 3/95, Washington DC, 1995, US Department of Health and Human Services.

---

ventilator-dependent patient run approximately $21,570 in the hospital setting as opposed to $7,050 in the home setting.[11] In this case, home health services represent a monthly dollar savings of $14,520.

A contrary view of this savings is held by some experts who maintain that home health care will eventually cost the government more because of increased participation.[4,10,11] There may be some truth to this belief. According to HCFA, over 3 million persons were projected to receive reimbursable home health services under Medicare and Medicaid during 1993.[5] In addition, the real costs of providing home care may well go beyond direct financial costs. Real costs include human and in-

direct costs of home care. The human costs include the psychosocial, physical, and health burden borne by patients/caregivers who utilize home health services.[14] Indirect costs include medications, respite services, health of the caregiver, family stability, and psychosocial burden in providing home care.[14] All things considered, the overall savings in keeping the patient at home appears greater and more beneficial to society than unnecessary and preventable hospitalizations.[4,10,14]

Along with government monies came regulations and public policy-making that changed the nature of the home care industry. As the following sections demonstrate, this also influenced home health nursing practice.

HCFA: DUTIES OF HOME HEALTH PERSONNEL

Duties of the physician. The physician reviews and directs the plan of care. The plan of care is reviewed by the attending physician as often as the severity of the patient's condition requires, but at least once every 62 days.

Duties of the registered nurse. The registered nurse makes the initial evaluation visit, regularly reevaluates the patient's nursing needs, initiates the plan of care and necessary revisions, provides those services requiring substantial and specialized nursing skill, initiates appropriate preventive and rehabilitative nursing procedures, prepares clinical and progress notes, coordinates services, informs the physician and other personnel of changes in the patient's condition and needs, counsels the patient and family in meeting nursing and related needs, participates in inservice programs, and supervises and teaches other nursing personnel.

Duties of the licensed practical nurse. The licensed practical nurse furnishes services in accordance with agency policies, prepares clinical and progress notes, assists the physician and registered nurse in performing specialized procedures, prepares equipment and materials for treatments observing aseptic technique as required, and assists the patient in learning appropriate self-care techniques.

Duties of the therapist. The qualified therapist assists the physician in evaluating level of function, helps develop the plan of care (revising as necessary), prepares clinical and progress notes, advises and consults with the family and other agency personnel, and participates in inservice programs.

Duties of the medical social worker. The social worker assists the physician and other team members in understanding the significant social and emotional factors related to the health problems, participates in the development of the plan of care, prepares clinical and progress notes, works with the family, uses appropriate community resources, participates in discharge planning and inservice programs, and acts as a consultant to other agency personnel.

Duties of the home health aide. The certified home health aide is assigned to a particular patient by a registered nurse. Written instructions for patient care are prepared by a registered nurse or therapist as appropriate. The certified home health aide participates in observation, reporting and documentation of patient status and the care or service furnished; reads and records temperature, pulse and respiration; uses basic infection control procedures; is knowledgeable of basic elements of body functioning and changes in body function that must be reported to an aide's supervisor; maintains a clean, safe and healthy environment; recognizes emergencies and knowledge of emergency procedures; is knowledgeable of the physical, emotional and developmental needs of and ways to work with the populations served by the HHA, including the need for respect for the patient, his or her privacy and his or her property; utilizes appropriate and safe techniques in personal hygiene and grooming that include (a) bed bath, (b) sponge, tub or shower bath, (c) shampoo, sink, tub or bed, (d) nail and skin care, (e) oral hygiene, and (f) toileting and elimination; uses safe transfer techniques and ambulation; uses normal range of motion and positioning; is knowledgeable of adequate nutrition and fluid intake; and performs any other task that the HHA may choose to have the home health aide perform.

From Health Care Financing Administration: *Home Health Insurance Manual,* Pub No 11 -Thru T273, Rev 3/95, Washington DC, 1995, US Department of Health and Human Services.

THE IMPACT OF GOVERNMENT REGULATIONS AND PUBLIC POLICY ON HOME CARE

The following chronology describes government regulatory and public policy issues that influenced home care and home health nursing. Historically, home care has been synonymous with nursing. As a result, patient care outside the hospital was strongly influenced, managed, and controlled by nurses. Before the enactment of the Medicare program, the emphasis of care was focused on health promotion and restoration therapies. During the 1960s this would change.

Although home care needs are viewed as primarily nursing in nature, the American Medical Association insisted on a medical framework that directs home health services in return for lending support to the Medicare program.[9] As a result the government mandated physician certification as a requirement for all Medicare services, including home health.[9] Therefore home care beneficiaries (patients) were assigned to the care of a physician, with the plan of care established and reviewed by

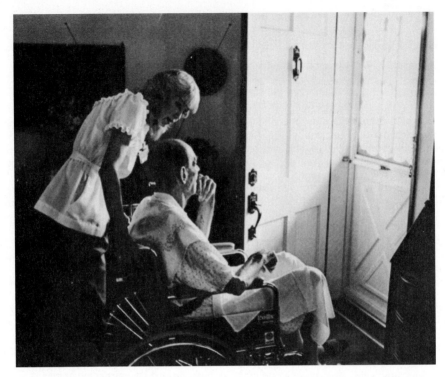

Figure 1-5 The hospice nurse offers a ray of sunshine. (Courtesy Anne Allen.)

the physician. Disease and disability, with an increasing emphasis upon home technology in service delivery, became fundamental to the plan of care. Consequently, traditional home care nursing was brought under the auspices of medicine. As a result the primary focus of home health nursing practice is now directed toward restorative, rehabilitative, and palliative (hospice) therapies (Figure 1-5). At present, health promotional behaviors are primarily viewed as a consequence of care as influenced by government regulations for reimbursement of home visits. Chapter 4 discusses current Medicare documentation guidelines for reimbursement of home health services.

Government regulation of health care continues to be felt throughout the home care industry. The Omnibus Budget Reconciliation Act (OBRA) removed a prior 3-day hospitalization stay requirement and provided reimbursement for increased numbers of visits, financing home health as a practical alternative to inpatient hospital care.[3] Consequently, proprietary agencies increased their participation in Medicare-reimbursed home health care services. In 1985 new summary forms appeared from Medicare—HCFA 485, 486, 487, and 488—as a means of providing documentation guidelines for reimbursement and quality control. With electronic billing the 486 is now being phased out. Reorganization and restructuring of home health agencies such as the development of quality patient care programs occurred.

As described, the arrival of diagnostic-related groups in the 1980s had far-reaching effects on the growth of the home care industry. DRGs are determined by medical diagnosis, extent of illness, and average length of stay for a specified illness, along with other statistical data.[2] As a result of the prospective payment system (PPS) for DRGs, hospitals are awarded predetermined amounts of money for patient care. In terms of financial gain, it remains in the hospital's interest to facilitate early discharge. Increased referrals to home health services resulted. In response to this growing home care population, home health agencies ex-

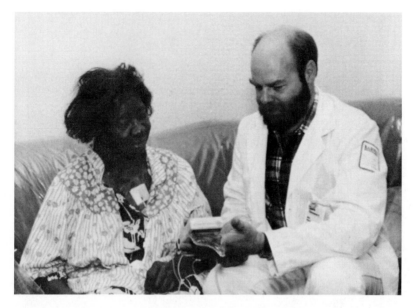

Figure 1-6 Intravenous therapy in the home. (Courtesy Barnes Hospital, St Louis.)

panded staff, resources, and technological services. Home care—traditionally nonproprietary—was now becoming a big business,[9] a growing and very competitive business.

In the mid-1980s major growth in the home care industry was experienced by proprietary agencies and hospital-based home care departments that could provide a vast array of services, such as respiratory, home medical equipment, and pharmacy departments, and whose financial resources could withstand Medicare regulations and public policy making.[10] Traditional home care agencies such as the VNAs that provided many free visits continued to inherit the indigent patient population, while experiencing a loss of "paying" patients to these proprietary and hospital-based agencies. It is believed that the current decline in voluntary or nonprofit agencies is related to an inability to compete with the tremendous resources and facilities of hospital-based agencies, along with difficulties in adhering to the numerous Medicare and state regulations.[10] However, the quality of VNA services and their dedication to their communities continue to be well respected and much emulated.

Federal regulations in the late 1980s and early 1990s mandated new requirements for quality control and expanded the coverage of home health services. Home health aide training and competency requirements, the establishment of a state home health hotline for patient complaints, and an increase in Medicare hospice and home intravenous therapy programs (Figure 1-6) resulted. A federal requirement for advance directives that specify patient/caregiver wishes regarding durable power of attorney for health care, as well as living will requests, occurred.

As related to Medicare regulations for reimbursement of home health services, the majority of patients seen in home health are elderly (Figure 1-7). However, in the 1990s postpartum and pediatric home health services have also grown (Figure 1-8). Mental health services, assisted living programs, homemaker services, maternal-child programs, and related community and traditional public health services are also current trends in marketing strategies. According to the most recent statistics from NAHC, as of 1994 there were a total of 15,027 home care agencies in the United States.[11] This number consisted of 7521 Medicare-certified home health agencies; 1459 Medicare-certified hospices; and 6047 home health agencies, home care aide organizations, and hospices that did not participate in Medicare.[11]

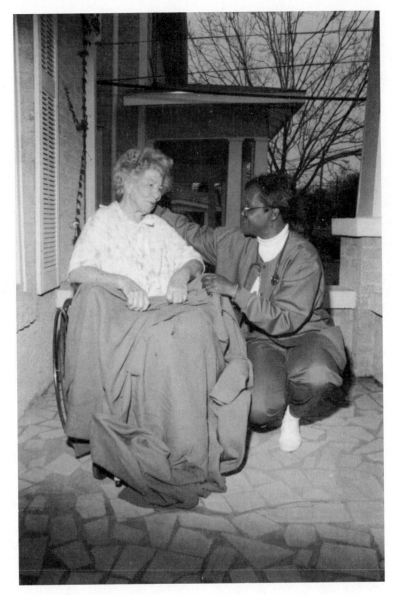

Figure 1-7 Caring for the older adult. (Courtesy Ruth Constant and Associates, Beaumont Home Health Services, Inc., Beaumont, Tex.)

Government regulations and public policy making continue to affect the home care industry and, ultimately, home health nurses. For example, the Omnibus Reconciliation Act of 1987 also required that HCFA implement a demonstration project to test prospective payment as a means for reimbursing Medicare-certified home health agencies for the services they provide. Prospective payment trials are now ongoing and are expected to end in 1998.[6] The trials will determine whether prospective payment is preferable to the current reimbursement system.

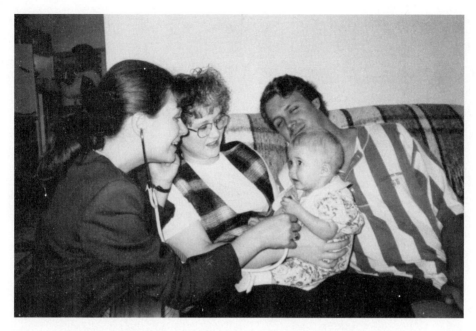

Figure 1-8 Pediatric nurse caring for the family. (Courtesy The Family Services and Visiting Nurse Association of Alton, Ill.)

Reimbursement of home health services currently occurs through a cost-based, retrospective payment system. Prospective payment entails setting a rate or a set of rates for a specific amount of service (e.g., a skilled nursing visit, or an entire episode of home health care) that is known before the service is provided.[6] Potential advantages of a prospective payment system include a reduction in administrative and staff burden in processing lengthy claims and excessive paperwork, both notorious to home care. In addition, the program allows home health agencies to retain profits generated by increases in efficiency.[6] Potential disadvantages that a prospective payment system may have for home health nurses may include an underutilization of services as home health agencies are driven to maximize profit.

The physician's role in managing home care and hospice patients is now recognized in economic terms by Medicare. As of 1995, physicians will receive some reimbursement for care plan oversight services for certain home care and hospice patients under Medicare Part B physician payment provisions.[12] The 1990s will likely see a consolidation of home care agencies into managed care systems as discussed in Chapter 8.[4]

The 1990s also reflect changes in the fundamentals of home health nursing practice. Although there is lively debate in academia regarding where home health fits into nursing curriculum, schools of nursing are increasing their emphasis upon home visits in curriculum planning. This is viewed as important in preparing students for the realities of nursing practice in the twenty-first century (Figure 1-9). Chapter 3 describes the process of working with student nurses in home health agencies. In 1993 the American Nurse's Credentialing Center (ANCC) administered the first examination recognizing home health nursing as a specialty practice, a specialty practice that blends with, yet is distinct from, community and public health nursing. The American Nurse's Association has also established standards of care for home health nursing practice.[1]

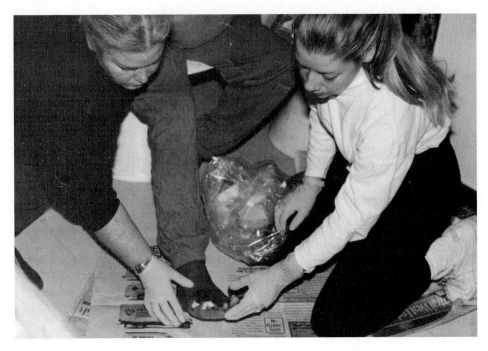

Figure 1-9 Working with student nurses in home care. (Courtesy Robyn Rice.)

As described in this chapter, historical, social, and government regulatory demands for alternative health care delivery systems have resulted in a renaissance of nursing care within the patient's environment. It is also clear that home health nursing practice will continue to evolve and be shaped by (1) increased patient acuity levels at home, (2) increased medical technology use outside the hospital, (3) social and economic restructuring of health care services, (4) the tremendous variation of patient problems when health care needs are managed at home, and (5) home health nurses, endeavors to maximize the quality of patient care within the home milieu.

CONTEMPORARY HOME HEALTH NURSING: A PHILOSOPHY OF PRACTICE

Home health nursing is the delivery of quality nursing care to patients in their home environment; it is provided on an intermittent or part-time basis. The patient's caregiver or family and home environment (which includes community resources) are viewed as critical elements of a successful plan of care. Therefore a focus upon a holistic assessment of patient/caregiver needs within the home milieu is emphasized.

Principles of home health nursing practice are directed toward providing cost-effective, quality health care in a setting that is often more conducive to health restoration and patient contentment than the hospital setting. It is recognized that patient/caregiver cooperation and self-determination for optimal health or best level of functioning are important to achieving successful self-care management at home.

Furthermore, home health nursing practice should reflect the current state of knowledge in the field of patient care. Individual state Nurse Practice Acts dictate the activities that nurses may legally carry out in the home. Agency policy and procedures and standards of care will also influence the delivery of patient care, as will the availability of resources such as equipment, supplies, funding, and patient family systems.[5]

Quality patient care is accomplished through a multidisciplinary approach whereby home health nurses, as case managers, orchestrate the plan of care. The patient care plan or clinical pathway, based on the nursing process of assessing, diagnosing, planning, implementing, and evaluating, is directed toward:

- Providing health restorative, rehabilitative, and palliative (hospice) therapies; health promotional behaviors are viewed as a very important consequence of these therapies.
- Educating the patient/caregiver about the illness or disability and mutually identified health care needs; recommendations to promote optimal health or best level of functioning and self-care management follow.
- Developing patient/caregiver competence, decision making, and judgment in self-care management at home.
- Fostering positive patient/caregiver adjustment to and coping mechanisms for changes in lifestyle, role, and self-concept as a result of illness or disability.
- Reintegrating the patient/caregiver back into the family, community, and social support systems.

Home health nursing is both science and sensitivity in practice, dedicated to quality patient care. Such a philosophy reflects a commitment to ongoing educational programs that promote a knowledge base and clinical expertise; to clinical research to validate home care as a preferred alternative to hospitalization; to driving home health agency clinical policy and decision making; and to fostering political strength and solidarity of the nursing profession in order to provide for the health care needs of our nation today and tomorrow.

SUMMARY

Home health care will continue to be a growth industry shaped by government regulations and social pressures for economically viable alternatives in health care. As home health continues to evolve, home health nurses will very likely network with hospitals, outpatient services, public health services, school nurse services, and a variety of community-based health services in providing efficient and equitable ways to deliver quality health care to the public. As described in subsequent chapters in this book, such responsibilities will require home health nurses to be expert clinicians, managers, and leaders in health care.

REFERENCES

 1. American Nurses' Association: *Standards of home health nursing practice,* Kansas City, Mo, 1986, The Association.
 2. Balinsky W, Starkman J: The impact of DRGs on the health care industry, *Health Care Manage Rev* 12:61-74, 1987.
 3. Brault G: Home health care nursing: the changing picture. In Bullough B, Bullough V, editors: *Nursing in the community,* St Louis, 1990, Mosby.
 4. Dee-Kelly P, Heller S, Sibley M: Managed care: an opportunity for home care agencies, *Nurs Clin North Am* 29(3):471-481, 1994.
 5. Health Care Financing Administration: *Bureau of management and strategy* (HCFA Pub No 03341), Washington, DC, 1993, HCFA.
 6. Health Care Financing Administration: *The home health agency prospective payment demonstration,* Cambridge, Mass, 1995, HCFA.
 7. Health Care Financing Administration: *Home health insurance manual* (Pub No 11 Washington, DC, US Department of Health and Human Services Thru T273, Rev 3195), 1995.
 8. Irwin T: *Home health care: when a patient leaves the hospital.* Speech given before the Public Affairs Committee for the City of New York, 1978.
 9. Kilbane IK: The demise of free care, *Nurs Clin North Am* 23(2):435-442, 1988.
10. Mundinger M: *Home care controversy: too little, too late, too costly,* Rockville, Md, 1983, Aspen Systems Corp.
11. National Association For Home Care: Basic statistics about home care. In *Homecare,* Washington, DC, 1994, The Association.
12. National Association For Home Care: *NAHC reviews new physician billing for oversight regulations,* Washington, DC, Jan 13, 1995, The Association.
13. Stanhope M and Lancaster J: *Community health nursing: process and practice for promoting health,* ed 3, St Louis, 1993, Mosby.
14. Varricchio C: Human and indirect costs of home care, *Nurs Outlook* 42(4):151-157, 1994.

2 Understanding Home Health Care: Applying Theory to Clinical Practice

Robyn Rice

Every discipline faces the challenges of how to implement professional responsibilities. How is the job to be done? What direction or focus should be taken to accomplish the goals of work? What are these goals and how should they be determined? For nursing, these questions are complicated by the fact that quality patient care and professional standards of practice are significantly influenced by political, social, cultural, and economic factors within this country. For example, state and government regulations for reimbursement of home health services significantly influence the plan of care.[7] Likewise, differences among nurses in their level of educational preparation, work experience, and personal work ethics are additional variables that affect the delivery of quality patient care.

Home health nurses will probably face some of the greatest demands for change and innovation as health care continues to move away from traditional hospital settings and into the community. For this group of nurses, the challenges of providing quality patient care will likely involve caring for increased numbers of sicker patients across the life span. For example, in today's economic climate frequency of visits and the amount of time allocated to get the job done will likely be compressed. In addition, home health nurses may well experience an expansion of their role, reflecting increased responsibilities for assisted living programs, personal care homes, and a variety of alternative health care delivery systems in the community. Yet in the community these nurses will continue to attend to the very real and enormous health care needs of our multicultural society, (i.e., health care needs that are not always

matched by adequate family and environmental resources). Nurses who work in the challenging milieu of home health care need to consider the following questions: What is the purpose of home health care? What responsibilities do home health nurses' have to their patients? What, if any, are the patients' responsibilities for their plan of care? How are clinical services to be determined, implemented, and evaluated? With the changing regulatory and economic restructuring of health care in this country, how can home health nurses ensure quality patient care yet maintain professional standards of practice?

There are no simple answers to these questions. However, it is clear that the spectrum of illness and health care is so broad and expansive that responsibilities for care must be shared by nurses, patients, and caregivers as needed. It is also clear that innovations in health care must support quality patient care yet maintain professional standards of practice, lest finances become the **one and only** consideration that drives the plan of care.[1,2] Most important, nurses who can articulate their role have a base from which to maintain professional standards of practice.

The purpose of this chapter is to provide home health nurses with a practical framework for home health nursing practice and service delivery. A brief overview of major nursing theory relevant to home care is discussed. The role of the home health nurse is defined. In addition, a theoretical framework or conceptual model for home health nursing practice is presented at the end of the chapter. There are many theories and models useful in understanding home care. To cover all of them is beyond the scope of a single chapter. Refer to the reference list at the end of the chapter for further resources in theory development.

THEORY DEVELOPMENT

Theories begin with assumptions about nature and human behavior. They are researched-based concepts that explain *relationships.* Theories are derived from conceptual frameworks or models that serve as a link in theory development.[3,4]

Conceptual frameworks or models (also referred to as paradigms) identify relationships among concepts and allow the user to visualize diagrammatically how concepts are linked and connected to one another.[19] They can be used to direct ways of thinking and behaving. A statement or proposition expressing the relationships proposed in the model can be tested for accuracy and truthfulness. Such a statement or proposition is called a hypothesis. If research shows the hypothesis proposed in the model to be true, then theory development can proceed.[6]

Theories and conceptual frameworks or models are important to nurses because they define the boundaries of professional practice and identify nurse-patient-caregiver relationships as they relate to quality patient care. Nursing theories build on each other and contribute to individual and professional perceptions of illness and wellness. They promote insights into professional practice and serve as a basis for inquiry and research.[3,4,6,13,16] Moreover, a general understanding of nursing theory assists home health nurses in establishing their role in home care.

NURSING THEORY

Theories and research of many nursing theorists have had a tremendous impact upon nursing. The following section highlights those nursing theories that the author has particularly found useful in understanding home care. Again, the reader is referred to the reference list at the end of the chapter in pursuing further information on nursing theory and theory development.

Nightingale

In her book *Notes on Nursing,* Florence Nightingale described disease as a reparative process, not necessarily accompanied by suffering.[14,23] Nightingale, the first nursing and environmental theorist, considered disease to be an effort of nature to remedy a process of poisoning or decay. She believed that nurses should primarily focus their interventions on causes and symptoms of suffering, not on the symptoms of the disease.

Nightingale emphasized the impact of environment and sanitation on patient recovery. She cited five essential points in securing "the health of houses": pure air, pure water, efficient drainage, cleanliness, and light.[11] To this day her beliefs are reflected in basic infection control practices such as handwashing and infectious waste disposal.

Orem

Dorothea Orem's self-care deficit theory of nursing describes three concepts basic to nursing practice: self-care, self-care deficits (dependent-care deficit), and nursing systems.[15] The health focus of Orem's self-care theory is for individuals and families to maintain a state of wellness. Self-care encompasses the basic activities that aid health promotion, well-being, and health maintenance.[15]

Self-care deficits occur when individuals can no longer meet their self-care requisites.[15,19] Self-care requisites include the need for food, air, rest, social interaction, and other components of human function. They are categorized by Orem as universal, developmental, or health deviation self-care requisites.[15,19] These self-care requisites are the focus of health-related behaviors of individuals, families, and communities.

Nursing systems, the third concept of Orem's theory, are multidimensional and viewed as wholly compensatory, partly compensatory, or supportive-educative.[15,19] If the patient requires complete nursing care and is unable to assist with health needs, care is categorized as wholly compensatory. Care that can be performed by both patient and nurse is termed partly compensatory. Care is categorized as supportive-educative when nurses are able to assist patients to make their own decisions and take actions to fulfill self-care requisites.

Orem's theory views care as something to be performed by both nurses and patients.[15] The role of the nurse is to provide education and support that help patients acquire the necessary abilities to perform self-care.[15]

Leininger

Madeline Leininger's transcultural nursing theory proposes that cultural care provides the broadest and most important means that nurses can use to promote health and well-being. Leininger suggests that nursing is an inherently transcultural profession. Transcultural care knowledge is seen as essential if nurses are to give competent and necessary care to people from different cultures.[11,12]

Leininger views care as the essence of nursing. Care is regarded as the means to help patients recover from illness or unfavorable life conditions. Leininger links care and culture together and proposes that they should not be separated in nursing actions and decisions. Regardless of cultural background, all people are seen as dependent on human care for growth and survival.[11] Leininger suggests that the ultimate goal of cultural care nursing is to assist, support, or enable all individuals to maintain well-being, improve life, or face death.[11,12,19]

Watson

Jean Watson's theory of human caring in nursing is metaphysical in nature and proposes human caring as the moral ideal of nursing.[21,22] Nurses participate in human caring (1) to protect, enhance, and preserve humanity by assisting individuals to find meaning in illness, pain, and existence, and (2) to help others gain self-knowledge, self-control, and self-healing.[21]

Illness is seen not as disease but rather as disharmony within a person's inner self. Watson's theory views health as unity and harmony within body, mind, and soul. Attainment of harmony generates self-knowledge, self-reverence, self-healing, and self-care processes.[21,22] Watson suggests that when nurses assist patients to find meaning to their existence, patients gain self-knowledge, self-control, self-love, choice, and self-determination in health decisions and lifestyle management.[21,22]

A THEORETICAL FRAMEWORK FOR HOME CARE: THE RICE MODEL OF DYNAMIC SELF-DETERMINATION

Home health nurses can offer extensive support, education, and resources, but unless the patient/caregiver actively manage their health care needs at home, the plan of care is unlikely to succeed. Consider the patient standing on the corner of a busy street trying to sell the battery from his IV pump for illicit drug money. Consider the patient

with congestive heart failure who tells the home health nurse, "I don't care what you or the doctor say, I am going to eat my salt!" These examples are realities for nurses working in home care across this country. They call for a shift in theoretical thinking for nurses who, for too long, have shouldered the entire responsibility for patient/caregiver health. They call for nursing strategies that promote patient/caregiver participation with the plan of care. This relates to the fundamental purpose of home health.

The purpose of home health is not to make patients well. Wellness is certainly a deserved for consequence of nursing actions in the home milieu, but it is not guaranteed. *Rather the purpose of home care is to provide patients/caregivers with the support, treatment, information, and understanding they need to successfully manage their health care needs at home.* For out of active self-care management will optimal health or best level of functioning arise.[9]

Building on the previously mentioned nursing theories, as well as on concepts of motivation and culture described in Chapter 6, the author proposes a professional model, unique to home care, called the Rice Model of Dynamic Self-Determination.[9,10,14,15,21] It is a patient-focused model for home health nursing practice.

Dynamic self-determination is derived from patient/caregiver motivational factors which include interpersonal perceptions of health beliefs and world view, sociocultural influences, support systems, and disease process. The goal of dynamic self-determination is for patients to successfully manage their health care needs at home and thus to achieve a state of intrapersonal harmony and optimal health. The home health nurse's role is that of *facilitator* of home independence through patient education, patient advocacy, and case management. The Rice Model of Dynamic Self-Determination is shown in Figure 2-1.

Patients are viewed as holistic units of care that include the patient and the caregiver as they interact in the home environment. Health care needs are related to disease or altered states of wellness and are seen as subjective. Patients' perceptions of disease and wellness are related to a continuum of intrapersonal harmony. Intrapersonal harmony is acquired when mind, body, and spirit are without need and frustration; it is the patient's

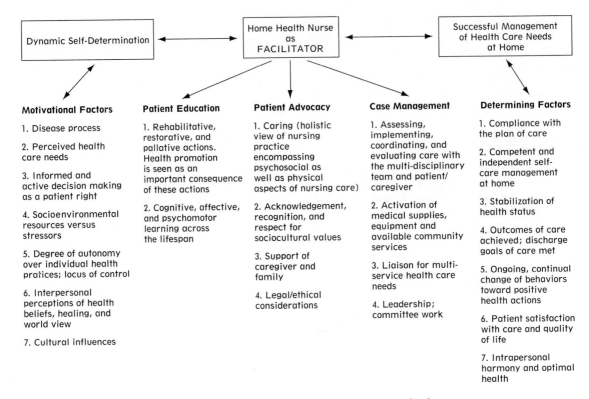

Figure 2-1 The Rice Model of Dynamic Self-Determination.

optimal level of health. Simply stated, optimal health refers to the patient's best level of functioning.

Dynamic Self-Determination allows patients to bridge the gap between need and goal attainment. The relationship between nurse-patient-caregiver moves through stages of dependence, interdependence, and independence when attaining goals. Exacerbation of illness or complications from disease process may cause patient/caregiver regression to a previous phase. Likewise, disease process or disability may predispose the patient to plateau at a certain phase. The three phases of the nurse-patient-caregiver relationship are as follows:

Dependence. Initially the home health nurse performs the majority of care and initiates patient/caregiver instruction for self-care.

Interdependence. As skills, knowledge, and confidence are gained, the patient/caregiver performs the majority of care, reinforced and guided by the home health nurse.

Independence. The patient/caregiver is able to perform and sustain self-care, successfully managing health care needs at home with no or little intervention by the home health nurse.

The Rice Model of Dynamic Self-Determination has the following premises:

- The processes of medical treatment and health teaching do not guarantee patient/caregiver optimal health because home care is administered by home health nurses on an intermittent basis.
- The patient/caregiver *shares responsibility* for managing health care needs at home, supported and *facilitated* by the home health nurse.
- The role of the home health nurse as *facilitator* of self-determination is multidimensional and focuses on the patient's cultural, intrapersonal, spiritual, technological, environmental, and educational needs for goal attainment.

- Successful management of health care needs at home *depends* on the patient/caregiver's participation in the plan of care.
- Participation occurs by collaboration among the patient/caregiver, the nurse, and the multidisciplinary team in mutual goal setting and decision making. The patient/caregiver's roles are *active* roles.
- Participation in the plan of care results from dynamic self-determination to manage health care needs at home. It is primarily achieved by rehabilitative, restorative, and/or palliative actions as influenced by government regulations for reimbursement of home health services. Health promotional behaviors are seen as an important consequence of these actions.
- The caregiver is viewed as an extension of the patient and the patient's needs. The role of the caregiver is to provide social and physiological support to the patient and becomes an integral part of the plan of care. Therefore the caregiver must be supported and cared for; for example, consider respite services when faced with caregiver burnout.
- Dynamic self-determination is an ongoing, reflective process and is necessary to achieve intrapersonal harmony and optimal health. It arises from motivation for goal achievement and involves the process of goal attainment. It reflects the patient's disease process, health beliefs, and cultural considerations, as well as socioenvironmental and community resources necessary for self-care management.
- It is recognized that some patients are not ideal candidates for home health. Chapter 7 discusses the legal and ethical issues involved in such decisions. However, dynamic self-detemination is *not intended* to be an avenue for premature patient discharge from home health services when nurses are faced with problems of patient/caregiver nonparticipation in the plan of care. Rather, principles of dynamic self-determination can be applied by home health nurses in identifying patient/caregiver insecurities with self-care management in order to strengthen the patient/caregiver's desires and abilities for home independence.

The Rice Model of Dynamic Self-Determination can be useful to home health nurses in a variety of ways. The model can be incorporated into an admission assessment tool in assisting staff to organize and develop the plan of care. For example, after the initial assessment, the following questions are asked:

1. What are the patient/caregiver's educational needs?
2. What are the patient/caregiver's advocacy needs?
3. What are the patient/caregiver's case management needs?
4. Is the patient willing and able to participate in the plan of care? If the patient is unable to learn health teaching or manage self-care, is there a caregiver or family member who can assume some of these responsibilities? Does the home environment support safe delivery of services (e.g., adequate housing, resources, neighborhood issues)? If the answer is an absolute "no" to the three previous questions, consider alternate methods of service delivery and approaches. The patient *may not* be an appropriate candidate for home health; this is particularly true for high-tech home health care services such as home ventilator management, which will require active patient/caregiver involvement and environmental support.
5. What does the patient/caregiver want to learn or know to manage home health care needs? (Prioritize health teaching based on patient/caregiver *self-perceived* survival needs.)

The model can be used as a theoretical framework for clinical pathways that emphasize patient/caregiver participation with the plan of care. For example, wound care or diabetic teaching may well be assessed from patient/caregiver self-determined health care needs and incorporated into the patient care plan or clinical pathway. It can also provide a basis for discharge goals of care. See Chapter 8 and Appendixes 8-1 and 8-2.

The Rice model's greatest strength is that it provides a commonsense approach to home health care. It would be particularly helpful as an orientation tool for staff new to home care. It could also be used to familiarize student nurses with their role expectations in home health. It provides concepts for theory development in home care.

Research supporting the Rice Model of Dynamic Self-Determination is qualitative in nature and derived from 10 years of practical working experience in home health. The model has been supported by anecdotal evidence.[8,17,20] The author has received both verbal and written communication from home health nurses and educators on both a national and an international level that the model is consistent with practice needs in home care.[18,20] The author is currently conducting re search to further test the model as to its applicability to home health and theory development; data will be available when the studies are completed.

The Rice Model of Dynamic Self-Determination emphasizes *shared* responsibility for interpersonal harmony and optimal health between the nurse, patient, and caregiver. It is proposed as an emerging professional model for home health nursing practice—a model that will continue to be shaped by government, political, and social reforms for health care.

SUMMARY

As home health care continues to evolve within the medical and economic restructuring of this country, its purpose and implementation will continue to reflect the health care needs of our nation and home health nurses' endeavors to provide quality patient care. This chapter has presented ideas and concepts that give home health nurses direction and guidance to achieve the complex tasks they face. Theories, questions, and ideas serve to generate thinking. And therein lie the real answers to our many challenges.

REFERENCES

1. American Nurses' Association: *A social policy statement*, Kansas City, Mo, 1981, Author.
2. American Nurses' Association: *Nursing's agenda for healthcare reform*, Kansas City, Mo, 1991, Author.
3. Campbell J, Bunting S: Voices and paradigms: perspectives on critical and feminist theory in nursing, *ANS* 16(3):39-56, 1993.
4. Clarke P, Cody W: Nursing theory-based practice in the home and community: the crux of professional nursing education, *ANS* 17(2):41-53, 1994.
5. Easton KL: Defining the concept of self-care, *Rehabil Nurs* 18(6):384-387, 1993.
6. Fawcett J: *Analysis and evaluation of nursing theories*, Philadelphia, 1993, FA Davis.
7. Health Care Financing Administration: *Health insurance manual* (Pub No 11), Washington, DC, US Department of Health and Human Services, 1995.
8. Huck S, Cormier W, Bounds W: *Reading statistics and research*, New York, 1974, HarperCollins Publishers. (Note: this book gives a good overview of statistical analysis, yet is easy to read.)
9. Jopp M, Carroll MC, Waters L: Using self-care theory to guide nursing management of the older adult after hospitalization, *Rehabil Nurs* 18(2):91-94, 1993.
10. Leininger M: Transcultural care diversity and universality: a theory of nursing, *Nurs Health Care* 6(4):209-212, 1985.
11. Leininger M: Quality of life from a transcultural nursing perspective, *Nurs Sci Q* 7(1):22-28, 1994.
12. Leininger M: *Transcultural nursing: concepts, theories, and practices*, ed 2, Philadelphia, 1995, FA Davis.
13. Levine M: *Nursing knowledge: improving education and practice through theory.* Paper presented at Sigma Theta Tau Theory Conference, Chicago, 1992.
14. Nightingale F: *Notes on nursing: what it is and what it is not*, New York, 1969, Dover, Appleton & Co.
15. Orem D: *Nursing: concepts of practice*, ed 5, St Louis, 1995, Mosby.
16. Randall BP: Nursing theory: the 21st century . . . a panel discussion on theory development, *Nurs Sci Q* 5(4):176-184, 1992.
17. Rice R: A conceptual framework for nursing practice in the home-the Rice Model of Dynamic Self-Determination, *Home Health Care Nurs J* 12(2):51-53, 1994.
18. Rice R: *The Rice Model of Dynamic Self-Determination*, Anecdotal presentation at the Indiana Association for Home Care State Conference, May 17, 1995.
19. Riehl-Sisca J: *Conceptual models for nursing practice*, ed 3, Norwalk, Conn, 1989, Appleton & Lange.
20. Universite' De Moncton in New Brunswick, Canada: Conversation and communication with Assistant Professor Monique Cormeir-Daigle regarding adapting their assessment tool for home health to the Rice Model of Dynamic Self-Determination, Fall 1994.
21. Watson J: *Nursing: human science and human care: a theory of nursing*, Norwalk, Conn, 1985, Appleton-Century-Crofts.
22. Watson J: Window on theory of human caring. In O'Toole M, editor: *Miller-Keane encyclopedia and dictionary of medicine, nursing, and allied health*, ed 5, Philadelphia, 1992, WB Saunders.
23. Widerquist J: The spirituality of Florence Nightingale, *Nurs Res* 41(1):49-55, 1992.

3 Role Preparation and Implementation

Robyn Rice

Virtually every aspect of nursing offers certain attractions to professionals wishing to work in that specialty area. Why would one choose home health nursing? Most nurses electing to practice in this specialty do so because they enjoy working within the community. Compared to traditional hospital settings, practice in the home environment offers nurses an expanded role associated with increased power and autonomy of practice. Community networking and socialization, independent time management, and more "normal" working hours are additional incentives (although home health agencies operate 24 hours a day, 7 days a week, the majority of working hours *are* weekdays with periodic on-call and weekend duties).

This chapter describes role preparation and implementation for home health nurses. Issues influencing responsibilities of clinical field staff are reviewed. Home health agency guidelines for orientating new field staff are presented. In addition, the role of the clinical nurse specialist (CNS) as a support system for the home health agency staff is also discussed. The chapter concludes with a section on working with students in home care because they, too, have a future in this exciting and challenging field of nursing.

A PROFILE OF HOME HEALTH NURSES

Home health nurses are not merely critical care or hospital-based nurses who "just run into the home to do a procedure." Such an attitude is disparaging to home health nurses who work closely with patients and their families, sometimes in environments with few resources. Like other specialty areas of practice, nursing care in the home setting does require special preparation and knowledge.

Ideally, nurses entering the home health field should be educated at the baccalaureate level. This background provides a basis for nursing practice that involves management skills, family and community concepts, and expanded clinical experiences in community health settings. In addition, baccalaureate graduates have an in-depth exposure to the nursing process with an emphasis on critical thinking and decision making.

Home health nursing practice is very complex, requiring independent decision making and precise assessment. Therefore the author recommends that after graduation, a minimum of 1 year of medical-surgical experience should usually be required as a basis for entry into home care. Specialty assignments such as pediatric or high-tech home care should be reflected in the staff member's work history. Exceptions to this recommendation would be for those new graduates whose past work experiences and level of maturity will enable them to fulfill role expectations.

CLINICAL FIELD STAFF: ROLE EXPECTATIONS

In facilitating patient/caregiver self-care management as discussed in Chapter 2, clinical field staff function in multiple roles. They must be expert clinicians and educators who are comfortable working within the home milieu. Role expectations also require individuals to function as case managers who are willing to assume leadership responsibilities for an autonomous nursing practice that directs multidisciplinary care. Qualities and characteristics that address these role expectations include advanced assessment and evaluation skills, effective communication skills, sound judgment, effective documentation skills, flexibility and creative problem solving, and self-direction.

Advanced assessment and evaluation skills

The home health nurse must be able to perform an in-depth holistic assessment of the patient, family, and home environment. An assessment of available community services as a source of referral for patient/caregiver needs is also important. This is followed by an ongoing evaluation that determines the patient's progress (or lack of progress) in meeting outcomes of care. The home health nurse's assessment and evaluation provides guidelines for changes in the plan of care or the frequency of visits. Last and most important, assessment and evaluation are the basis for offering patients/caregivers alternative choices in their health care such as changes in the plan of care, referral to specialty services, placement in a long-term care facility or hospice, homemaker or assisted living services, rehospitalization, or discharge from home health services.

Effective communication skills

Since the patient, the physician, and the home health agency are separated by distance, home health nurses must maintain open communication channels to implement the plan of care and coordinate the services of the multidisciplinary team. Effective communication skills are also essential for case conferencing with the multidisciplinary team. Furthermore, in the home milieu, nurses will find themselves teaching patients who have unique ways of doing things and personal convictions. (See Chapter 6.) Effective communication fosters good working relationships with the patient/caregiver despite differences in educational levels and religious and/or ethnic backgrounds.

Sound judgment

Moving away from the institutional setting and working in the patient's home affords certain freedoms in practice and entails different responsibilities. Although the physician is just a phone call away, the plan of care and number of visits are frequently adjusted by the home health nurse. If the home health nurse determines that the patient needs immediate medical attention, a trip to the emergency room or physician's office may be necessary. Home health nurses must use sound

judgment and decision making skills when determining what actions to take. For example, sound judgment is also required when differentiating between a safe housing area/situation and an unsafe one. Home health nurses must know when to proceed and when to stop and confer with their patient service managers regarding questionable, possibly unsafe, situations.

Effective documentation skills

Most home health nurses will work in Medicare-certified home health agencies. Government regulations outlining reimbursement of home health services, as described in the Home Health Insurance Manual publication number 11 (HIM-11), highly influence clinical documentation guidelines.[2] Home health nurses must have a current and accurate knowledge of these regulations when documenting patient care because documentation is the basis for payment. In addition, as case managers, home health nurses must effectively document patient/caregiver progress in meeting outcomes and goals of care in accordance with the agency's quality improvement program. (Refer to Chapter 4, for a discussion of documentation guidelines and to Chapter 9, for a discussion of clinical elements of program evaluation.)

Flexibility and creative problem solving

Some nurses feel comfortable practicing home health care and view visiting various neighborhoods and working in the patient's home as both challenging and rewarding. Other nurses may have difficulty adjusting to home environments that differ from their own. Home health care does not take place in a controlled environment. Improvisation of supplies, equipment, or therapies in the home setting is necessary and requires flexibility and creative problem solving. Creative problem solving is also needed for essential committee work which directly influences clinical practice issues.

Self-direction

Home health nurses are largely self-directed. They set up their own daily and weekly schedules, adding patients to their caseload as requested and adjusting their schedules accordingly. They must familiarize themselves with the patient service area and orient themselves to the location of each patient's home. In addition (as indicated previously), changes in the plan of care and the frequency of visits are typically initiated by the home health nurse as part of case management.

FIELD STAFF: ROLE PREPARATION AND IMPLEMENTATION

Once employed by a home health agency, new field staff should receive an orientation to the agency to prepare them to work in home care. This preparation is usually done by staff development through a formal orientation schedule and periodic in-service programs.

Home health agency orientation

Visits by the home health nurse are based on patient needs. As discussed in Chapter 2, the ultimate goal of home care is successful patient/caregiver management of health care needs at home. Universal factors influencing self-care management at home include the following:

- Age-related and cultural factors (specific patient needs that may vary with the age and cultural preference of the patient)
- Psychobiological factors (mental, emotional, spiritual, and physiological needs)
- Specific disease manifestation (chronic, congenital, short-term, or terminal)
- Socioeconomic and environmental factors (availability of family support systems to assist with the plan of care, availability of medical supplies, adequate food and housing, and access to the medical system)

The orientation program should acquaint new field staff with these factors and provide them with the knowledge needed to practice comfortably and competently within the community. The formal orientation should include (but not be limited to) the following:

Review of documents stating the agency's philosophy of care, scope of services, and program evaluation. These documents indicate how the agency regards patient care, the agency's place within the community, the agency's limits of practice, and standards of care. The agency's organizational structure should be reviewed at this time. The purpose and function of the various home health agency committees as well as the quality improvement (QI) program should also be dis-

cussed. The patient care plan or care path can serve as an orientation tool to the QI program and outline nursing care for patient groups frequently encountered in home health.

Review of the agency's policy and procedure manual. The home health agency should have a manual, updated yearly, that provides guidelines for all aspects of patient care, including infection control.[4] This manual should be reviewed with field staff during orientation. Policies regarding reporting through the chain of command and on-call as well as weekend service delivery should also be discussed.

Review of documentation forms and procedures. The paperwork in home care is voluminous but necessary because it serves as a primary source for validating services. At the end of the shift in a hospital, documentation reflects patient stability or implementation of corrective actions. The focus of documentation in home care is influenced by Medicare guidelines and is quite different from that seen in the institutional setting. The HIM-11 and related government regulatory guides for reimbursement of clinical services should be shown to new field staff. Clinical documentation requirements should be reviewed. It is important to emphasize that, at present, home health is financed by retrospective reimbursement and that documentation is the basis for payment.

The use of all agency forms, including the visit report, patient care plan or care path, time cards, daily/weekly itinerary logs, and the field chart, should be explained during orientation.

Principles of case management. See Chapter 8, Case Management and Operational Strategies for Home Health Nurses.

Introduction to the multidisciplinary team and ancillary services. It should be emphasized that multidisciplinary conferences and patient referrals to specialty services strengthen the plan of care, and are expected of home health nurses as case managers. The purpose and roles of the multidisciplinary team and ancillary services should be explained. New field staff should know when and how to refer patients to specialists such as the home health aide; registered dietitian; physical, occupational, or speech language pathologist; hospice nurse; social worker; or clinical nurse specialist. Medicare guidelines for reimbursement of specialty services and documentation requirements in making the referral should be reviewed with new field staff. It should be emphasized that all referrals must be approved by the physician.

If individuals from each specialty service can personally participate in the orientation, new staff members can place a name with a face. The following box describes clinical indicators for multidisciplinary referrals. In addition, familiarity with local medical suppliers, wound-care vendors, and commodity representatives enhances home health nurses' abilities to recommend products. Interagency networking on a local, regional, and national level also should be introduced and encouraged. (See Appendix 3-1.)

Instruction on community safety and map reading. Commuting to patients' homes in a safe manner is a concern for all staff working within the community. Some areas may be unsafe and declared off-limits. Safety precautions such as those listed in the box on p. 30 should be reviewed.[3] The local police department may be willing to give a yearly "safety in the community" in-service for field staff. A street guide or road map is recommended for field staff. Likewise a car or cellular phone is also recommended to enhance communication when out in the field.

Although perspectives on wearing a uniform in the field vary, the author believes that staff members should be taught to view uniforms and name badges as an important part of identification to the public. From the author's past experience as a Visiting Nurse Association (VNA) nurse, the traditional navy uniform worn by many VNA and public health nurses is a recognized symbol of respect and professionalism within the neighborhood.

Introduction to the home milieu. During orientation, it is also important to discuss the concept of home milieu. Home milieu refers to working in the patient's home environment, which may include family and/or caregivers, pets, friends, farms, and communities.

In the home milieu, home health nurses could find themselves working in the cities or in the countryside (Figure 3-1). Patient populations, practice needs, and transportation issues will vary in these areas. As applicable, staff orientation should support role implementation in both urban and rural settings.

In addressing the home milieu, it should be emphasized that the patient's home environment, within a sociocultural context, may be drastically different from that of the home health nurse. Although professional standards of practice should be maintained, new staff should be reminded that in going into a patient's home "they are the guest" and should behave accordingly. Although healthy sanitation and health practices are to be encouraged, new staff must realize that roaches and dirty dishes are a way of life for certain families. Consequently it is important that home health nurses leave their personal prejudices and convictions at home.

When working in the home milieu, sensitivity to ethnicity and the fact that people ultimately have the right to "live their own lives" should be stressed.

Instruction on home improvisation. Creative intervention is often a part of home health nursing. Inadequate supplies need not always prevent delivery of needed care. Home improvisations such as using a coat hanger attached to a door hook for an IV pole, making a robe by pinning a blanket, preparing homemade normal saline or acetic acid for irrigation fluids, and using newspapers covered with cheesecloth for a bed pad should be reviewed.[4]

Ethical considerations. Ethical issues arise in the many stressful patient/caregiver situations that home health nurses encounter. Ethical concerns with which home health nurses will be involved include patients with insufficient or inadequate food, housing, or medical supplies; patients who lack proper support systems; and patients who choose to die at home.[3]

It is important to support new nurses coming into home care by reviewing some of the legal and ethical concerns they may encounter, along with suggestions for resolution. It is important to identify home health agency staff that field staff can turn to should they experience problems in the field. Chapter 7 discusses the nurse's responsibilities when working in the sometimes overwhelming home milieu.

In addition to "in-house" orientation, patient service managers should plan for joint field visits as a part of the orientation program. This allows new staff to observe their peers coordinating and giving care in the home. Staff expertise is also fostered by ongoing in-service training that reviews pharmacology, medical-surgical and psychosocial issues,

CLINICAL INDICATORS FOR MULTIDISCIPLINARY REFERRALS[4]

Clinical indicators for: clinical nurse specialist (CNS) referral

Consider a referral to the CNS in the following circumstances:
• Complex patient care issues
• Lack of patient response to the medical treatment plan
• Staff needs for support, advocacy, and encouragement

Clinical indicators for: home health aide referral

Consider a home health aide referral when assisted or complete personal care services are needed to include:
• Bathing
• Grooming
• Preparing meals
• Eating
• Oral hygiene
• Skin and/or nail care
• Toileting and elimination
• Ambulating
• Exercises
In addition to personal care, consider home health aide services for:
• Light housekeeping
• Washing clothes
• Grocery shopping
• Procedural care within the auspices of the job description

Clinical indicators for: hospice referral

Consider a hospice referral for the following situations:
• Palliative care needs
• Respite care needs for the patient/caregiver
• Patient care needs are "stable" but the patient/family has ongoing needs for counseling/coping, etc. that wouldn't be covered by "routine home care benefit"
• Extensive patient care needs not able to be met by usual home care coverage. For example, extensive pain management, psychological, or spiritual care needs
• Patient/family needs for extra assistance that could be helped with volunteers (e.g., picking up medications, groceries, or other supplies; talking to and being with someone)
• The home health agency/organization is unable to provide the extent of services that the patient/family needs or requests
• At patient and/or family request in preparation for what to expect at the time of death and after

Clinical indicators for: nutritional therapist

Consider a nutritional therapist referral for the following:
• Special diet orders
• Failure to thrive; pediatric growth and development issues
• Certain disease processes such as COPD, diabetes, CHF
• Obesity
• Anorexia

Continued

CLINICAL INDICATORS FOR MULTIDISCIPLINARY REFERRALS—cont'd

Clinical indicators for: psychiatric home health nurse referral

Consider a psychiatric home health referral for the following:
- Unrelieved stress or high anxiety states
- Continued noncompliance with the plan of care
- Depression
- Hallucinations
- Delusions
- Dementia
- Unrealistic or unreasonable thought patterns
- Thoughts of suicide
- Prolonged grief
- Maladaptive coping
- Manipulative patients
- Chronic, debilitating illnesses
- Inability to sleep, rest, or eat
- Bizarre dress or behavior
- Sexually seductive patients
- Patient abuse and/or neglect
- Confusion or emotional lability
- No physical limitations but is unsafe outside of the home due to mental/emotional state
- When the patient has an active psychiatric diagnosis
- Management and evaluation of a patient care plan

Clinical indicators for: skilled nursing (RN or LPN under RN supervision)

Consider a referral to SN in the following circumstances:
- Observation and assessment of the patient's condition when only the specialized skills of a medical professional can determine the patient's status
- Management and evaluation of a patient care plan
- Teaching and training activities
- Administration of medications (review specific Medicare regulations)
- Tube feedings
- Nasopharyngeal and tracheostomy aspiration
- Catheter care
- Wound care
- Ostomy care
- Nutritional needs
- Medical gases
- Rehabilitation nursing (includes bowel and bladder programs)
- Venipuncture

Clinical indicators for: rehabilitation referral

Consider a rehabilitation referral and evaluation for the following circumstances:

Physical therapy
- Patients who have decreased ability to roll, move about, or come to a sitting position in bed
- Patients who have decreased ability to transfer
- Patients who have impaired balance and/or coordination
- Patients who have decreased gait ability or who require special devices or gait aids; patients who are unable to ascend/descend stairs or enter and exit the home
- Patients who have functional loss of range of motion or strength in any extremity

CLINICAL INDICATORS FOR MULTIDISCIPLINARY REFERRALS—cont'd

- Patients who require therapeutic intervention for pain or edema control
- Caregivers who require instruction in methods of assisting patients with any of the above losses or who require instruction in the establishment of a home exercise program
- Patients or caregivers who require equipment recommendations to enhance the functional abilities of patients or increase the ease of caring for patients
- Management and evaluation of a patient care plan

Occupational therapy
- Patients who have decreased ability to perform the activities of daily living (ADL), i.e., bathing, dressing, toileting, cooking, eating
- Patients who require instruction in one-handed techniques (fire motor treatment)
- Patients who have impaired cognition, perception, or awareness of body parts (sensory, perceptual, and neurodevelopmental treatment)
- Patients who require joint protection techniques, pain/edema control, and/or splinting
- Patients who require instruction in energy conservation techniques
- Patients who require equipment recommendations or adaptations to their environment to enhance their functional ability

Speech language pathologist
- Patients with decreased ability to express and/or receive communication
- Patients with impaired cognition and/or memory
- Patients with impaired ability to phonate
- Patients with dysphagia who thus require swallowing instructions
- Patients who are apraxic

Clinical indicators for: social service referral
Consider a social service referral for the following:
- Discord between the patient-caregiver-family-home care team
- Severely impaired vision and/or hearing
- Living alone with the diagnosis of functional or organic brain syndrome (dementia or Alzheimer's)
- Malnutrition
- Terminal conditions (except certified hospice patients who usually receive the services of the hospice social worker)
- Possible or probable child/adult abuse or neglect
- Depression, manic depression, anxiety reaction, or schizophrenia for basic counseling (refer to the psychiatric home health nurse for problems with thought disorders)
- Recent amputees
- Newly diagnosed diabetics
- Multiple sclerosis (MS)
- Stroke or paralysis
- Patients requiring high-tech home care services
- Patients with AIDS
- Counseling for long-range planning and decision making
- Inadequate housing conditions (includes the need for air conditioning or any other assistance with heating and cooling)
- Stress management
- Patient/caregiver noncompliance with the plan of care
- Need for long-term care placement
- Inadequate financial resources
- Inadequate caregivers or caregivers who are "overwhelmed" with the patient's many health care needs
- Community resource planning

SAFETY IN THE COMMUNITY[3]

Precautions to take prior to visits
- Wear a name badge and uniform that clearly identifies you as a representative of the home health agency. Wear shoes that you can run in if necessary.
- Call patients in advance and alert them to the approximate time of your visit. Confirm directions to their residence.
- Request that unruly or overfriendly pets be properly secured before making visits. Back away, never run from a dog. Walk slowly around farm animals so as not to frighten them.
- Keep change for a phone call in your shoe or pocket. Do not carry a purse. Before leaving the agency, lock your purse in the trunk or cover your purse with a blanket if it will be visible.

Precautions when traveling
Car
- Keep your car in good working order with plenty of gas. Obtain an automobile club membership for possible car problems.
- Consider use of a personal cellular phone to maximize communication.
- Store a blanket in the car in the winter and a thermos of cool water in the summer. Keep a snack in the glove compartment.
- If your car fails, turn on emergency flashers, put a CALL POLICE sign in the window, and wait for the police. Do not accept rides from strangers.
- Keep your car locked when parked or driving. Keep windows rolled up if possible.
- Park in full view of the patient's residence (avoid parking in alleys or deserted side streets).

Walking on the street
- Have nursing bag/equipment ready when exiting from the car. Keep one arm free.
- Walk in a professional, businesslike manner, directly to the patient's residence.
- When passing a group of strangers, cross to the other side of the street, as appropriate.
- When leaving the patient's residence, carry car keys in your hand (pointed ends of keys between fingers may make an effective weapon).

Precautions during visits
In the home environment
- Use common walkways in buildings; avoid isolated stairs or darkened (unlit) areas.
- Always knock on the door before entering a patient's home.
- If relatives or neighbors become a safety problem, consider the following:
- Discuss the problem with the patient and schedule a visit time when the relative or neighborhood is quiet.
- Make joint visits with another home health nurse or arrange for escort services.
- Close the case if the problem is not able to be resolved.

Defense strategies
- Run, scream, or yell "fire" or "stranger"; kick shins, instep, or groin; bite or scratch; use a whistle attached to your key ring, chemical sprays, or nursing bag for defense.

Nursing considerations
Visit neighborhoods with questionable safety or gang/drug related problems in the morning. Some areas may have to be declared unsafe and therefore not serviced by your home health agency. In the event of robbery, never resist to keep your nursing bag. It can easily be replaced. When on duty, notify the home health agency clinical service manager of any car trouble, auto accident, or incident when personal safety is in question for further instructions. **Never** go into or stay in a home if you feel personal safety is in question. Always respect and listen to your "gut feelings."

A

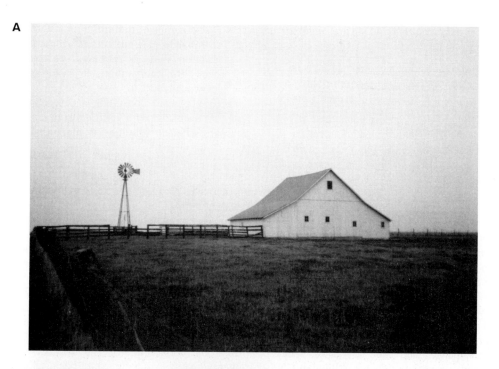

B

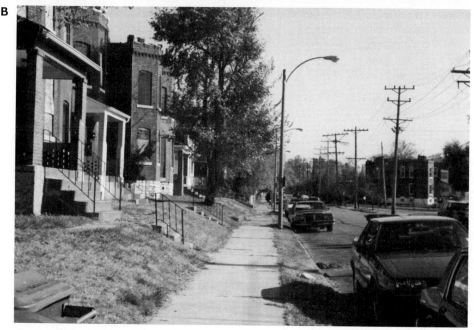

Figure 3-1 Rural *(A)* vs. urban *(B)* areas of practice. (Photographs by Robyn Rice.)

quality improvement, and Medicare regulations that influence the delivery of patient care.

THE CLINICAL NURSE SPECIALIST IN HOME CARE: ROLE EXPECTATIONS, PREPARATION, AND IMPLEMENTATION

Home health clinical nurse specialists (CNSs) should be prepared at the master's level so that they can assist home health agency staff in dealing with complex patient needs and home health agency support requests. In addition, CNSs who work with high technology in home care do well with a critical care background.

In order to enhance staff utilization of the CNS, it is important to review the role and function of the CNS. Clinical nurse specialists are master's level nurses who, as agents of change, facilitate quality patient care. They are more highly trained, skilled care providers than staff nurses. According to Roy and Martinez, CNSs are individuals with innate and acquired abilities to deal with the changing world.[5]

In home health care, CNSs serve as educators, consultants, patient and staff advocates, speaker bureaus, and community liaisons. Although CNSs may have many duties (e.g., writing policies and procedures, serving on product evaluation/quality assurance/forms committees), their primary focus should be patients and staff.

The art of consultation is "to help." Therefore in order to be available to staff on an as-needed basis, CNSs should avoid taking on a large caseload or being assigned to administrative desk duties that could consume the majority of their time. The multidimensional nature of home care demands that CNSs focus on a holistic nursing practice that encompasses patients, caregivers, and the home environment. This viewpoint moves the staff from task-oriented to outcome-oriented care. Instead of "What are we doing?" the question becomes "Where are we going?" and "How are we getting there?" The CNS's support of staff includes the following:

- Sharing information, research, and resources pertinent to patient care via orientation sessions, in-service training, service area or district meetings, and writing for publication
- Role modeling by performing direct patient care when co-visiting with staff
- Committee work

- Participating in multidisciplinary conferences to enhance staff problem solving and communication skills as concerns, frustrations, and needs for interventions in case management are vocalized
- Serving as a consultant and resource person by assisting with data collection/assessment and offering solutions or alternative answers

CNSs should help staff make difficult clinical and ethical decisions by jointly assessing patient problems, formulating the interventions, and evaluating the outcomes. Co-visits with staff provide an arena where information is exchanged and working relationships are defined. This establishes patterns of problem solving that home health nurses can recall for use in meeting future patient needs. As a result, co-visits with CNSs build the confidence of home health nurses in their own assessment and decision making abilities.

The relationship between CNSs and home health nurses should be one of mutual respect, trust, and collaboration.[1] Therefore CNSs should openly avoid criticizing staff because they may become reluctant to ask for help or seek referrals. The preferred approach is not "What you are doing wrong?" but rather "What can we do to improve the situation?" Resources in home care are often scarce. Home health nurses, when working with their patients and families, may find themselves in some very stressful situations. Consequently when consulting with staff, the CNSs should present a very supportive persona.

IMPLEMENTING STUDENT LEARNING IN HOME CARE
Role expectations and preparation of nursing instructors in home care

Faculty work history and experience will largely determine the nursing instructor's ability to lead a successful home health rotation. The demands of the rotation are great. This is one of the few clinical areas where student visits, under the supervision of the instructor, are directly billable to Medicare.[2] Therefore home health instructors must be expert clinicians, knowledgeable of the Medicare regulations for reimbursement of services, capable of collaborating with case managers, and appreciative of family and caregivers when working in the home milieu. A master's degree in community health, home health, medical-surgical nursing, or a related specialty in nursing is recommended; *work experience in home health is the key.* If these conditions are met, students are very likely to have a positive learning experience in home care.

Guidelines for working with students in home care

Home health agencies provide an excellent clinical practicum for educating students about home care (Figure 3-2). Through home health, students learn basic concepts of case management and how to work with patients and their families in the home setting. It is important to clarify with field staff up front exactly what their responsibilities are toward the students and exactly what the students will be doing with the patients. Field staff will need support in promoting student learning. (See the box on p. 35.)

Student learning in home health can be fostered in many ways. Independent student home visits with periodic instructor co-visits to guide learning is one of the most rewarding methods to teach students about home care. Not only does it foster student responsibility to learn, but it also enhances self-direction for time management and accountability for patient care—the realities of nursing practice. Initially students will require a lot of contact with their instructor. However, as skills and confidence are gained, students become comfortable in making home visits without the instructor right there looking over their shoulder. Students should follow the dress code and safety recommendations given earlier in the chapter. Jewelry, "big hair," and excessive makeup are to be discouraged.

Organizing students to work in home health takes planning. Senior nursing students are recommended for independent home visits; cars are required. No more than eight students are advised for the rotation. It is recommended that students be paired into teams of two. This serves two functions: (1) it enhances student safety and (2) it maximizes efficiency of clinical time as instructors will split their visit time up among the student teams. Most clinical rotations involve 2 days at the agency. So as not to overload the instructor, it is recommended that each student carry two patients as his or her caseload. This patient load may vary

with clinical time and availability of patients. Hopefully, students will be able to follow the same patients during their rotation.

As with new field staff, it is a good idea to structure a 1-day classroom orientation for students, covering safety in the community, infection control, map reading, and documentation. Students' observational visits with staff on the second clinical day in home health is recommended so they can become better acclimated to the home milieu. This should be followed with a postconference that allows for a debriefing of their experiences. *It is highly recommended that home health instructors carry cellular phones because this reassures students, their families, and the home health agency staff that the instructor is readily available for student needs.*

Co-visits with student teams should be planned so that all patients are seen by the instructor. In other words, if clinicals are on Tuesdays and Wednesdays, the instructor would see half of the patients with students on Tuesdays and the other half on Wednesdays. In planning their schedules, instructors *must* be available to supervise students performing certain procedural care (such as blood draws) and as needed. A daily visit schedule for all teams, given out to students and the home health agency supervisory staff, is recommended. It is important to list all pertinent phone numbers on the schedule. This way everyone knows where everyone else is, what time they should be there, and how to get in contact. In consideration of patient needs and requests, instructors should spread visit times out over the day. Students should not be allowed to vary the visit time because instructors must have a schedule that reasonably accesses them to all students.

Students often have a tendency to focus on the procedural aspects of care when making home visits. Instructors should make a point of role modeling the "art" of conversation with patients and their families as a way of assisting students to overcome their fears and initial awkwardness in the home setting. Aside from assessment and procedural skills, instructors should stress the importance of developing therapeutic relationships with the household. Frankly, most patients enjoy the extra time and attention that their student nurse gives them. In assisting students to conceptualize the relationships between the patient, family,

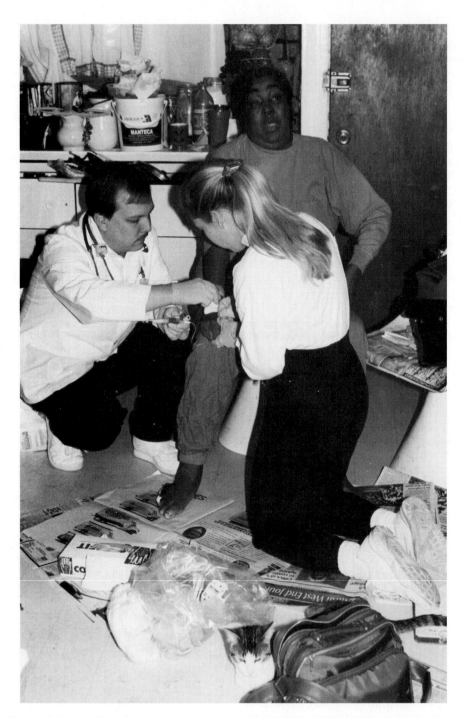

Figure 3-2 Student nurse performing venipuncture in the home. (Photograph by Robyn Rice.)

TIPS FOR FIELD STAFF WHO ARE WORKING WITH NURSING INSTRUCTORS AND STUDENTS

- Meet with the nursing instructor. Ask for a copy of the students' course syllabus and clinical schedule. Determine the following:
  1. What days of the week will the students be in clinical? What are their clinical hours? How long will the students be in home health?
  2. What will the students be doing in clinical? What are their learning objectives? How does home health fit into their learning objectives?
  3. Will the students be doing procedural care? If so, how will they be supervised? Who is responsible for supervising the students?
  4. How is the paperwork going to be handled? Who is going to be responsible for processing the students' paperwork and ensuring its accuracy?
  5. Who will be responsible for notifying the physician of changes in the patient's status? Who will be responsible for taking physician orders?
  6. What will be the procedure for the school of nursing should weather get bad? (How will the instructor let you know if clinical is cancelled for any reason?)
- Exchange beeper and/or cellular phone numbers with the nursing instructor. In addition, obtain the instructor's office or work number.
- Request that the nursing instructor and/or students call or page you with any concerns. As a backup, encourage them to talk to your supervisor or the desk manager for assistance in decision making.
- Request that the home health agency have a bulletin board or mailbox where you can leave notes or information for the nursing instructor and students.
- Assign students to patients who are challenging yet not overwhelming for the student; consult with the nursing instructor as to the appropriateness of the assignment. Wound care and blood draws provide good learning experiences. *Don't be stingy with patients!*
- Conference with students when possible. Be friendly; find out how things are going. Ask the students to tell you how they are assisting their patients to meet their outcomes of care. Quiz the students on assessment findings. This is a good time to build assessment skills.

  Often students want to report to the physician everything they find that deviates from the norm. Explain that patients in home care often have wide variances in vital signs. Tell them to immediately report abnormal vital signs and findings to you and/or their instructor; stress that you and/or their instructor will be available to assist them in further decision making.
- Remember that students usually go by the book. As realities set in, home health care can be scary for them at first. Be supportive of the students and nursing instructor. When the students and/or nursing instructor tell you something about a patient's condition, *listen* to what they have to say. It may be necessary to make an extra home visit to evaluate the nursing instructor's and/or students' concerns.
- Address any concerns directly to the nursing instructor. Let the nursing instructor work out problems with students. Consult with your supervisor regarding unresolved problems with nursing instructors and/or students.
- Don't forget to give praise when it is deserved. Remember, we were all in nursing school once.

---

neighborhood, and community, instructors should increase student awareness of all resources available to their patients. Afternoon clinical activities could be planned to enhance student learning of community resources for patients. For example, a visit to the American Lung Association or similiar organization, a visit to the local neighborhood association, or a trip to the nearby Kmart to identify economical patient resources can provide fun and rewarding learning experiences for students.

Course-related assignments are advised to direct student learning when students are not out in the field. Required clinical textbooks and reading assignments are suggested. Afternoon conferences should be planned with the multidisciplinary services in order to better acquaint students with principles of case management. Likewise, afternoon conference time should be set aside in order to review patient care issues and student documentation. Require students to complete a weekly log describing how they are meeting clinical objectives. In evaluating their learning experience, instructors could require students to type a 3-page paper describing their learning experience in home care. Creativity with writing should be encouraged because creativity and visionary thinking are fundamental to an autonomous profession and the essence of home health nursing practice.

Instructors should not put themselves in a position whereby they are trying to take physician orders all day long. This will tie them up in one home and make them unavailable to the other student teams. For the most part, instructors should let supervisory staff and case managers handle the physician orders.

Instructors should be respectful of supervisory staff and case managers; let them know what is going on. If there are patient care problems or concerns, instructors and students should report them as a way of mutual decision making. Methods of "reporting off" will vary. It is a good idea for instructors to request that students leave copies of the patient visit report and related documentation in the case managers' mailboxes at the end of the clinical day.

The conditions of student performance and instructor responsibilities should be clearly documented when initially contracting with the agency for clinical placement. To emphasize a previous point, instructors should make sure that these guidelines are shared with the respective case managers. Student assignments must be mutually worked out between the agency and instructor because some home health patients are not appropriate learning experiences for students. Also, student assignments should be made in the relatively safer areas of the community. Likewise it is not recommended that students open or close the case for safety as well as documentation issues. Instructors should respect the home health agency's input on these matters; however, instructors should never forget that they are ultimately responsible for the quality of the student's learning experience and for the student's safety.

The success of a home health clinical rotation really depends on the cooperation of the home health agency. From an economic point of view, some home health agencies may be reluctant to provide student observational experiences or mentor students because this can tie up staff time. The school of nursing may wish to consider the possibility of *service sharing* with the home health agency as a means of compensating the agency for use of its staff. Service sharing could involve the school of nursing offering free tuition, in-services, or a physical assessment course for home health agency staff.

SUMMARY

The role of the home health nurse clearly encompasses elements that are outside the realm of traditional views of nursing. Confidence and competence are essential qualities that are required when working in a variety of environments with patients who have diverse sociocultural backgrounds and health care needs. In preparing nurses for this role, it is clear that these qualities should be fostered early on in basic training.

Home health nurses function with a high degree of independence and personal accountability for multidisciplinary service. Their influence over the quality of patient care is *significant*. Consequently, home health nurses have an intriguing opportunity to enhance the vision of what nursing really can be.

REFERENCES

1. Bellman G: *The consultant's calling: bring who you are to what you do,* San Francisco, 1990, Jossey-Bass Publishers.
2. Health Care Financing Administration: *Home health insurance manual* (Pub No 11), Washington, DC, 1995, US Department of Health and Human Services.
3. Johnson T: Personal communication, Visiting Nurse Association of Greater St Louis, September 1989.
4. Rice R: *Manual of home health nursing procedures,* St Louis, 1995, Mosby.
5. Roy C, Martinez C: A conceptual framework for CNS practice. In Hamric A, Spross J, editors: *The clinical nurse specialist in theory and practice,* New York, 1983, Grune & Stratton.

Appendix 3-1

National Community Resources and Services

AIDS Action Council
729 Eighth Street, SE, Suite 200
Washington, DC 20003

Alcoholics Anonymous (AA)
General Service Office
PO Box 459, Grand Central Station
New York, NY 10164

Al-Anon/Alateen Family Groups
Headquarters, Inc.
PO Box 862, Midtown Station
New York, NY 10018-0862

Alzheimer's Disease and Related Disorders
70 East Lake Street
Chicago, IL 60601

American Association of Diabetes Education
3553 West Peterson Avenue
Chicago, IL 60659

American Association of Retired Persons
1909 K Street, NW
Washington, DC 20006

American Cancer Society
777 Third Avenue
New York, NY 10017

American Diabetes Association
1 West 48th Street
New York, NY 10017

American Heart Association
44 East 23rd Street
New York, NY 10010

American Legion National Headquarters
PO Box 1055
Indianapolis, IN 46206

American Lung Association
1740 Broadway
New York, NY 10019

American Parkinson's Disease Association
147 East 50th Street
New York, NY 10022

American Red Cross National Headquarters
17th and D Streets, NW
Washington, DC 20006

Amyotrophic Lateral Sclerosis Association
21021 Ventura Blvd, Suite 321
Woodland Hills, CA 91364

Arthritis Foundation
221 Park Avenue South
New York, NY 10003

Asthma and Allergy Foundation of America
1717 Massachusetts Avenue, NW, Suite 305
Washington, DC 20036

Dystonia Foundation
8383 Wilshire Blvd, Suite 800
Beverly Hills, CA 90211

Easter Seal Society for Crippled Children
and Adults
2023 West Ogden Avenue
Chicago, IL 60612

Epilepsy Federation of America
4351 Garden City Drive
Landover, MD 20785

Juvenile Diabetes Foundation
23 East 26th Street
New York, NY 10010

Leukemia Society of America, Inc.
211 East 43rd Street
New York, NY 10017

Lupus Foundation of America
PO Box 12897
171 Massachusetts Avenue, NW, Suite 203
Washington, DC 20036

Manic Depressive Association
53 West Jackson Blvd, Suite 618
Chicago, IL 60654

Mental Health Materials Center
419 Park Avenue South
New York, NY 10016

Muscular Dystrophy Association, Inc.
810 Seventh Avenue
New York, NY 10019

National Aid to Retarded Citizens
(formerly NAR Children)
2709 East Street
Arlington, TX 76011

National AIDS Information Clearing House
PO Box 6003
Rockville, MD 20850

National Alliance for the Mentally Ill
2101 Wilson Blvd, Suite 302
Arlington, VA 22201

National Association for Down's Syndrome
628 Ashland Avenue
River Forest, IL 60305

National Association for Mental Health, Inc.
1800 North Kent Street, Rosslyn Station
Arlington, VA 22209

National Association for Sickle Cell Disease, Inc.
945 South Western Avenue, Suite 206
Los Angeles, CA 90006

National Association for Visually Handicapped
305 East 24th Street
New York, NY 10010

National Asthma Center
875 Avenue for the Americas
New York, NY 10001

National Center for the Prevention of Child
Abuse
332 South Michigan Avenue, Suite 1250
Chicago, IL 60604-4357

National Council on the Aging
1828 L Street, NW
Washington, DC 20036

National Cystic Fibrosis Research Foundation
3379 Peachtree Road, NE
Atlanta, GA 30326

National Epilepsy League
6 North Michigan Avenue
Chicago, IL 60602

National Foundation-March of Dimes
1275 Mamaroneck Avenue
White Plains, NY 10605

National Genetics Foundation
250 West 57th Street
New York, NY 10019

National Hemophilia Foundation
Soho Building
110 Green Street, Room 406
New York, NY 10012

National Hospice Organization
1901 North Moore, Suite 901
Arlington, VA 22209

National Kidney Foundation
116 East 27th Street
New York, NY 10016

National Paraplegia Foundation
333 North Michigan Avenue
Chicago, IL 60601

Nutrition Foundation, Inc.
489 Fifth Avenue
New York, NY 10017

Paralyzed Veterans of America
7315 Wisconsin Avenue, NW
Washington, DC 20014

Parents of Down's Syndrome Children
11507 Yates Street
Silver Spring, MD 20902

Shriner Hospital for Crippled Children
323 North Michigan Avenue
Chicago, IL 60601

Stroke Clubs of America
805 12th Street
Galveston, TX 77550

United Cerebral Palsy Association, Inc.
66 East 34th Street
New York, NY 10066

United Ostomy Association
1111 Wilshire Blvd
Los Angeles, CA 90017

4 Developing the Plan of Care and Documentation

Robyn Rice

The complexities of managing patient care at home demand a scientific as well as a caring approach. In the hands of knowledgeable and caring nurses, the nursing process provides an organized, step-by-step approach to patient care. It is a process that lends integrity and direction to professional nursing practice in the home. As reflected throughout this book, it is a process that coordinates and evaluates multidisciplinary care.

The intent of this chapter is to help home health nurses develop a plan of care for their patients based on the nursing process. Steps in the process, as well as guidelines for writing outcomes of care, are reviewed. Medicare regulations that influence clinical documentation are also discussed along with tips for completing paperwork.

PREPARING FOR THE HOME VISIT

After formal admission of the patient by a home health agency, the referral is sent to the patient service manager in the appropriate service area within the agency. Patient assignments are determined by where the patient lives (such as zip code) or by the patient's requirements for specialty services (such as intravenous therapy). The patient service manager reviews the referral information and assigns the patient to a home health nurse.

Before the initial home visit, the home health nurse should examine the information on the referral to determine the purpose of the visit. The patient's address and home telephone number, along with any specific orders, should be listed on the referral. It is advisable for the nurse to review the patient's medical record, if available, before the initial visit.

Initial preparation for care will focus on the medical diagnosis as identified by the referral. Once the nurse has assessed the patient and home, subsequent preparation will be directed toward both nursing and medical diagnoses. Nurses should use current research and professional literature, policy and procedure manuals, and resource individuals when preparing the plan of care.

A phone call to the patient is strongly recommended before making the visit. This allows the home health nurse an opportunity to give the patient an approximate time for the visit, to validate or clarify directions to the patient's house (maps should be available from the agency), to request that pets be restrained if necessary, and to inquire about any need for medical supplies. Most important, the phone call allows the home health nurse to begin to assess patient/caregiver needs in developing the plan of care. Once these activities have been completed, stocked nursing bags and any other needed supplies or forms should be obtained.

CONDUCTING THE HOME VISIT

Patients in home care are viewed in the context of their household and community. Home health nurses focus not only on patient health care needs but also on familial, sociocultural, economic, and environmental factors that may affect care (Figure 4-1).

Assessing phase

Data collected during the assessing phase are used to provide the physician with further guidelines for the plan of care and to develop the nursing care

FAMILY SERVICE AND VISITING NURSE ASSOCIATION
DATA BASE I

I. GENERAL INFORMATION

Name:_____ Age:_____ Date of birth ___/___/___ Sex:_____ Race:_____

Address:_____ SS#_____ Source of income_____

City / State /Zip_____ Religious preference_____

Phone #_____ Directions to home:_____

_____

Medicare #_____ Effective Date_____ **Medicaid #**_____ Effective Date:_____

Private Insurance (name)_____ Address_____

Phone #_____ Policy #_____ Insured's name:_____

Insured's SS# :_____ Insured's Place of employment:_____

M.D. Name:_____ Phone #_____ Fax #_____

Address/ zip_____ DME:_____ Phone #_____

Last MD contact:_____ Pharmacy:_____ Phone#_____

Other MD:_____ Address:_____ Phone#_____

Other MD:_____ Address:_____ Phone #_____

II. SOCIO-ECONOMIC DATA:

Housing: ☐Rent ☐Own Occupation:_____ Retired: ☐ Yes ☐ No Date of retirement_____

Place of employment:_____ Education_____ Able to read: ☐ Yes ☐ No Marital Status: M S D W O

Family / home situation:_____

Other members in the household	Name	Relationship	Participates in care
			☐ Y ☐ N
			☐ Y ☐

Emergency Contact:

Name:_____ Relationship:_____

Address_____ Phone #:_____

III. MEDICAL:

Diagnosis	Date of Onset	Recent Surgery & date

ADLs	ASSISTANCE				COMMENTS
	Independent	Minimal	Maximal	Unable to do	
Toileting					
Personal care					
Meal preparation					
Eating					
Transfers					
Dressing					
Ambulation					
Stairs					
Household Chores					
Laundry					
Telephone					
Assistive Devices					
Sleep					
Money Management					

HOMEBOUND STATUS:_____

_____

Figure 4-1 Database collection. (Courtesy The Family Services and Visiting Nurse Association of Alton, Ill.)

FAMILY SERVICE AND VISITING NURSE ASSOCIATION
DATA BASE II

Assessment	Code	Describe or measure	Assessment	Code	Describe or measure
Neuro:			**GI Tract/ Nutrition:**		
Pupils			Appetite		
LOC / Orientation			Changes in wt.		
Fainting / dizziness			Special diet		
Spasticity / paresis			Fluid intake		
Paresthesias			Alcohol intake		
Coordination / balance			Caffine coffee/tea		
Seizures / tremors			Swallowing		
Speech			Nausea /vomiting		
Pain			Abdominal distension		
Smell, touch, taste			Abdominal pain		
Knowledge Deficit ☐ Yes ☐ No			Eructation		
EENT:			Hemorriods		
Vision			Bowel sounds		
Last eye exam			Ulcers		
Glasses			Use of antiacids		
Teeth and gums			Knowledge Deficit ☐ Yes ☐No		
Dentures			**Elimination:**		
Throat			BM frequency		
Hearing			Melena		
Knowledge deficit ☐ Yes ☐No			Constipation		
Respiratory:			Laxatives (frequency)		
Respiratory rate			Enemas (frequency)		
Rhythm			Incontinent of stool / urine		
Lung sounds			Frequency		
Abdominal breathing			Dysuria		
Cough			Hematuria		
Sputum (color/cosistency)			Nocturia		
Barrel chest			Retention		
Symmetry			Catheter: size:		
Wheezing			☐ Foley ☐ straight		
Dyspnea (on exertion)			Date last changed:		
Pillows			Type:		
Smoking habits			Knowledge Deficit ☐ Yes ☐No		
Knowledge Deficit ☐Yes ☐ No			**Musculoskeletal /Motor:**		
			Joint pain		
			Muscle cramps		
Cardiovascular:			Movement limitations		
Radial pulse ☐ Reg ☐ Irreg			Range of motion:		
Apical pulse ☐ Reg ☐ Irreg			A-ROM ☐ P-ROM		
Pedal pulse ☐Rt. ☐ Lt			Drop foot		
Capillary refill (in seconds)			Contractures		

B/P	lying	sitting	standing
Rt			
Lt			

Assessment	Code	Describe or measure
Chest pain		
Phlebitis		
Varicose Veins		

Edema (measure in inches)	Rt.	Lt.
Pedal		
Ankle		
Calf		
Knowledge Deficit ☐Yes ☐ No		

Assessment	Code	Describe or measure
Prosthesis		
Gait		
Equilibrium		
Atrophy		
Knowledge deficit ☐Yes ☐No		
General:		
Sleep pattern		
Aids (sleep/ pain) freq.		
Pain		
Night sweats		
Frequent infections		
Fatigue		

Code: WNL - Within normal limits   P - Problem   DNA - Does not apply

Patient Name: _____

Continued

Figure 4-1, cont'd. For legend see opposite page.

FAMILY SERVICE AND VISITING NURSE ASSOCIATION
DATA BASE III

ASSESSMENT	Code	Describe or measure	ASSESSMENT	Code	Describe or measure
Emotional / Mental:			**Sexuality/ Reproductive:**		
Attention span / grasp			Breasts: lumps/discharge		
Health status/ insight			Self breast exam		
Adaptation to diagnosis			Last pap smear		
Anxiety			Menses LMP (date)		
Depression			Number of children		
Body image			Birth control		
Relates to others			Discharge vagina / penis		
Hobbies interests/activities			Last prostate exam		
Knowledge Deficit ☐Yes ☐No			Sexual problems		
Safety:			Knowledge Deficit ☐Yes ☐No		
Dwelling, structure			**Integumentary:**		
Hazards			Color		
Heat			Rash (describe)		
Bathroom /communal			Decubitus		
Fire plan			Incisions		
Smoke detectors			Turgor		
Emergency numbers			Hair		
Knowledge Deficit ☐Yes ☐No			Nails		
Equipment:			Bruising		
			Jaundice		
Other services			Temperature: O R A		
			Knowledge Deficit ☐Yes ☐No		

Fingerstick B/S: **Last meal**

Medications present: ☐Yes ☐No **Compliance:** ☐Yes ☐No
Understanding ☐Yes ☐No
Teaching Initiated:
Medicare, Medicaid, Pvt. Ins. payment discussed ☐Yes ☐No
Conditions for home health care   ☐ Yes ☐ No
Care Plan / MD orders   ☐ Yes ☐ No
Proposed length of visits   ☐ Yes ☐ No
Other disciplines referred:
☐ PT   ☐ OT   ☐ ST   ☐ MSW   ☐ HHA

Use coding system below to help describe wounds:
1. Rash   6. Pressure area (intact skin)
2. Lesions   7. Open wound
3. Petechiae   8. Surgical wound
4. Bruise   9. Scar
5. Abrasion   10. Other

Comments:

R.N. Signature   **Date:**

Code: WNL - Within normal limits   P - Problem   DNA - Does not apply

Figure 4-1, cont'd. For legend see p. 42.

plan. At this point it is important to distinguish between the plan of care and the patient care plan. According to the Health Insurance Manual publication number 11 (HIM-11), the plan of care (previously called the plan of treatment) is the medical treatment plan that is established by the treating physician.[2] In addition, Medicare expects that a discipline-oriented patient care plan be established, where appropriate, by a home health nurse regarding nursing and home health aide services and by skilled therapists regarding specific therapy treatment. Medicare states that these plans of care may be incorporated within the physician's plan of care on the Medicare forms 485, 486, and 487 or prepared separately.[2] From a quality point of view, the author recommends that the patient care plan be done in a care path format described later in this book.

A holistic approach in care plan development is recommended. Components of the assessment phase include (1) the initial telephone call, (2) the assessment interview, (3) the assembly of a historical database (including socioenvironmental and family assessment), (4) the nursing health history, (5) the medication assessment, and (6) the physical assessment (including spiritual, mental, and functional status).

Initial phone call. The assessment phase of the patient begins with telephone contact. During this time the home health nurse receives feedback about the patient's situation and current health status. Most important, the phone call can be utilized to ask patients how they are doing. This information is invaluable when planning visits. It also prevents dramatic surprises when the home health nurse arrives at the patient's home.

Assessment interview. The assessment phase next moves to the initial formal assessment interview. The purpose of this interview is to collect data and obtain other information. Even though a printed form, checklist, or outline is usually followed, nurses should be receptive to all information offered by patients, families, or caregivers. The assessment interview primarily collects subjective data from the patient's responses to questions, but nonverbal cues should also be noted. The assessment interview is an important step in the establishment of nurse-patient-caregiver therapeutic relationships.

Historical database. An important element of the historical database is the socioenvironmental assessment, which should present a clear picture of the patient in the home. In addition to identifying the patient's economic status and living conditions, the home health nurse should focus on factors such as the cooperation of the patient/caregiver, and the availability of environmental resources needed to implement care.

In addition, a family assessment is also recommended in recognizing all support systems available to assist with patient care. Learning, communication, and coping styles of patients, families, or caregivers should be identified. Each person's role in the household should be considered when developing the plan of care. This is of particular importance when working with pediatric cases. (See Chapter 20, which reviews family systems theory.)

Nursing health history. The nursing health history deals with patients' responses to and perceptions of their health status. It focuses on patients' feelings regarding their need for health care and their expectations regarding this care. Clues to patients' abilities to deal with current health problems are sought. The nursing health history also helps to identify past patterns of health and illness, the presence of risk factors, and the availability of resources to the individual.

If a complete *medical* health history is not available, additional information should be sought. This additional information should include a description of the patient's present health status, past medical and surgical history, family medical history, and a review of body systems. The review of body systems consists of the patient's responses to questions concerning each body system. It is not the same as the physical assessment, which seeks objective data.

Medication assessment. Information should be gathered about all prescription and nonprescription medications. Home health nurses should ask to see **all** of the patient's medicines, including over-the-counter medications. A complete medication assessment provides nurses with the opportunity to verify the name, dosage, and frequency of administration for each medicine. As described in Chapter 24, this can provide some invaluable insights as to the patient's learning needs. The purpose of the

MEDICATION SHEET

Patient Name: _____   RN Signature/Date: _____

Admission Date: _____

Diagnosis: _____   Change/Update: _____

Allergies: _____

Physician Name/Office Number: _____   RN Signature/Date: _____

MEDICATION	Start	Stop	Dosage, Time, Route	PATIENT EDUCATION
1.				Date:_____ ☐Action ☐Purpose ☐Prior Review Side Effects (list) _____ _____ _____ ☐ Administration: _____
2.				
3.				
4.				
5.				
6.				
Non-prescription Medications:				

Figure 4-2 Medication sheet.

medicine, adverse reactions, allergies, side effects, and therapeutic effects should be determined. Figure 4-2 is an example of a medication form used for recording this information.

Medications should be reviewed on each visit to note changes in dose, frequency, or type. These findings should be prescribed by the physician in the patient's record. Consequently, changes in the medication regimen become a basis for new teaching.

Physical assessment. The physical assessment is another major source of information. It consists of an evaluation of the patient's health status through the use of the nurse's specially trained senses of sight, hearing, touch, and smell. Patients can be examined in a head to toe, systematic manner or according to body systems. Nurses should develop their own approach and should be ready to adapt their assessment skills to the particular patient.

The physical assessment should identify any functional limitations that the patient may experience when ambulating or performing activities of daily living (ADLs). As described in Chapter 16, this becomes a basis for a further evaluation by the rehabilitation therapists.

Spiritual assessment. As described more fully in Chapter 23, the mental health assessment is typically performed in conjunction with the physical assessment. As depicted in Figure 4-3, the database may also include a spiritual assessment. This will be especially important for hospice home health nurses because issues of hope and faith play a major role in patient care.

Initially, home health nurses should do a complete physical assessment. On later visits it may be necessary to assess only specific problem areas. Any changes noted in later assessments should be reflected in the chart. This serves to keep the database current and up-to-date.

In reporting assessment findings to the physician, home health nurses primarily report deviations from the patient's baseline status. In home care, it is not unusual to find patients with fluctuating vital signs or blood glucose levels. Many physicians, as they continue to adjust medical treatment, may feel it is unnecessary for the nurse to report this information after each visit. When in doubt, home health nurses should obtain written guidelines from the physician regarding when he or she wants to be notified of the patient's status. These guidelines should be placed in the medical record. Home health nurses should **never** hesitate to notify the physician of assessment findings or to send the patient to the emergency room for medical evaluation when your "gut feelings/common sense" tell you to do so.

Diagnosing phase

Once the assessment is completed, the nurse interprets the data and develops nursing diagnoses. A nursing diagnosis is a clear, concise statement of the patient's health status. It reflects the patient's healthy and unhealthy response(s) and the supporting factor(s) for each response.[6]

Nursing diagnoses commonly used in home care include knowledge deficit (identify subject), activity intolerance, and self-care deficit.[5] Of note, as documentation systems are moving toward multidisciplinary needs, many home health agencies are utilizing nursing diagnosis to lead multidisciplinary care (i.e., nursing diagnosis/identified patient problem).

Planning phase

Plan of care. Trends in health care, such as care paths, are merging nursing care plans with multidisciplinary needs. In addition, with increasing emphasis upon patient participation in the plan of care, nursing care plans are now more commonly being referred to as patient care plans.

Patient care plan. The patient care plan is established by the home health nurse and the multidisciplinary team, which includes the physician. It reflects the medical treatment plan, interventions, projected outcomes of care, and long-term goals. The plan has a specific aim or purpose regarding patient care. It is recorded to maximize quality patient care, to ensure appropriate utilization of resources, to evaluate the delivery of services, and can provide documentation to validate Medicare reimbursement of services.[2,3,9]

The first step in the planning phase is the establishment of priorities. The nurse, the multidisciplinary team, and patient/caregiver should work together to identify the immediate concerns and patient/caregiver needs. Nursing diagnoses are then derived and outcomes of care *mutually* determined. Priorities are constantly changing. As the patient's medical condition changes, the "ranking" of the nursing diagnoses will also change.

Outcomes of care. The next step in the planning phase is the identification of goals and outcomes of care. Goals and outcomes of patient care should reflect the nursing diagnosis and overall plan of care (POC). They give direction to nursing interventions and pace activities within the patient care plan.[1,6] They both should be written as patient-centered rather than nurse-centered statements. In other words, goals and outcomes of care should contain verbs that reflect responses to be observed in the patient, not activities to be performed by the nurse.

Goals are generalized long-term outcomes of care that should occur by discharge. Statements of long-term goals do not describe the exact process necessary to reach the goal. For example, "the patient's appetite will improve in 4 weeks" is a long-term, patient-centered goal.

Outcomes of care are precise and measurable. They reflect steps leading to the accomplishment

Hospice Spiritual Assessment   **Client Name:** _____

1. Client's current and past religious affiliation.
2. Clergy   Name: _____ Address: _____ Phone: _____
3. What is the religious affiliation of immediate family members, significant other, or caretaker.
4. Which religious/spiritual practices are meaningful to the client (e.g., prayer, sacraments, rosary, Bible readings, hymns, yoga)?
5. Which aesthetic interests enhance the client's life (e.g., art, music, nature)?
6. Which relationships are most important and meaningful to the client?
7. Which holidays, family events, or rituals are significant to the client and family?
8. What are the client's sources of strength in life?
9. How does the client describe his/her life in relation to its meaning, successes, and joys?
10. Is the client at peace? If not, describe.
11. What meaning does pain/disease/terminal illness and death have for the client?
12. What does the client usually do to cope with fear/anger? Stress?
13. Are there relationships where forgiveness/reconciliation is sought?
14. What legacy or message would the client like to leave to others?

Signature: _____   Date: _____

S.M. Hatch/H.L.L.

Figure 4-3 Spiritual assessment. (Courtesy Suzanne Hatch, West Stockbridge, Mass.)

of the long-term goal. For example, "the patient will eat 800 calories per day by the end of the week" is a short-term, patient-centered outcome of care. See the box on writing outcomes of care. As with priority setting, patients should be involved in setting their own goals and outcomes of care.

Implementing phase

Once long- and short-term goals have been identified, home health nurses, in partnership with the patient/caregiver and multidisciplinary team, can identify specific interventions, actions, or therapies that will help patients achieve outcomes of care and goal resolution. Although directed by the physician and initiated by home health nurses, intervention within the patient's environment is, by nature, frequently improvisational. What works well for one patient may or may not work well for another. Therefore recommendations for care may be determined by trial and error.

Implementation of the patient care plan by home health nurses functioning in the role of case managers involves exchanging information with patients/caregivers, coordinating referrals, facilitating multidisciplinary conferences, and—as the patient's advocate—seeking resources within the community. Specific home health nursing interventions involve a great variety of procedural skills such as dressing changes, medication administration, intravenous therapy, and foley catheter changes, to name a few.[2,3]

The implementation phase should integrate the plan of care and patient care plan into the patient's environment. Patients/caregivers then are able to take on the responsibilities for self-care management which will involve learning, assessment, task achievement, evaluation, and decision making. They acquire knowledge, judgment, and confidence as home health nurses support and encourage this process. The following principles govern implementation of the patient care plan:

1. Formal guidelines as to what the nurse can and cannot do are determined by the home health agency's scope of services, and its policies and procedures.
2. Implementation should be inclusive of the multidisciplinary team and patients/caregivers because all will participate in effecting the plan of care.

3. The relationship between home health nurses, physicians, the multidisciplinary team, and patients/caregivers should be a collaborative and cooperative one, based on a mutually derived plan of care.
4. Improvisation and individualization of interventions and outcomes of care are a fact of life when working in the home milieu.
5. Medicare regulations strongly influence documentation and services rendered and are the basis for reimbursement of Medicare-certified home health agencies.

Documentation

Careful attention must be paid to documentation. Accurate, precise documentation reflects the quality of patient care, validates the need for services rendered, and serves as a basis for reimbursement by Medicare.

Medicare guidelines. As discussed in Chapter 1, Medicare—administered by the Health Care Financing Administration (HCFA)—influences the financial operation of Medicare-certified home health agencies. The Health Insurance Manual publication number 11 (HIM-11) and Federal Register identify conditions to be met for coverage of home health care services. In addition, each state's Department of Health and Home Health Licensing Bureau regulates the delivery of services. These conditions periodically change pending federal and state review. The federal and state requirements to be met for the coverage of home health services include but are not limited to:[2,3,9]

1. A physician-certified POC which must be periodically reviewed and signed for the duration of services; this is called the certification period. (Currently, certification periods are approximately 9 weeks or 62 days.) Any change in the plan must be signed and dated by the physician. A verbal order may precede the signed order. All oral orders must be countersigned and dated by the physician before the agency bills for the care.

   Oral orders are put into writing and signed and dated upon receipt by the home health nurse or therapist responsible for providing or furnishing the ordered services. Oral orders are only accepted by

WRITING OUTCOMES OF CARE TO DOCUMENT PATIENT/CAREGIVER RESPONSE TO THERAPY

Definition

Outcomes of care are objective measurements of the patient's health status to be achieved or worked toward during home care services. They represent a change in the patient's health status from one time frame to another. The main purpose in using outcomes is to guide planning, implementation, and evaluation of the plan of care (POC). Outcomes of care support discharge goals of care. In documenting patient/caregiver response to therapy, outcomes of care should:

1. State the expected behavioral performance.
   Specific performance verbs:
   - Write
   - List
   - Cite
   - Verbalize
   - Accomplish
   - Perform
   - Demonstrate
   - Explain
   - Utilize
   - Achieve
   - Identify
   - Assist
2. State the criteria or measurable level of performance specified. Criteria include concepts such as amount and accuracy.
   Examples:
   "Patient cites correct medication regimen."
   "Patient identifies complications of disease process (such as, *list in narrative of visit report, on POC, or on care path*) to report to case manager, physician."
   "Patient achieves optimal response to the physical treatment plan as evidenced by wound healing."
   "Patient agrees to the plan of care by explaining treatment principles, use of multidisciplinary services, and estimated length of service(s) without the prompting of the nurse."
3. Reflect the treatment plan and identified primary nursing diagnoses/patient problems.
   Example:
   Medical treatment plan: Decubitus ulcer
   Standard of care: Skin/integumentary
   Primary nursing diagnoses/patient problems:
   - Impaired skin integrity
   - Impaired physical mobility
   - Knowledge deficit: disease process, risk complications, nutrition, procedural care, infection control, socioeconomic resources, etc.
4. Occur within an expected time frame. Set a specific date for outcome achievement.
5. Evaluate the POC using skilled observation, oral questioning, or written measurement. Did the patient's health improve? Were outcomes met? **Was there a positive change in patient behaviors enabling self-care management and promoting best level of function?** If no, why not? Outcomes that are not met should be coded as variances. Identify any variance(s) and determine a corrective plan of action with the physician, the multidisciplinary team, and patient.

Be aware that quality outcome measures are used to evaluate many aspects of service delivery. See Chapter 9 for more information about outcomes.

personnel authorized to do so by applicable state and federal laws and regulations as well as by the home health agency's internal policies.

The plan of care is considered to be terminated if the patient does not receive at least one covered skilled nursing, physical therapy, speech language pathology service, or occupational therapy visit in a 62-day period unless the physician documents that the interval without such care is appropriate to the treatment of the patient's illness or injury.

2. Services that are viewed as reasonable and necessary, and documented on the HCFA 485, 486, and 487. (See Figures 4-4 to 4-6.) Key issues that determine what is reasonable and necessary include (a) whether the skills of a nurse or physical, occupational, or speech therapist are needed to treat illness and/or injury, (b) whether the condition of the patient will improve in a reasonable and predictable period of time, and (c) whether the patient is confined to home for medical or psychiatric reasons.

3. Objective clinical evidence supporting the patient's needs for intermittent skilled care. The need for management and evaluation of patient care, as well as intermittent procedural care (tube feedings, ostomy care, venipuncture), patient/caregiver teaching/training activities, and abnormal or fluctuating vital signs, or symptoms of drug toxicity, or changes in cardiopulmonary or mentation status, or changes in the medication regimen are conditions that validate the necessity for home care visits. (See Chapter 2 for multidisciplinary indicators for service.)

4. Homebound status should be documented each visit. (See the box on guidelines for documenting homebound status.) In addition, some states require that patients notify the home health agency of any homebound status change.

5. All visit orders on the plan of care must state the treatment, the discipline, and the visit frequency for the 9-week period. The following are examples of visit orders:

a. Home health aide—3 wk 4; 2 wk 5 to assist with bath and personal care.
b. Social services—2 visits q 60 days to help the family identify community resources to pay bills and buy food.
c. Skilled nurse—3 wk 4; 2 wk 5 to assess patient with infected dermal wound, change wound dressing, instruct patient/caregiver on wound care, and evaluate healing.

Ranges of 1-2 visits may be used in stating the frequency of visits within the certification period. For example, skilled nurse 4-5 wk 1; 3-4 wk 2; 1-2 wk 4; 1 wk 2; for home intravenous therapy management and two visits prn for problems with central venous catheter leakage (note: a specific reason and a description of the patient's vital signs or symptoms that would occasion the visit must be documented for prn visits). If a range of visits is ordered, the upper limit of the range is considered the specific frequency.

Review fiscal intermediary guidelines for reimbursement when using ranges to specify visit frequencies. **Any** changes in the visit frequency or new orders must be authorized and signed by the physician.

6. The patient's rehabilitation potential, goals/outcomes of care, and discharge status must be stated on the plan of care. This should reflect the desired outcome and an estimated discharge time. For example, wound to heal by 01/96. Discharge to self/physician care. (Note: for anticipated prolonged admissions, as with a severe decubitus ulcer, estimate the discharge by stating the month and year. This period may be reused upon recertification as needed.)

7. If the patient has not achieved stability at the end of the certification period and requires continued home care, identify which discipline will provide what services, and the frequency/duration of visits. At this time, the physician should receive, review, sign, and return an updated HCFA 485 prior to the start date of the recertification period. (Typically recertifications are sent about 2 weeks before the current certification period ends.) Of note, the period of time

Department of Health and Human Services
Health Care Financing Administration

Form Approved
OMB No. 0938-0357

HOME HEALTH CERTIFICATION AND PLAN OF TREATMENT

1. Patient's HI Claim No.	2. SOC Date	3. Certification Period From: To:	4. Medical Record No.	5. Provider No.

6. Patient's Name and Address

7. Provider's Name and Address.

8. Date of Birth:	9. Sex	M	F	10. Medications: Dose/Frequency/Route (N)ew (C)hanged

11. ICD-9-CM	Principal Diagnosis	Date

12. ICD-9-CM	Surgical Procedure	Date

13. ICD-9-CM	Other Pertinent Diagnoses	Date

14. DME and Supplies	15. Safety Measures:

16. Nutritional Req.	17. Allergies:

18.A. Functional Limitations

1 Amputation
2 Bowel/Bladder (Incontinence)
3 Contracture
4 Hearing
5 Paralysis
6 Endurance
7 Ambulation
8 Speech
9 Legally Blind
A Dyspnea With Minimal Exertion
B Other (Specify)

18.B. Activities Permitted

1 Complete Bedrest
2 Bedrest BRP
3 Up As Tolerated
4 Transfer Bed/Chair
5 Exercises Prescribed
6 Partial Weight Bearing
7 Independent At Home
8 Crutches
9 Cane
A Wheelchair
B Walker
C No Restrictions
D Other (Specify)

19. Mental Status:
1 Oriented
2 Comatose
3 Forgetful
4 Depressed
5 Disoriented
6 Lethargic
7 Agitated
8 Other

20. Prognosis:
1 Poor
2 Guarded
3 Fair
4 Good
5 Excellent

21. Orders for Discipline and Treatments (Specify Amount/Frequency/Duration)

22. Goals/Rehabilitation Potential/Discharge Plans

23. Verbal Start of Care and Nurse's Signature and Date Where Applicable:

24. Physician's Name and Address	25. Date HHA Received Signed POT	26. I ☐ certify ☐ recertify that the above home health services are required and are authorized by me with a written plan for treatment which will be periodically reviewed by me. This patient is under my care, is confined to his home, and is in need of intermittent skilled nursing care and/or physical or speech therapy or has been furnished home health services based on such a need and no longer has a need for such care or therapy, but continues to need occupational therapy.
27. Attending Physician's Signature (Required on 485 Kept on File in Medical Records of HHA)	Date Signed	

Form HCFA-485 (C4) (4-87)

PROVIDER

Figure 4-4 HCFA form 485, home health certification and plan of treatment. (From *Health Insurance Manual,* Pub No 11 -Thru T273, Rev 3/95, Washington, DC, 1995, US Department of Health and Human Services.)

Department of Health and Human Services
Health Care Financing Administration

Form Approved
OMB No. 0938-0357

MEDICAL UPDATE AND PATIENT INFORMATION

1. Patient's HI Claim No.	2. SOC Date	3. Certification Period		4. Medical Record No.	5. Provider No.
		From:	To:		

6 Patient's Name	7. Provider's Name

8. Medicare Covered: ☐ Y ☐ N | 9. Date Physician Last Saw Patient: | 10. Date Last Contacted Physician:

11. Is the Patient Receiving Care in an 1861 (J)(1) Skilled Nursing Facility or Equivalent? ☐ Y ☐ N ☐ Do Not Know

12. ☐ Certification   ☐ Recertification   ☐ Modified

13. **Specific Services and Treatments**

Discipline	Visits (This Bill) Rel. to Prior Cert.	Frequency and Duration	Treatment Codes	Total Visits Projected This Cert.

14. Dates of Last Inpatient Stay: Admission _____ Discharge _____ | 15. Type of Facility:

16. Updated Information: New Orders/Treatments/Clinical Facts/Summary from Each Discipline

17. Functional Limitations (Expand From 485 and Level of ADL) Reason Homebound/Prior Functional Status

18. Supplementary Plan of Treatment on File from Physician Other than Referring Physician: ☐ Y ☐ N
(If Yes, Please Specify Giving Goals/Rehab. Potential/Discharge Plan)

19. Unusual Home/Social Environment

20. Indicate Any Time When the Home Health Agency Made a Visit and Patient was Not Home and Reason Why if Ascertainable	21. Specify Any Known Medical and/or Non-Medical Reasons the Patient Regularly Leaves Home and Frequency of Occurrence

22. Nurse or Therapist Completing or Reviewing Form	Date (Mo., Day, Yr.)

Form HCFA-486 (C3) (4-87)

PROVIDER

Figure 4-5 HCFA form 486, medical update and patient information. (From *Health Insurance Manual,* Pub No 11 -Thru T273, Rev 3/95, Washington, DC, 1995, US Department of Health and Human Services.)

Department of Health and Human Services
Health Care Financing Administration

Form Approved
OMB No. 0938-0357

ADDENDUM TO: ☐ PLAN OF TREATMENT ☐ MEDICAL UPDATE

1. Patient's HI Claim No.	2. SOC Date	3. Certification Period		4. Medical Record No.	5. Provider No.
		From: To:			

6. Patient's Name	7. Provider Name

8. Item
   No.

9. Signature of Physician	10. Date

11. Optional Name/Signature of Nurse/Therapist	12. Date

Form HCFA-487 (C4) (4-87)

PROVIDER

Figure 4-6 HCFA form 487, addendum to plan of treatment/medical update. (From *Health Insurance Manual,* Pub No 11 -Thru T273, Rev 3/95, Washington, DC, 1995, US Department of Health and Human Services.)

GUIDELINES FOR DOCUMENTING HOMEBOUND STATUS[9]

Be as specific as possible. Indications of homebound status include:

1. Restricted mobility from disease process such as unsteady gait, draining wounds, depressed immunity, or pain.
2. Poor cardiac reserve, shortness of breath, or activity intolerance secondary to unstable or exacerbated disease process.
3. Bed or wheelchair bound patients who require physical assistance to move any distance.
4. Patients who require caregiver help with assistive devices such as a cane, walker, wheelchair, or other special device to leave home.
5. Failure to thrive, low birth weight infants.
6. A tracheostomy, abdominal drains, foley catheter, or nasogastric tube that restricts ambulation.
7. Home ventilator dependence or a patient who is unable to ambulate with portable oxygen.
8. Psychotic ideation, confusion, or impaired mental status that restricts functional abilities outside of the home.
9. A new colostomy or ileostomy that complicates ambulation.
10. Fluctuating blood pressures or blood sugars that predispose patients to syncope or dizziness.
11. Patients who cannot ambulate stairs or uneven surfaces without assistance of caregiver.
12. 5 day or less post-op eye surgery where the physician has restricted patient activity.
13. Patients who are legally blind or cannot drive.
14. Natural disasters or geographic barriers such as dirt roads or islands that restrict patient activity or make it a taxing effort for the patient to leave.

before recertification begins on the day of the initial visit.

8. A psychiatrist must direct the plan of care for patients requiring the services of a psychiatric home health nurse. (Note: HCFA is currently reviewing a proposal which would allow a physician to direct the plan of care for patients requiring the services of a psychiatric home health nurse.)
9. Complete a visit report each time the patient is seen (Figure 4-7). Each visit report

should stand on its own merit regarding Medicare guidelines for reimbursement (Table 4-1). In addition, documentation on the visit report should directly reflect the medical treatment plan, related nursing diagnosis, interventions, and outcomes of care as identified on the patient care plan.

Subsequent visit reports must document procedures or skilled care which concurrently reflect **changes** in medical treatment in order to support continued or increased services.

10. Obtain physician's orders for multidisciplinary services and follow home health agency policy for consultation services. The orders for multidisciplinary services should identify which discipline is requested, for what purposes, and the frequency/duration of visits needed.

Review home health agency policy when consulting with the clinical nurse specialist. A copy of the patient's HCFA form 485 may be attached to the referral for further clarification of patient needs. After the consultation is completed, the original request for consultation should be placed in the chart along with the consultant's visit report and subsequent recommendations.

Multidisciplinary conferences should be held for each patient at least every 60 days (many states require conferencing for each patient every 30 days) to review management of patient care (Figure 4-8). Consider updating the patient care plan during the multidisciplinary conference. In advocating a mutually determined plan of care, share this information with patients/caregivers so they too are able to identify their progress with the plan of care and recognize needed areas of improvement. Likewise this information should be summarized and sent to the physician for care plan oversight.

11. Obtain physician orders for all medical supplies and home medical equipment (HME). Documentation showing that supplies and equipment are reasonable and necessary for the patient's treatment and recovery is required in order for Medicare to reimburse the expense. For example, if requesting a bedside commode, document

BARNES

VISIT REPORT

DISCIPLINE: ☐ SN ☐ PT ☐ ST ☐ OT ☐ MSS ☐ NT

LAST NAME	FIRST	INITIAL	DATE OF BIRTH	ID #	BRANCH/ZIP

TEMP.	PULSE	RESP.	B.P. R/L		

HOMEBOUND STATUS: ☐ AMBULATION ☐ ENDURANCE ☐ VISION ☐ INFECTION ☐ RESPIRATORY ☐ OTHER _____

SN	PT	ST

SN

Weight _____ LBM _____
Foley Change ☐ Yes ☐ No Size _____
Fingerstick Glucose _____
Lab Test _____
Medications Administered/Route _____
Caregiver Present ☐ Yes ☐ No ☐ Self
Comprehension of Instructions ☐ Yes ☐ No
☐ Uncertain

PT

Training	Device/Assistance	Exercise	Extremity (ies)
☐ Gait		☐ Active	
☐ Stairs		☐ Passive	
☐ Prosthetic		☐ Resistive	
☐ Transfer		☐ Ultrasound	
		☐ Other	

ST

Training In:
☐ Oral-facial Exercises ☐ Esophageal Voice
☐ Compensatory Techniques ☐ Voice Therapy
☐ Language Therapy ☐ Dysphagia
☐ Use of Electrolarynx ☐ Other _____
☐ Augmentative Communication

OT	MSS	NT

OT

☐ ADL/IADL Instructions ☐ Environmental Modifications
☐ U.E. Muscle Re-education ☐ Home Safety Instructions
☐ Functional Mobility Training ☐ Other
☐ Energy Conservation/Work Simplification

MSS

Problems Effecting Recovery _____
Contributing factors _____
☐ Financial Assistance ☐ Housing Assistance
☐ Support Services ☐ Hospice
☐ Counseling ☐ Other _____
Codes _____ Visit Number _____

NT

Usual Weight _____
Current Weight _____
Ideal Body Weight _____
Calorie Intake _____
Diet Order _____
Supplements _____

HOME HEALTH AIDE SUPERVISORY VISIT   ☐ Yes ☐ No

Aide/Patient/Caregiver Rapport _____
Goals Met ☐ Yes ☐ No _____
If assignment changed: ☐ New assignment completed ☐ Communicated to Aide

Aide Present   ☐ Yes ☐ No
Need for Continued Service ☐ Yes ☐ No
Aide Assignment Change   ☐ Yes ☐ No
☐ Communicated to Patient/Caregiver

STANDARDS OF CARE   P = PROBLEM   NPN = NO PROBLEM NOTED   NA = NOT APPLICABLE

STANDARD	P	NPN	NA	STANDARD	P	NPN	NA	STANDARD	P	NPN	NA
1. SENSORY				6. ELIMINATION				11. SEXUALITY			
2. SKIN/MUCOUS MEMBRANE				7. ACTIVITY/EXERCISE				12. COGNITIVE RESPONSE			
3. RESPIRATORY				8. COMFORT				13. SOCIAL SYSTEM			
4. CIRCULATORY				9. IMMUNE/INFECTION COMMUNICABLE DISEASE ☐ FAMILY ☐ PATIENT				14. HEALTH MANAGEMENT			
5. NUTRITION				10. NEURO/CEREBRAL FUNCTION				15. SAFETY			

STD #	ASSESSMENT/INTERVENTION/EVALUATION/PLAN

Patient Rights and Responsibilities Reviewed ☐ yes ☐ no   Educational Materials Given ☐ yes ☐ no

OTHER SERVICE NEEDS ASSESSED ☐ Yes ☐ No   **ORDERS RECEIVED** ☐ Yes ☐ No ☐ NA

CASE CONFERENCE
☐ SN ☐ PT ☐ ST ☐ OT
☐ MSS ☐ NT ☐ AIDE ☐ DOCTOR
☐ OTHER _____

PROGRESS NOTE (_____ – _____)

Patient Signature _____

Signature/Title _____
Date _____ Time In _____ Time Out _____

White copy—Chart   Yellow copy – Control   Pink – Employee   3995-75 rev. 7/92

Figure 4-7 Multidisciplinary visit report. (Courtesy Barnes Home Health Services, Barnes Hospital, St Louis, Mo.)

Table 4-1 Guidelines for Medicare documentation to validate the need for home care services[10]

Avoid the following words	Use instead
Monitor, supervise. Denotes a stable patient.	**Assess, evaluate.** *Monitor* may be used when managed care is ordered and the skilled nurse is supervising paraprofessionals to ensure safe delivery of the therapeutic regimen.
Healing well. Suggests that visits are unnecessary, and supports patient discharge from home health services.	Objectively describe the wound in terms of size, depth, drainage, color, and odor.
Discussed. Does not require the skills of a professional; anyone can discuss.	**Teach, educate, instruct, demonstrate**
Prevent/prevention. Not covered. Must be done incidental to a skilled service such as assessment, teaching, and treatment.	Focus on **restorative, rehabilitative,** and/or **palliative** (hospice) interventions.
Stable, independent. Negates medical necessity and supports patient discharge from home health services.	Document response to treatment.
Feeling better. Subjective and supports patient discharge from home health services.	Focus on the patient's physical assessment, functional ability, and problems/needs.
Noncompliant/uncooperative	Document specific problems with coping or refusal to follow the plan of care as source of referral to psychiatric home health nurse or social worker. Document refusal to follow the plan of care as a justification for a learning contract or per home health agency policy, patient discharge.
Went to the market/going to church, etc. Negates homebound status.	Document equipment, manual assistance, and number of people required for patient to leave home. Verify homebound status each visit. If the patient leaves the home, explain why trips were taken as related to lifestyle or medical necessity.
Patient not at home	**Not available for visit** or **no answer to locked door.** Document on next visit why patient was not available for visit. "At community appointment," for example.
Continue care plan	Describe what your next visit plans are based on, e.g., "assess cardiopulmonary status of CHF patient."
Maintenance. Never use this word because it negates the necessity of visits, and supports patient discharge from home health services.	Document response to the plan of care or case management needs.
Confused	Describe disorientation to person, place, or time. Describe ability to follow commands, short- and long-term recall.
Chronic condition. Is indicative of a stable condition.	Describe exacerbation of the chronic condition that requires the services of a skilled nurse.
Reinforce, reinstruct. Repetitive instruction will not be covered unless learning difficulties are documented.	Document comprehension difficulties, attention deficit, or other problems that hamper ability to learn and necessitate repeating instructions. Use words such as **demonstrate, teach, instruct,** or **educate.**
Observed. Anyone can observe.	Use **assess** or **evaluate.** Skilled observation may be used as a component of patient education to document patient/caregiver return demonstration.

Date: _____ Patient Name: _____
Attendees: _____
_____
Patient progress in meeting outcomes of care:
_____
_____
_____
_____
_____
_____
_____
_____

Recommendations: _____
_____
_____

Figure 4-8 Multidisciplinary conference form.

"patient is unable to stand" rather than "patient has limited mobility." The plan of care (HCFA 485) must reflect any HME already in the home.

12. As discussed in the previous section, establish the patient care plan. Many states require that a patient care plan be established by the home health nurse or therapist reflecting all services and disciplines involved in the patient's care in addition to the POC (485, 486, 487).

   Document and update patient/caregiver response to the plan of care and any changes in the plan of care weekly. Patient problem areas or resolution of identified problems should be summarized at least every 60 days. Many home health agencies use the 485, 486, 487 at recertification to summarize the patient's progress with the plan of care.

13. Establish the Patient's Bill of Rights with patient/caregiver signature acknowledging that they have received this information. HCFA requires that each patient be made aware of the bill of rights upon admission to the home health agency. At this time consider establishing the home health agency's bill of rights or patient responsibilities for care. This can have profound implica-

tions for service delivery as discussed in Chapter 7.

14. Review and document the patient's or legal guardian's wishes regarding HCFA's requirement for advance medical directives. Special issues to consider are the patient's wishes regarding "Do Not Resuscitate" (DNR) orders, organ donation, and request/refusal of specific treatments such as tube feedings and other medical procedures. Follow individual state laws regarding implementation of advance medical directives and durable power of attorney for health care.

15. As applicable, document the home health aide supervisory visit every 14 days to include:
   a. Patient/caregiver satisfaction with the home health aide service
   b. Continued need for home health aide service
   c. Recommendations to continue or change visit frequency
   In addition, home health aide assignment sheets (care plans) must be completed by home health nurses. They should give home health aides specific instructions regarding patient care, as shown in Figure 4-9. No dependent services (home health aide) may be covered by Medicare after the final qualifying service has been furnished.

16. Document pertinent conversations regarding the patient's care on appropriate home health agency forms such as the visit report, addendum notes, telephone communique, or multidisciplinary conference forms.

17. When services are no longer required, complete the appropriate patient discharge summary form. The discharge summary must include the patient's medical and health status at discharge. The home health agency must notify the physician of the availability of the discharge summary and send it to him or her upon request. Consider written patient/caregiver discharge instruction guidelines to include:
   a. Special diet orders
   b. Activity orders
   c. Medication orders
   d. When to call 911 or the physician
   e. Follow-up appointment with the physician

AIDE CARE PLAN (INTERMITTENT VISITS)

☐ ARCADIA VALLEY HOME CARE ☐ DePAUL HOME CARE ☐ ST. ANTHONY HOSPITAL HOME HEALTH AGENCY

☐ ST. JOSEPH HEALTH CENTER and ST. JOSEPH HOSPITAL WEST, HOME HEALTH ☐ ST. MARY'S HEALTH CENTER; HOME HEALTH CARE AGENCY

☐ ST. MARY'S HEALTH CENTER, HOME HEALTH AGENCY (J.C.) ☐ S.S.M. HOME CARE

Pt name _____ Pt # _____ Diagnosis _____

Mental Status: _____ oriented _____ disoriented _____ confused _____ forgetful _____ agitated

    Comments _____

Mobility Status: _____ SBA _____ walker _____ cane _____ transfer bed/chair _____ w/c _____ reposition/bedbound _____ Hoyer lift _____

    Comments _____

Functional Limitations: ___vision _____ hearing _____ swallowing _____ endurance _____ unsteady gait _____ incontinence

    Comments _____

Significant other: _____ Able & willing to assist in care ☐ Yes ☐ No

Code status _____ Food Allergies _____ Pt's DOB _____

Goals: _____ Maintain personal hygiene _____ Respite to family _____ Progress to independent care

Visit frequency _____

INTERVENTIONS ORDERED

	each visit	range		each visit	range		each visit	range
Vital Signs	___	___	set hair	___	___	**Elimination**		
Weight	___	___	shave	___	___	catheter care	___	___
			fingernails: clean/file	___	___	question bowel status	___	___
General Hygiene			toenails: clean/file	___	___			
complete bath	___	___	assist to dress	___	___	**Mobility**		
assisted bath	___	___	assisted tub bath	___	___	ROM	___	___
assisted shower	___	___				ambulate w/assist	___	___
assisted tub bath	___	___	**Nutrition**			**Other:**		per request
skin care/lotion	___	___	encourage fluids	___	___	clean work area	___	___
oral hygiene	___	___	prepare light meal	___	___	linen change	___	___
comb/brush hair	___	___	feed patient	___	___	make bed	___	___
shampoo/dry hair	___	___	assist at meal	___	___	light laundry	___	___

Special precautions: _____ oxygen _____ bleeding _____ diabetic _____ seizure _____ Other: _____

Special care needs: _____

_____

_____

ANY CHANGE IN PATIENT'S CONDITION MUST BE DOCUMENTED AND REPORTED TO YOUR SUPERVISOR

Initial RN signature _____ Date _____

PLAN OF CARE UPDATE/RECERTIFICATION		
Date	Changes	RN signature
_____	_____	_____
_____	_____	_____
_____	_____	_____
_____	_____	_____

Home Health Aide Signatures

Name	Date	Name	Date	Name	Date
_____	____	_____	____	_____	____
_____	____	_____	____	_____	____

Figure 4-9 Guidelines for home health aide assignments. (Courtesy DePaul Home Health Department, DePaul Health Center, Bridgeton, Mo.)

Additional components of the medical record.
All telephone conversations pertinent to the care
of the patient and the performance of the home
health nurse should be documented. It is recommended that home health nurses keep a copy of all
documented telephone conversations or conversations pertinent to work performance. Documentation should reflect what was discussed, the time
and date, and who took part in the conversation.

Always write neatly and legibly. The medical
record is a legal document that describes not only
patient outcomes but also the type of care given.
The medical record is a reflection of the expertise
of the home health nurse and that of the agency.
(Refer to Chapter 7.)

Complete records in a timely manner consistent
with agency policy. It has been said, "If it is not
documented, it probably did not happen." This
saying may be applied to home health care as: **"If
it is not documented, it is not reimbursed by
Medicare."**[4] Intermediary denials of payment are
processed and documented on the HCFA 488.
Home health agencies may contest unpaid claims
with their intermediaries.[7,8]

Evaluating phase

Evaluating is the fifth step in the nursing process.
Evaluation measures the effectiveness of medical
treatment (nursing actions as well as multidisciplinary care) and appropriate utilization of resources. It is the act of determining the patient's
progress in meeting outcomes of care and achieving long-term goals.[1]

Some patient care plan formats have preplanned
outcomes of care based on major patient groups or
related patient classification topology; they have
been referred to as care paths, critical pathways,
and clinical pathways. Chapter 8 discusses the
uses of care paths as evaluation tools for case
management. Once goals and outcomes of care are
achieved, or it has been determined that the patient
no longer requires home care or is no longer
appropriate for home health services, discharge
from the home health services occurs.

SUMMARY

Developing the plan of care and precise documentation provides nurses with systematic and scientific
methods for delivering patient care. Consequently
the patient care plan becomes a virtual care map,
whereby nursing implements and directs cost-
effective services, and guides patient/caregiver actions in the management of health care needs at
home. In summary, careful attention to documentation provides a method for evaluating the quality of
care, serves as a basis for reimbursement of services,
and creates an enormous database for nursing research.

REFERENCES
1. Antone T, Davis P: Outcomes measurement: fact vs fiction,
   HomeCare 16(10):107-108, 1994. (Note: this issue has a
   number of good articles on using outcomes in home care.)
2. Health Care Financing Administration: Medicare conditions of participation, *Federal Register* 59(243):December
   20, 1994.
3. Health Care Financing Administration: *Home health insurance manual* (Pub No 11), Washington, DC, 1995, US
   Department of Health and Human Services.
4. Magliozzi H: Home care: charting that makes it through
   the Medicare maze, *RW* 6:75, 1990.
5. North American Nursing Diagnosis Association: NANDA
   nursing diagnoses: definitions and classification 1995-
   1996, 1995, The Association.
6. Pinnell N, DeMeneses M: *Nursing process: theory, application and related processes,* Norwalk, Conn, 1986, Appleton & Lange.
7. Randall D: The role of the medicare fiscal intermediary
   and the regional home health intermediary, part I, *JONA*
   22(6):47-53, 1992.
8. Randall D: The role of the medicare fiscal intermediary
   and the regional home health intermediary, part II, *JONA*
   22(7/8):24-29, 1992.
9. Rice R: Medicare documentation guidelines for reimbursement, *Home Health Care Nurs* 11(6):57-59, 1993.
10. Rice R: The home milieu. In Rice R, editor: *Manual of
    home health nursing procedures,* St Louis, 1995, Mosby.

5 Infection Control in the Home

Robyn Rice

The specter of illness moving out of the hospital and into the community has profound implications for home health nursing practice today. Increasingly virulent microorganisms coupled with greater numbers of a sicker as well as an immunocompromised population in home care pose real concerns regarding the transmission of infectious disease. In addition, the community is experiencing expanding poverty, transcultural migration, and environmental changes that have the potential to spread disease. In fact, the United States is experiencing a reemergence of several infectious diseases once thought to be eradicated.[6] As a result, infection control policies and procedures, both for patients and staff, are more important to clinical practice than ever before.

FROM PAST TO PRESENT: UNDERSTANDING THE NEED

History is replete with outbreaks of disease such as the bubonic plague, influenza, polio, and now, acquired immune deficiency syndrome (AIDS). Humans have always been, and most likely will continue to be, exposed to the destructive forces of disease and infection. An example from the 1300s provides insights as to the impact that a plague can have on the community.

In October 1347, Genoese merchant ships landed at Messina, Sicily, with dead and dying men at the oars. The ships had reportedly come from the Crimea. The sick and dying sailors had an infection that manifested itself as black swellings in the armpits and groin that oozed foul smelling blood and pus. Their skin was covered with the boils (buboes) and black blotches caused by internal bleeding. The infection was very painful and the sick died quickly, within a week or less after the symptoms first appeared.[25]

The disease was the bubonic plague, a contagion that reportedly killed approximately 10 million people, one third of the population of the known world in the fourteenth century.[25] Caused by the bacillus Yersinia pestis, the plague was transmitted by infected rats and fleas. Poor nutritional status and unclean living conditions characteristic of medieval society were felt to contribute to morbidity and mortality rates. The plague was particularly ferocious in cities where there was close contact between people, and usually took from 4 days to a week to kill. Of note, a more lethal and infectious airborne pneumonic variation of the plague bacillus developed. The victims of pneumonic plague usually died within 48 hours. Coughing of blood either by itself or as an additional symptom was reported by medieval physicians and scholars. It is also believed that a third variant of the bacillus caused septicemia and rapid death within hours.[25]

The black death obliterated entire communities. Physicians, clergy, and sisters of the convents who tried to assist plague victims were literally wiped out; some died at their patient's bedside.[25] Ignorance of the cause, rapid transmission of the infection, gruesome symptomatology, and high mortality rates served to further terrify the people. Confronted with the horror of the black death, communities in western Europe attempted to isolate themselves from outsiders or strangers who represented the source of the contagion. If this was impossible, contact with the plague-struck victims was discouraged. Those who were able fled their homes as the plague approached. In trying to find a "reason" or scapegoat for the plague, the Jews were blamed and accused of poisoning the water.[27] As the black death raged across western Europe from 1347 to 1350, so did the massacre of the Jewish communities.[27] From all accounts it was a time when brother turned away from brother and parents abandoned children, when brutality and chaos reigned. Hope seemed all but lost. Chronicling the historical accounts of the plague in medieval times, Philip Ziegler describes:[27]

" 'Father abandoned child;' wrote Agnolo di Tura of the plague at Siena, 'wife, husband; one brother, another; for this illness seemed to strike through the breath and the sight. And so they died. And no one could be found to bury the dead for money or for friendship... And in many places in Siena great pits were dug and piled deep with huge heaps of the dead... And I, Agnolo di Tura, called the Fat, buried my five children with my own hands, and so did many others likewise. And there were also many dead throughout the city who were so sparsely covered with earth that the dogs dragged them forth and devoured their bodies.' "

One may ask, what does the black death have to do with infection control in the home? In fact, historical accounts of the bubonic plague during the fourteenth century have meaningful implications for today's home health nurses. Today's home health nurses are caring for patients with a variety of infectious diseases including AIDS. Ideally, when faced with a disease such as AIDS, the community response should be an informed one based on scientific principles. In looking at our history, however, fear of the unknown all too often replaces rational thought. This irony holds true for today. Although the situation is improving, many patients with HIV-1 infection have found that no one wants to be near them, much less provide physical care. This avoidance is partly a result of public fear of contracting a disease for which there is no cure, with death as the end result. It is also due to the fact that, like our medieval ancestors, we still have much to learn about infectious diseases and their transmission. These fears of the unknown and public misconceptions regarding the transmission of infection make it difficult for home health nurses to call on resources within the community when coordinating care for immunocompromised patients.

From an historical perspective, some additional points are made. Originally a bloodborne pathogen, the bacillus causing the plague during the 1300s, changed into a more lethal respiratory form. Home health nurses should be aware that bacteria and viruses can and do mutate. One has only to follow the historical development of hepatitis A (an oral/fecal pathogen) to hepatitis B (a bloodborne pathogen) to realize that this is true (Figure 5-1). In addition, in implementing infection control precautions, it is important to recognize that bloodborne pathogens are not the only infectious agents in the community.

In trying to isolate himself from the plague, medieval man understood that it was something outside of his home that was bringing the contagion to his family. Today we also recognize that patients are not likely to become infected by agents in their home environment; the threat arises as the nurse moves from home to home. When caring for populations at risk for communicable disease, home health nurses should be aware that they have the potential to become carriers and therefore, are potential sources of infection.

Sound infection control policies and procedures, for both patients and staff, will resolve some of these concerns. Regulations and recommendations for accreditation and licensure specified by the Centers for Disease Control and Prevention (CDC), the Joint Commission on Accreditation of Healthcare Organizations (JCAHO), and the Occupational Safety and Health Administration (OSHA) are useful to direct home health organizational infection control policies and procedures.[12,16,20,22]

In addition, community education about disease transmission and basic infection control practices benefits the patient, the family, and society in coping with epidemics. Education *can* change behavior so that fears of the unknown are overcome. As a result the community response to people with infectious disease becomes an informed and humane one. The purpose of this chapter is to describe how and why disease is transmitted and to provide current recommendations for infection control precautions in the home setting.

EPIDEMIOLOGY

Epidemiology is the study and explanation of the interrelationships among the host, the disease

HEPATITIS - by year, United States, 1965-1993

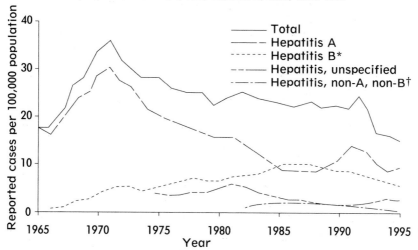

* The first hepatitis B vaccine was licensed June 1982.
† Cases reported as acute, non-A, non-B hepatitis may include many chronic hepatitis C virus (HCV) infections because the test for antibody to HCV (anti-HCV) does not distinguish acute infections from chronic infections.

Figure 5-1 Hepatitis as a changing disease. (From CDC summary of notifiable diseases - 1993, *MMWF,* 1994, p. 32.)

agent, and the environment in disease causation.[3] The CDC publishes many reports on the prevalence and mortality rates of communicable disease.[4-13] In addition to summarizing the reported cases of various communicable diseases in the United States, these reports reveal several points of interest. First, almost all communicable diseases are actively being reported in the United States. Table 5-1 provides a historical summary of reported cases of notifiable diseases in the United States.[8] Of interest, since 1991 there has been a steady increase in the incidence of meningococcal infections reported each year. The polio vaccine has almost eradicated polio, but isolated cases are still reported. Cases of hepatitis A continue to be reported in significant numbers. However, the incidence of reported hepatitis B has been decreasing since the 1980s. It could be speculated that the hepatitis vaccine and public education regarding transmission of infectious disease might be the cause of this.

According to the CDC, AIDS cases continue to be reported in increasing numbers. In 1984, 4,445 cases of AIDS were first reported as opposed to

103,533 cases reported in 1993. The 1992 revision in the CDC surveillance case definition of AIDS, which went into effect in 1993, may account for the dramatic jump in reported AIDS cases from 1992 to 1993.[5] This trend is expected to plateau.[5] As of 1995, the CDC estimates that over one million Americans are infected with HIV-1.[13]

In terms of respiratory disease, tuberculosis (TB) has reemerged in the United States. As a result, the CDC recommended tuberculosis control laws in 1993 requiring health care agencies to report cases of TB to local or state health departments and direct observational therapy for patients who were noncompliant with the medication regimen.[7,12] The CDC now recommends special air purifying masks when caring for patients with TB.[11,12]

It is interesting to note that isolated cases of the bubonic plague are still reported worldwide. In 1994 the CDC reported outbreaks of bubonic and pneumonic plague with numerous deaths in India.[10] To the extent that this summary represents an accurate profile of infectious disease in the

Table 5-1 Notifiable diseases—summary of reported cases, United States, 1984-1993

Disease	1993	1992	1991	1990	1989	1988	1987	1986	1985	1984
U.S. total resident population (in thousands) 1990 census; July 1 est. 1984–1989, 1991–1993.	257,908	255,082	252,177	248,710	248,239	245,807	243,400	241,078	238,740	236,158
AIDS	103,533	45,472	43,672	41,595	33,722	31,001	21,070	12,932	8,249	4,445
Amebiasis	2,970	2,942	2,989	3,328	3,217	2,860	3,123	3,532	4,433	5,252
Anthrax	–	1	–	–	–	1	1	–	–	1
Aseptic meningitis	12,848	12,223	14,526	11,852	10,274	7,234	11,487	11,374	10,619	8,326
Botulism, total (including wound and unsp.)	97	91	114	92	89	84	82	109	122	123
Foodborne	27	21	27	23	23	28	17	23	49	19
Infant	65	66	81	65	60	50	59	79	70	99
Brucellosis	120	105	104	85	95	96	129	106	153	131
Chancroid	1,399	1,886	3,476	4,212	4,692	5,001	4,998	3,756	2,067	665
Cholera	18	103	26	6	–	8	6	23	4	1
Diphtheria	–	4	5	4	3	2	3	–	3	1
Encephalitis, primary*	919	774	1,021	1,341	981	882	1,418	1,302	1,376	1,257
Post-infectious*	170	129	82	105	88	121	121	124	161	108
Gonorrhea	439,673	501,409	620,478	690,169	733,151	719,536	780,905	900,868	911,419	878,556
Granuloma inguinale	19	6	29	97	7	11	22	61	44	30
Haemophilus influenzae	1,419	1,412	2,764	⋯	⋯	⋯	†	⋯	⋯	⋯
Hansen disease (leprosy)	187	172	154	198	163	184	238	270	361	290
Hepatitis A	24,238	23,112	24,378	31,441	35,821	28,507	25,280	23,430§	23,210§	22,040
Hepatitis B	13,361	16,126	18,003	21,102	23,419	23,177	25,916	26,107§	26,611§	26,115
Hepatitis, non-A, non-B‖	4,786	6,010	3,582	2,553	2,529	2,619	2,999	3,634§	4,184§	3,871
Hepatitis, unspecified	627	884	1,260	1,671	2,306	2,470	3,102	3940§	5,517§	5,531
Legionellosis**	1,280	1,339	1,317	1,370	1,190	1,085	1,038	948	830	750
Leptospirosis	51	54	58	77	93	54	43	41	57	40
Lyme disease	8,257	9,895	9,465	⋯	⋯	⋯	†	⋯	⋯	⋯
Lymphogranuloma venereum	285	302	471	277	189	185	303	396	226	170
Malaria	1,411	1,087	1,278	1,292	1,277	1,099	944	1,123	1,049	1,007
Measles (rubeola)	312	2,237	9,643	27,786	18,193	3,396	3,655	6,282	2,822	2,587
Meningococcal infections	2,637	2,134	2,130	2,451	2,727	2,964	2,930	2,594	2,479	2,746
Mumps	1,692	2,572	4,264	5,292	5,712	4,866	12,848	7,790	2,982	3,021
Murine typhus fever	25	28	43	50	41	54	49	67	37	53
Pertussis (whooping cough)	6,586	4,083	2,719	4,570	4,157	3,450	2,823	4,195	3,589	2,276
Plague	10	13	11	2	4	15	12	10	17	31

Poliomyelitis, paralytic[††]	3	6	9	6	9	9	9	9	7	8
Psittacosis	60	92	94	113	116	114	98	224	119	172
Rabies, animal	9,377	8,589	6,910	4,826	4,724	4,651	4,658	5,504	5,565	5,567
Rabies, human	3	1	3	1	1	–	1	–	1	3
Rheumatic fever, acute	112	75	127	108	144	158	141	147	90	117
Rocky Mountain spotted fever	456	502	628	651	623	609	604	760	714	838
Rubella (German measles)	192	160	1,401	1,125	396	225	306	551	630	752
Rubella, congenital syndrome	5	11	47	11	3	6	5	14	–	5
Salmonellosis, excluding typhoid fever	41,641	40,912	48,154	48,603	47,812	48,948	50,916	49,984	65,347	40,861
Shigellosis	32,198	23,931	23,548	27,077	25,010	30,617	23,860	17,138	17,057	17,371
Smallpox	Last documented case occurred in 1949									
Syphilis, primary and secondary	26,498	33,973	42,935	50,223	44,540	40,117	35,147	27,883	27,131	28,607
total, all stages	101,259	112,581	128,569	134,255	110,797	103,437	86,545	68,215	67,563	69,888
Tetanus	48	45	57	64	53	53	48	64	83	74
Toxic-shock syndrome	212	244	280	322	400	390	372	412	384	482
Trichinosis	16	41	62	129	30	45	40	39	61	68
Tuberculosis	25,313	26,673	26,283	25,701	23,495	22,436	22,517	22,768	22,201	22,255
Tularemia	132	159	193	152	152	201	214	170	177	291
Typhoid fever	440	414	501	552	460	436	400	362	402	390
Varicella (chickenpox)	134,722	158,364	147,076	173,099	185,441	192,857	213,196	183,243	178,162	221,983
Yellow fever	Last indigenous case reported 1911; last imported, 1924									

*Beginning in 1984, data reflects change in categories for tabulating encephalitis reports that were recorded by date of report to state health departments. Data for previous years are from surveillance records reported by onset date.

†Not previously notifiable nationally.

§Reports from New York City are not available.

¶The number of reported cases of non-A, non-B hepatitis is misleading because in some states, reported cases included persons positive for antibody to hepatitis C virus (anti-HCV) identified in routine screening programs but who did not have acute hepatitis.

**Data are recorded by date of report to the state health department. Data for all years previous to 1982 are from surveillance records reported by onset date.

††Annual case reports from state health departments; numbers may not reflect changes based on retrospective case evaluations or late reports (see *MMWR* 1986;35:180–2).

From CDC Summary of Notifiable Diseases, *MMWR*, 1994, p. 67.

community, the following conclusions that affect home health nursing may be drawn:[2,3,8,13,24]

- Infectious disease exists in many forms in the community.
- Although vaccines and increased public awareness of cause and treatment of infectious disease have drastically reduced rates of transmission and incidence of infection for many communicable diseases, cases continue to be reported.
- AIDS and hepatitis B infection are continuing to be reported, and both are associated with high mortality rates.[8] The increasing incidence of AIDS cases is of particular concern because at present there is no known vaccine or cure.
- The presence of the human immunodeficiency virus (HIV-1) in home care is being felt. One study showed that 2 of 22 health care workers who acquired HIV were apparently infected in the home care setting.[4] Household transmissions of HIV-1 among family members, although rare, are now being reported.[9]
- Common infectious diseases seen and treated in the home include tuberculosis (TB); pneumonia; scabies; pediculosis; streptococcal pharyngitis; impetigo; urinary tract infections; a variety of skin, fungal, and gastrointestinal infections as related to HIV-1 infection; and methicillin resistant Staphylococcus as well as pseudomonas in wounds.[14,24]

The immediate recognition and identification of infection may be difficult as many infectious diseases are relatively "silent" in initial manifestation of clinical signs and symptoms. It is likely that many such cases go unreported and the CDC statistics may well represent only the tip of the iceberg (Figure 5-2). The lesson for home health workers in the community is: IF YOU DON'T SEE IT, IT DOESN'T MEAN IT'S NOT THERE.

A careful, ongoing patient evaluation for infectious disease should be a part of everyday nursing therapies in home care. In addition, infection control tracking should be used as a component of the quality improvement program (Figure 5-3).

MECHANISM OF INFECTION

Understanding how communicable disease is transmitted is the first step in the implementation and management of infection control. First, an

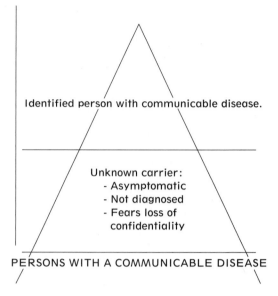

Figure 5-2 Unreported/unknown versus identified cases of communicable disease.

infectious agent must exist. Infective bacteria and viruses, as well as a variety of microbial, plant, and parasitic sources, exist—all with the potential to infect. Second, the infectious agent must have a reservoir within which it can live and multiply in such a manner that it can be transmitted to a host. Any person, animal, plant, or substance capable of sustaining life can serve as a reservoir. Finally, what is needed for infection to occur is a mode of transmission and a susceptible host.[2]

A susceptible host is a person or other living animal that has no specific immunity against the infectious agent. The lack of immunity caused by a compromised immune system is particularly relevant for those who work in home care because the majority of their patients are older adults who have compromised immune systems as a result of aging.[2,3]

Mechanisms of transmission vary, the most common types being contact, droplet, airborne, and vector-borne transmission.[3,12]

Contact transmission

Contact transmission includes direct and indirect contact transmission.[2,12] Infectious agents may be contracted by direct contact between persons, as

Infection Control Report

Complete this form: (check where appropriate)
__ The employee has signs/symptoms of infectious disease.
__ The patient/caregiver has signs/symptoms of infectious disease.
__ The physician has ordered a culture to be done.
__ The physician has ordered an antibiotic for the patient.
__ The patient has expired or been rehospitalized with suspect infectious disease.

Employee/Patient/Caregiver Name_____

Site of Infection	Signs/Symptoms of Infection
__ Respiratory system	__ Adventitious lung sounds
__ Blood	__ Green/yellow/copious sputum
__ HEENT	__ Dyspnea
__ Integumentary system	__ Pain/tenderness
__ Gastrointestinal system	__ Elevated temperature
__ Genito-urinary system	__ Purulent drainage
__ Musculoskeletal system	__ Erythema
__ Other (specify)_____	__ Edema
_____	__ Diarrhea
	__ Cloudy/foul urine
	__ Dysuria
	__ Other (specify)_____

Culture	Lab Specimen
Date ordered:_____	Date ordered: _____
Source: _____	Source: _____
Results:_____	Results:_____

Comments: (e.g., more specific description of infection, any other diagnostic tests ordered by the physician)

Professional Signature:_____ Date: _____

Figure 5-3 Tracking infectious disease in the home.

by sexual intercourse, touching, and biting (including animal bites). Direct contact may also occur with exposure of susceptible tissue to dust or contaminated soil (fungus/spores).[2,12]

Transmission by indirect contact occurs when an infectious agent is introduced into a susceptible host via food, water, blood products (blood transfusion, for example), medical equipment, dressings, or anything that serves as an intermediate source.

Droplet transmission

In droplet transmission, a droplet containing the infectious agent is emitted by an infected host and contaminates a susceptible host.[2,12] A proximity of 3 to 4 feet is usually required for droplet transmission. A cough is a good example of this type of transmission.

Airborne transmission

Airborne transmission requires the entry of microbial aerosols into the respiratory tract. In this type of transmission the infectious agent could be spread by humidifiers or fans in the ventilation system of the home.[2,3,12]

Vector-borne transmission

Vector-borne transmission occurs when the infectious agent is passed from a nonvertebrate host such as an arthropod (for example, a mosquito) to a susceptible host (a human).[2] The infection is transmitted when the arthropod bites, regurgitates, or deposits feces or other material containing the infectious agent through the bite wound or an open area of the skin.

To summarize, infection occurs as a result of transmission of an infectious agent to a susceptible host. Home health nurses must keep in mind that an infected individual will not necessarily show signs or symptoms of the infection but may nonetheless be capable of infecting others. Understanding mechanisms of transmission provides insight into the management of communicable diseases. The following principles are recommended:[12,23]

- Clean and sanitary living conditions will reduce the incidence of infection and communicable disease.
- Good nutrition, personal hygiene, and health will reduce the incidence of infection and communicable disease.
- The routine use of infection control precautions will reduce the incidence of infection and communicable disease.
- The prevalence of the infectious agent is reduced by means of immunizations and antibiotic administration.
- The practice of consistent handwashing is to be emphasized.

These principles, incorporated with a philosophy that all patients should be treated as though they have an infectious disease, are elemental to nursing practice in the home. In addition, they support the following infection control guidelines recommended by the CDC.[12]

STANDARD PRECAUTIONS FOR HOME CARE

In 1995 the Centers for Disease Control and Prevention (CDC) issued new isolation guidelines called *Standard Precautions* that contain two tiers of approach. The first tier uses major features of universal precautions and principles of body substance isolation (BSI). (See the box titled Standard Precautions.)[18] Standard precautions apply to (1) blood, (2) all body fluids regardless of whether

---

STANDARD PRECAUTIONS (tier one)

- Standard precautions apply to blood, all body fluids, secretions, excretions, nonintact skin, and mucous membranes.
- Hands are washed if contaminated with blood or body fluid, immediately after gloves are removed, between patient contact, and when indicated to prevent transfer of microorganisms between other patients or environment.
- Gloves are worn when touching blood, body fluids, secretions, excretions, nonintact skin, mucous membranes, or contaminated items. Gloves should be removed and hands washed between patient care.
- Masks, eye protection, or face shields are worn if patient care activities may generate splashes or sprays of blood or body fluid.
- Gowns are worn if soiling of clothing is likely from blood or body fluid. Wash hands after removing gown.
- Patient care equipment is properly cleaned and reprocessed and single use items are discarded.
- Contaminated linen is placed in leakproof bag and handled as to prevent skin and mucous membrane exposure.
- All sharp instruments and needles are discarded in a puncture-resistant container. CDC recommends that needles be disposed of uncapped or use a mechanical device for recapping.
- A private room is unnecessary unless the patient's hygiene is unacceptable. Check with Infection Control Professional.

Table 5-2 Transmission categories (tier two)

Category	Disease	Barrier protection
Airborne precautions	Droplet nuclei smaller than 5 microns; measles; chickenpox (Varicella); disseminated varicella zoster; pulmonary or laryngeal TB	Private room, negative airflow of at least six exchanges per hour, mask or respiratory protection device (see CDC TB Guidelines)
Droplet precautions	Droplets larger than 5 microns; Diphtheria (pharyngeal); Rubella; Streptococcal pharyngitis, pneumonia, or scarlet fever in infants and young children; Pertussis; mumps; mycoplasma pneumonia; meningococcal pneumonia or sepsis; pneumonic plague	Private room or cohort patients; mask
Contact precautions	Direct patient or environmental contact; colonization or infection with multidrug-resistant organism; respiratory syncytial virus; shigella and other enteric pathogens; major wound infections; herpes simplex; scabies; varicella zoster (disseminated)	Private room or cohort patients; gloves, gowns

they contain blood, (3) non-intact skin, and (4) mucous membrane.[12]

The CDC also proposes a second tier disease-specific approach (Table 5-2). This approach provides isolation guidelines with new transmission categories based on airborne, droplet, and contact transmission of infectious disease.

Standard precautions which reflect the Occupational Safety and Health Administration's (OSHA) bloodborne pathogen standard, promote handwashing and use of gloves, masks, eye protection, or gowns when appropriate for patient contact. These guidelines are based on the theory that all patients should be treated as though they have a communicable disease. This reinforces the idea that all body substances (oral and body secretions, breast milk, blood, feces, urine, droplet or airborne spray from a cough, tissues, vomitus, wound, or other drainage) including non-intact mucous membranes are to be treated as a potential source of infection regardless of whether the patient has a communicable disease.[18,23] The following guidelines reflect adaptation of (1) the CDC standard precautions, (2) the JCAHO standards for home care, and (3) OSHA's bloodborne pathogen standard:[12,16,20]

Recommended equipment

1. Personal protective equipment provided to the employee by the home health agency should include the following:
   a. Disposable nonsterile/sterile gloves and utility gloves
   b. Disinfectants
      i. Chemical germicides that are approved for use as agency disinfectants and are tuberculocidal when used at recommended dilutions
      ii. Products registered by the Environmental Protection Agency (EPA) as being effective against human immunodeficiency virus (HIV) with an accepted HIV label
      iii. A solution of 5.25% sodium hypochlorite (household bleach) diluted to 1:10 with water (Mix a fresh supply of bleach every day for effective disinfection.)
   c. Masks, cardiopulmonary resuscitation (CPR) masks, air purifying masks, goggles, moistureproof aprons/gowns, shoe covers, and caps
   d. Leakproof and punctureproof specimen containers

e. Sharps containers

f. Liquid soap, soap towelettes, dry hand disinfectants (alcohol based), sodium hypochlorite wipes or dry bleach

g. Paper towels

h. Bottled sterile water for eye irrigation

i. Extra uniform kept in a plastic bag in the car

j. Box or container to store nursing bag when in the car, newspapers

Recommended clinical policies[11,12,15,20,23,24]

1. **Handwashing.** Hands should be washed before and after patient contact. Wash hands during patient care if soiled. Wash hands with soap and water immediately after removing gloves. *The wearing of gloves does not eliminate the necessity for handwashing.*[17,21,26] If soap and water are not available, antiseptic hand cleanser or towelettes may be used. Then wash hands with soap and water as soon as possible.

2. **Gloves.** Wear gloves if the possibility of contact transmission may occur. Change gloves between each patient procedure. Wear nonsterile latex gloves when performing any clinical procedure that may expose staff to the patient's blood or other body substances (e.g., with venipuncture and during perineal care).

    Sterile latex gloves are to be worn during certain clinical procedures that require sterile technique (e.g., during certain dressing changes or inserting a urinary catheter). Utility gloves are used to clean up equipment, the work area, or spills.

    Sterile and nonsterile latex gloves are to be disposed of after each use in a leak-resistant waste receptacle such as a plastic trashbag. Utility gloves are to be issued to each household. Utility gloves may be disinfected and reused. Dispose of and replace utility gloves that show signs of cracking, peeling, tearing or puncture, and other signs of deterioration.

3. **Gowns/aprons, shoe covers, caps.** Wear moistureproof, disposable gowns or aprons, shoe covers, or caps when there is reasonable expectation that contact transmission may occur. After use, remove and dispose of personal protective equipment in a plastic trashbag in the work area.

4. **Masks.** Disposable face masks are to be worn whenever there is a reasonable expectation that droplet transmission may occur. Dispose of masks after each use in a plastic trashbag in the patient's home.

5. **Disposable CPR masks.** Use disposable CPR masks if required to provide artificial mouth-to-mouth or mouth-to-stoma ventilation.

6. **Air purifying masks.** Use an air purifying mask able to filter particles 1 micron in size with a filter efficiency of $\geq 95\%$ given flow rates of up to 50 liters per minute when caring for patients with tuberculosis; a fitting test is recommended.[11,12]

    When airborne precautions are required, post a homemade "STOP" sign outside the patient's room.[18] Instruct the household to wear masks when entering the room and caring for the patient. The "STOP" sign should alert visitors including children of the necessity to wear a mask when entering the patient's room.

7. **Goggles.** Goggles or safety glasses with side shields are to be worn when there is a reasonable expectation that droplet transmission may occur to the eyes. Clean goggles with soap and water after each use. Discard in a plastic trashbag in the patient's home if goggles become cracked or heavily contaminated.

8. **Sharp objects and needles.** Place sharp objects and needles in a punctureproof disposable container. A needle shall not be bent, sheared, replaced in the sheath or guard, or removed from the syringe after use.[18,19] Do not recap used needles.

9. **Sharps containers.** Sharps containers shall have the following properties: punctureproof, red in color, labeled with a biohazard sign on the outside, and leakproof. Never fill sharps containers to where contents protrude out of the opening. *Do not fill sharps containers over two-thirds full.* Store sharps containers on top of the refrigerator in the home or some place out of reach from children. Bring the containers into the home health agency when nearly full for commercial waste disposal unless intrave-

nous therapy services collect the containers for disposal. Review local and state ordinances regarding disposal of sharps containers.

10. **Specimen collection.** Blood or other body substance specimens shall be placed in a leakproof bag and secured in a punctureproof container during collection, handling, storage, and transport. Place a biohazard symbol on the outside of the punctureproof container whose sole purpose will be to transport laboratory specimens.

    Label specimens with the patient's name and identifying data. Handle all specimens carefully to minimize spillage. Place the punctureproof container on the floor of the car during transport. According to home health agency policy, a courier service may be called to pick up laboratory specimens left at the patient's home.

11. **Personal.** Eating, drinking, smoking, applying cosmetics or lip balm, and handling contact lenses are prohibited in patient care areas where there is reasonable likelihood of occupational exposure to blood or body substances. Food and drinks are not to be kept in patient care areas where blood or other potentially infectious materials are present.

12. **Miscellaneous.** All clinical procedures shall be performed in such a manner to minimize splashing, spraying, splattering, or generating droplets of blood or body substances. Mouth pipetting/suctioning of blood or other body substances is prohibited. Change a soiled uniform as soon as is possible. Keep the nursing bag stored in a container or in a designated clean area in the car when traveling.

13. **Exposure incident.** In the event of eye or body contact with the patient's blood or body substances, (1) irrigate the eye with water (use sterile water stocked in the nursing bag if running water is not available), (2) wash the exposed body part with soap and water, and (3) contact the home health agency clinical supervisor for follow-up instructions. If the uniform is contaminated, put on an alternate uniform kept in the car.

14. **OSHA regulations.** Infection control standards and policies published by OSHA will be accessible to all home health employees for reference.[20] A copy of these regulations shall be placed in the infection control manual or appropriate policy/procedure manual located in an easily accessible place in the home health agency office.

15. **Patient education and documentation.** Notify the physician of any signs or symptoms of patient or caregiver infection. Instruct the patient/caregiver in applicable infection control precautions in the home.

    Document standard precautions, patient/caregiver instructions regarding infection control and compliance with precautions, and pertinent findings on the visit report. Update the patient care plan. Complete a report for an exposure as appropriate.

HOME CARE APPLICATION

The recommendations in this section are practical home care adaptations of standard precautions and may be individualized to meet specific patient needs.

Provision of care for patients with communicable diseases[11,23,24]

- Explain all procedures and their rationale to patients. Respect patients' rights to privacy and confidentiality.
- Do not replace any contaminated equipment in the nursing bag until it has been disinfected. Contaminated equipment that cannot be cleaned in the home should be placed in a plastic bag and transported to the agency for disinfection or left in the patient's home for exclusive use with that patient. (Disposable equipment should be used whenever possible.)
- Place disposable contaminated items (dressings, etc.) in a plastic bag, seal the bag, and place it in the trash.
- Pour contaminated liquids (urine, stool, vomitus) into a toilet, followed immediately with full-strength bleach and flushing.
- Visit patients with communicable diseases last or at the end of the workday.
- **Take only needed equipment/supplies into the home.**

Bag technique and handwashing

Proper technique should be observed at all times. The inside of the nursing bag should be regarded as a clean area.[23] The bag should be transported in the car on top of a supply of newspapers. Once in the patient's home, select the cleanest or most convenient area and spread newspaper. Place the bag on the newspaper. Prepare a receptacle (trash-bag) for disposable items. Open the nursing bag, and remove items needed to wash hands. Hand-washing supplies should be placed at the top of the bag. Close the bag. Go in and out of the nursing bag as few times as possible. Take items to wash hands (liquid soap/paper towels) to the sink area. *Remember, this is the patient's home. Ask the patient where you should wash your hands.*

When at the sink, use one paper towel upon which to place other items. A second and third towel are used for washing and drying hands before and after care has been given. Remove watch. Wet hands and forearms and then lather using vigorous friction, starting at fingertips and working toward forearms. Hold the hands lower than the elbows when washing hands. Hold hands under running water for at least 10 seconds. Rinse and dry the hands from the fingers toward the forearm. Turn the faucet off with a paper towel (return liquid soap to nursing bag when care has been given). Apply lotion as needed. To prevent cross-contamination between patients and staff, wash hands *before* and *after* care of patient. If wearing gloves, *wash hands after removal of gloves.*[23,26] Avoid using cloth towels or bars of soap; these may become a haven for bacteria. If running water or clean facilities are not available, hands should be cleaned with an antiseptic foam or rinse. If providing care for a patient on specific isolation orders, consider use of a Betadine scrub.

Return to the bag, open it again, and remove necessary items for the visit. Keep the bag closed during the visit. Leave all plastic containers in the bag. Do not reenter the bag unless your hands are clean. If a plastic apron is worn, do not return it to the nursing bag. Remove the apron by folding the exposed side inward and discard it along with newspaper and other used, disposable items in the patient's waste receptacle. The nursing bag should not be exposed to extreme temperatures or left in the car for long periods of time. Nursing bags should be cleaned, disinfected, and restocked weekly at the home health agency.

Disinfection and cleaning

Disinfection methods in the home setting vary. All items to be disinfected should be cleaned first with a detergent and running water. The following are cited as disinfectants used in home care: bleach, white vinegar, hydrogen peroxide, boiling water, phenolics, and isopropyl alcohol.[23,24] The item to be disinfected will primarily determine the disinfectant to be used. Bleach corrodes metal but is cited as an all-purpose disinfectant in the home for blood and body fluid contamination.[23,24] White vinegar (acetic acid) may be used to disinfect respiratory therapy equipment, although home medical equipment (HME) vendor guidelines for cleaning respiratory therapy equipment should be reviewed.

Routinely wipe down the bell/diaphragm of the stethoscope with a disinfectant between patients. If using a baby scale, wipe the scale down with disinfectant between uses or use a fresh disposable plastic sheath/pad underneath the baby on each visit. For glucose meters, follow specific manufacturer's guidelines for cleaning. If patients do not have their own thermometer, wipe the thermometer with an antiseptic pad before and after use and place a plastic/protective sheath over the thermometer before administration to a patient.

Disposal of soiled dressings

Place contaminated dressings and disposable supplies in a plastic bag for disposal.[23] Disinfection with a 10% bleach solution before disposal is recommended. Seal the plastic bag and place it in the trash. In most states, the patient is responsible for waste disposal in the home setting. The home health nurse is responsible for educating the patient regarding neutralization of infectious waste and safe disposal procedures. Review local ordinances regarding infectious waste disposal in the home.

Contaminated wound precautions

Wash hands. Wear a disposable apron to protect clothing from contamination by drainage or body secretions. Use disposable gloves on both hands. With aseptic technique, follow wound care protocol per physician orders. When procedure is completed, remove apron and gloves and discard into a plastic bag, secure the top, and seal. Wash hands.

PATIENT EDUCATION

As stated previously, patient education is a major focus for home health nurses when providing care. (See the box listing patient education guidelines for infection control.) Home health nurses should instruct the patient and caregiver about infectious disease; mechanisms of transmission; signs and symptoms of infection to report to the physician; environmental, health, and personal hygienic habits that reduce the incidence of infection; as well as specific infection control precautions such as proper techniques in handwashing, needle disposal, and infectious waste disposal. For example, patients should be instructed to cover their mouths when they cough; this prevents the spread of germs.

Although home health nurses should primarily use a sterile technique when performing most procedural care, clean technique is usually taught to the patient and caregiver. Information must be imparted so that the patient and caregiver can safely manage infectious disease in the home. With this in mind, the following guidelines are recommended.

Bathroom. When others must share a bathroom with a patient whose disease is spread by stool, request that the patient cover the faucet and handles with tissue paper before touching them. The patient should also use a separate toothbrush and drinking glass. The person cleaning the bathroom should wear rubber gloves, the gloves should be disinfected with a 10% bleach solution after use, and cracked or torn rubber gloves should be discarded. Damp towels and washcloths should be removed as quickly as possible. Recommend that the family use a liquid soap. If the patient has an outdoor toilet, 3 to 4 cups of lime should be placed in the toilet weekly.[24]

Kitchen. Instruct the family to keep the refrigerator clean and set the temperature at 45° F.[23,24] Weekly cleaning of the inside of the refrigerator with regular household cleaning agents will help control microbial growth.

There is no need to prepare the patient's food with separate cooking utensils, but patients should

be discouraged from sharing the food off their plate with other members of the household. The patient's utensils and dishes do not necessarily need to be isolated from those used by other household members if they are washed thoroughly with hot, soapy water. However, the use of common or unclean eating utensils should be avoided. Instruct household members to wash the patient's dishes last and then disinfect the sink with a 10% bleach solution.

Laundry. Soiled linen should be handled as little as possible and should be bagged at the location where it was used.[23,24] Caregivers should be instructed to store infected linen in a separate, leakproof plastic bag and to keep the bag tied shut. Hands should be washed immediately after handling soiled laundry to prevent spread of infection.

Contaminated linens should be washed separately from household laundry in extremely hot water (160° F for 25 minutes).[23,24] One cup of household bleach in addition to the detergent should be added to each load of laundry. The wash cycle should be run through twice, and then the laundry should be dried. To clean the washer, the caregiver should run the empty machine through a complete cycle using a commercial disinfectant or 1 cup of full-strength bleach. Rubber gloves should be worn when handwashing soiled laundry and then disinfected with a 10% bleach solution.

Patient's room. Encourage daily cleaning of the room. Items such as toys, books, and games may be cleaned with soap and water or wiped down with alcohol.[23,24] Trash containers should be washed with soap and water and sprayed with commercial disinfectant. Floors and furniture should be washed with germicidal solution. The room should be aired out, if possible.

Personal hygiene. Patients should be taught to wash their hands in soap and water before and after evacuating bowels or bladder and before handling food. They should cover their mouth when coughing or sneezing and then wash their hands. Paper or tissues used by a patient experiencing a productive cough need to be discarded into a plastic garbage bag.

Caregivers should wash their hands before and after delivery of patient care. The patient's body

---

PATIENT EDUCATION GUIDELINES: INFECTION CONTROL IN THE HOME

1. If possible, have your own room.
2. Clean your room daily. Items such as toys, books, and games may be cleaned with soap and water or wiped down with alcohol. Wash trash containers with soap and water; then spray the containers with a commercial disinfectant. Wash the floors and the furniture with a commercial disinfectant. Follow manufacturer's guidelines for cleaning medical equipment. Usually soap and water are fine. When it is possible, open the windows and air out your room.
3. Clean up spills of blood or urine with a 10% bleach solution. Mix 1 part of bleach to 10 parts of water daily. Throw away unused bleach solution at the end of the day.
4. The family should wear disposable gloves if contact with the patient's blood, wound drainage, feces, urine, open areas of the skin, or other bodily fluids is a possibility. The family members should wear utility gloves if they are handling soiled linens, cleaning the patient's living area, or cleaning up spills of blood, urine, or feces.
5. Clean utility gloves with hot soap and water; then disinfect the gloves with a 10% bleach solution. Throw away and replace cracked or torn utility gloves.
6. Bag your trash separately (from that of the family) in a plastic leakproof bag. Double bag as needed to prevent leakage of soiled bandages or disposable items. Keep animals and pets out of your trash.
7. Place needles, syringes, lancets, and other sharp objects in a hard-plastic or metal container with a screw-on lid or with a lid that fits securely. Don't use a glass container. If you use a coffee can, be sure to reinforce the plastic lid with heavy-duty tape. Keep containers with sharp objects out of children's reach.
8. Family members should maintain personal cleanliness by washing their hands before and after using the bathroom and before handling food. Family members should wash their hands before and after giving patient care. (Keep patient as clean as possible.)
9. Use a liquid soap in the bathroom. Cover the faucet and the handles with tissue paper before touching them. Each family member should use his or her own toothbrush and drinking glass. If you have an outdoor toilet, place 3 to 4 cups of lime in the toilet weekly.
10. Cover your mouth and nose when coughing or sneezing to prevent the spread of germs. Turn your head to avoid droplets from coughs or sneezes.
11. Refrigerate milk and other perishable foods. Drink safe water. The household may use the same cooking pots and utensils; however, commonly used or unclean eating utensils should be avoided. Do not share food from the same plate. Wash your dishes last, or use disposable dishes.
12. Maintain health at a high level by eating a balanced diet and getting adequate amounts of sleep, rest, sunshine, fresh air, and exercise.
13. Obtain and maintain protection against the diseases for which there are no known immunizing agents. Talk to your physician about your immunizations.
14. Call your physician and home health nurse when you have complaints of frequent cough; sudden weight loss; diarrhea; vomiting; increased drainage, increased size, or increased redness of any wounds; elevated temperature; areas of skin breakdown; lethargy; night sweats; aching; rashes; sore throat; headache; burning during urination; painful urination; or stiff neck.
15. Keep in mind the following regarding infection control in the home: (1) good common sense usually provides the best solutions to many situations, and (2) the liberal use of soap and water is still one of the best ways to prevent the spread of infection.

From Rice R: *Manual of home health nursing procedures,* St Louis, 1995, Mosby.

---

should be kept clean with soap and water baths. *Gloves should be worn by caregivers whenever there is a possibility of touching a patient's blood or body substances.*[12]

Pets. Pets sometimes harbor organisms (in excreta or hair) that may pose a threat of serious illness to someone with a compromised immune system. AIDS patients in particular should not be responsible for cleaning the bird cage, cat litter box, or fish tank.[24]

Other. Soiled bedpans and commodes should be cleaned with bleach or household detergent and hot water. Disposable supplies used during patient care should be placed in a separate plastic bag from the rest of the family trash and sealed. Sharps containers should be stored in an area that is inaccessible to children or to others who may be injured. Plastic bags and needle containers should be disposed of in compliance with local public health department and community waste disposal regulations. Usually the regular trash disposal system can be used, but local authorities should be consulted if there are any questions.

ADMINISTRATIVE CONSIDERATIONS

In developing specific procedures regarding infection control, home health agencies must ensure employee cooperation and safety. The CDC and OSHA suggest that this can be accomplished by doing the following:[12,20]

- Conduct an initial orientation program for employees, explaining epidemiology, modes of transmission, and agency policies regarding infectious disease. The need to recognize that all patients may have a potentially infectious disease should be emphasized, and universal/BSI precautions should be taught. Provide yearly in-service training in infection control to reinforce the initial program.
- Issue supplies and clean equipment and bags to minimize transmission of disease. It is recommended that nursing bags be turned in weekly for cleaning and disinfection.
- Managers should monitor staff during field visits to evaluate staff technique and compliance. This gives managers an indication of when staff retraining or counseling is needed.
- Clearly define the agency's procedures for internal processing of infectious waste. A local waste hauler may be contracted to remove the agency's infectious waste (e.g., sharps containers) as deemed necessary.[15]
- Instruct employees to report home-acquired infections to the agency for follow-up, surveillance, and evaluation. In addition, infection and communicable disease are to be reported according to individual state law.

The agency's infection control program should also have written follow-up procedures—including testing, counseling, and appropriate medical intervention—for possible exposure of staff to HIV or HBV. The hepatitis B vaccine, a series of three injections, should be made available to those health care workers who are frequently exposed to blood or blood products on the job.[20]

SUMMARY

The planning and implementation of infection control policies in home care is no easy task because of the scope of services provided. In formulating such policies, it would be well to remember a few simple rules. First, soap and water are still highly recommended because good handwashing is a proven step in basic sanitation.[17,21] Second, an infection control program should focus on behaviors rather than barrier precautions. Therefore explain precautions clearly and completely, for unless staff and patients find such recommendations meaningful, compliance is unlikely. Historically, mankind has always experienced the destructive forces of plague and communicable disease. A strong educational focus on staff and public awareness of infection control precautions contributes to the welfare of our communities. In this manner we will all be ready to effectively deal with the plagues of today and the ones that will surely come tomorrow.

REFERENCES

1. Andrist L: Taking a sexual history and educating clients about safe sex, *Nurs Clin North Am* 23(4):959, 1988.
2. Bean J: Plague, population and economic decline in the middle ages, *EcHR*, April 1963.
3. Berenson AS: *Control of communicable diseases in man,* Washington, DC, 1985, American Public Health Association.
4. Centers for Disease Control and Prevention: Update: universal precautions for prevention of transmission of human immunodeficiency virus, hepatitis B virus, and other bloodborne pathogens in health care settings, *MMWR* 37:377-382, 387-389, 1988.
5. Centers for Disease Control and Prevention: 1993 revised classification system for HIV infection and expanded surveillance case definition for AIDS among adolescents and adults, *MMWR* 41-RR. 17:1-19, 1992.
6. Centers for Disease Control and Prevention: Addressing emerging infectious disease threats: a prevention strategy for the United States, *MMWR* 43-RR.5:1-18, 1993.
7. Centers for Disease Control and Prevention: Tuberculosis control laws-United States, *MMWR* 42-RR.15:1-15, 1993.

8. Centers for Disease Control and Prevention: Summary of notifiable diseases-1993, United States, *MMWR* October 21, 42(53):1-73, 1994.

9. Centers for Disease Control and Prevention: Human immunodeficiency virus transmission in household settings-United States, *MMWR* 43(19):347-356, 1994.

10. Centers for Disease Control and Prevention: Human plague-India, *MMWR* 43(38):690, 1994.

11. Centers for Disease Control and Prevention: Guidelines for preventing the transmission of tuberculosis in health care facilities, *Fed Reg* 59(208):54242-54303, 1994.

12. Centers for Disease Control and Prevention: Draft guidelines for isolation precautions in hospitals, *Fed Reg* 59(214):56552-56570, 1994.

13. Centers for Disease Control and Prevention, Statistics Department: Personal Communication, March 1995.

14. Czurglok P et al: MSRA: dealing with a hidden hazard, *Nursing* 12:68-69, 1991.

15. Hedrick E: Infectious waste management—will science prevail? *Infect Control Hosp Epidemiol* 9(11):83, 1988.

16. Joint Commission on Accreditation of Healthcare Organizations: *Accreditation manual for home care,* Oakbrook Terrace, Illinois, 1995, The Commission.

17. Larson E: A causal link between handwashing and risk of infection? *Infect Control Hosp Epidemiol* 9(1):28, 1988.

18. Lynch P et al: Implementing and evaluating a system of generic infection precautions: body substance isolation, *Am J Infect Control* 18(1):42, 1990.

19. McCray E et al: Cooperative needlestick surveillance group: occupational risk of the acquired immunodeficiency syndrome among health care workers, *N Engl J Med* 314(17):1127, 1986.

20. Occupational Health and Safety Administration: *29 CFR Part 1910.1030 occupational exposure to bloodborne pathogens,* Washington, DC, 1991, US Department of Labor.

21. Reingold A, Kamp M: Failure of gloves and other protective devices to prevent transmissions of hepatitis B virus to oral surgeons, *JAMA* 259:2558, 1988.

22. Rice R, Jorden J: Implementing an infection control program for the community facility, *JONA* 4(5):37, 1992.

23. Rice R: *Manual of home health nursing procedures,* St Louis, 1995, Mosby.

24. Simmons B et al: Infection control for home health, *Infect Control Hosp Epidemiol* 11(7):362-370, 1990.

25. Tuchman B: *A distant mirror—the calamitous 14th century,* New York, 1978, Ballantine Books.

26. Yangco BC, Yangco NF: What is leaky is also risky, *Infect Control Hosp Epidemiol* 10(12):553-556, 1989.

27. Ziegler P: The black death, New York, 1971, Harper and Row Publishers.

6 Patient Education in the Home

Robyn Rice, Karen Balakas, Virginia Drake, Patricia Freed,
Irene Kalnins, Anne Schappe, and Gail Wilkerson

Patient education is a very important component of home health nursing practice. As home health nurses visit patients on an intermittent basis, either the patient or caregiver must be able to manage health care needs *after* the nurse has left the home. Therefore a primary focus of patient care in the home is teaching and learning.

Home health nurses also recognize that the patient's "right to know" is intrinsic to quality patient care.[8,49] Patients have the right to know about their illness, treatments, and available resources in the community in order to achieve and maintain their best level of health. This relates to the purpose and goals of patient education in the home.

The goal of patient education in the home is to teach patients how to assume responsibility for their health; the emphasis is self-care management. Self-care management in health (discussed throughout this book) refers to those positive patient activities and health behaviors that keep the patient at home and out of the hospital. The home health nurse and home care team facilitate patient self-care management by utilizing teaching strategies that promote patient decision making, competence, and judgment in achieving home independence.

The process of patient education in the home can be quite challenging for home health nurses. What and how patients learn will be shaped by their beliefs concerning their own health, by cultural considerations, by age, by the patient's personal desire to achieve the best level of health, by the disease process or disability, and many other variables reflecting the home milieu.

The purpose of this chapter is to present home health nurses with useful concepts and practical information when providing patient education in the home. A vast amount of literature addresses patient education; to comprehensively discuss all of it is beyond the scope of a single chapter. However, the authors give an overview of information felt to be pertinent to clinical needs of field staff. The reader is referred to the rather extensive reference list at the end of the chapter for further information on individual subject matter.

Teaching and learning

Teaching is defined as methods of communication that facilitate learning.[1] *Learning* is defined as a primarily purposeful activity that often results in a change in the patient's thinking, behavior, or both.[1]

Learning occurs in three domains: the cognitive domain, the affective domain, and the psychomotor domain. In promoting a change in the patient's thinking or behavior, all are important to consider.[1,42]

Cognitive learning. Cognitive learning refers to intellectual activities such as thought, recall, decision making, drawing inferences, and arriving at conclusions. Applications of cognitive learning involve giving information to patients/caregivers about the disease process, medications, and treatments. Cognitive applications of learning may also include problem solving, empowering patients/caregivers to deal with the health care system, and strategizing lifestyle alterations to maintain household functioning.

Affective learning. Affective learning addresses the patient/caregiver's attitudes, feelings, and beliefs. Feelings, attitudes, and beliefs are often neglected aspects of patient education. Home health nurses may lack confidence in addressing these needs. Patients and their caregivers may be reluctant to share this information unless trust and rapport have been well established. Miscommunication, cultural misunderstandings, and divergent therapeutic goals between the nurse and patient/caregiver may result when these aspects of learning needs are not fully explored and addressed. Establishing a trusting and caring relationship with patients/caregivers is an essential prerequisite to affective learning. Encouraging and accepting expression of feelings and exploring health-illness beliefs are simple applications of this type of learning.

Psychomotor learning. Psychomotor learning refers to learning physical skills, tasks, or procedures such as a dressing change. Psychomotor learning is the most concrete type of learning; it is therefore frequently the easiest to teach and evaluate. This type of learning is best done in a step-by-step fashion, beginning with the more simple aspects of care and proceeding to the more complex aspects of the procedure.[1] For example, in home IV therapy patients are first taught how to hook up IV fluids to the tubing and then move on to the more complicated aspects of IV pump operation.

CONCEPTUAL BASIS

Concepts and theoretical frameworks provide working guidelines for home health nurses in answering the question, How do we teach? Concepts and theory are also useful in answering the question, How do patients learn?

Behavioral learning theory

Behavioral theorists such as Guthrie, Skinner, and Thorndike propose a stimulus-response(behavior) reinforcer in associative learning and behavior modification.[20,47,51] In using principles of behavioral modification, home health nurses should plan teaching strategies that elicit the desired behavior. If an undesirable behavior persists, then a more desirable reward must be substituted. Several principles of behavioral modification would be helpful to consider in designing a teaching-learning plan for patients and their families. These include the following:[50]

- Behavior that is not reinforced will decrease or cease.
- Reinforcement (reward) is a personal issue; a reward for me may not be a reward for you.

- Frequent and consistent reward is required during initial behavior change.
- With demonstrated behavior change, intermittent and variable reward is more sustaining.
- Reinforcement can involve administration of some positively perceived reward or removal of a positive or pleasurable activity.
- Behavioral learning is not aversive (punishment).
- To break the cycle of undesired behavior, the nurse may need to identify the reinforcement the individual is receiving and work toward removing it.

Cognitive-developmental learning theory

Cognitive-developmental learning reflects the work of theorists such as Erickson, Koehler, Koffka, Lewin, and Piaget.[14,19,29,30,32] Cognitive-developmental theories of learning take into account all the individual's life experiences and perceptions. Changes in perception are believed to result in a reorganization of thinking, referred to as the development of cognitive structures. Motivation to learn is derived from a need to make sense of the world, solve problems, and develop more cognitive structures in order to process life experiences.

Cognitive-developmental theorists believe that intellectual development is a gradual process that occurs over the life span. As the individual matures, comprehension moves from the concrete to the abstract. As a result, individuals are able to develop more extensive and integrated ways of thinking and understanding. Therefore learning is viewed as an ongoing intellectual evolution of insights (or perceptions) and understanding that guides human behavior.

Home health nurses must have extensive knowledge of human growth and development. Applications of developmental theory would include devising a learning plan for a skill involving small incremental steps that build over the course of several scheduled visits, designing age appropriate activities for a homebound child, and reorganizing the home milieu so that the patient with mild dementia can continue to function as independently as possible.

Humanistic learning theories

Elements of humanistic psychology take a holistic viewpoint in understanding when, how, and under what circumstances individuals learn. Elements such as love, creativity, self-growth, self-esteem, autonomy, and self-direction are emphasized as motivators in the learning process. An active patient role in determining what will be learned is emphasized.

Abraham Maslow's theory of human motivation has served as a framework for a humanistic approach to learning.[35] His theory is based upon a hierarchy consisting of physiological, security and safety, love and belonging, self-esteem, and self-actualization needs. As shown in Figure 6-1, these needs are arranged in order of priority for satisfaction. Maslow believed that lower-level needs must first be satisfied before individuals attempt to satisfy higher-level needs. Basic physiological needs (such as food, water, oxygen, elimination, rest, and comfort) that are essential for survival were seen as first-level needs that take precedence over other needs. According to Maslow's theory, the patient's basic physiological needs must be

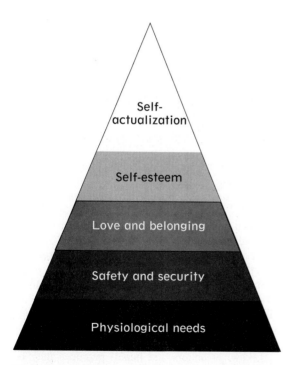

Figure 6-1 Maslow's hierarchy of needs. (Reprinted with permission from Potter P, Perry A: *Fundamentals of nursing: concepts, process, and practice,* ed 3, St Louis, 1993, Mosby.)

met before patient education is attempted. Otherwise, patient anxiety over unmet basic needs is so great that learning is almost impossible. Self-actualization occurs after all other needs are met and is seen as the point at which individuals are capable of truly creative processes.

Davis-Sharts' research into Maslow's theory suggests that a hierarchy of basic human needs may be transcultural.[11] In her study of 60 cultural units, she tested levels of physiological and security needs. Her findings suggest empirical evidence to support the concept that basic human needs are primary motivating forces underlying all human behavior.

Home health nurses can apply this information by recognizing that survival needs for home independence are priorities of health teaching for all patients, regardless of ethnic background. For example, when teaching home ventilator-dependent patients, learning how to operate and troubleshoot equipment may well take precedence over understanding the disease process.

Social-cognitive learning theories

According to social-cognitive theorists such as Kohlberg and Rotter, the process of learning occurs as individuals acquire knowledge, values, moral judgments, and standards of behavior by observing others.[31,44] Moral development is believed to occur as individuals proceed through life experiences. Likewise, behavior is thought to be influenced by perceived effects of consequences of actions. In addition, proponents of social-cognitive learning suggest that much behavior is regulated by both internal and external cues for action.

Locus of control. Locus of control relates to patient willingness to take action and readiness to learn. Based on Rotter's social learning theory, locus of control theory depicts people as primarily internally or externally influenced to take health actions.[44] Wallston et al. (1978) developed this construct further, suggesting that reinforcement for health-related behaviors is primarily internal, a matter of chance, or under the control of powerful others.[53]

"Externals" believe that they are at the mercy of fate, luck, or social environment and have little influence over what happens to them.[7,28,48] In contrast, "internals" believe that they can master their own environment and thus take an active approach toward their own health decisions.[37] Externals are seen as more compulsive and may need more assistance and guidance for health care, such as a learning contract.[37]

Locus of control in the elderly appears to be influenced by the environment and physical constraints. Research suggests that as the health of the elderly declines, their locus of control orientation becomes more external as dependence on the caregiver is increased.[6,33] Activity is also negatively correlated with an external locus of control, suggesting that health and activity are strong influences on locus of control.[25] Finally, locus of control may also have negative psychological consequences such as depression and learned helplessness; these, in turn, may lead to detrimental physical changes.[24,40,48]

In general, internals are more likely to desire mutual goal setting and decision making in developing the plan of care while externals may need more structure and guidance in their therapeutic regimen, perhaps relying on the assistance of a caregiver.

Self-efficacy. Self-efficacy refers to the belief that one can sucessfully perform a behavior that is necessary in order to achieve a certain outcome.[42] It relates to the patient's confidence level that the required task or change in behavior can be accomplished. Home health nurses can use principles of self-efficacy to build confidence levels in their patients. In using principles of self-efficacy, home health nurses should recognize that the first step in promoting change is to get the patient to believe that they *can* learn new skills and ways of doing things.

Health promotion model. Like the locus of control theory, Pender's health promotion model proposes that an individual's cognitive-perceptual status as well as other modifying factors are important determinants of participation in health-promoting behaviors. According to Pender, health promotion is directed toward increasing the level of well-being and self-actualization of the individual.[38] Pender's model provides a framework for predicting health practices (Figure 6-2).[38] It suggests that the patient's participation in the plan of care is based upon the following:[38,42]

- Perceived importance of health
- Perceived control (described as the relationship between one's beliefs about internal/

external control and one's decisions regarding health care)
- Severity of disease
- Perceptions of benefits associated with actions to reduce the threat of illness
- Perceptions of potential barriers (physical, psychological, or financial) associated with health actions
- Demographic characteristics
- Interpersonal and situational factors
- Behavioral factors

This model helps explain why and in what circumstances people will assume responsibility for their health. Research indicates that modifying factors such as demographic, structural, and sociocultural influences will also determine the likelihood of health-promoting behaviors.[37]

Home health nurses can use conceptual applications of learning to (1) develop a plan of care that is realistic for the patient's abilities, desires, and resources, (2) promote compliance by evaluating the patient's perceptions of disease and determination for best level of health as a baseline for participation in the plan of care, and (3) understand complex human behavior in finding better ways to teach.

SOCIOCULTURAL CONSIDERATIONS AND HEALTH BELIEFS

Motivation of health practices and willingness to learn are best understood within a sociocultural context. In examining different ethnic groups, research indicates that compliance with the plan of care is not achieved solely by health teaching.[16,39,40] For realistic working relationships to occur, the plan of care must fit the patient's value and belief systems. (See the box on p. 82.)

Certain beliefs and health practices are unique to ethnic group and class. For example, many patients have a strong belief in religion as a means of healing.[16,43] Evil may be seen as the cause of illness.[16,43] Certain patients and their families may consider prayer and religious worship to be paramount to recovery.[1,16]

Likewise, beliefs and health practices may be influenced by *geographic ethnicity.* For example, people residing in rural areas tend to rely on informal sources such as family, relatives, and friends for health-related concerns. Research indicates that rural people tend to define health as the

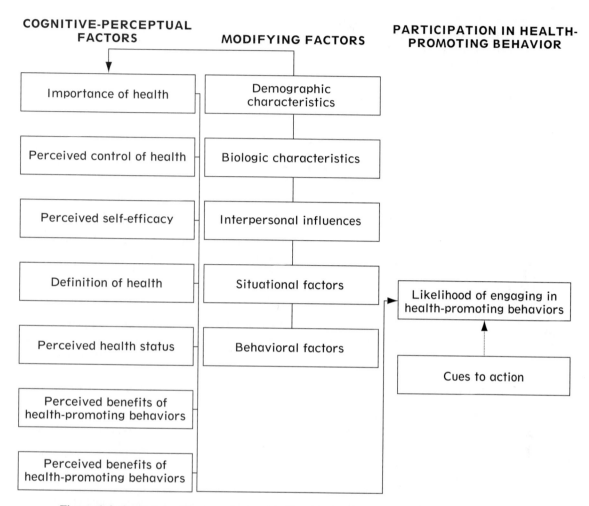

COGNITIVE-PERCEPTUAL FACTORS

MODIFYING FACTORS

PARTICIPATION IN HEALTH-PROMOTING BEHAVIOR

Importance of health

Perceived control of health

Perceived self-efficacy

Definition of health

Perceived health status

Perceived benefits of health-promoting behaviors

Perceived benefits of health-promoting behaviors

Demographic characteristics

Biologic characteristics

Interpersonal influences

Situational factors

Behavioral factors

Likelihood of engaging in health-promoting behaviors

Cues to action

Figure 6-2 Pender's health promotion model. (Reprinted with permission from Pender N: *Health promotion in nursing practice,* ed 2, Norwalk, Conn, 1987, Appleton & Lange.)

ability to work or function in one's role.[9] Rural people may view a loss of health as dependency or inability to work. Therefore a focus on promoting self-reliance and sustaining functional abilities would be an important part of the plan of care for rural patients.

Certain ethnic groups may seek advice from elder family members, community leaders, or faith healers respected for their knowledge of healing. Likewise, some patients may rely on folk medicine.[43] Popular folk medicine may include getting extra rest, traditional dietary changes such as special soups, over-the-counter medications, herbs, poultices, amulets, and religious practices and rituals.[16,43,52,54]

Home remedies are one type of folk medicine. They are found in almost every household and are given various degrees of importance by patients. Table 6-1 lists some common home remedies. Depending on the patient's values and beliefs and the nurse's and physician's assessment of the *safety* of the remedies, certain home remedies may be incorporated into the plan of care. In these matters, home health nurses may well become mediators between patients and physicians.

To the greatest extent possible, home health nurses should respect ethnic and religious beliefs. For example, when encouraging dietary changes, home health nurses should be careful not to recommend

> **PROVIDING CULTURALLY
> SENSITIVE HOME HEALTH CARE
> IN A PLURALISTIC SOCIETY**
>
> 1. Have an understanding of one's own values and beliefs about health and illness.
> 2. Seek information and understanding about the specific cultural group's health care practices and associated values and beliefs.
> 3. Establish a mutual, collaborative relationship with the patient and family.
> 4. Explore the patient/family's perception of what is wrong and contributing factors.
> 5. Determine what action the patient/family would like to take.

foods that are restricted by the patient's religion. The following guidelines may assist home health nurses gain acceptance into any family:

1. Respect the patient/family's right to refuse your services.
2. Remember that you are a guest in the patient's home and behave accordingly.
3. Recognize and respect the family's communication and decision making channels.
4. Be courteous and respectful at all times to caregivers and all family members (and their pets).
5. Call before visiting to let the patient know you are coming whenever possible.
6. Leave your professional agency's identification card with the patient.

Understanding cultural diversity within the home milieu (Figure 6-3) as well as individual health beliefs permits home health nurses to provide a realistic and achievable plan of care.[16,52] This helps people from all ethnic backgrounds to better care for themselves.

PRINCIPLES OF ADULT LEARNING

Adult learners have their own characteristics which must be considered when teaching. These include more varied life experiences, stressful economic and family responsibilities, specific goals and desires for learning, a slower pace in learning style, a preference for self-directed prob-

lem solving approaches to studies, and increased physical limitations (such as declining vision and hearing, or poor circulation).[17]

Adults learn best when the problems they study are important to their own interests. In working with adults, it is important to address what they believe to be their immediate problem. Therefore the home health nurse should provide adult patients with material or information that has personal relevance for the patient. Home health nurses should acknowledge the adult learner's experiences and draw from them when using examples to illustrate a point during teaching. Ignoring or devaluing adult learners' experiences or questions may be perceived as a rejection of their personhood or life's work. This phenomenon may be one reason why adults express deep resentment when they return to school or learning situations; they may feel they are not treated like professionals or "grown-ups."[1]

Patient education and the nursing process

Although the majority of home care patients are elderly, home health nurses are likely to encounter patients and caregivers of all ages with diverse ethnic backgrounds and educational needs. Age, developmental stage, cognitive level, and focus of care (rehabilitation versus terminal care) will all influence educational content and teaching strategies. The nursing process of assessment, diagnosis, planning, implementing, and evaluation provides a general framework for patient education. Consider the following guidelines:[17,27]

Assessing (data collection). Identify who will receive teaching and include caregivers or family members who will assist patients with care and thus also require teaching. Determine readiness to learn (recognize motivational, developmental, and sociocultural background). Mutually assess learning needs with the patient/caregiver; identify appropriate learning strategies and tools.

Next identify availability of resources, supplies, or equipment needed for undertaking the therapeutic regimen at home. Initiate referrals and/or consultations as needed. Determine whether the patient's environment is conducive to learning or appropriate for the recommended therapeutic regimen; make adjustments as needed.

Identifying nursing diagnoses/patient problems. Nursing diagnoses commonly used in home

Table 6-1 Common home remedies

Common ailments	Internal remedies			External remedies	
	Teas	Syrups	Other oral remedies	Poultices	Topical remedies
Boil or "rising"				Tobacco	Membrane of an egg
					Fatback, salty meat
					Flaxseed, tansy, or jimsonweed
Chest cold			Vaseline and sugar		Mutton or beef tallow (covered with flannel)
Colds	Tansy Ginger Catnip	Onion and sugar (whiskey) Lemon and honey	Castor oil Patent medicines		
Constipation	Comfrey or sage		Castor oil		
Cough		Onion and sugar (whiskey) Lemon and honey Horehound leaf and sugar Wild cherry bark and sugar	Vaseline and sugar		
Diarrhea	Black pepper Cinnamon or nutmeg		Flour water Blackberry juice or wine		
Earache					Molasses, honey, or sweet oil Warm chamber water Pipe smoke (blow into ear)

Adapted with permission from Roberson M: Home remedies: a cultural study, *Home Health Care Nurs* 5(1):36, 1987.

Continued

care include those of knowledge deficit, self-care deficit, and activity intolerance. (See Chapter 4 for further information on nursing diagnoses.)

Planning (assigning priorities to learning needs). Mutually plan learning goals and outcomes of care with the home care team and the patient. Give priority in health teaching to the patient's immediate self-perceived survival needs in the home.

Implementing (actions). Initiate and implement activities designed to meet learning outcomes; activities should focus upon cognitive, affective, and psychomotor learning.[21] (See Chap-

ter 4 for information regarding writing behavioral outcomes of care.)

Evaluating (determining whether outcomes and goals of care were met). In recommending discharge from home health services, evaluate the patient's participation in self-care and the patient's ability to make appropriate decisions regarding health care needs. Is there a change in the patient's behavior toward positive health actions?

Determine if the patient has knowledge of the therapeutic regimen (e.g., treatments, procedures, medications) and disease process. Determine if the

Table 6-1 Common home remedies—cont'd

| Common ailments | Internal remedies | | | External remedies | |
	Teas	Syrups	Other oral remedies	Poultices	Topical remedies
Fever		Onion and sugar (whiskey) Lemon and honey	Niter, quinine	Cabbage leaf (bruised) Onion, raw (cut and bind in place) Potato, raw (slice and bind in place)	
Headache			Coca-Cola Patent medicines	Cabbage leaf (bruised)	
Rash	Ginger Catnip				Vaseline, oatmeal, or burned flour
Sore throat		Horehound leaf and sugar			
Splinters					Fatback, salty meat
Swellings				Mullein weed	
Thrush					Vaseline, urine, or boric acid
Toothache					Lemon extract, perfume, tobacco, or red pepper seed Heat, hot salt bag
Upset stomach	Tansy Peppermint, nutmeg, Jerusalem oak, or clove		Calamus root (chew) Soda and vinegar		
"Wind colic" (babies)	Catnip				

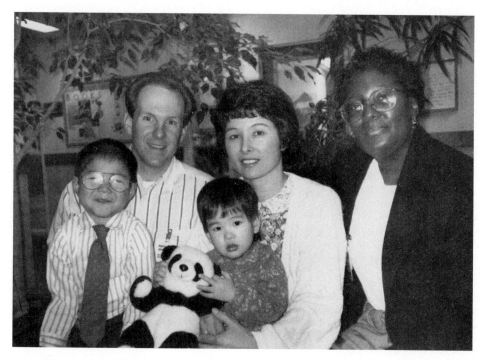

Figure 6-3 An image of our multicultural community. (Photograph by Robyn Rice.)

patient is satisfied with the teaching plan and home health services; provide this feedback to the QA/QI committee.

Encouraging patient/caregiver active participation in the plan of care

Successful management of health care needs at home requires the patient's *active participation* with the plan of care.[8,27] Patients are taught to recognize problems with equipment as well as detrimental changes in health status that should be reported to the nurse and physician. For example, COPD patients are taught the importance of reporting the first signs of a cold because the immediate use of antibiotics can prevent respiratory infections and hospitalization. Likewise, treatments specific to the health care needs at home (e.g., medication regimen, wound care), use of equipment and supplies (IV pump, walker, home whirlpool, dressings), and personal care (diet, elimination, mobility, bathing, and dressing) all become part of active patient tasks through the process of patient education.

If the patient is not able to learn, the home health nurse must identify a caregiver, family member, or friend who will receive health teaching. It may be necessary for patients with extensive health care needs and no available caregiver to consider alternate health care strategies such as homemaker services or long-term care placement.

Medicare documentation guidelines for patient education

As stated in Chapter 4, Medicare considers teaching to be skilled care and reimbursable. The box on p. 86 provides guidelines for teaching and training activities considered reimbursable by Medicare. Since reimbursement is based on documentation, the documentation of patient education should be very specific. Describe what was taught and to whom, state goals of teaching activities that were met, give an evaluation of the patient's or caregiver's ability to learn, and present plans for future teaching sessions.[23]

Duplication of teaching provided by other disciplines should be avoided because Medicare will

---

GUIDELINES FOR TEACHING AND TRAINING ACTIVITIES

Teaching and training activities which require the skills of a licensed nurse include, but *are not limited to* the following:

- Teaching the self-administration of injectable medications, or a complex range of medications
- Teaching a newly diagnosed diabetic or caregiver all aspects of diabetes management, including how to prepare and to administer insulin injections, to prepare and follow a diabetic diet, to observe foot-care precautions, and to observe for and understand signs of hyperglycemia and hypoglycemia
- Teaching self-administration of medical gases
- Teaching wound care where the complexity of the wound, the overall condition of the beneficiary or the ability of the caregiver makes teaching necessary
- Teaching care for a recent ostomy or where reinforcement of ostomy care is needed
- Teaching self-catheterization
- Teaching self-administration of gastrostomy or enteral feedings
- Teaching care for and maintenance of peripheral and central venous lines and administration of intravenous medications through such lines
- Teaching bowel or bladder training when bowel or bladder dysfunction exists
- Teaching how to perform the activities of daily living when the beneficiary or caregiver must use special techniques and adaptive devices due to a loss of function
- Teaching transfer techniques, e.g., from bed to chair, which are needed for safe transfer
- Teaching proper body alignment and positioning, and timing techniques of a bedbound beneficiary
- Teaching ambulation with prescribed assistive devices (such as crutches, walker, cane, etc.) that are needed due to a recent functional loss
- Teaching prosthesis care and gait training
- Teaching the use and care of braces, splints and orthotics and associated skin care
- Teaching the proper care and application of any specialized dressings or skin treatments (for example, dressings or treatments needed by beneficiaries with severe or widespread fungal infections, active and severe psoriasis or eczema, or due to skin deterioration from radiation treatments)
- Teaching the preparation and maintenance of a therapeutic diet
- Teaching proper administration of oral medication, including signs of side effects and avoidance of interaction with other medications and food

Adapted from Health Care Financing Administration: *Health insurance manual* Pub No 11 -Thru T273, Rev 3/95, Washington, DC, 1995, Department of Health and Human Services.

---

deny payment.[23] Thus it is important for home health nurses to coordinate educational activities with the multidisciplinary team.

Last, Medicare does not pay for reinstruction unless documentation verifies the need. Home health nurses should document what the learner did not understand or comprehend to justify revising the teaching plan to more adequately suit the learner's needs and abilities. Home health nurses should document a short attention span, cognitive deficits, or learning difficulties as a reason for repetitive teaching.

TEACHING STRATEGIES

Teaching strategies in the home primarily include discussion, storytelling, and demonstrations. Ample time should be allowed for comments and patient questions. In leadership roles, home health nurses may find that they are occasionally requested to lecture to groups of people or for organizations. (See the box titled Group Teaching Strategies on p. 89).

TEACHING TOOLS

Teaching tools provide visual and audio guides for learning. Examples of teaching tools useful for patient education include videos, models, audiocassette tapes, flip charts, pamphlets, posters, photographs, checklists, and cartoons. (See Table 6-2 for features of various teaching materials and Figure 6-4, using symbols as teaching tools.)

Preprinted patient education guides regarding disease process, procedures, and treatments are a

Table 6-2 Using teaching tools in home care

Type	Advantages	Disadvantages	Helpful hints
Video recordings	Best possible substitute for actual experience Easily obtainable Easy to remake and update Can be stopped and rerun Familiar to many	Patient/caregiver may not have a VCR/TV Technical skill with film-making helpful Expensive initial investment	Must be compatible with the VCR Can take three times longer than you expect to make a tape
Objects and models	Depict the real thing as closely as possible Can be handled and studied at the patient's pace Replicas—static Analogues—dynamic Appeal to kinesthetic learners	Can be bulky and heavy Inconvenient to transport Time consuming Expensive Analogues—demand conceptual sophistication	Require advance planning if borrowed
Audiocassette tapes	Can be used with individuals or groups Good for developing listening skills Accessible Cheap Can be tailor-made, erased, or remade Good for enhancing stress management skills	Patient/caregiver may not have a cassette player Can be dull if used by itself Can be damaged easily	Must be protected from temperature and moisture extremes Should be of high quality Must be long enough
Pamphlets and posters	Portable, attractive, and attracting Can be used before, during, and after a presentation Can be studied at patient's pace Readily available Often free Posters can be used to clarify the patient's medication regimen or aspects of procedural care	Time consuming to make Need a prop Bulky to carry and store Pamphlets—may overwhelm patient if too many	Pamphlets—must be checked for currency and must be passed out at the most propitious time Should contain few words and lots of space Posters—figures and drawings can be placed on the poster
Photographs and cartoons	Easily personalized Can elicit emotions Can portray many more thoughts than words alone Allow the patient to control the pace	Inappropriate for large groups Can be distracting if passed during talk Yellow with age Cartoons—can inadvertently offend or confuse	Should be tried out on people of similar ages and backgrounds as your patients Look more lively if in color May require explanations

Adapted from Babcock D, Miller M: *Client education: theory and practice,* St Louis, 1994, Mosby, pp. 224-225.

Continued

Table 6-2 Using teaching tools in home care—cont'd

Type	Advantages	Disadvantages	Helpful hints
Computer-assisted instruction (CAI) programs	Allow the patient to control the pace Reinforce correct responses immediately Good for sequential thought processes Allow the patient to repeat the lesson if necessary	Patient/caregiver may not have necessary equipment for home CAI programs Time consuming to monitor and do Are of a limited value if the teacher is not available Require patients who are visual learners and computer literate Can be boring	Allow the teacher to select the more user-friendly software available Work best if the teacher spends enough time with the patient to ensure that he or she is comfortable with the program
Flip charts	Versatile, portable, used like a chalkboard May be prepared before the presentation or spontaneously during presentation	Require artistic talent and good handwriting	Teacher should have a good supply of black and colored pens and should use masking tape or soft, gummy adhesive to affix flip charts to the wall
Patient education guides	Versatile, portable. Easy to leave in the patient's home health agency folder	Require patients who are visual learners and who are literate	Develop patient education guides to correspond to the clinical pathway

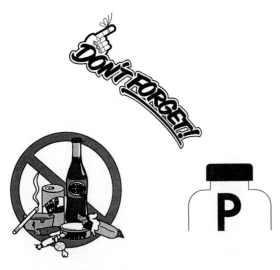

Figure 6-4 Using pictures and symbols as teaching tools.

useful learning resource and an upcoming trend in home care. In addition, they free the home health nurse from the burden of documenting in the narrative of the visit report what was taught. Keep a copy of the education guide in the patient's folder at the home and a copy in the medical record. (See p. 90 for the box that provides an example of a patient education guide.) As will be discussed in Chapter 8, consider developing patient education guides for each care path.

In evaluating the usefulness of teaching tools, ask yourself the following questions:[54]

- Is the teaching tool accurate?
- Can the teaching tool help the learner meet behavioral outcomes of care?
- Is the material relevant to the learning needs of the patient?
- Do the materials reflect the developmental and functional needs of the patient?

GROUP TEACHING STRATEGIES

1. Relax! They want to hear what you have to say.
2. Dress the part and look professional.
3. Mentally rehearse the sequence of your presentation. Make sure you have practiced your session beforehand!
4. Arrive at least one half hour early so you can settle in and troubleshoot the room setup or equipment.
5. Use your prepared session notes but do not read from them.
6. Check your session notes and transparencies/slides for correct sequencing before you start your presentation.
7. Establish credibility at the beginning of your presentation. Tell them a little about yourself. A joke or humorous story will capture your audience's attention early on.
8. Tell your audience when they can expect their break or lunch before you begin your presentation. Also, tell them where the bathrooms and phones are.
9. Give your audience an outline of events and topics. Go over handouts as needed.
10. Move around. Do not stand in one spot.
11. Keep eye contact with your audience.
12. Use all the principles of adult learning. Ask questions. Be comfortable answering questions. Use brainteasers. Be enthusiastic. Use relevant storytelling to capture and recapture your audience's attention. *Work your audience.*
13. Plan for a morning and afternoon interactive learning experience if giving an all-day program. For example, have the audience get into groups and do some group work relevant to the presentation topic.
14. Understand the psychology of the group and use it to your advantage. Find out in advance who your participants are. The group will have individuals from varying backgrounds. Some individuals in the group will have very little knowledge of your subject matter while other individuals will feel that they are experts on all subject matter. Serve the majority. Recognize that you cannot meet everyone's needs.
15. Do not let one person take over your program. Some individuals are needy for attention. Make time for them during breaks or at lunch. Give them a leadership role during the interactive experience but limit it to that. Be aware that security can remove disruptive individuals.
16. Get feedback from your audience.
17. The key to a successful presentation is to entertain as well as educate. Share your knowledge and creative talents with your group, so that when they leave you they are energized and empowered by your subject matter!

• Is the teaching tool written at a level the patient can understand?

TEACHING STRATEGIES FOR SPECIAL PATIENT GROUPS IN HOME CARE
The older adult patient

It has been shown that with normal aging there is little change in intelligence. However, with chronic disease there does appear to be a slight decrease in intelligence.[4] Likewise, older adult patients often require more time to learn. Psychomotor skills in particular may take longer to master.[54] However, the old adage, "you can't teach an old dog new tricks" is false; adults maintain the ability to learn throughout life (Figure 6-5).

The normal changes associated with aging described in Chapter 24 will certainly affect teaching strategies. (These changes are summarized in Table 6-3.) This will require an adjustment of teaching techniques to accommodate specific age-related physical and psychosocial changes.[54] It is important that home health nurses be aware of these normal aging changes when developing an educational plan.[12]

As many standard teaching tools are devised for younger patients, it is important that home health nurses be creative in their approach to health education for the older adult. (Figure 6-6 summarizes effective teaching techniques for the older adult patient.)[36] Be aware that older adults don't like to be patronized any more than younger adults, so don't tell them information they already know.

The noncompliant patient

Noncompliance by patients with their prescribed health care regimen remains one of the most

PATIENT/CAREGIVER EDUCATION GUIDES WOUND CARE

1. Always wash your hands before and after changing your dressing because good handwashing will help your wound stay clean and prevent the spread of germs.
2. Keep all your medical supplies in a clean area; boxes of dressings, gloves, and other medical supplies may be stored in a clean plastic trashbag.
3. Throw away wound care solutions after 1 week or sooner if you see particles forming in the container or if the solution changes color or becomes cloudy.
4. Notify the home health agency if you are running out of supplies.
5. Gather up your supplies. Prepare a plastic bag for disposal of dirty dressings and supplies.
6. Prepare your new dressing as your case manager has instructed you. All caregivers should wear gloves when assisting you with your dressing changes.
7. Carefully remove your old dressing and inspect your wound. Any noticeable differences in size, color, or drainage should be reported to your case manager or aide at the next visit.
8. Apply your new dressing as your case manager has shown you. See below for specific steps to put on your new dressing. Your dressing should be changed according to schedule or if it comes off or becomes soggy.
9. Place your dirty dressings/supplies in a plastic trashbag. Seal and dispose of the bag in your family trash.
10. Call your case manager if you have an elevated temperature or problems with pus or excessive wound drainage or if swelling or pain occur with your wound.

Specific steps to clean your wound and change your dressing:

Patient/caregiver signature: _____   Date: _____
Case manager signature: _____   Date: _____
Care Path number: #1; wound management _____
white copy-patient's home record; yellow copy-medical record

Reproduced courtesy of American Nursing Development of Maryville, Ill.

challenging and frustrating behaviors with which home health nurses contend. Frequently, noncompliant behavior is interpreted by the home health nurse as personal rejection by the patient. Internally the nurse is thinking, "don't you realize I am trying my best to help you, and you (the patient) won't even cooperate with me." Home health nurses may feel angry, discouraged, frustrated, hopeless, and helpless that their offerings of care are being rebuffed by the patient. These feelings may lead the nurse to interpret the patient's uncooperative behavior as a rejection of the nurse's competency, professional acumen, and personhood. This sets the stage for an adversarial relationship with the patient rather than one of advocacy. Home health nurses may unconsciously

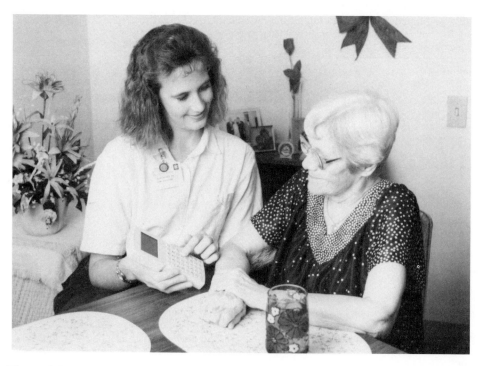

Figure 6-5 Using a handheld computer to teach patient care to the older adult. (Courtesy Saint Anthony's Health Center, Alton, Ill.)

retaliate against the presumed ungrateful or unco-operative patient by ignoring, rejecting, or prematurely discharging the patient from services.

Remember, all behavior is purposeful and all behavior has meaning.[15] Consider that noncompliant patients and/or caregivers cannot be helped unless the reasons for their behavior are understood. In trying to alter maladaptive or unhealthy behaviors, consider the term *nonparticipation.* Why is the patient not participating with the plan of care? What behaviors underlie nonparticipation?

It is *crucial* to be nonjudgmental; accept the patient's behavior while working to change it. Likewise do not view nonparticipation and noncompliance as de facto negative, uncooperative behavior on the part of the patient; but rather the patient's way of trying to communicate that there is something unacceptable, uncomfortable, or unsatisfactory about the plan of care. It is important to assess what the patient is trying to convey by the noncompliant behavior.

By working together, the home health nurse and patient can identify a mutually satisfactory plan of care with which the patient will be *willing* and *able* to comply. Once this task is achieved, the home health nurse and patient will both feel less distressed and be better able to partner together in future health care situations.

In working with noncompliant patients, begin with a comprehensive assessment focusing first on the positive behaviors of the patient, and then moving to the noncompliant behavior. To establish rapport it is important to acknowledge those behaviors with which the patient has complied.

It may be surprising to learn that the patient is unaware of any intentional noncompliance. This information indicates a knowledge deficit which can be corrected by additional patient education. Perhaps the patient did not understand the directions, the importance of following the directions, or some other part of the process. The patient may have misplaced the directions and not known who

Table 6-3 Age-related changes and alterations in teaching techniques

Age-related changes	Teaching techniques
Reaction time Lengthens	• Slow pace of presentations • Do not rush client response • Provide liberal practice time • Give small amounts of information at each session • Repeat information frequently • Use analogies • Reinforce teaching with videos, practice
Vision Lens yellows and thickens Decreased lens accommodation	• Avoid blue and green paper • Use white paper • Use nonglossy paper • Make sure eyeglasses are worn • Use 12- to 16-point type • Use bold type • Use black or red ink • Use simple sentence structure • Use magnifying mirror • Make sure eyeglasses are worn • Use large graphic illustrations
Hearing Ability to discriminate sounds decreases	• Speak slowly • Use short sentences • Do not shout • Face patient when speaking, make sure lighting allows your face to be seen clearly • Use slightly louder tone • Eliminate background noise • Have client wear hearing aid • Use amplifier • Determine whether client hears better with one ear • Allow time for client to repeat information
Memory Decreased short-term memory	• Teach one concept at a time • Use oral, written, demonstration techniques

Adapted from McCaffrey B, Boyle D: The elderly patient with cancer: teaching/learning considerations for ostomy, wound, and continence management, *Progressions* 6(1):18, 1994. Weinrich S, Boyd M: Education in the elderly, *J Gerontol Nurs* 18(1):17, 1992.

to contact for help. The point is that home health nurses *must not* assume the patient is being noncompliant just to be rebellious or uncooperative.

Noncompliance may also be influenced by the family or friends. Others may genuinely believe they are contributing to the patient's best interests and be unaware that their "helping" efforts are undermining the patient's well-being. Unfortunately, there are situations when others interfere as a result of their own agendas which are *not* in the best interest of the patient. If such a situation exists, the involved persons must be confronted

Teaching the Elderly

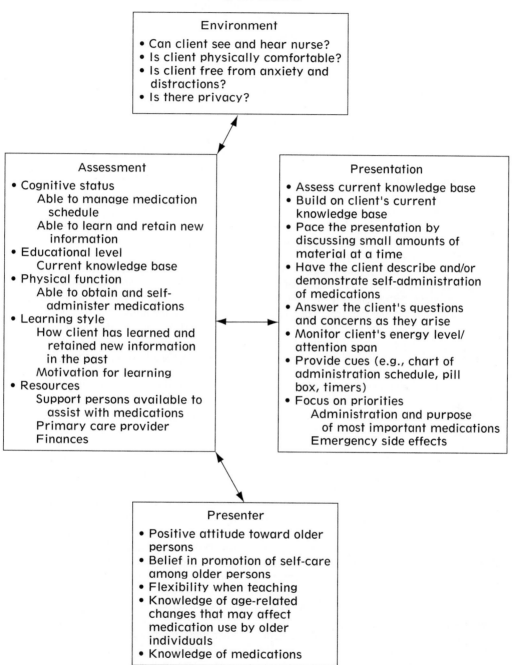

Figure 6-6 Teaching the elderly. (Adapted from Dellasega C, Clark D, McCreary D, Helmuth A, Schan P: Nursing process: teaching elderly clients, *J Gerontol Nurs* 20(1):31-38, 1994.)

about their detrimental effects on the patient's welfare.

There are many varied reasons for noncompliance. These include knowledge deficits related to the plan of care, lack of financial resources to comply, lack of support systems to assist the patient with compliance, lack of trust in the home care team and physician, negative side effects of treatment, insecurities with self-care management, ethnic barriers, value differences, disease process, or cognitive aberrations (such as dementia, depression, or psychosis) that impair the patient's ability to comply.

Home health nurses have the responsibility to supportively inquire about all issues which have bearing on noncompliance including sensitive, personal issues such as sexuality, family problems, or financial concerns. The home health nurse might say, "As your nurse I am concerned that you have not been following your plan of care. I am willing to help you find a way to do whatever is best for your health. What can you tell me about the things that are preventing you from complying with the recommendations for your plan of care?" By asking the patient for specific information, the home health nurse increases the chances of obtaining useful data.

Proceed by asking the patient to share his or her understanding of what behaviors are necessary to achieve compliance with the plan of care. Encourage the patient to weigh and discuss the advantages and disadvantages of the requested change.[39]

Inquire about possible side effects of medication, fear and anxiety about managing illness at home, lack of resources or other forms of support, or other factors interfering with compliance. At this point the home health nurse may state, "It has been my experience with some other patients having difficulty following the treatment regimen, that they experienced (state side effect of medication or problem). I'm wondering if perhaps the same thing is happening to you?" This gives the patient the knowledge that the nurse understands some of the problems and will be comfortable hearing them and discussing them with the patient. This approach encourages the patient to identify reasons for noncompliance. Until all the reasons are understood, minimal (if any) progress will be made toward compliance.

If patients are unable to change with information alone, consider behavioral strategies. Pfister (1993) offers the following recommendations:[39]

- Identify the behavior to be changed.
- Analyze the behavior. (Consider the meaning of the behavior to the patient and socioenvironmental factors or events that influence the behavior.)
- Identify environmental factors or events that would facilitate the desired behavior.
- Gradually add behaviors that enhance the accomplishment of the new behavior.
- Assist the patient to find new ways to meet needs that old behaviors previously met.
- Help the patient identify means within his or her own environment to build continuous reinforcement

Complying with the therapeutic regimen can be difficult. Step-by-step planning—focusing on incremental changes—may be more successful than expectations for immediate and drastic changes in behavior (for example, diet modifications).[2,3] It is very important to encourage patients for the positive things they have done since the last visit. In giving praise, focus on achievements; stress the difficulty of the level of accomplishment.

As a matter of routine home health agency policy, it should be made clear to the patient during the admission process that compliance with the plan of care is expected. It should also be made clear that failure to work with the home care team could result in termination of home health services. If the patient demonstrates continued unacceptable health behaviors, a learning contract is recommended. (See the following box.) If the patient fails to comply with the learning contract, consult with supervisory staff and follow home health agency policy; these situations will have legal as well as ethical implications. (See Chapter 7.)

Unless a patient is consciously or unconsciously self-destructive, it is rare to find a person who totally refuses to comply with the plan of care once the significance is understood and the obstacles removed. When working in the home milieu, home health nurses focus on those patient behaviors they can change and accept that there may be certain behaviors that the patient will not

---

ELEMENTS OF THE LEARNING CONTRACT

1. Date
2. People in attendance (it is recommended that the social worker or supervisor attend this session with the nurse and patient/caregiver)
3. Identified problematic behavior
4. Identified interventions for problem resolution:
   a. Nursing actions/therapies
   b. Patient/caregiver actions
5. Method of evaluation of care
6. Time frame for problematic behavior to resolve (in most cases give the patient/caregiver one visit to turn things around)
7. Home health agency course of action should the problematic behavior continue or resurface during the course of the patient's care (consult with your legal team, consider discharging the patient to the physician's care if problems continue)
8. Signatures and dates

---

change. In delivering services, a middle ground of patient adherence with the plan of care is usually acceptable (*how* acceptable will ultimately be up to the professional judgment of the home health nurse).

The illiterate patient

Low literacy indicates a lack of reading skills but also limits the patient's ability to organize perceptions and thoughts about the therapeutic regimen. Patients with low literacy skills may react to a complicated, fast-paced learning situation by withdrawing from or avoiding the experience because their process of interpretation is slow.[26] If questioned about understanding, the patient may well smile and nod that the information was understood while mentally wishing the home health nurse to be gone. Such a response may be due to low self-esteem and a lack of vocabulary, comprehension, or problem solving ability to verbalize what was not understood. Teaching strategies for the illiterate patient include:[26]

- Simplified therapeutic regimens, medication schedules
- Techniques such as cuing (combining timing with the situation that reminds the patient to

perform the task, for example, teach a patient with diabetes to examine the feet during morning care) and tailoring (allow the patient to decide on a schedule that is acceptable to the patient and is within the realm of the physician's orders, for example, the patient may wish to schedule medications around mealtimes)
- Simplified teaching tools, use of pictures or stick figures
- A slow-paced teaching style, lots of reinforcement, information repeated as needed
- A warm, nonjudgmental approach (foster patient self-esteem by acknowledging that academic degrees and advanced levels of education are not always equated with good common sense nor are they a requirement for learning or a desire to better one's life)

The mental health patient

Since many individuals today have dual diagnosis (that is, a physical and mental illness), it is likely that home health nurses will be providing care to these patients and their families. Therefore it is essential that home health nurses be able to provide information about the disease, medication, and treatment; information to help patients cope with the illness in their daily lives; and information to help them live with the stigma of mental illness.[18,34] In addition, patients may experience emotional needs that take priority over physical needs. Anxiety, fear, distrust, and misperception are not uncommon behaviors in patients/caregivers experiencing health alterations. Therefore home health nurses need relational skills to decrease anxiety, provide security, and promote trust.

In some instances, patients in the home experience profound alterations in thought, feeling, and behavior that are associated with mental illness. These patients should routinely be seen by the psychiatric home health nurse or by an advanced practitioner in mental health. (See Chapter 23.)

Educational approaches to patients with mental illness should aim at empowerment and active decision making within an egalitarian patient-nurse relationship.[45,55] Patients and their caregivers need to learn to recognize when the patient's behavior warrants immediate medical attention or hospitalization. In addition, home health nurses should educate the patient and family about the importance of forming alliances within the community as a part of discharge planning. Several general guidelines may be helpful for home health care nurses to consider when planning teaching-learning activities in the home for patients with mental illness. These include the following:

- Make assessments, not assumptions.
- Avoid challenge and confrontation; build trust and acceptance.
- Demonstrate a positive attitude that improvement/change can occur and support this attitude in the patient/family.[22]
- Foster self-esteem, share goals, and teach about self-esteem.[18]
- Use relevant, brief, clear, and nonmoralistic teaching strategies.
- Avoid overload and overstimulation.
- Set a slow pace to decrease stress and promote concentration.
- Provide verbal and written information (remember that psychotropic medications can affect vision).
- Balance teaching about compliance with teaching about self-care practices.[41]
- Find additional resources in the community for the patient and family.

The pediatric patient

As individuals become more responsible for their own health care, the role of the home health nurse in home pediatric care becomes even more important. Children, if given information which is accurate and delivered at their level of understanding, can learn to make appropriate decisions regarding their own health, as well as participate in their own care. Whether the nurse is making a well-baby visit and discussing immunizations, caring for an acutely or chronically ill child or family member, or preparing the family for death, children need to be included in the health teaching. Children listen attentively and observe behaviors. They will piece together bits of information and use their imagination to draw erroneous conclusions if their teaching needs are not met. Education needs to be directed in a very specific manner to ensure the child's understanding of the information.

A child's thinking and reasoning abilities mature over time. At most stages of development, children are capable of some participation in their own care. Home health nurses need to be able to determine what the child can understand, what can be remembered, what skills are possible for the child, and what should not be included in the teaching.

Home health nurses will need to draw on their knowledge of growth and development, as well as theories related to personality and cognitive development, when planning teaching strategies for children. A child's current ability to cope with illness will affect his or her level of comprehension. For example, during periods of stress and illness, many children will regress to earlier, more familiar patterns of behavior.

Caring for children involves working closely with the family. Since the home health nurse will need to design a teaching plan that will provide for at least two people—the child and the caregiver—it is helpful to ask the children or parents how they best learn. The following descriptions of personality and cognitive stages of development will give home health nurses a general framework which will be helpful in planning individualized teaching.

Infants and toddlers (birth to 3 years). According to Piaget, an infant in the *sensorimotor* period develops behaviors and responses to stimuli in the environment that will be the base for perceptive and intellectual development. Children in this age group learn through their senses: seeing, hearing, smelling, tasting, and touching. Simple explanations regarding how something will feel, look, smell, taste, or sound can be understood by the child. Infants and young children are also acutely aware of the parental response to any situation. For this reason, it is important that home health nurses initiate health teaching with the parent prior to any procedure which involves the child. Teaching for the toddler should occur just before or during the nursing intervention.

Preschoolers (3 to 6 years). The preschool period is characterized by *preoperational* thought. Children of this age have beginning memory and begin rudimentary problem solving, relying more on their own perceptions than on logical reason.[56] Preschoolers have a very active imagination and little understanding about how the body works. Health teaching needs to be delivered in language

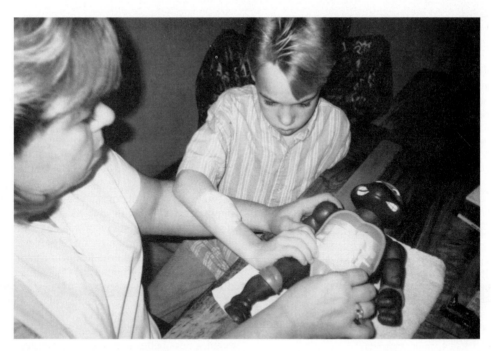

Figure 6-7 Using a model to teach a child about dressing changes. (Photograph courtesy Robyn Rice.)

they can understand. For example, the nurse might tell a child the blood pressure cuff is going to "hug your arm."

When teaching young children, home health nurses should be very careful with the words that are used. These children take words literally. When someone speaks of a CAT scan, the child may imagine a huge cat looking them over; a voice box may be perceived as a boom box in the neck.

During these years, children have many fears concerning the intactness of their body. Band-aids can help heal real or imagined injuries. If a child's parent or someone in the household is sick, children may wonder if they too will become ill. Children should be reassured about who will care for them when they or someone in their home is sick.

An effective strategy for teaching preschoolers may be to use dolls or stuffed animals for "practice" (Figure 6-7). Letting children handle equipment before using it will often decrease the child's fear. Videos may also help explain things to children in language they comprehend. Make-believe play and fantasy storytelling work well with small

children. Home health nurses may wish to use puppets, models, stuffed toys, or coloring books as teaching tools.

In make-believe play (see box) the child assumes the characteristics and desired behaviors of a caregiver and a doll/puppet represents the child. Anticipated stressors or problems are identified in the process as a means of teaching the child positive coping strategies with illness or disability.

Storytelling with children is different than with adults. For adults, real-life situations may be used to make a point or share an experience. With children, the nurse begins a fantasy story and lets the child finish the story. This identifies insecurities and provides a means to establish positive coping for the child.

School-agers (6 to 12 years). During the school-age years, children are in the stage of cognitive development Piaget termed *concrete operations.* Problem solving now occurs through a process of systematic operations during which logical reasoning is applied to concrete problems.[19] Children are able to use their thought processes to experience events and actions. Their

---

MAKE-BELIEVE PLAY

Suggested equipment:
- Doll, puppet, stuffed animal
- Bandages
- Syringes
- Splints
- IV tubing and bags
- Any other medical equipment used for the child

Procedure:
- Invite the child to pretend a puppet/doll/stuffed animal is "sick."
- Invite the child to be the caregiver (e.g., nurse, doctor, therapist).
- Ask the child what is wrong with "Teddy" (generally it will be the same thing that is wrong with the child).
- Ask appropriate questions, e.g., "how did Teddy get sick?", "what are you going to do to make Teddy feel better?", "how does Teddy feel when he has to get _____(e.g., an IV, his dressing changed), "what is important for the caregiver (e.g., nurse, doctor, therapist) to tell Teddy?"
- Use the information that the child gives you to clarify misperceptions over the course of the next few visits. (Keep in mind that children's ability to understand reasons for treatment is limited by their cognitive development.)

---

developing cognitive abilities now allow them to understand and accept another's viewpoint.[56] However, this understanding is still limited to immediate reality. These children cannot conceptualize abstract or hypothetical reality.

Since the child is still unable to understand concepts such as infection or the function of the neuroendocrine system, health teaching will need to be delivered using concrete examples. A newly diagnosed diabetic child may be able to use the analogy of gasoline in an automobile to understand the need for insulin. Pictures, models, books, and videos are very helpful for these children. School-agers learn best when they are able to see and handle equipment as they are being taught how to use it.

School-agers enjoy being productive and will usually participate in care when given the oppor-

tunity. They also may use medical terminology that is not clearly understood. Misconceptions and inaccuracies are common and home health nurses will need to clarify the child's understanding of the information. Providing children with knowledge will help them gain a feeling of mastery and control over their health.

Adolescents (12 to 18 years). Around the time of adolescence, individuals develop a more sophisticated type of thinking. Piaget termed this phase *formal operations* and identified it as involving the transformation of thought and the assumption of adult roles.[19] Part of this transformation includes being able to imagine possibilities. Through their study of science and biology, adolescents have an understanding of the physiology of the internal body. They understand cause and effect, so a concept such as bacteria causing a disease can be processed. Illness, however, thwarts adolescents in thinking about the possibilities of their adult roles.

Although an adolescent can intellectually understand illness better than a younger child, it is very difficult on an emotional level. Illness is contrary to everything that is important to an adolescent: the future, independence, and physical prowess. Individuals in this age group should be increasingly more involved in decisions concerning their health. They need truthful information. Occasionally adolescents will test reality concerning their health. For example, adolescents may stop taking medication or stop following a certain diet to see if these treatments really do affect their health. Information on substance abuse and sexuality is very important to this age group.

The caregiver

There is scant literature on educating caregivers in the home setting. It is estimated that 50% of American adults will at some point be caregivers for an ill or disabled friend or loved one.[5] As caregivers, these adults will need to learn new skills and knowledge required to provide a variety of physical and emotional interventions.

Research indicates that caregivers' expressed needs for assistance from professionals are markedly similar across studies.[10] They want (1) information and skill training for managing the requisite tasks and activities of caregiving, (2) affordable and accessible community resources, and (3) recognition and reassurance that the care they provide is important.

Davis (1992) presents a model of professional interventions with caregivers which include the following:[10] (1) caregiver education: content-defined teaching programs designed to increase caregiver knowledge about the patient's problems, symptoms, prognosis, and available resources, (2) caregiver support: problem-focused counseling and supportive actions that encourage or enable the caregiver to express feelings and concerns, (3) caregiver skill training: structured activities designed to enable a caregiver to master new skills, and (4) caregiver substitution: the provision of day care or respite services. All of these may be used by home health nurses to maintain an effective caregiving unit in the home.

Specific techniques for teaching caregivers have been described in relation to hospital-based units that simulate a home environment and allow the caregiver to practice care activities with the support of nursing staff.[46] Consider the following suggestions:

- Assess caregiver knowledge and abilities prior to beginning any teaching. Caregivers may be unable to perform part or all of certain tasks because of diminished vision, arthritic deformity of hands, poor upper body strength, or cognitive deficits. Home health nurses need to break down new tasks into their component parts and assess the caregiver's ability to perform each part; other caregivers or adaptive equipment may be able to compensate for specific steps in a sequence that the primary caregiver is unable to perform.
- Provide instructions in writing for teaching caregivers, with each step clearly, concisely stated. (The caregiver receives a copy for reference, and another copy becomes a part of the patient's medical record.)
- Document outcomes of teaching.

Home health nurses must be aware that failure to carry out the activities taught may not always be a case of "Diagnosis: Knowledge Deficit." Work with caregivers to mutually achieve reasonable goals, and to keep expectations to a manageable level.[13]

Observe for signs of caregiving unit breakdown, burnout, and a need for respite which include[13] (1)

feelings of exhaustion and resentment, (2) feelings of inadequacy, (3) loss of loving and caring feelings, (4) lack of pride in care activities, (5) destructive coping methods, (6) refusal to think of self, (7) shutting out others who offer help, (8) breakdown in family relationships because of caregiving pressures, (9) continuing in a no-win situation to avoid being a failure, even if the situation is detrimental to the patient, and (10) feelings of being alone. If the patient's needs overwhelm the abilities of the caregiver, consult with social services; alternate assistance including long-term care placement may need to be considered.

The intermittent visits of the home health nurse to teach and support caregivers often cannot meet all their educational and support needs, 24 hours a day, over the course of a chronic progressive illness. An innovative strategy that may become widely accessible to caregivers in the future is described by Brennan, Moore, and Smyth (1991).[5] In a randomized field experiment, caregivers of Alzheimer's patients were assigned to a telephone support group or a ComputerLink group. The 22 caregivers in the ComputerLink group received a computer, modem, and training. The computer system provided three kinds of resources: (1) an electronic encyclopedia with 200 factual entries about Alzheimer's, (2) a decision support system, helping caregivers select among alternative actions, and (3) a communications pathway, with access to a caregiver-to-caregiver discussion group and access to a nurse expert.

This innovative approach to caregiver education and support utilizes the principles of adult learning, making information available when the learner needs and wants the information, at the pace the learner selects.

As caregiver needs for education increase and nursing time becomes a scarce commodity, home health nurses need to use all available and appropriate teaching methods described in this chapter. It is also important to recognize that when fostering learning about patient care, caregivers will also need nurturing and lots of hugs in the process (Figure 6-8).

SUMMARY

The unique role of home health nurses is to help patients and their caregivers learn new behaviors

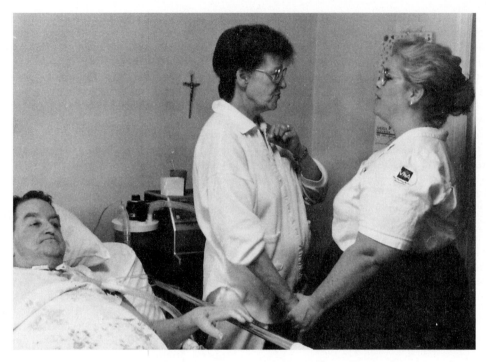

Figure 6-8 Caring for the caregiver. (Photograph courtesy Robyn Rice.)

that have a positive impact on their health and their lives. Much of this is accomplished through patient education. As we enter the patient's world, we work with the patient in mutually deciding what to teach, when to teach, and how to teach. Disease process, age, family, sociocultural background, and other elements of the home milieu will influence the process.

Success in patient education is primarily achieved when patients accept responsibility for their own quality of life, actively participate in the plan of care, and are self-determined to manage health care needs at home. The true measure of the value of patient education lies in the patient's ability to sustain positive health behaviors after discharge from the home health agency and to avoid unnecessary hospitalizations. When these goals are achieved, we close our nursing bags and move on.

REFERENCES

1. Babcock D, Miller M: *Client education: theory and practice,* St Louis, 1994, Mosby.
2. Becker M, Maiman L: Strategies for enhancing patient compliance, *J Community Health* 6(2):113-131, 1980.
3. Blackwell B: Treatment adherence, *Br J Psychiatry* 129:513-531, 1976.
4. Botwinick J: *Aging and behavior,* ed 2, New York, 1978, Springer Publishing, p. 48.
5. Brennan PF, Moore SM, Smyth KA: ComputerLink: electronic support for the home caregiver, *Adv Nurs Sci* 13(4):14-27, 1991.
6. Brothen T, Detzner D: Perceived health and locus of control in the aged, *Percept Mot Skills* 56:946, 1983.
7. Burgess C: Application of the rotter scales of internal-external locus of control to determine differences between smokers, non-smokers and ex-smokers in their general locus of control, *J Adv Nurs* 19:699-704, 1994.
8. Chaisson M: Patient education: whose responsibility is it and who should be doing it? *Nurs Admin Q* 4(2):1-11, 1980.
9. Davis C et al: An interactive perspective on the health beliefs and practices of rural elders, *J Gerontol Nurs* 17(5):11-16, 1991.
10. Davis LL: Building a science of caring for caregivers, *Fam Community Health* 15(2):1-9, 1992.
11. Davis-Sharts J: An empirical test of Maslow's theory of need hierarchy using hologeistic comparison by statistical sampling, *Adv Nurs Sci* 9(1):58-72, 1986.
12. Dellasega C et al: Nursing process: teaching elderly clients, *J Gerontol Nurs* 20(1):31-38, 1994.
13. DeMeneses M, Perry G: The plight of caregivers, *Home Health Care Nurs* 11(4):10-14, 1993.

14. Erickson E: *Childhood and society,* New York, 1963, WW Norton.
15. Freud A: *The ego and mechanisms of defense,* New York, 1958, International Universities Press.
16. Germain C: Cultural care: a bridge between sickness, illness, and disease, *Holistic Nurs Practice* 6(3):1-9, 1992.
17. Gessner B: Adult education: the cornerstone of patient teaching, *Nurs Clin North Am* 24(3):589-595, 1989.
18. Gordon V, Tobin M: Facilitator's manual. In Maynard C: Psychoeducational approach to depression in women, *J Psychosoc Nurs* 31(12):9-14, 1993.
19. Gruber H, Voneche J, editors: *The essential Piaget,* New York, 1977, Basic Books Inc.
20. Guthrie E: *The psychology of learning,* New York, 1935, Harper and Row.
21. Hafstad L: Outcome factors in patient education, *Physician Assistant* 16(2):37-41, 1992.
22. Hayes R, Gantt A: Patient psychoeducation: the therapeutic use of knowledge for the mentally ill, *Social Work in Health Care* 17(1):53-66, 1992.
23. Health Care Financing Administration: *Health ins man,* Pub No 11 -Thru T273, Rev 3/95, Washington, DC, 1995, US Department of Health and Human Services.
24. Horgan P: Health status perceptions affect health-related behaviors, *J Gerontol Nurs* 13(12):30-33, 1987.
25. Hunter K et al: Discriminators of internal and external locus of control orientation in the elderly, *Res Aging* 2(1):49-60, 1980.
26. Hussey L: Overcoming the clinical barriers of low literacy and medication noncompliance among the elderly, *J Gerontol Nurs* 17(3):27-29, 1991.
27. Johnson E, Jackson J: Teaching the home care client, *Nurs Clin North Am* 24(3):687-693, 1989.
28. Kist-Kline G, Lipnicky S: Health locus of control: implications for the health professional, *Health Values* 13(5):38-47, 1989.
29. Koehler W: Gestalt psychology, *Am Psychol* 14:727-734, 1958.
30. Koffka K: *Principles of gestalt psychology,* New York, 1935, Harcourt, Brace and World.
31. Kohlberg L: Moral development. In *International encyclopedia of science,* New York, 1968, McMillan.
32. Lewin K: *Field theory in social sciences,* New York, 1957, Harper and Row.
33. Lumpkin J: Health versus activity in elderly person locus of control, *Percept Mot Skills* 60:228, 1985.
34. Manderino MA: Social skill building: with chronic patients, *J Psychosoc Nurs* 25(9):18-23, 1987.
35. Maslow A: *Motivation and personality,* New York, 1970, Harper & Row.
36. McCaffrey B: The elderly patient with cancer: teaching/learning considerations for ostomy, wound, and continence management, *Progressions* 6(1):11-21, 1994.
37. Nemcek M: Health beliefs and preventative behavior, *AAOHN* 38(3):127-138, 1990.
38. Pender N: *Health promotion in nursing practice,* ed 2, Norwalk, Conn, 1987, Appleton & Lange. *(Note:* A third edition is expected during 1996 with revisions in Pender's model.)
39. Pfister-Minogue K: Enhancing patient compliance: a guide for nurses, *Geriat Nurs* 14(3):124-132, 1993.
40. Pollock S, Christian B, Sands D: Responses to chronic illness: analysis of psychological and physiological adaptation, *Nurs Res* 39(5):300-304, 1990.
41. Redman B: Patient education at 25 years: where we have been and where we are going, *J Adv Nurs* 18:725-730, 1993.
42. Redman B: *The process of patient education,* ed 7, St Louis, 1993, Mosby.
43. Roberson M: Home remedies: a cultural study, *Home Health Care Nurs* 5(1):35-40, 1987.
44. Rotter JB: Generalized expectancies for internal versus external control of reinforcement. In Rotter J, Chance J, Phares E, editors: *Applications of a social learning theory of personality,* New York, 1972, Holt, Rinehart & Winston.
45. Ryglewicz H: Psychoeducation for clients and families: a way in, out, and through in working with people with dual disorders, *Psychosoc Rehabil J* 15(2):80-89, 1991.
46. Shivley S, Djupe A, Lester P: Lessons in caring: a care by caregiver program, *Geriatr Nurs* 14(6):304-306, 1993.
47. Skinner B: *Beyond freedom and dignity,* New York, 1972, Random House.
48. Smith R: Who is in control-an investigation of nurse and patient beliefs relating to control of their health, *J Adv Nurs* 19:884-892, 1994.
49. Storch J: Consumer rights and health care, *Nurs Admin Q* 4(2):107-114, 1980.
50. Swenson L, Skinner B: Reinforcement or operant conditioning. Chpter 4, In *Theories of learning: traditional perspectives/contemporary developments,* Belmont, Calif, 1980, Wadsworth Publishing.
51. Thorndike E: *Animal intelligence,* New York, 1911, Macmillan.
52. Tripp-Reimor T, Anna L: Cross-cultural perspectives on patient teaching, *Nurs Clin North Am* 24(3):613-619, 1989.
53. Wallston K, Wallston B, DeVillis R: Development of the multidimensional health locus of control (MHLC) scales, *Health Educ Monogr* 6:161-170, 1978.
54. Weinrich S, Boyd M: Education in the elderly, *J Gerontol Nurs* 18(1):15-20, 1992.
55. Williams C: Patient education for people with schizophrenia, *Perspect Psychiat Care* 25(2):14-21, 1989.
56. Wong D: *The essentials of pediatric nursing,* ed 4, St Louis, 1993, Mosby.

7 Legal and Ethical Issues in Home Care

Gayle H. Sullivan, Joanne P. Sheehan, and Robyn Rice

- An elderly home care patient who has clearly stated his wish to not be resuscitated arrests at his home while the home health nurse is present, but there is no DNR order in his medical record.
- A home health nurse who has been threatened by a patient's family member refuses to provide care in the home, and the patient later dies from lack of care.
- The spouse of a patient falls, suffering possible injury while the home health nurse is in the home, but refuses any assistance.
- A patient's condition is deteriorating, but attempts to reach her physician fail.
- A home health nurse is requested to perform a procedure that she or he does not feel qualified to do.

Home health nurses are likely to encounter at least one of these dilemmas in the course of their work. While home care has been confronted with ethical and legal issues since the early 1900s,[9] the practice of home health nursing has become increasingly complex and the corresponding ethical and legal accountability has increased as well. Consequently a heightened awareness of the legal requirements and ethical guidelines that direct nursing practice within the home milieu is critical.

UNDERSTANDING OUR LEGAL SYSTEM

Home health nurses should be aware of three types of actions in our legal system: criminal actions, administrative law actions, and civil actions. All three are important to consider.

Criminal actions

Criminal actions are brought by the state against the defendant accused of crimes as defined by the state. While health care providers are not typically involved as defendants in criminal actions, they have been prosecuted for crimes such as negligent homicide, insurance fraud, falsification of a business record, and theft of narcotics. The consequences of being found guilty generally involve some restriction on conduct, such as a jail sentence or probation, and sometimes a fine payable to the state.[15] The victim is not compensated in a criminal proceeding.

Administrative law actions

Administrative law actions are brought by state agencies empowered by the legislature to investigate complaints and take specified actions. The State Board of Nursing in each state and the Department of Health may investigate complaints against nurses. Complaints may be filed by patients or their families. Many health care organizations, and in some cases individual practitioners, have obligations under state law to report instances of misconduct, revocation or suspension (including voluntary suspension) of privileges, disciplinary action, or termination. Pursuant to any investigation, a hearing may be held. As part of this process, the State Board of Nursing is empowered to take actions including revoking, suspending, or restricting the nurse's license; requiring the nurse to undergo treatment; requiring the nurse to pursue continuing education in certain areas; and publicly censuring the nurse.

A nurse's license is a property right and cannot be taken without due process of law. Therefore nurses have constitutional rights in the administrative law process. To ensure that their rights are adequately protected, home health nurses should retain experienced counsel if they suspect that their conduct is being investigated.[1,2,15]

Home health nurses should also be aware that the typical malpractice insurance policy is not designed to provide coverage for administrative law actions. However, considering that the end result of such an action could be the revocation of the nursing license, retaining the advice of an attorney is a small price to pay.[6]

Case example: Administrative law action. A complaint was filed against a home health nurse alleging failure to initiate CPR in a timely fashion. After an investigation and a hearing, the actions taken by the state board included requiring the nurse to successfully complete an adult CPR training course and placing the nurse on probation for one year. This action limits the nurse's ability to change employment because she may not do so without written permission of the state board.

Civil actions

Civil actions are designed to resolve disputes between individuals. Home health nurses, by virtue of their familiarity with patients and their families, may become entangled in many types of civil actions, including personal injury suits, workers' compensation claims, and divorce and custody proceedings. One of the most common types of civil actions in which home health nurses and their agencies can be involved is a malpractice or professional negligence suit. Malpractice (discussed later in this chapter) is a specific type of negligence. Anyone can be negligent, but only a professional can commit malpractice.

The purpose of civil action is to compensate with money for injuries caused, not to punish the person who committed the harm. Therefore the consequence of being found liable in a negligence or malpractice claim typically involves the payment of money damages to the injured party.

Case example: Civil law action. A home health nurse administered an injection of Demerol and Vistaril IM to the right deltoid of an elderly patient with poor muscle mass. The patient developed erythema which developed into a third degree burn

and was accompanied by severe pain. According to the home health agency's policies, the deltoid was not a site approved for this type of IM injection. A civil suit was brought against the home health nurse and the home health agency, alleging negligent administration of medication. $200,000 was demanded for settlement purposes. The case is pending.

UNDERSTANDING MORE ABOUT MALPRACTICE

Malpractice is defined by four distinct elements, all of which must be proven by the plaintiff. Elements of malpractice include the following:

1. Duty: established by a professional relationship
2. Breach of duty: an act or omission in violation of the standard of care
3. Injury
4. Causation: nurse's breach of duty caused the patient's injury

A duty is created by a professional relationship. With that in mind, consider the following example:

Case example: Establishing a duty. A home health nurse stops at a grocery store on her way home from work. She sees that an elderly gentleman is lying on the sidewalk just in front of the store and a small crowd has gathered. The spouse of a former patient recognizes the home health nurse and calls out for her to help. The home health nurse does not want to become involved, and even though she can initiate lifesaving action, she shouts back, "I'm not a nurse anymore," and then enters the store to shop. The elderly man dies.

Will the family of the deceased be successful in an action against the home health nurse if they claim that she had an obligation to stop and help, and her failure to do so caused his death? Conflicting answers to this question illustrate a difference between what the law and ethical codes require. Here, while ethical codes dictate that home health nurses should assist,[3] the law does not require it. A malpractice claim against home health nurses under these circumstances will surely fail because the first element, duty (a professional relationship), is lacking.

Suppose that in this case, a home health nurse does attempt to help. However, after determining that the patient has no pulse, she announces that there is nothing more she can do and leaves the scene. How does this change the analysis of liability? This represents a Good Samaritan situation, generally referred to as an emergency located away from the provider's place of employment. Each state has a Good Samaritan statute, and while these laws generally do not require nurses to assist at the scene of an emergency, immunity for negligence is provided if they do. Gross negligence is not protected, however, and abandoning a patient under these circumstances would most likely rise to that level, eliminating the Good Samaritan shield. Consider the following Good Samaritan guidelines:

- If you choose to stop at the scene of an emergency, stay until the ambulance arrives or someone of equal or greater skill takes over for you.
- Do not accept payment for services rendered.

The establishment of a professional relationship in the home care setting is created by the home health agency's contract to provide care to the patient. The duty is to meet the standard of care or, put another way, to act like a reasonably prudent nurse under the same or similar circumstances. The standard of care is determined by evaluating a variety of sources including the home health agency's policies and procedures, the individual state nurse practice acts, other state statutes and regulations, clinical guidelines promulgated by professional organizations, job descriptions, pertinent literature, and expert witness opinions.

It is particularly important for home health nurses to be aware of the significance of the home health agency's policies and procedures. The plaintiff's attorney will review the medical record, request copies of applicable policies and procedures, and then compare what the policy says should have been done with what is documented. Discrepancies provide an opportunity to argue that nonadherence with policies and procedures is evidence of malpractice.[8] A lay jury will find this compelling.[12] Consider implementing the following guidelines for policies and procedures:

- All employers should have written policies and procedures.

- Policies and procedures should be accessible to all staff members.
- Beware of mandatory language (such as, "the nurse shall . . .", "in every case . . .").
- Encourage discretionary language (such as, "when appropriate . . .", "in the nurse's professional judgment . . .").
- In-services should be provided on changes or additions to policies and procedures.
- Policies and procedures should be reviewed annually for accuracy.
- Annual reviews should be documented.

In addition to establishing the duty, the plaintiff must show that a breach of duty or violation of the standard of care occurred. Failing to use correct procedural technique when indicated, delegating specialized functions to untrained assistants, failing to notify a physician about significant changes in the patient's condition, and failing to teach the patient/caregiver how to operate home medical equipment, can all constitute a breach of duty.

A successful malpractice claim also requires that the plaintiff suffer an injury. Generally, this must be a physical injury such as paralysis, brain damage, fracture, or scarring. Emotional damages may be claimed in connection with the physical injury. In malpractice actions, damages based on purely emotional injuries are prohibited in most jurisdictions.

Causation, the last element of malpractice, can be the most problematic. There must be evidence that the nurse's breach of duty caused the patient's injury.

Case example: Elements of malpractice. A 40-year-old male patient was visited by a home health nurse at 10:00 AM, 1 day after discharge from the hospital and 5 days post gallbladder surgery. The home health nurse noted signs of infection at the incision site and an elevated temperature. The home health nurse left a message with the attending physician's answering service requesting the doctor to return the call but did not document this. The physician never called back and the home health nurse forgot to follow up. At 4:00 PM that day, the patient suffered a massive cardiac arrest and died. The autopsy report indicated myocardial infarction as the cause of death.

This case example can best be analyzed by considering each of the four elements of malpractice:

Duty. A professional relationship existed by virtue of the home health agency agreement to provide services to the patient.

Breach of duty. The home health nurse should have followed up with the physician and documented these efforts. A failure to do so is arguably a breach of duty. If there was a question regarding medical coverage, the patient service manager should have been contacted.

Injury. Cardiac arrest and death are physical injuries.

Causation. It would be difficult to argue that the home health nurse's omission was the cause of the patient's injury in this case. However, note that if the patient had become septic and died, the outcome would likely be different.

WHAT ALL HOME HEALTH NURSES SHOULD KNOW BEFORE ACCEPTING EMPLOYMENT

Prior to accepting employment with any home health agency, home health nurses should ascertain the following information regarding future employment: (1) Will the home health nurse be an employee of the home health agency or an independent contractor? (2) Is the home health nurse familiar with the type of care and treatment patients require and the type of equipment that will be used? (3) Has the home health nurse been properly oriented and familiarized with his or her responsibilities to the patient and the home health agency? (4) Will the home health nurse be provided with a safe environment in which to work? (5) Is the home health nurse familiar with requirements to report to state agencies?

Employee of home health agency or independent contractor?

Whether home health nurses function as independent contractors or as employees may determine whether the home health agency will provide malpractice insurance, unemployment compensation benefits, and workers' compensation benefits; make social security payments (FICA); withhold income tax; and whether the Fair Labor Standards Act would apply. The ultimate question is whether the employer has the right of general control over the means and method of work of the employee. The employer of an independent contractor is ordinarily not liable for the negligence of the contractor; however, the employer can be liable when the employer has selected an incompetent independent contractor.[7]

If the patient reasonably believes that the home health nurse, even though an independent contractor, was acting on behalf of the home health agency, the home health agency faces potential liability for the conduct of the home health nurse.

Nursing malpractice coverage. Home health nurses should be aware of the dollar amount of the professional liability coverage provided by their employer. The home health agency's policy should provide coverage for its employees within the scope of employment. It would not, then, apply to situations arising outside of work (assisting at the scene of an emergency or administering an injection to a neighbor, for example). Therefore home health nurses should consider purchasing an individual policy to ensure coverage for any situation that may arise. Home health nurses should also determine the type of policy that is in effect.

A professional liability policy can be either a *claims made* or an *occurrence* policy. The claims made policy will cover home health nurses for incidences which occur *and* result in a claim during the policy period. If the policy includes a retroactive date, incidents which have occurred prior to purchase of the policy may also be covered.

An occurrence policy will provide coverage if a negligent act occurs during the time period that the policy is in effect, and if that negligent act gives rise to a claim for malpractice at any time in the future, even after the policy has expired. Home health nurses who change employers and liability coverage may experience a period of time in which they are uninsured. It is important to avoid this. Only by knowing the type of policy in force, its expiration date, and limits of liability can nurses be prepared to protect themselves from gaps in coverage.

Other insurance. Prior to accepting employment, home health nurses must also determine whether or not they or their employer will provide automobile liability insurance for the motor vehicle that will be used during the course of employment to get to patients' homes. Typically it is the nurse who provides this insurance.

Familiarity with type of care, treatment, and equipment required by patient

Prior to accepting employment, home health nurses should inquire as to the orientation provided by the home health agency for new hires. They should inquire whether a supervisor or a preceptor will be assigned to them for any period of time. If so, home health nurses should especially request experiences which are a requirement for work that is unfamiliar to them.

A standard checklist should be completed both preorientation and postorientation to document exposure to different situations and devices that are used in the home. A thorough review of the job description and the state's Nurse Practice Act should be part of any orientation. The home health agency's policies and procedures should also be reviewed.[19] In addition, the home health agency should provide staff with in-services and educational offerings designed to build clinical skills and foster competence with work expectations.

Home health agency responsibilities to patient

Once the home health agency admits the patient, no matter how complex the care, the agency is obligated to provide reasonable and competent care to that patient. If the patient's care needs progress beyond the ability of the home health agency, the agency is obligated to assist the patient to identify an acceptable alternative health care provider.

Appropriate supervision must be available during all service hours. In addition, the home health agencies should provide access to qualified consultation when supervisors have neither appropriate clinical training nor experience for clinical practice needs.[10]

Provision of safe work environment

Home health nurses must know how to protect their patients and themselves from harm. (See Chapter 3, which discusses safety in the community.) As an employer, the home health agency should provide staff with a safe working environment. Any form of sexual or physical harassment or abuse of staff should be reported to the nurse's supervisor and the Director of Nursing. Such problems may also be a matter for review by the professional consultation or ethics committee.

Home health nurses should adhere to their agencies' policies and procedures in documenting and reporting such incidents. In the event of assault, the nurse should consider filing a complaint with the local police department.

Familiarity with requirements to report to state agencies

Home health nurses must be familiar with the requirements in their state for reporting suspected abuse or neglect. Every state has a law that specifies a state agency to which suspected cases of child abuse/neglect and elder abuse/neglect must be reported. Neglect can be defined as not providing for necessary physical, emotional, medical, or surgical needs, thereby endangering the person's health. Abuse is a form of cruelty to an individual's physical, moral, or mental well-being. In most states it is mandated that an RN or LPN who has reasonable cause to suspect or believe that an elderly person has been abused, neglected, exploited, or abandoned, or is in the need of protective services, *shall* report such information to the Commission on Aging. It is also mandated in most states that an RN or LPN who has reasonable cause to suspect or believe that any child under the age of 18 has been subjected to physical injury, maltreatment, sexual abuse or exploitation, deprivation of necessities, emotional maltreatment or neglect, must report the same to the applicable state agency and the local police department. Failure of home health nurses to file such reports will subject them to an imposition of a fine and to disciplinary action within some states. Any and all observations of suspected abuse or neglect should be documented in the patient's medical record. Appropriate home health agency forms should be completed. If the person suspected of being abused or neglected is not a patient, the home health agency should have specific policies and procedures to follow and forms to document clinical concerns and actions taken. In most states, if the reporting of abuse and/or neglect is done in good faith, the reporter will be immune from civil and criminal liability. However, any individual who willingly makes a false abuse and/or neglect report may be liable for civil and criminal penalties as provided in the state's statutes.[4]

If home health nurses observe and/or suspect a coworker or supervisor of abuse or neglect, the same reporting procedures should be taken. Additionally, home health nurses and/or home health agencies should report the professional misconduct to the State Department of Public Health and/or the State Board of Nursing.

Reporting communicable diseases. Home health nurses must also report communicable diseases to the appropriate state and community agencies. If a home health nurse is exposed to a communicable disease, the agency's appropriate policies and procedures should be followed. Additionally, the home health nurse should consider filing a workers' compensation claim, which will put the employer and local workers' compensation commissioner on notice of the potential injury. (See Chapter 5 for information on infection control in the home.)

DOCUMENTATION ISSUES

The medical record has become an increasingly public document open to review by state surveyors, insurance carriers, attorneys, and jurors as circumstances warrant. The home health nurse's documentation constitutes the bulk of the record, and serves as a crucial piece of evidence in ethical dilemmas and legal proceedings.

The medical record can prevent malpractice suits from being brought. If the record is complete and legible, and documents that the standard of care was met, the case will be of less interest to the plaintiff's attorney.

The medical record can also protect home health nurses in the event suit is brought. Years may pass between the time of an incident and the time the defendants are even aware of the potential for liability. However, the medical record is written at the time the events take place, while the events are clear and fresh in the writer's mind. It is sometimes referred to as "the witness that never dies."

Record keeping in home care

Complete, accurate, and truthful documentation is the cornerstone of the defense of any malpractice claim. The following are some important guidelines for recording assessments, and documenting treatments and other actions taken in the home care setting:

- Document all assessments objectively. Objective documentation states the nurse's assessment based on facts, observations, patient's statements, and other measurable criteria. Subjective documentation states the nurse's conclusions without supporting facts and should be avoided. (See Table 7-1.)
- Date and time each visit report at the time it is written, even if it is well after the visit has taken place. Indicate the time of the visit on the report. The visit report is often used to determine the chronology of events. Therefore accurate dating and timing of visit reports are critical.
- Sign all entries. The visit report should be signed with the home health nurse's first name or initial, last name, and title. Certain documentation may be initialed, such as an IV flow sheet or medication administration record. This is legally acceptable provided there is a space for each writer to initial and sign the document.
- Be certain that the patient's name appears on each page of the medical record.
- Accurately document all patient/caregiver teaching. In malpractice litigation, health care providers often face claims that they provided insufficient information to patients regarding

Table 7-1 Subjective vs objective documentation

Subjective documentation	Objective documentation
Skin good	Right hand and fingers pink and warm to touch. No complaints of pain or tingling. Nail beds blanch well.
Appears depressed	Client is tearful. States, "I have never been this depressed in my life."
Teaching client to give own insulin	Client able to give own insulin, demonstrates correct technique, and has no additional questions.

use of equipment, techniques for procedures, recognizing signs and symptoms, side effects of medications, and so forth. Without supporting documentation, it's the patient's word against the home health nurse's word. To fully protect yourself, document all patient and family teaching done, including what was told, who was present, any return demonstrations given and by whom, that an opportunity to ask questions was given, and instructions to follow in the event of a problem.

- Maintain professionalism in documentation, particularly with regard to patients and their families. Remember, patients have a right to the information contained in their record. Documentation that subjectively characterizes a patient as "uncooperative," "obnoxious," "rude," or "snotty" (all examples from real charts), may be so offensive to the patient and family that they seek legal counsel. In a malpractice action, this type of documentation will allow the plaintiff's attorney to argue that the nursing staff did not like the patient, and substandard care was delivered as a result. Therefore if a patient is truly uncooperative, be certain to document the objective reasons for this conclusion. (For example: patient is noncompliant with medication regimen or diet, refuses to perform range of motion exercises, or does not follow instructions for dressing change.)
- Use approved home health agency abbreviations.
- Properly correct mistakes on the visit report and other parts of the record. A failure to do so could constitute an alteration of the record, rendering a case indefensible. Every agency should have a written policy on how to correct a mistake, add information, and make late entries. Although the law does not require that nurses document perfectly, it does require corrections to be made pursuant to policy. (See the box titled Corrections, Additions, and Late Entries.)
- Do not rewrite notes, even to obtain reimbursement for the patient or agency. This is an unethical practice which can create significant legal exposure for both the home health nurse and the home health agency. Insurance fraud

---

CORRECTIONS, ADDITIONS, AND LATE ENTRIES

To correct a mistaken entry:
- Draw a single line through the entry, date and initial it, and continue your documentation.

To enter an addendum to an existing note:
- Write the date and time of the new entry on the next available space in the record (even if several days have passed), and state "addendum to note of [*date and time of prior note*]."

To make a late entry:
- Late entries can be made in situations where no note was written at all; for example, the nurse forgot to document a home visit.
- Write the date and time of the new note on the next available space in the record or on a visit report, and state "late entry for visit of [*date and time of visit*]."

---

allegations, loss of credibility in a malpractice action, and investigation by the State Board of Nursing are but a few of the problems a nurse who participates in this practice could face.

Physician orders and nursing implications

Although home health nurses have a duty to follow physician orders, there are five major exceptions to this general rule: (1) the order is illegible, (2) the order is illegal, (3) following the order could cause harm to the patient, (4) the order is against the policy of the home health agency, and (5) the home health nurse is not trained to carry out the order. In any of these situations, the home health nurse's ethical and legal obligation to protect the patient rises above the duty to follow the physician's orders.

Home health nurses should first confer with the physician who wrote the order, and document this in the record. For example, "Discussed lasix dose with Dr. Smith, no changes ordered." If the home health nurse is still not comfortable with the order, he or she should not hesitate to invoke the home health agency's chain of command and document this as well. The documentation could read, "Supervisor Jones notified of above conversation with

Dr. Smith. Medication not given." Bear in mind that collaborative decision making to resolve complex ethical and legal issues can protect home health nurses from making erroneous choices.[16]

It is important to remember that the nurse always has the right to refuse to carry out an order. Although disciplinary action may be threatened, the nurse should prevail provided the chain of command is followed and documented.

Incident reports

A patient falls out of bed while the home health nurse is in the home. Assessing him and initiating treatment for any injury are obvious priorities, but eventually an incident report must be completed. Situations requiring completion of an incident report will vary from agency to agency, but the usefulness of these forms in detecting and preventing recurring problems is universal.

While incident reports are intended exclusively for home health agency use, they can be important in legal proceedings as well. The plaintiff's attorneys can gain access to incident reports, which often contain valuable information such as names, phone numbers, and addresses of witnesses; the cause of the incident; and corrective actions taken. It is important therefore to report information factually. Avoid making statements that affix blame, express opinions, or draw conclusions. The facts should be documented as follows:

- Date, time, and location of incident
- Family member notified (name, time, and by phone or in person)
- Name of physician notified and time
- Facts of the occurrence (for example, in the case of medication that was not ordered for the client, "10 mg Inderal given PO," not "10 mg Inderal given PO, by mistake because I picked up the wrong med.")
- Direct quotes from third parties (the patient, for example)
- Assessment of the patient, using objective documentation
- Action taken

Incidents involving staff members, such as needlestick injuries, may also require completion of an incident report, and should be documented in the same fashion. Every home health agency should have written procedures for completing incident reports and seeking medical treatment for on-the-job injuries.

Patient incidents should be documented on the visit report as well. Since the record is the place an attorney would look to determine whether the standard of care was met, include the details of any follow-up care and the patient's response to treatment. Do not document that an incident report was completed, however. At the least, this is a red flag to the plaintiff's attorney who could argue that reports mentioned in the record are part of the record and must be disclosed.[18]

Keeping incident reports confidential can be facilitated by implementing a few basic security procedures. First, stamp all incident reports "confidential." Be certain incident reports are completed and routed to the appropriate persons within 24 hours. Limit distribution to those involved in reviewing the incident, and store reports in a locked file cabinet. Do not make copies of incident reports for patients or their family members, because this would surely destroy any hope of preserving confidentiality. Home health nurses should not make copies of incident reports for personal use. Not only would this constitute a breach of confidentiality, but it would likely be a violation of home health agency policy as well.

Patient rights and responsibilities

Home health nurses must be familiar with the patient's bill of rights and the patient's responsibilities, and review them with the patient. (See the boxes titled Patient Rights and Patient Responsibilities.)

It should be documented in the medical record that the patient's bill of rights and the patient's responsibilities have been given to and reviewed by the patient, and the patient has acknowledged an understanding of each. Signed copies are to be maintained in the patient's medical record.

With this information in the record, the home health agency may be better positioned to discharge abusive and noncompliant patients from care without exposing the home health nurse and home health agency to allegations of abandonment. Home health agencies do have the right to discharge patients from home care. To terminate this relationship effectively, a certified letter should be sent to the patient (return receipt re-

Statement of rights

A person who receives home care services has these rights:

1. The right to receive written information about rights in advance of receiving care or during the initial evaluation visit before the initiation of treatment, including what to do if rights are violated.
2. The right to receive care and services according to a suitable and up-to-date plan, and subject to accepted medical or nursing standards, and to take an active part in creating and changing the plan and evaluating care and services. *The provider must advise the recipient in advance of the right to participate in planning the care or treatment.*
3. The right to be told in advance of receiving care about the services that will be provided, the disciplines that will furnish care, the frequency of visits proposed to be furnished, other choices that are available, and the consequences of these choices, including the consequences of refusing these services.
4. The right to be told in advance of any change in the plan of care and to take an active part in any change *and the planning before any change is made.*
5. The right to refuse services or treatment.
6. The right to know, in advance, any limits to the services available from a provider, and the provider's grounds for a termination of services.
7. The right to know, *and to be advised, both orally and in writing,* in advance of receiving care whether the services are covered by health insurance, medical assistance, or other health programs, the charges for services that will not be covered by Medicare, and the charges that the individual may have to pay. *The provider must advise the recipient of home care services, both orally and in writing, of any changes in such coverage and the recipient's liability for charges as soon as possible, but no later than 30 calendar days after the provider becomes aware of a change.*
8. The right to know what the charges are for services, no matter who will be paying the bill.
9. The right to know that there may be other services available in the community, including other home care services and providers, and to know where to go for information about these services.
10. The right to choose freely among available providers and to change providers after services have begun, within the limits of health insurance, medical assistance, or other health programs.
11. The right to have personal, financial, and medical information kept private, and to be advised of the provider's policies and procedures regarding disclosure of such information.
12. The right to be allowed access to records and written information from records in accordance with section 144.335.
13. The right to be served by people who are properly trained and competent to perform their duties.
14. The right to be treated with courtesy and respect, and to have the client's property treated with respect.
15. The right to be free from physical and verbal abuse.
16. The right to a reasonable, advance notice of changes in services or charges.
17. The right to a coordinated transfer when there will be a change in the provider of services.
18. The right to voice grievances regarding treatment or care that is, or fails to be, furnished, or regarding the lack of courtesy or respect to the client or the client's property.
19. The right to know how to contact an individual associated with the provider who is responsible for handling problems and to have the provider investigate and attempt to resolve the grievance or complaint. *The provider shall document in writing all complaints, as well as document, in writing, any resolution of the complaint against anyone furnishing services on behalf of the provider.*
20. The right to know the name and address of the state or county agency to contact for additional information or assistance.
21. The right to assert these rights personally, or have them asserted by the client's family or guardian when the client has been judged incompetent, without retaliation.

I have reviewed and understand my responsibilities as described above.

Signature of client: _____ Date: _____

Relationship if not
signed by client: _____ Date: _____

Case manager: _____ Date: _____

Source: Carla Scheffert, RN, Minneapolis, Minn, 1995.

PATIENT RESPONSIBILITIES

Statement of responsibility

A person who receives home care has the following responsibilities:

1. Every client shall provide accurate and thorough information regarding his/her health history, mental health history, hospitalizations, present status, allergies, medications, and any other information pertinent to his/her well-being.
2. Every client shall report any significant or unexpected change in his/her status.
3. Every client shall participate and adhere to the development and update of the Home Health Plan of Care with the health team or collaboration with the attending physician.
4. Every client shall have the right to refuse treatment, programming, and/or instructions as well as the responsibility for his/her actions and consequences.
5. Every client, to the best of his/her ability, shall make it clear that he/she comprehends requests and expectations. The client will request further information concerning anything he/she does not understand.
6. Every client shall adhere to the stipulations of the Home Health Care Admissions Agreement.
7. Every client will inform the home health services when unable to keep a home health care visit.
8. Every client will assist in developing and maintaining a safe environment.
9. Clients are responsible for fulfilling the financial obligations of their health care as promptly as they are able.

I have reviewed and understand my responsibilities as described above.

Signature of client: _____ Date: _____

Relationship if not
signed by client: _____ Date: _____

Case manager: _____ Date: _____

Source: Carla Scheffert, RN, Minneapolis, Minn, 1995.

quested), and a copy should be placed in the record. It is always advisable to consult legal counsel before discharging patients with conditions requiring regular medical attention. A sample letter for discharging a noncompliant patient is shown in Figure 7-1.

ADVANCE DIRECTIVES

The advance directive allows a competent patient to advise others of his or her choices and treatment in the event of future incapacity.

The Patient's Self Determination Act, which is part of the Omnibus Budget Reconciliation Act (OBRA), became effective December 1, 1991. In order to continue to be eligible for Medicare and Medicaid funds, health care facilities (including home health agencies) must determine at the time of admission whether the patient has an advance directive. If not, the patient must be provided with education concerning the applicable state laws on advance directives and the home health agency's policies on advance directives. If the patient has an advance directive, it should become part of the medical record.

Living will

The living will is one type of advance directive. It is a written statement of a patient's wishes regarding the use of medical treatment when the patient is in a terminal state or determined to be permanently unconscious. Although state laws vary, a terminal condition can generally be defined as one that is incurable or irreversible and, without the administration of life support systems, will result in death. The living will may list life support systems the patient does not want, such as artificial respiration, cardiopulmonary resuscitation, and artificial means of providing nutrition and hydration.

Health care agent or proxy

In addition to the living will, some state statutes provide for the appointment of a health care agent. If the patient's physician determines that the patient is unable to understand and appreciate the nature and consequences of health care decisions and to reach and communicate an informed decision regarding the treatment, the health care agent may be authorized to state the patient's wishes concerning medical care. Depending on the juris-

Dear Client:

The agency finds it necessary to inform you that as of (date), it will no longer provide home care services due to (reason). Since your condition requires continued attention from a home care provider, it is suggested that you place yourself under the care of another agency without delay. The above termination date should give you ample time to select an agency of your choice from the home care providers in this city. If you are not acquainted with another agency, you should consult with your attending physician or contact the (town agency or professional association and phone number). Should a medical emergency arise before the termination date indicated above, you should contact your attending physician, and may contact us as well. The agency will make your medical records available to the agency you designate below. Since your records are confidential, your written authorization is required. Please complete the enclosed form and return it to (agency) (enclose an authorization to transfer records).

Very truly yours,
AAA Agency

cc: (patient's attending physician)

Figure 7-1 Sample letter for discharging a noncompliant patient.

diction, this may include the withholding or removal of life support systems. The agent may also take whatever actions are necessary to ensure that the patient's wishes are given effect. It is imperative that the home health agency and the home health nurse know who the patient's appointed health care agents are and how to reach them in case of an emergency. This should be documented in the patient's medical record.

A patient may revoke the living will or appointment of health care agent at any time in any manner. If the patient does so, it should be well documented in the patient's medical record, and the physician should be notified so that the physician's record may also be documented.

Case example: Advance directives. The patient has executed a valid living will. The living will indicates that the patient does not wish CPR, artificial respiration, and artificial means of hydration and nutrition. The patient has appointed her son as her health care agent. A copy of the living will and appointment of health care agent is contained in the patient's medical record. The home health nurse assumes care of the patient, at which time the patient lapses into a coma and dies. Based on the patient's living will no CPR or artificial means of respiration are given by the home health nurse. The next day, the home health agency that employs the home health nurse is notified by the patient's son, that his mother had changed her mind and wanted to live as long as possible. However, this information was not given to the patient's health care providers. Is the home health nurse liable for malpractice and professional misconduct for not taking aggressive measures?

In the absence of knowledge of the revocation either of a living will or appointment of health care agent, a health care professional is not subject to civil or criminal liability or discipline for unprofessional conduct for carrying out the living will. If the health care provider or agent is unwilling to comply with the wishes of the patient, care of the patient should be transferred as promptly as possible to a health care provider who is willing to comply with the wishes of the patient within the confines of the applicable state law.

Do not resuscitate orders

Do not resuscitate orders may differ from state to state. The order must be written by the patient's physician. In addition, "do not treat" or "do not hospitalize" orders should also be written by the physician and kept in the patient's medical record.

Informed consent

Prior to initiating any medical intervention, valid consent of the patient and/or the legally authorized substitute decision maker must be obtained. Lack of informed consent that proximately causes an injury to a patient may give rise to a claim of professional negligence and/or malpractice.

Historically it has been up to the clinician, typically physicians who perform the procedure, to discuss treatment with the patient and obtain required consent. Thus far no duty to obtain informed consent has been established for home health nurses, and no home health agency has been successfully sued for a failure to obtain informed consent. However, it is the home health nurse's obligation to speak up when the patient appears not to understand, seems to be incompetent, or may have been coerced into agreeing to a procedure. Although not required in most instances, *written* informed consent is preferable to a conversation that is not documented.[5] The consent must be given voluntarily from an informed competent person. In providing informed consent, the elements of disclosure should include (1) the nature of the procedure, (2) the risks and hazards of the procedure, (3) the alternative to the procedure, and (4) the anticipated benefits of the procedure.[13]

Right to confidentiality in medical records. As with all patients, home health care patients have the right to confidentiality of medical records. The patient's medical records may not be released to a third party without the written consent of the patient. Authorizations should be scrutinized carefully to determine the scope of the allowed disclosure. Limitations which may be included in the authorization include time frames of treatment, reference to a particular injury and/or disease entity, and to whom the records may be released. The authorizations should not be more than 1 year old. If the authorization does not provide for the disclosure of psychiatric treatment, then the same should not be released. In some states a health care provider may not release records which make mention of the HIV virus and/or its related symptoms without the express consent of the patient.

Confidentiality and security of the field or travel chart should be addressed by home health agency policy. The practicalities of delivering quality patient care dictate that certain patient information must be available to caregivers in the home. The confidentiality and security of this information should be discussed with the patient and/or family pursuant to home health agency policy.

COMMON AREAS OF LIABILITY AND HOW TO AVOID THEM
Inadequate staff training for assigned tasks

Case example. An inexperienced home health nurse was assigned a patient on a portable ventilator. The home health nurse was worried about her lack of training and experience with ventilator-dependent patients, but as a new grad, she felt pressured to take the assignment and talked herself out of these concerns. She thought it best not to question her superior's judgment and accepted the case.

Guidelines to avoid liability

- Before you accept or refuse a client you think you are untrained to competently handle, determine precisely what type of care will be required and whether you will receive any supervision.
- Be thoroughly familiar with the care your patient requires. You must know how to operate any equipment in use, provide associated care, make relevant clinical assessments, and detect potential problems.
- Be certain that you are not being asked to perform a function that violates your home health agency's policies and procedures.
- Refuse to perform any treatment not permitted by your state's Nurse Practice Act. If you do not know whether a particular procedure is beyond the scope of nursing practice in your state, contact the state board to find out.
- Insist on proper training and information before you accept an assignment of a patient with whose care you are unfamiliar. Request an in-service as necessary prior to implementing care.
- Refuse to accept an assignment if you are not familiar with the care the patient requires.
- Put the reasons for your refusal in writing in a memo to your supervisor. State your objections factually. For example, "I have never irrigated a patient's colon using traditional equipment without supervision and my training was over 10 years ago," as opposed to "I'm not comfortable using traditional equipment to irrigate a patient's colon."
- Express a willingness to take a comparable assignment in the future provided you receive appropriate training and supervision.
- If you are the supervisor, you are responsible to ensure that employees to whom you delegate have the proper training and authority to perform assigned tasks. If you knew or should have known the employee was not sufficiently trained, you could be liable for negligent delegation.

- Familiarize yourself with the skills and abilities of anyone you supervise, nurses and nursing assistants included.
- The supervisor or primary care nurse should discuss the proper care for each patient with the nursing assistant who will be involved in the care. Clarify circumstances under which the case manager is to be notified.
- If you are forced to make an assignment you think may be unsafe, or you are unable to properly supervise another, put someone in your chain of command on notice before you take this action.
- Implement an annual criteria-based performance evaluation that documents clinical abilities and skills of all nursing staff members.

Patient falls

Case example. The patient is an 88-year-old male with poor eyesight. He ambulates with a walker. While the home health nurse leaves the room to get something for the patient, he gets out of his chair and attempts to ambulate to the bathroom. Unfortunately, his walker is nowhere near his chair and he walks unaided. The patient falls and fractures his hip.

Guidelines to avoid liability

- Evaluate the patients who are at risk for falling at home due to impaired senses, decreased physical capabilities, side effects of medications, or their environment. Initiate a referral to rehabilitation services as necessary.
- Document your assessment and the fall prevention plan, including all patient and family teaching.
- Keep all ambulating devices and corrective lenses within reach of the patient.
- Routinely educate and remind the patient how to avoid falls and document this completely.
- Evaluate the patient's environment for potential risks, such as loose carpeting, poor lighting, and steep stairs.
- When environmental hazards exist or a patient is noncompliant with the fall prevention plan, consider having the patient and/or family sign a statement indicating their understanding that a fall resulting in serious injury is possible in these circumstances. Keep a copy in the patient's medical record.

Medication errors

Case example. A home health nurse is assigned to a cardiac patient. The home health nurse notes that the patient's blood pressure is lower than usual, and that the patient is complaining of being tired all of the time. The home health nurse reviews the patient's medication record and sees that the patient is taking 2 antihypertensive medications. She phones the patient's physician and reviews the medication orders. The order for the first antihypertensive medication had expired when the second medication was ordered. However, the first medication was never discontinued; therefore the home health nurse continued to give the medication.

Guidelines to avoid liability

- Prior to administering medication, check and double-check the patient's name, route of administration, the correct dosage, the correct medication, and the time(s) of administration.
- Be familiar with the medication administered, its side effects, and its compatibility with other medication the patient may be taking.
- Observe the patient for potential side effects of the medication; document and report the same to the patient's physician.
- Adhere to the home health agency's policies for medication renewal by the physician.
- Immediately report medication errors to the patient's physician and your supervisor. Complete an incident report form as required.
- Validate patient self-reported changes in medications with the physician's office.
- Report instances of patient self-medication error or dangerous home remedy to the physician and follow home agency policy regarding this matter.

Faulty equipment

Case example. Your patient is a 69-year-old male with chronic obstructive pulmonary disease, and he is on a portable ventilator. You routinely check the flow rate during your visits and document this. The patient complains that for the past 3 days, he has awakened with a headache. You wonder whether the ventilator is properly calibrated and whether the patient is receiving too much oxygen.

Guidelines to avoid liability

- Be thoroughly familiar with any equipment used in the care of your patient. You must know how to operate the equipment, monitor it, provide associated care, and detect potential problems.
- Insist on proper training and information before you accept an assignment of a patient whose care involves the use of equipment you are not familiar with.
- Refuse to accept an assignment if you are not familiar with all applicable medical devices and their operation.
- Be certain that nursing assistants providing care to your patients are thoroughly familiar with any equipment in use.
- Provide the patient and the patient's caregivers with complete instructions on the use of all equipment.
- Carefully document in the record all teaching you have done with the patient and caregivers on the equipment in use.
- Request and observe patient/caregiver return demonstrations with procedural care and equipment and document this in the record.
- Ensure that the manufacturer's instruction manual is attached to the equipment in the home.
- Contact the company "Write it Right"* for assistance in evaluating and preparing medical device user instructions.[11]
- If equipment failure could be life-threatening, determine the availability of a backup generator and/or backup equipment in the home. Provide specific instructions to follow in the event of equipment failure and keep a copy in the record.
- If you suspect that a device is malfunctioning, call for immediate service, notify your supervisor and the patient's attending physician, and document in the record the steps you have taken.
- Complete an incident report detailing any equipment malfunction or failure.

- If you plan to use any of your own equipment on the job, have it inspected by the home health agency and get the home health agency's written approval for its use. This may protect you from liability if a problem occurs.
- The Safe Medical Devices Act of 1990 requires the reporting of any equipment malfunction resulting in serious injury, illness, or death. The suspected malfunction and details of the occurrence should be reported by the home health agency within 10 weekdays to the FDA and the equipment manufacturer.[21]

Communication and safety problems

Case example. You have accepted assignment of a new patient, an 86-year-old female stroke victim who lives with her daughter and 27-year-old grandson, a chronic schizophrenic with a history of violence. At 7:30 PM on the day after your first home visit, you receive a call from the daughter, who thinks her mother has had another cerebral vascular attack. You arrive at the home and are met by the grandson, who threatens to harm you if you enter.

Guidelines to avoid liability

- If you feel your safety is threatened, immediately leave the home and notify your patient service manager of the problem.
- All home health agencies should have an administrator or patient service manager on call 7 days a week, 24 hours a day to assist with clinical decision making. This person should carry a beeper and be available immediately by telephone to consult and advise you.
- Before you accept your first patient assignment know your chain of command, including names and phone numbers of your supervisor, Director of Nursing, Agency Administrator, and Medical Director. If you cannot reach your immediate supervisor, call the Director of Nursing and so on. If your immediate supervisor is not responsive to your clinical needs, continue to follow the chain of command for assistance in appropriate decision making.
- Nonclinical emergencies should be covered in the home health agency's policy, but even if they aren't, invoke the chain of command when you need assistance.

---

*Small Manufacturers Assistance Office and Health and Industry Program Center for Devices and Radiological Health Food and Drug Administration HF2220, 1350 Piccard Drive, Rockville, MD 20850.

- Be assertive enough to initiate the chain of command. Remember, it is your legal duty, and a failure to do so could result in patient injury and professional liability.
- Carry the name and telephone number of the patient's attending physician with you on all home visits. Do not hesitate to involve the patient's doctor.
- Factually document in the record your efforts to communicate with others. Specify who was called and the time.
- If you are the supervisor, know who is available to you before you start your shift, including names and phone numbers. If you contact the Agency Administrator or Medical Director in response to a problem, document this in a memo and keep one copy for your files.
- Remember, whether you are a manager or primary care nurse, putting someone in authority on notice of the problem is critical.
- If you are unable to reach anyone in your organization, use your best judgment in response to the situation, bearing in mind that in most instances it is better to be overcautious. Documenting all efforts to obtain assistance and acting in good faith should serve to protect you in the event of litigation.

Inadequate medical response

Case example. An 83-year-old patient suffers an apparent transient ischemic attack while you are in the home. You do not want to leave without speaking to the patient's physician who you suspect will want to see the patient and probably adjust the medication orders. By the time you are ready to leave, the doctor has not returned your call. This physician is known to ignore nurses' calls and then complain to administration that he has not been kept informed.

Guidelines to avoid liability

- Note in the record every attempt to reach the patient's physician, including the time, content of messages left, the facts conveyed in each conversation, and efforts you have made to go up the chain of command.
- If the patient's condition is rapidly deteriorating, do not hesitate to get medical treatment for the patient. Invoke your chain of command; in an emergency, call EMS.

- When a particular physician routinely ignores nurses' calls or provides otherwise inadequate care, bring it to the attention of your supervisor in a memo. Document factually, noting, for example, instances in which you attempted to reach the doctor, but did not receive a timely response. Keep one copy of the memo for your files.
- If a doctor's response rises to the level of incompetence, report it to your supervisor in a memo.
- Contact the patient's physician whenever you detect more than a minor exacerbation of the patient's condition, or whenever the physician has asked to be notified.
- Always alert a doctor whose patient is en route to the hospital.
- Trust your instincts when the patient's condition seems serious. You have a duty to be an assertive advocate when the physician does not respond appropriately to your patient's needs.

Admitting inappropriate patients into home care

Case example. The home health nurse is assigned to a patient with a history of mental health problems. The patient is continually changing residences to various shelters. Often the home health nurse cannot locate the patient, or the patient is not home at the time of the scheduled visit.

Guidelines to avoid liability

- Carefully screen patients, including their home environment for equipment needs, prior to accepting them.
- Consider whether home health services can reasonably be expected to meet the needs of the patient. Review government regulations for reimbursement; Medicare will not reimburse home visits in which the patient is noncompliant or no longer homebound. (See Chapter 4.)
- Document all of the patient's noncompliance in the medical record. Be specific by using actual examples of noncompliance and report the same to the physician. Let the physician know that the patient is in jeopardy of discharge.
- Request a multidisciplinary conference to evaluate the patient's needs and whether a

referral to a different agency may be appropriate.

- Provide the patient with a written letter indicating that he is discharged from the agency (Figure 7-1). If possible, have the patient sign the letter and return it to the agency. If you cannot locate the patient, send a letter (with return receipt) to the last known address. Be sure to inform the patient's physician prior to the patient's discharge and copy the physician with the discharge letter.
- Maintain a copy of any correspondence with the patient in the patient's medical record.

SUMMARY

Home care is growing and will continue to become increasingly complex in service delivery. For home health nurses, this means caring for more acutely ill patients and using the associated technology within the sometimes unpredictable environment of the home milieu. In these circumstances, careful attention to legal and ethical ramifications of patient care is a *must*.

REFERENCES

1. Aiken T, Catalano J: *Legal, ethical and political issues in nursing,* Philadelphia, 1994, FA Davis.
2. The American Association of Nurse Attorneys, 420 Light Street, Baltimore, MD 21230-3816, (410-752-3318).
3. American Nurses Association: *Code for nurses with interpretive statements,* Kansas City, 1985, ANA.
4. Brendt N: The home health care nurse and suspected child abuse and/or neglect, *Home Health Care Nurs* 12(4):10-11, 1994.
5. Cat M, Bigot A: *Geriatrics and the law: patient's rights and professional responsibilities,* New York, 1985, Springer Publication.
6. Catalano J: *Ethical and legal aspects of nursing,* Springhouse, Pa, 1991, Springhouse Corp.
7. *Darling v Burrone Brothers, Inc,* 162 Conn 187, 1972.
8. De Marzo D: Policies and procedures: protection or peril? *RN* 56(7):61-65, 1993.
9. Haddad A, Kapp M: *Ethical and legal issues in home health care,* Norwack, Conn, 1991, Appleton & Lange.
10. Joint Commission on Accreditation of Health Care Organizations: *Home health standards,* 1989, Chicago, JCAHO.
11. Kingsley P, Backinger C, Brady M: Medical device user instructions: the patient's need, the nurse's role, *Home Health Care Nurs* 13(1):27, 1993.
12. Laska L, editor: *Medical malpractice verdicts, settlements & experts,* 11(2):19, 1995. Case reported: *Ballon v St. Joseph Hospital and Janet Reyes, RN,* Passaic County (NJ) Superior Court, Case No PAS-L-3271-90.
13. Meisel, Kabnick: Informed consent to medical treatment: an analysis of recent legislation, *UPitt Law Review,* 41:407, 427, 1980.
14. Northrop CE, Kelly ME: Legal issues in nursing, St Louis, 1987, Mosby.
15. *People v Coe,* 131 Misc 2d 807, 1986.
16. Rubsamen DS, editor: A fatal case of aspiration pneumonitis, *Professional Liability Newsletter* 24:10, 1994.
17. Sullivan G: Home care: more autonomy, more legal risks, *RN* 57(5):63-68, 1994.
18. Sullivan G: The right way to fill out an incident report, *RN* 57(12):53-55, 1988.
19. Sullivan G: When assignments don't match skills, *RN* 58(4):57-60, 1995.
20. Sweeney M: Your role in informed consent, *RN* 54(8):55-60, 1991.
21. Tammelleo A: Who's to blame for faulty equipment? *RN* 53(10):67-72, 1990.

8 Case Management and Leadership Strategies for Home Health Nurses

Robyn Rice

Learn to make a body of a limb
—Shakespeare, Richard II

The cost of health care in America has skyrocketed out of control. The rise in health care expenditures demonstrates this increase in costs. For example, in 1992 total health care spending rose by 11.5% to $838.5 billion.[24] Home health expenditures alone, as a percent of total Medicare expenditures, rose from 2.4% in 1988 to a projected 8.3% in 1996.[19] In 1994 total health care spending was approximately 14% of the gross national product (GNP).[24] Within this economic climate of spiraling expenditures, the public is demanding cost-effective, quality patient care. As a result, professional accountability for efficient and effective utilization of health care services is being emphasized in all areas of practice.

How is accountability for efficient and effective patient care to be addressed by a caring profession such as nursing? In dealing with the regulatory and economic restructuring of health care in this country, home health nurses *must utilize innovative approaches* to patient care that maximize efficiency and utility of service. They must also maintain professional standards of practice. These challenges will be met as home health nurses assume both management and leadership responsibilities for patient care. In balancing economics with a professional commitment to serve the public, home health nurses must not only implement patient care but also have a *say* in how patient care and clinical policies are determined, implemented, and evaluated.

Refer to Chapters 1-7 and the clinical chapters in this book which build on principles of case management. The purpose of this chapter is to provide an overview of case management andlead-ership strategies that empower home health nurses to address issues of fiscal accountability of services, to deliver quality patient care, and to maintain professional standards of practice.

MANAGEMENT AND LEADERSHIP STRATEGIES

More patients, sicker patients, regulatory issues influencing the availability of resources, and increasing professional responsibilities for patients are realities for home health nurses. Yet the milieu of home care is rewarding to those nurses who enjoy the tremendous amount of freedom and autonomy of nursing practice that home care offers. For these nurses, their experience is not "Nurse, do this," but rather "Nurse, what do we do?" In other words, in addition to delivering patient care, home health nurses often consult with physicians to make recommendations for service coordination and treatment. In order to rise to this expectation and maintain the public's trust that quality patient care will be given, home health nurses must be expert clinicians. As a result, familiarity with disease processes, medical treatments, wound-care products, community resources, and a working knowledge of the home milieu are required. In preserving professional standards of practice, home health nurses must have a strong voice in governing clinical policies. They must be managers and leaders.

Management vs leadership

Bennis and Goldsmith differentiate management and leadership in the following manner, "A good manager does things right. A good leader does the right things."[3] In the management role, home health nurses are concerned with the implementation, organization, structuring, and evaluation of systems, procedures, and policies. In the leadership role, home health nurses are not only concerned about providing quality patient care but have definite ideas and opinions about how patient care and home health agency policy should be determined.[5] The implication is that a leadership role is more likely to involve visionary, innovative, and inquiry-based approaches. Management is about implementing and evaluating policy. Leadership creates policy.[3] In the following sections, clinical applications of how home health nurses can be effective managers and leaders are presented.

TRENDS IN MANAGEMENT: CASE MANAGEMENT
Historical perspectives

Home health and community-based nurses have traditionally utilized principles of case management when providing and coordinating services for their patients. However, models of case management continue to be shaped by government and privately owned companies. Historically, case management models have been around since the turn of the century when Visiting Nurse Associations emphasized service coordination of patient care. The term *case management* first appeared in social welfare literature in the 1970s.[17]

Case management broadly refers to the process of delivering patient care according to patient "case type" or individual needs. Case type refers to groups of patients who share a common medical or nursing diagnosis. Case management focuses on the achievement of patient outcomes of care within an effective and appropriate time frame (length of stay). As a cost containment initiative, case management operates under the umbrella of managed care.

Managed care became a popular term in the 1980s. Managed care refers to the systems that provide the structure, regulations, and guidelines for implementing cost-effective patient care. These systems link the provider with the public in managing cost, access to resources, and quality patient care.[23] Examples of public managed care systems include Medicare and Medicaid. Examples of private managed care systems include health maintenance orga-

nizations (HMOs) and preferred provider organizations (PPOs).

Reimbursement of health care services is intricately tied to the principles of case management and managed care. Medicare's reimbursement of home health services differs from its reimbursement of hospitals. In the early 1980s the Omnibus Budget Reconciliation Act (OBRA) mandated that Medicare pay for hospitalizations at a fixed rate or a prospective payment determined by diagnostic-related groups (DRGs). At present, Medicare reimbursement of Medicare-certified home health agencies is based upon a renewable certification period with retrospective reimbursement of services. As a result, Medicare-certified home health services are allotted more freedom in billing for fees and services as compared to hospitals. However, this will probably change as government policy imposes tighter controls regulating reimbursement of home care services. Using utility screens, HMOs and PPOs are already limiting the number of home visits nurses can make. Prospective payment seems a likely trend for home care. Hence the current emphasis within the home care industry is upon more efficient utilization of services through the process of case management as well as care path development. Home health agencies are now focusing their attention upon case management models in which care is structured by patient care plans that are based on a working knowledge of case type, anticipated outcomes, and resource utilization.[10,12,21,26] Additionally, in order to improve continuity of care and decrease fragmentation of services, trends in documentation systems in home care agencies are moving toward multidisciplinary notation.

Home health definitions of a case manager and case management

The case manager is an expert clinician who is responsible for maintaining standards of care, coordinating multidisciplinary services, utilizing community resources, and ensuring that patient/caregiver outcomes of care are met within a reasonable time frame. The Commission on Insurance Rehabilitation Specialists provides certification for case managers, and the National Association of Case Managers serves as a support and accreditation organization for case managers.[6] The registered nurse (RN) serves as the case manager

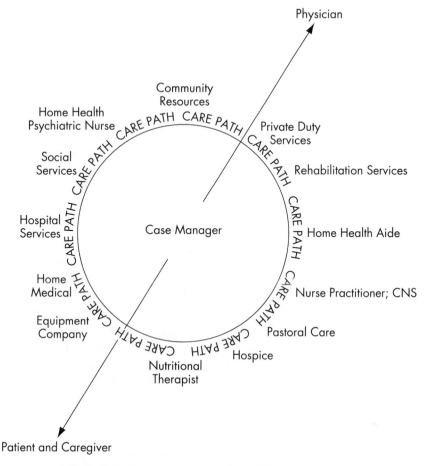

Figure 8-1 The case manager and multidisciplinary resources.

in home care. The only exception to this would be if the patient is receiving only rehabilitation services. In this case, the therapist would serve as case manager.

There are many models of case management. This chapter will present a home health agency point of service case management model. In this model, case management is broadly defined as a process of multidisciplinary care in which nursing coordinates its services with those of other disciplines.[1,2,7,17,18,22] (See Figure 8-1.)

In this model, home health nurses work with many different physicians and care for patients with a variety of diseases and functional disabilities. Therapeutic interventions are based upon a patient classification system or case type. Docu-

mentation systems with predetermined patient goals, outcomes of care, and anticipated learning needs for patient case types are emphasized. The result is a standardized, high quality, cost-effective plan of care.[15,17,28] Elements of case management in a home health-based case management model include the following:[1,10,11,14]

- Autonomy in practice as decision making of case managers and support services is encouraged; an emphasis upon decentralized decision making
- Accountability for practice as case managers are vested with the authority and responsibility for clinical and financial outcomes for their caseload; an emphasis upon risk management

strategies that decrease the probability of incurring adverse outcomes

- Decreased fragmentation of services as the patient is followed by an individual or group of individuals who are responsible for assisting the patient/caregiver through the system; an emphasis upon coordination of care
- Outcome evaluation; expected outcomes are determined during the admission process and compared with actual outcomes in identifying opportunities for improvement of services
- Satisfaction of customers and consumers (including the patient/caregiver, physician, and home health staff); improved patient outcomes, improved coordination of services, decreased rework, recognition of service and accountability for role, consistency in policy implementation, and increased satisfaction for all
- The use of the primary nurse (RN) as case manager; an emphasis upon full-time salaried field staff as case managers
- Efficient and effective resource utilization; an emphasis upon multidisciplinary referrals for service
- A collaborative practice between case manager, physician, and the multidisciplinary team; the case manager merges each discipline's plan of care into one collaborative plan with mutually agreed upon goals; an emphasis upon increased communication systems via the plan of care
- A comprehensive patient/caregiver assessment
- An emphasis upon patient/caregiver education
- An emphasis upon active patient/caregiver participation with the plan of care
- Caseload organization

Clinical applications of case management: Implementing service and organizing the caseload

As discussed in Chapter 4, outcomes of care are derived from the admission assessment. In the role of case manager, it will be important for home health nurses to meet with the patient/caregiver and mutually develop the plan of care. For example, when identifying outcomes of care, the patient/caregiver's perceptions of learning needs should be assessed. This information would then be incorporated into the plan of care (Figure 8-2).

Typical questions regarding the implementation of home care services and caseload organization often involve the number of patients to be seen and the time that the home health nurse should spend in the patient's home. The information in the box on p. 124, may provide insights in answering these questions.

The caseload will require basic organization so that all the patients are seen and services rendered as ordered by the physician. Home visits are primarily made from 8 AM to 4 PM during the workweek. However, additional staff coverage is provided for after hours and weekend visits.

Many nurses carry a field chart for each patient. Information in the field chart includes the physician's up-to-date orders for treatments and medications, a copy of the plan of care, and a calendar to indicate patient/caregiver visit frequency as well as dates for specimen collection, specific procedural requirements, physician office visits, or when recertification orders should be sent in.

A calendar outlining visit frequency services of all disciplines is advised (Figure 8-3). As case managers, home health nurses should use calendar planning to ensure that multidisciplinary visits are spread across the workweek. This way everyone does not show up at the patient's home on the same day, which can be exhausting and inconvenient for the patient/caregiver.

Field charts are typically placed in a mobile file cabinet that may go with the nurse from office to car. A folder including basic service information about the home health agency, a copy of the plan of care or care path, and related information is usually kept in the patient's home.

As technological advances increase, trends in organizing the caseload include the use of mobile cellular phones and dictaphones to maximize efficiency of communications, and the use of laptop computers with a modem to record and transmit patient data from the car. (See the box titled Tips for Organizing the Caseload.)

Teamwork is very important in home care because patients are often visited by many disciplines. A collaborative relationship is fundamental to teamwork so that everyone understands their role and gives the best effort toward achieving patient/caregiver outcomes of care.[23] This includes the patient/caregiver.

Patient's Name: _____   Yes   No   Comments

1. Patient is under the care of a physician.   __   __
2. A reasonable expectation exists
   that the patient's
   medical needs   __   __
   nursing needs   __   __
   rehabilitation needs   __   __
   social needs   __   __
   can adequately be met by the home
   health staff in the patient's home.
3. The home health agency has adequately
   trained staff to provide services to the patient. __   __
4. The home environment is safe for visiting staff.   __   __
5. The home environment supports required
   technology for home health services.   __   __
6. A home evaluation is needed prior to discharge.   __   __
7. The patient is willing to work with the
   home health agency staff in learning self-care
   management at home.   __   __
8. The patient is trainable.   __   __
9. If the patient is unable to assist home
   health agency staff with self-care management,
   a caregiver or family member is willing and
   able to do this.   __   __
10. The patient/caregiver understands
    their rights and responsibilities for home
    health services.   __   __

11. Primary nursing diagnosis/patient problems:

12. Patient/caregiver educational needs: (include patient/caregiver self-perceived learning needs)

13. Patient/caregiver advocacy needs: (procedural care? Psychological and spiritual support?)

14. Patient/caregiver case management needs: (multidisciplinary referrals for service?
    Community resources? Recommended Care Path Standard?)

Professional's Signature:_____ Date: _____

Figure 8-2 Questions to use during admission planning to the home health agency. (Theoretical framework: The Rice Model of Dynamic Self-Determination.)

Medicare will deny payment for duplication of services.[15] Home health nurses should work with the multidisciplinary team so there is no duplication of services between disciplines. For example, if the patient requires instruction on energy conservation techniques, this should either be done by the occupational therapist or skilled nursing but *not* by both disciplines. Multidisciplinary conferences are one way for case managers to bring the team together.

A multidisciplinary conference for each patient is recommended once a month in order to review

---

RESEARCH IN HOME CARE:
A National Survey [27]

During 1994, while giving a national lecture series for home health nurses, the author surveyed seminar attendees regarding average caseload and visit frequency.[27] The results of the survey may have useful applications in planning the caseload.

An average caseload for home health nurses ranged from 15 to 46 patients. It was noted that some of the patients in the nurse's reported caseload were only seen monthly (for example, patients receiving services for a monthly indwelling foley catheter change).

Patient acuity levels and service area (or expected miles driven) influenced the size of the caseload. For example, nurses who reported a smaller caseload stated that they "drove great distances" or cared for patients who received high-tech services such as intravenous (IV) therapy. Also, nurses in Florida and Texas reported increases in caseload during the winter months when older adults migrated to areas with milder climates.

Patient acuity levels, mileage, extra time required with patient admissions, work with student nurses, and planned office time were also cited as factors that influenced the number of patients that the nurses were able to see in 1 day. Typical daily visits fell in the range of 3 to 9 patients with a mean of 5.6 patients, again depending on patient needs and other work-related expectations the home health nurse may have had. For example, nurses providing high-tech services such as home IV therapy reported daily visits in the range of 2 to 5 patients with a mean of 3.4 patients. It was interesting to note that home health nurses in New York City reported an average daily visit schedule higher than nurses in most other parts of the country. This could possibly be related to the fact that the New York City nurses who were surveyed, reported that they typically walked to work and that most of their patients were located in one apartment building or on a city block.

In terms of length of visits, nurses surveyed reported a mean of 45 minutes for a Medicare repeat visit (this included time allotted for paperwork) with a mean of 2 hours required for Medicare openings or patient admissions (this included time allotted for paperwork). High-tech services such as an initial TPN visit or an initial visit for a ventilator-dependent patient took longer. Reported estimates varied with a mean from 3.8 hours (this included time allotted for paperwork).

Average driving time or average miles driven in the course of a day by home health nurses was not assessed in the survey.

---

patient/caregiver progress toward meeting identified outcomes of care. Conferences should make use of present day electronic communication systems (such as telephone conferences, e-mail communications, and electronically recorded care plans) to increase efficiency in service. During the conference, the role of each team member should be reviewed relative to achieving patient/caregiver outcomes of care. Progress toward goals of care, as well as variances or identified problems, should be reviewed. An action plan would be implemented for problem resolution. (See the Outcome Failure Analysis box.) Variances would then be tracked in the quality improvement (QI) program (refer to Chapter 9). If the patient's physician is unable to attend the conference, the case manager should send the physician a copy of the conference summary and seek feedback as appropriate. It would also be important to share the conference summary

with the patient/caregiver in order to identify those outcomes of care which had been accomplished and those which required further work.

Adjusting the visit frequency during services and planning for patient discharge are also part of case management for home health nurses. Typically the patient will require more visits at the beginning of services. Once initial needs are met and the patient is stabilized, the visit frequency should decline as the patient/caregiver becomes more comfortable with self-care management of health care needs at home. Fluctuations in visit frequency, the need for increased visits during services, and the need for patient/caregiver recertification must be supported by clinical documentation indicating outcomes of care not met or instability of the patient/caregiver's health status in order to obtain Medicare reimbursement for services.[15] (See the box titled Patient Discharge Criteria.)

Patient's Name _____
Current Certification Period _____
Recertification orders required by _____

Sunday	Monday	Tuesday	Wednesday	Thursday	Friday	Saturday
	SN (AM FBS) hha	PT	SN hha	PT MSW	SN hha	
	SN hha	PT	SN hha *hha supervisory visit	PT	SN hha	
	hha	SN PT	hha	SN MSW	hha PT	
	hha	SN PT	hha *hha supervisory visit	SN (AM FBS)	hha PT	
	hha	SN PT	hha	SN (no SN visit as patient has MD office appointment)	hha PT	

SN=RN   PT=physical therapy services
hha=home health aide   MSW=social worker

Figure 8-3 Using a calendar to plan home visits.

An operational model for service delivery

Many home health agencies are moving toward an evaluation system whereby nurses have a set number of efficiency points to earn each week rather than "numbers of patients seen." In this model, field staff are not only evaluated on clinical expertise but on service to the agency. As described later in this chapter, service could take on the form of committee work. In this model, part-time and LPN staff would typically cover Thursday afternoon visits while the case managers would come into the agency to attend to paperwork; participate in committee work, conferences, or in-services; and set up the next week's visits.

These quotas or point systems, mutually determined by staff and administration, would be based on the miles that the home health nurse must drive each day, patient acuity levels, the mentoring of student nurses, and the amount of committee work or service that the home health nurse has agreed to take on. Overtime pay typically would be discouraged. Operational models, like the one described,

---

TIPS FOR ORGANIZING THE CASELOAD

- Plan patient visits to maximize efficient mileage. Look at the patient's address and find the location of the residence on the street map; avoid unnecessary driving.
- Plan to visit patients requiring lab work in the morning as test results are usually requested by the afternoon.
- Use the travel chart or calendar as a reminder of when certain procedures, lab work, or recertification orders are due.
- If possible, visit patients with a communicable disease last or at the end of the day.

PATIENT DISCHARGE CRITERIA

- Goals of care met
- Outcomes of care achieved
- Stabilization of disease process
- Maximal potential with rehabilitation program achieved
- Moved outside of service area
- No longer homebound
- Noncompliant
- At the patient's or physician's request
- Rehospitalization
- Death
- Other

OUTCOME FAILURE ANALYSIS

1. Identify the outcome(s) that was not met.
2. Identify all possible causes.
3. Evaluate the likelihood of each.
4. Select the most probable cause(s) of outcome failure.
5. Identify all possible corrective actions.
6. Select the optimal corrective action(s).
7. Evaluate the efficacy of the action plan.

---

tend to promote efficient operation of clinical services as expectations of job performance are clearly defined and *talents of staff fully utilized.*

How can case managers implement and track multidisciplinary care? Described as "the road map to home care" and as "the critical tool of case management," **care paths** are becoming an increasingly popular means of bringing managed care to home care.[8,25]

The tool of case managers: Care paths

A care path is a standardized multidisciplinary plan of care that enables home health nurses to plan, implement, coordinate, and evaluate the care for certain groups of patients based on a shared medical or nursing diagnosis or some form of patient classification system based upon a standard of care.[2,8,28] Originally described as a critical

pathway by Zander, its purpose is to evaluate whether quality patient care is being delivered in a cost-effective and timely manner.[30] The term *care path* is recommended for home health agencies instead of *clinical pathway* or *critical pathway* because patients at home provide self-care management that is neither clinical nor critical.[19] Care paths in home care are used as follows:[8,14,18,22,25]

- Patient care plans
- Standards of care
- Orientation tools for staff in learning home care
- Educational tools for student nurses in learning home care
- Multidisciplinary conference guides
- Documentation and tracking tools for the QI program
- A patient database for purposes of research in future decision making

Care paths in home care involve standardized patient outcomes based on patient groupings that allow for individualization of content, which would be determined by the multidisciplinary team and the patient/caregiver during the admission process. It is important to share the content of the care path with the patient/caregiver so that the delivery of services, as well as patient/caregiver expectations with the plan of care, are clearly understood by all. Patient/caregivers should be able to articulate who they are being seen by, the purpose of each discipline, what *they are supposed to accomplish* during home health services, and an expected date of discharge. Care paths can be very specific in format and outline day-to-day care, or they can be more general in describing the overall course of service. A care path outlining care on a per visit or weekly basis is recommended for home health agencies.

The care path model in Appendix 8-1 is designed to replace the patient care plan and multidisciplinary conference guide.[2,6,14,16,20,22] For ease and simplicity of use, the care path is designed to fit front to back on an 8 1/2 by 11 inch piece of paper. Specific dates for achieving outcomes of care designated on the pathway would be selected by the case manager, the patient/caregiver, and the multidisciplinary team (including the physician) after initial patient assessment. In this particular form, outcomes also serve as critical events or actions the nurse would take in order to facilitate patient home independence and discharge. Daily visits would be documented on the visit report (Chapter 4). The case manager would be responsible for updating the care path each week with documented input from the multidisciplinary team at least once a month. A new form would be used each recertification period that would carry over outcomes yet to be achieved.

Note that the care path presented in Appendix 8-1 has predeveloped patient education guides that would be issued with the form. (See Chapter 6.) A patient edition of the care path can be found in Appendix 8-2. Patients would be provided with a stamped self-addressed envelope and encouraged to complete their care path survey and mail it back to the agency after discharge.

TRENDS IN LEADERSHIP: EMPOWERMENT

In striving toward innovation in health care, philosophies of leadership and management are changing. Trends in leadership suggest a flattened hierarchy within organizational systems where a shared governance is represented by councils, committee work, and internal restructuring for creative and inquiry-based change.[3] Innovative leadership builds an environment where staff feel free to voice recommendations or dissent. Innovative leadership utilizes the creative talents of staff to create a work environment that fosters trust, integrity, compe-

tence, and a vision of shared objectives or outcomes. Innovative leaders lead creative people. Creativity is a basis for empowerment.

Empowerment, within the context of this chapter, refers to those partnerships within the home health agency that emphasize innovative and creative approaches to the business of home care. It also promotes individual expression for quality patient care. For example, empowered home health nurses feel that they are at the center of things and that what they do makes a difference to the success of their home health agency. Empowerment obligates nurses to focus their attention not only to the patient's bedside, but also to the organization and operation of the home health agency. It obliterates a "pay per visit" mind-set where the nurse's only concern is to make the home visit and get paid. It discourages home health agencies from increasing daily visit frequencies to the point where it becomes impossible for staff to provide quality patient care. Likewise, empowerment puts aside autocratic managers who do not listen or care to listen to what their staff have to say. Through service such as committee work, home health nurses become more than bedside clinicians. They are given opportunities to apply their talents toward discovering the solutions to the complex problems facing health care today.[3] This is the essence of empowerment and the spirit of good business.

In order to effectively work within these changing organizational systems and govern clinical practice, home health nurses need to know how to be leaders as well as case managers.

Clinical applications of leadership: Committee work

Group work does not come easily to Americans; the United States is truly a country that values individualism. Yet active, organized committees with shared objectives can be one of the most politically effective means to determine and drive policy at the home health agency. Most important committee work allows home health nurses a platform from which to speak. The following questions are frequently asked by home health nurses: What types of committees should home health nurses be involved in? How do home health nurses get administration to support committee work? How does one chair a committee and run a meeting?

Committees your home health agency can't afford to be without

Clinical practice needs, economic constraints, regulatory issues, and the specter of legal/ethical issues in the milieu of home care drive the need for committee work. (See the box titled Recommended Committees for Home Health Agencies.)

Consider using a Professional Consultation Committee to assist staff in coping with some of the very difficult legal and ethical issues they face in home care. For example, abusive or noncompliant patients, inadequate medical treatment, and safety concerns may be very real problems for field staff. In these matters, the Professional Consultation Committee would become an advisory board for an appropriate course of action. In that

government and regulatory agencies seem to continuously redefine operational policy for home health agencies, consider the advantages of addressing changes in standards through the Professional Practice Committee. Who better able to determine clinical policies and procedures than field staff who practice them?

Consider this question: Does the home health agency have the best alcohol prep pad at the best cost? The Professional Research Committee could ensure this by evaluating different vendor brands of alcohol prep pads for cost efficiency. Committee members would squeeze each brand of prep pad and determine how many drops of alcohol were obtained. In this manner, the committee would be able to recommend that the home health agency purchase the lowest cost brand of alcohol prep pads that have the most drops of alcohol. In reality, the cost effectiveness of alcohol prep pads is a *little thing*. However, it is the little things that bespeak a mutual concern for quality when doing the *big things* such as patient care. The Professional Research Committee should meet with suppliers, evaluate products, and pass information along to field staff so that what is stocked in the medical supply room is relevant to clinical practice needs.

How do you get administrative support for committee work?

In approaching administration regarding the need for committees, it is important to present the benefits of committee work to the home health agency. What are the economic advantages? How can the home health agency strengthen services from committee work? Improved patient care, improved outcomes, improved employee satisfaction, improved working relationships, improved communications among the multidisciplinary services, and reduced liability are only a few of the benefits derived from committee work.

How to chair a committee and run a meeting

There are several ground rules that are important to understand when chairing a committee. First of all, the chair should be prepared to accept responsibility for the committee. Chairing a committee is definitely a leadership role and it will be necessary for home health nurses to handle the politics of leadership. It is important to understand one's role

---

RECOMMENDED COMMITTEES FOR HOME HEALTH AGENCIES

Professional standards committee
—QA/QI
—Staff preparation for state and regulatory review (mock survey)
—Care path development and implementation

Professional consultation committee
—Legal/ethical issues
—Staff safety
—Employee grievance

Professional research committee
—Product evaluation
—Research projects

Professional practice committee
—Policies and procedures
—Forms
—Technology
—Infection control

Professional service committee
—Educational in-services
—Fund raising
—Town hall
—Christmas party and summer picnic

as the chair, whether appointed or elected. Although committee member input is to be highly valued and expected, a primary role as chair is to keep the committee on track so goals are met. It is the chair's responsibility to ensure that the committee's designated assignments are achieved.

Second, the chair should consult with the administrator or director. As chair, it is important to find out the administrator's expectations of what the committee should be accomplishing. When meeting with the administrator, the chair should take notes as a matter for future reference. The chair should periodically review the committee's goals and progress with administration. There are some issues that may require the administrator's political clout or authority in order to get the committee work accomplished. For example, the chair may require administrative assistance in handling an uncooperative intraagency department or unresponsive committee member. Therefore the chair should keep administration informed and involved. When initially assuming the position of chair, the chair should make sure lines of authority are clearly understood. If the home health agency has made committee work mandatory as part of staff's job descriptions, the chair should find out up front from the administrator who is responsible for ensuring that staff attend the meetings. A chair should **never** accept the responsibility for ensuring member attendance or performance without some kind of authority to back this responsibility up. Such a situation will make a chair ineffectual and frustrated.

Third, the chair should meet with the committee. At this time, administrative ideas regarding the purpose and goals of the committee should be shared with the committee members. The administrative charge to the committee must be very clear and priorities must be set. It is important to mutually incorporate administrative assignments with goals that the committee members wish to achieve. A written action plan outlining committee goals and member responsibilities in meeting assignments with time lines for completion should be given to each committee member and the chair's administrator. At the end of the year (or whenever committee work is completed) the chair should report a summary of the committee's work and accomplishments to administration or to the home health agency's governing body. DeVries's

---

TIPS FOR CHAIRING A COMMITTEE AND CONDUCTING COMMITTEE WORK

- Arrange to reserve a room or place for all committee meetings.
- Consult with committee members in arranging times and dates to hold meetings; choose the most convenient meeting time for the group.
- Send out an announcement of the next committee meeting to all members at least 1 week before the meeting is scheduled; include an agenda on the announcement.
- Arrange to keep a record of the minutes of the committee meetings. Send out copies of the minutes to committee members and administration no later than 1 week after the meeting.
- Review the past minutes at the start of a new meeting to clear up old business.
- Consider providing refreshments; the sharing of food often relaxes the atmosphere and may enhance teamwork.
- Stick to time frames and schedules.

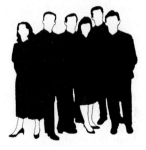

How to Run a Meeting, based on Robert's Rules of Order, provides some basic guidelines for running a meeting.[9] (See the box titled Tips for Chairing a Committee and Conducting Committee Work.)

Chairs should get to know the committee members and utilize their talents to the committee's advantage. For example, a particular committee member who enjoys research could perhaps be assigned to work that involves statistical analysis. As chair, it will be important to delegate committee assignments to the committee members. Issues will have to be thoroughly researched and analyzed before the committee makes recommendations to the home health agency. The chair should periodically touch base with committee members to make sure that assignments are being completed within the designated time frame.

Wess's *Victory Secrets of Attila the Hun* provides some interesting perspectives in leading groups and cultivating followers.[29] The literature also indicates that trust, integrity, enthusiasm, competence, consistency, and caring are qualities of leaders that followers appreciate and are drawn to.[4,13,20]

As chair, it is important to recognize that being a leader is no easy job. Leaders are often risk takers. The Japanese have a saying that, "the nail that sticks out is the one that gets hit." Job promotion, recognition, and professional achievements can, at times, make for jealous and hostile colleagues. If intraagency politics get rough, home health nurses should document any concerns they may have regarding their job and look to their *true colleagues,* as well as family, for support and guidance.

In advocating that the right things are done, it is important for home health nurses, as leaders, to understand that change can be an exhausting yet very rewarding process. It is also important to recognize that *hard work and dedication to improvement are the keys to success.*

SUMMARY

As managers and leaders, home health nurses appreciate that learning and competence are elemental to accountability for professional practice. In working with the public, such a philosophy is also essential for good business.

Where there is management, there is leadership. Where there is leadership, there is a team. As described in this chapter, through the process of teamwork, as well as individual expression for innovative approaches to service delivery, home health nurses can provide cost-effective, quality patient care *in caring ways.*

REFERENCES

1. American Nurse Association: *Nursing case management,* Kansas City, Mo, 1988, American Nurse Association.
2. Becker-Weilitz P, Potter P: A managed care system: financial and clinical evaluation, *JONA* 23(11):51-57, 1993.
3. Bennis W, Goldsmith J: *Learning to lead,* Reading, Mass, 1994, Addison-Wesley Publishing.
4. Brown H: *On success,* Nashville, 1994, Rutledge Hill Press.
5. Caserta J: Leadership, *Home Health Care Nurs* 13(2):6, 1995.
6. Cesta T: The link between continuous quality improvement and case management, *JONA* 23(6):55-61, 1993.
7. Cline K: Preparing for the first CM examination, *Case Management* 4:19-21, 1993.
8. Crummer M, Carter V: Critical pathways-the pivotal tool, *J Cardiovasc Nurs* 7(4):30-37, 1993.
9. DeVries M: *How to run a meeting,* New York, 1994, Penguin Books.
10. Eposito L: Home health case management: rural caregiving, *Home Health Care Nurs* 12(3):38-43, 1994.
11. Feldman C et al: Decision making in case management of home health care clients, *JONA* 23(1):33-44, 1993.
12. Goodwin D: Critical pathways in home health care, *JONA* 22:35-40, 1992.
13. Grohar-Murray M, DiCroce H: *Leadership and management in nursing,* Norwalk, Conn, 1992, Appleton & Lange.
14. Hawkins J, Goldberg P: Planning, implementing and evaluating a chemotherapy critical pathway, *Oncology Med* March/April:24-29, 1994.
15. Health Care Financing Administration: *Health insurance manual,* Pub No 11 -Thru T273, Rev 3/95, Washington, DC, 1995, US Department of Health and Human Services.
16. Jaffe M, and Skidmore-Roth L: *Home health nursing care plans,* ed 2, St Louis, 1993, Mosby.
17. Johnson K, Morrison E: Control or negotiation: a health care challenge, *NAQ* 17(3):27-33, 1993.
18. Lyon J: Models of nursing care delivery and case management: clarification of terms, *Nurs Econ* 11(3):163-165, 1993.
19. Marelli T: Care paths, *Home Care Nurs News* 2(4):1-3, 1995.
20. Marquis B, Huston C: *Leadership roles and management functions in nursing: theory and application,* Philadelphia, 1992, JB Lippincott.
21. Migchelbrink D et al: Population-based managed care: one hospital's experience, *NAQ* 17(3):45-53, 1993.
22. Molloy K: Defining case management, *Home Health Care Nurs* 12(3):51-54, 1994.
23. Mullahy C: Case manager and physicians: working associates, not adversaries, *Case Manager* 3(2):62-68, 1992.
24. Nurse Executive News Scan, 1993.
25. Nyberg D, Marschke P: Critical pathways: tools for continuous quality improvement, *NAQ* 17(3):62-69, 1993.
26. Packard N: The price of choice: managed care in America, *NAQ* 17(3):8-15, 1993.
27. Rice R: *Reported findings of average caseload and visit frequency.* Unpublished national survey of home health nurses conducted during 1994. Funded by American Nursing Development, Maryville, Ill, 1995.
28. Trinidad E: Case management: a model of CNS practice, *Clin Nurs Special* 7(4):221-223, 1994.
29. Wess R: *Victory secrets of Attila the Hun,* New York, 1993, Dell Publishing.
30. Zander K: Nursing case management: resolving the DRG paradox, *Nurs Clin North Am* 23(93):503-520, 1980.

Appendix 8-1

Care Path (CP) Standard: Skin/Integumentary System

Physician _____   Primary diagnosis_____

Case manager_____   Secondary diagnosis_____

ADM date_____   _____

DC date_____   Surgical procedure(s) and dates_____

Certification period from _____ to _____   _____

Admission assessment and initial visit forms completed □

Identified nursing diagnosis/patient or caregiver health care needs (check as appropriate)

_____ 1. Impaired skin integrity
_____ 2. Impaired physical mobility
_____ 3. Knowledge deficit re: disease process, risk complications, health management, infection control, socioeconomic resources
_____ 4. Pain
_____ 5. Other (list) _____
_____

CP standard utilized: #1; (list if adjunct CP utilized): _____

Multidisciplinary services utilized (check as appropriate)

RN	□	PT/PTA □	MSW	□	Other: (list) [volunteer, chaplain, _____
LPN/LVN	□	OT/COTA □	RD/NT	□	other agencies,vendors,
HHA/HMK	□	ST	□	Specialty nursing	□	suppliers, etc.]

SN total visits _____   Rehabilitation services total visits _____

Personal care total visits _____   Other disciplines/services total visits _____

Patient education guides utilized: (check as appropriate)

_____ 1. Patient/caregiver home CP
_____ 2. Wound care
_____ 3. Infection control
_____ 4. Medications
_____ 5. Home safety
_____ 6. Other (list):   [skin care] _____
_____
_____

**Pressure relief/reduction devices or home medical
equipment utilized: (list)** _____
_____
_____

CP treatment codes:

T1. Wet to dry NS	T3. Topical moisturizer	T5. Calcium aginate	T6. See medication record
T2. Dry dressing	T4. Hydrocolloid	Other: (list) [skin care] _____	

Care Path reproduced courtesy of American Nursing Development, Maryville, Ill.

Week 1   Progress toward meeting patient/
caregiver outcomes

Outcomes: [list code]   Variance(s): [list code-
Treatment: [list code]   OV; TV]

[Brief narrative of patient/caregiver progress with CP
including patient/caregiver learning, changes in
physician orders/treatments, or identified problems.
Utilize the variance tracking guide for problem
resolution or plan of action.]

Case manager's
signature:_____ Date: _____

Week 2   Progress toward meeting patient/
caregiver outcomes

Outcomes:_____ Variance(s):_____
Treatment:_____

Case manager's
signature:_____ Date:_____

Week 3   Progress toward meeting patient/
caregiver outcomes

Outcomes: _____ Variance(s):_____
Treatment: _____

Case manager's
signature: _____Date: _____

Week 4   Progress toward meeting patient/
caregiver outcomes

Outcomes: _____ Variance(s):_____
Treatment: _____

Case manager's
signature: _____Date: _____

Week 5   Progress toward meeting patient/
caregiver outcomes

Outcomes: _____Variance(s):   _____
Treatment: _____

Case manager's
signature: _____ Date: _____

Week 6   Progress toward meeting patient/
caregiver outcomes

Outcomes:_____ Variance(s):   _____
Treatment:_____

Case manager's
signature:_____ Date: _____

Week 7   Progress toward meeting patient/
caregiver outcomes

Outcomes:_____Variance(s):_____
Treatment:_____

Case manager's
signature: _____Date: _____

Week 8   Progress toward meeting patient/
caregiver outcomes

Outcomes:_____Variance(s):_____
Treatment:_____

Case manager's
signature: _____Date: _____

Week 9 Progress toward meeting patient/caregiver outcomes and discharge goals of care

Outcomes: _____Variance(s): _____

Treatment: _____

[*Brief narrative including medical reasons for patient discharge or need for recertification.
Were goals achieved? Were objectives or patient outcomes of care met?
Utilize the variance tracking guide for problem resolution or plan of action.*]

☐ Continue services

Identify outcomes with
related variances not met (list)_____
_____

Goals met? ☐ Yes ☐ No _____
_____

☐ Discharge
# of patient/caregiver outcomes_____
# of patient/caregiver outcomes met_____
% of patient/caregiver outcomes met _____
Goals met? ☐ Yes ☐ No
Discharge summary completed ☐

Case manager's
signature: _____ Date: _____

EVALUATION CRITERIA

Patient/caregiver discharge goal codes. The patient/caregiver:
G1. Will demonstrate knowledge of disease process and self-care management; skilled __ personal care __ other __
G2. Will stay outside of the hospital for three months
G3. Provide self-management for continued wound care; wound healed or no evidence of infection
G4. Will be satisfied with the CP and delivery of home health agency services
G5. Other (list) _____
_____

Patient/caregiver outcomes of care codes. The patient/caregiver:	Date/Week	Met	Not met	N/A
(Summarize at end of cert. period.)				
O1. Demonstrates correct medication regimen	—	—	—	—
O2. Demonstrates correct diet regimen	—	—	—	—
O3. Demonstrates correct wound and skin care regimen	—	—	—	—
O4. Identifies complication of disease process to report to case manager; physician	—	—	—	—
O5. Identifies community resources to buy food and pay bills; LTC placement				
O6. Verbalizes when to call 911 for help	—	—	—	—
O7. Demonstrates correct use of equipment and home safety precautions				
O8. Agrees to CP by explaining treatment principles, purpose/use of multidisciplinary services, and length of service(s) without prompting of nurse	—	—	—	—
O9. Achieves maximal rehabilitation potential: ADLS __ Ambulation __ Other __	—	—	—	—
O10. Achieves optimal response to treatment plan (physician) evidenced by wound healing	—	—	—	—
O11. Other (list)_____				

Variance codes:
V1. Learning difficulties/comprehension deficits
V2. Noncompliance; nonparticipation; self-neglect
V3. Exacerberation of disease process
V4. Lack of adequate response to medical treatment plan
V5. Lack of caregiver or family to assist with care
V6. Lack of socioeconomic resources to support home health care needs
V7. Infection
V8. Rehospitalization (state reason) _____
V9. Other (explain) _____
_____
_____

Variance Tracking Guide

CP standard# _____

Date	OV-TV	Problem resolution	Initials
	[*list codes*]	[*brief description of action plan*]	

Patient/Caregiver Care Path: Home Guide

Hello and **welcome** to_____ home health agency. The home health agency has been asked to visit you for _____ and related medical care so that you can reach your best level of health.

Our services will be approximately [*state visit frequency or projected length of service*]. During this time we will be following your physician's orders for your medical treatment. We will also be sharing information with you about how to get better and make the best decisions for your health!

During our services we will be following a plan of care designed specifically for your medical diagnosis. We call this plan of care a care path because it outlines all the important information, services, and medical treatment you will need to improve your health. We will periodically review your specific care path with you. This way you will always be updated and informed about your medical treatments, the delivery of the home health agency's services, and your progress with your care path.

A copy of your care path will be kept in a folder in your home to review at your convenience.

Your care path has specific tasks which we call outcomes of care for you and your nurse or therapist to accomplish in order to improve your health. These outcomes involve assisting you to manage your health care needs at home. For example, we will be teaching you how and when to take your medicines. Most important you will have an opportunity to add to your care path for your specific learning needs. Our philosophy is that **YOU HAVE A SAY IN YOUR HEALTH CARE!**

The care path is directed by your physician and carried out by your primary nurse or therapist. We call your primary nurse or therapist a case manager because they will coordinate all of your care including any additional services provided to you by the home health agency and your community. Your case manager's name is _____. Your case manager can be reached at _____.

Your case manager will go over your care path with you and update it each week. When you are ready for discharge, we will ask you to fill out a brief survey to let us know what you thought of your care while receiving our services. We appreciate your ideas and suggestions! Always call and speak with your case manager or physician if you have any questions or concerns regarding your health or the delivery of your health care services.

Thank you for choosing _____. We value you as an important customer and wish you great success with your care path!

Patient name:_____
Admission date:_____
Certification period: To: _____From:_____
Primary diagnosis or reasons for home visits: _____
_____
CP standard #:_____
Case manager's signature:_____ Date:_____

Care Path reproduced courtesy of American Nursing Development, Maryville, Ill.

Patient/Caregiver Guide: CP Standard#_____

Based on our assessment of your primary diagnosis and your individual needs, the following is a list of tasks which we call outcomes that we would like you to achieve during our services. We believe that achieving these outcomes improves your chances of getting better and being ready for discharge. The outcomes of care that we would like to help you accomplish during [*state visit frequency or projected length of service*] are: (list CP outcomes; consider revising them to the patient's level of understanding)

Patient/caregiver outcomes   **Date/Week met**

You may also benefit from other home health agency services such as the home health aide, physical therapist, or social worker. Talk to your case manager to see if these services are right for you. Services utilized: (list)

[*state discipline and visit frequency*]

Do you agree to work with us on your care path?   ❐ Yes   ❐No

Is there anything else you would like to learn or do in order to get better? If so, list them below and we'll try to help you with this.

Patient/caregiver signature:_____Date:_____
Case manager's signature:_____Date:_____

Patient/Caregiver Guide: CP Standard#_____

Date	Vital signs, treatments, progress meeting patient/caregiver outcomes	Initials

Patient/Caregiver Discharge Survey: CP Standard#_____

We would appreciate it if you would take a few minutes to complete the following survey. Check the boxes below as appropriate. Please mail the survey to us in the enclosed, preaddressed envelope at your earliest convenience.

Yes	No	
❐	❐	1. Did you feel that your care path helped you understand your medical treatment and the purpose of your home health services?
❐	❐	2. Did you feel that your care path allowed you to be involved in your own health care decisions?
❐	❐	3. Were you satisfied with your physician's care?
❐	❐	4. Were you satisfied with your patient care? Nursing __ Therapy __ Aide __ Other __
❐	❐	5. Were you satisfied with the medical supplies and equipment services you received?
❐	❐	6. Were your educational guides and the instructions given to you by your case manager helpful in assisting you to learn about your health?
❐	❐	7. Did you feel your case manager adequately answered your questions and addressed your health concerns?

If you answered "no" to any of the questions above, could you briefly tell us why? This is your opportunity to let us know what you liked or disliked about our services and let us know if there is anything we can do to improve our services.

Comments

We thank you for selecting_____as your home health agency. If we can serve you or your family in the future, please do not hesitate to let us know!

9 Quality Patient Care

Saundra J. Triplett and *Robyn Rice*

Thanks to the philosophies of Demming, Juran, and Crosby, American businesses (yes, home health is a business) are focusing their attention on *leading* as well as managing and *continually improving* standards for quality service.[8] This new focus is expanding the responsibility of quality patient care beyond the home health nurse to the collaborative work of the entire home health agency, from administration on down.

Home health nurses are a critical component in this movement, from assuring the presence of quality patient care (*quality assurance* or QA) to continually improving quality patient care (*quality improvement* or QI). Home health nurses have the knowledge, experience, and commitment needed to define, monitor, evaluate, and improve nursing patient care practices and outcomes.[22] Home health nurses also have experience working with both eager and uneager patients when teaching them how to manage their health care. These experiences and people skills are valuable resources to bring to the multidiscipline and multisystem QI committees or related work groups. Last, but not least, home health nurse involvement keeps patient care practices and outcomes realistic.

The purpose of this chapter is to take the mystery out of QI. It is not a new concept. We discuss how the concepts of QI build on professional expertise that requires a commitment to continually improve professional standards of practice and patient care outcomes.

This chapter introduces the home health nurse to this agencywide approach to QI by recognizing everyone's contribution to quality patient care. This approach puts the home health nurse and

multidisciplinary team who are responsible for the delivery and/or support of patient care, in charge of defining, monitoring, measuring, and identifying potential and real quality patient care problems. The home health nurse and multidisciplinary team are also responsible for solving the problems and evaluating improved practices or processes. The home health nurse, who is responsible for the delivery and coordination of patient care, contributes to this approach by **determining** *which* patient care services are needed, *how* patient care services are to be delivered, and *what* are the optimal patient care outcomes. This chapter builds on the groundwork laid in previous chapters that discussed service delivery and documentation issues, as well as case management and leadership strategies in home care. This chapter further empowers home health nurses to effect optimal outcomes of care yet maintain professional standards of practice.

CONCEPTS OF QUALITY IMPROVEMENT: BACK TO THE ROOTS

QI is not a new approach. Concepts of QI were utilized by Florence Nightingale during the Crimean War. In 1854 the British government sent Nightingale and 40 nurses to a 1,700 bed hospital in Scutari, Turkey. There they were to care for over 3,000 British soldiers who were dying of battlefield injuries and "contagious fever." Nightingale and her nurses saw the results of overcrowding and knew that care practice improvements were needed to prevent the deaths caused by poor sanitary practices. To gain the British government's support in improving the care practices and reducing the death rate, Nightingale reported the differences in practices and death rates between the Turkish military hospital and the military hospital in Manchester, England. The variances were astounding: a 42% mortality rate in Turkey, and a 2% mortality rate in England. Through Nightingale's persistence and success in gaining the government's support, the practice improvements were implemented and the hospital mortality rates in the Crimea matched those in Manchester.[21] The following summarizes Florence Nightingale's approach, which reflects the nursing process, as related to today's QI concepts:

1. Identify real *or potential* problem(s) by identifying and monitoring indicators or measures of patient care outcomes.
2. Define the care practices *or processes* being followed.
3. Use your own and others' knowledge and experience to identify ways to improve care practices or processes to improve results or outcomes.
4. Gain the necessary support to try new care practices or processes.
5. Use visual, not just written, descriptions to improve analysis and understanding (for example, flowcharts, graphs, surveys, case studies, pareto charts, fish-bone diagrams). Program evaluation then becomes both quantitative and qualitative in nature.
6. Compare the improved process results with previous results to identify the degree of improvement or variance.
7. Reach for and achieve increasing levels of performance, including those with other businesses (benchmarking).
8. Continue the process to continually maintain and/or improve outcomes.

This approach is the basis for QI and quality management, as discussed in Chapter 8. It recognizes the system in which we work (not individuals) as the primary barrier to quality patient care delivery and optimal outcomes. It focuses a review of problems, by those at all levels, to create better overall understanding, communication, and improvements that could not be achieved by one level working alone. It puts the power for change

---

QUALITY CONCEPTS

1. Quality can be defined and measured.
2. Quality is dynamic. It is not simply achieved and then disregarded.
3. Quality is the primary source of cost reduction.
4. Quality has to do with doing the "right" things right.
5. Quality relates to outcome.
6. Quality is everyone's responsibility.

Source: Katz J, Green E: *Managing quality: a guide to monitoring and evaluating nursing services,* St Louis, 1992, Mosby.

(improvements) into the hands of those involved in the process (empowerment).[8]

The box above lists concepts related to quality. In addition, there are six key elements to a successful home health QI program:

1. There must be acceptance and support by the home health agency administration—the leaders.
2. All others must know and believe #1.
3. Home health agency leaders must support and promote collaborative input and decision making from others.
4. Active involvement and teamwork are needed among home health agency clinical and support staff and nonagency workers involved in the services the agency provides (for example, community resources, patients, equipment suppliers, infusion companies, contract workers).
5. Commitment is needed from the top down to make customer satisfaction the agency's number one goal. Customers include patients, families, physicians, employees and ancillary staff, and related services/suppliers.
6. There must be a continuous drive to meet and improve all agency functions and a focus on improving industry quality goals.

Like Florence Nightingale and nurses of yesteryear, home health nurses of today are responsible for the delivery of quality patient care. Likewise, leaders in health care are responsible for supporting the nurse (and all others) in this ongoing effort.

Table 9-1 Comparing QA and QI paradigms [4,10,12,20]

Old QA paradigm	New QI paradigm
Leadership is vertical.	Leadership is horizontal with shared governance.
QA chairperson is responsible for the agency's quality program.	QA/QI chairperson facilitates and supports the QI program.
Problems are identified through failure reporting: deficiency chart audits, state and accreditation surveys, and patient complaints.	Systems and outcomes are monitored for immediate and overtime variances in appropriateness, effectiveness, and efficiency.
Problems are caused by people.	Problems are typically caused by systems (85%) rather than people (15%).
Management is responsible for creating new systems and fixing problems.	Customers and workers are a vital resource into the elimination of problems and the creation of effective systems.
Quality is attained when the standard is met.	A quality measure is an ever-increasing target.
Costs go up when QI is implemented.	Cost savings are made in improved systems, increased satisfaction of workers and patients, and elimination of rework.
Management knows best what *their* customers need.	Internal (workers) and external (patients, suppliers, etc.) customers provide valuable input into *our* home health programs.
Comparisons between home health and other businesses are not practical. Home health is too different.	Comparisons with other businesses that are known for prompt service, 24-hour availability, delivery exactness, customer satisfaction, and worker involvement give home health new ideas for problem solving.
Comparisons within the same industry are based on financial and volume data.	Quality outcome indicator testing, standardized data sets, and assessments provide home health agencies with quality care comparison tools.
Quality is hard to define and quantify.	Quality is defined and qualified by internal (workers) and external (patients, physicians, suppliers) customers.

SHIFTING PARADIGMS: QA TO QI

A shift in paradigms is occurring in the assessment of quality patient care (Table 9-1). The move is toward identification of indicators or criteria that help signal actual or potential patient care problems. Whereas QA monitored for compliance to standards, QI monitors for improvement opportunities.[6,12,15,20,23] The QI program builds on the QA program by *quantifying* and *qualifying* structure, process, and outcome standards. The result is the creation of indicators (measures and signals) of real or potential patient care quality problems.

Most home health QA programs originally focused on nursing or clinical services, as a means of ensuring compliance with Medicare's Home Health Conditions of Participation and, where required, annual state licensure. Initially the QA program reported the adherence to structure and process standards through deficiency (negative) ratings to minimum ratings of structure, process, or outcome standards. (See the Theoretical Framework section later in this chapter for definitions of structure, process, and outcome standards.) In its shifting, compliance ratings (positive) replaced deficiency ratings and 100% compliance replaced minimum standards. Outcome measures or indicators have gained significance over structure or process standards.[12,15,20,22]

The composition of the quality committee has shifted to represent agencywide services. Traditionally the QA committee was primarily composed of nursing staff (Figure 9-1). Current trends in QI now involve staff from all divisions. The philosophy of QI recognizes everyone's contribution in the delivery of quality patient care (Figure 9-2).

The key to a successful QI program is a shift to administration strategies that *provide* the vision and spirit for the new effort, *demonstrate* a belief that quality patient care is everyone's responsibility, and *create* an environment that encourages inquiry and the creative effort needed to achieve ever-increasing quality patient care goals.

In shifting from a QA to a QI paradigm, the QI program must be allowed to grow by both successes and failures. Involved staff must be empowered to address their own patient care practices and processes, and encouraged—through teamwork—to improve patient care outcomes.

QI COMMITTEE WORK

The QI committee's composition involves key individuals representing all agency divisions. To keep this program reality-based, emphasis is placed on the collaboration and involvement of (1) agency staff who are implementing and supporting patient care services, (2) patients who are receiving or have received services, (3) physicians who refer or may refer to the agency, and (4) suppliers who work with the agency to provide home medical equipment, medical supplies, infusion therapy products, or other services. (See Chapter 8 for tips in chairing a committee.)

A list of agency information and report sources is the best place for the committee to start. The QI committee should evaluate the source for its usefulness in its present state; update it to better reflect the defined measurements needed, or eliminate or replace it with a better information (data collection) source. Information sources include, but are not limited to, the following:

- Compliment/complaint files
- Deaths within 48 hours of admission
- Discharge status reports
- Financial reports for overall costs and for patient specific costs
- Medical record reviews reports
- Patient and staff incident reports

- Patient and staff new and continuing infection reports
- Patient demographics for diagnosis, services, supplies, length of stays, discharge codes, etc.
- Patient satisfaction surveys
- Peer clinical management reviews
- Physician satisfaction surveys
- Policies and procedures (easier to use when in a flowchart form)
- Recertification reports for goal achievement(s) of maintaining, progressing, or decreasing status
- Rehospitalization lists
- Service complications not recorded elsewhere (for example, hematoma after blood draws, UTI after catheterization, increasing wound size)
- Staff (employee) surveys
- Supervisor visit reports
- Team conference reports
- Other sources unique to the home health agency.

If the agency records are computerized, a data processing representative or knowledgeable computer person should serve on the QI committee or be available on an ad hoc basis. The data processing representative's knowledge and expertise to access available data, modify present systems, and improve available data, is a valuable resource to the QI program.

The QI Committee should develop a mission statement summarizing the agency's commitment to serving the public and the agency's goals of service. Standards of care will then flow from the mission statement and reflect service delivery. The committee can then *define, measure, evaluate,* and *improve* important aspects of patient care. The QI committee should also look at the *cost vs benefit* of patient care practice or process. (This will be discussed in greater detail later in this chapter.)

THEORETICAL FRAMEWORK

A number of theorists have conceptualized quality improvement. Deming, Juran, and Crosby emphasize quality improvement with a leadership open to change and ideas.[6,8] Goals of leadership are to involve all employees in agency policy and decision making. Customer-mindedness permeates such organizations.

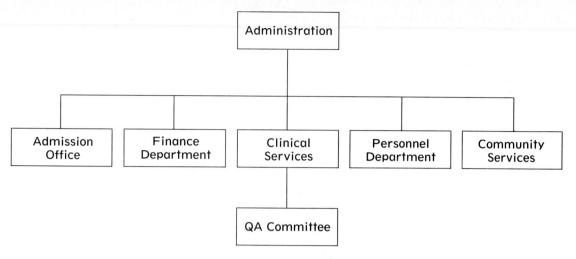

Figure 9-1 Historical QA program structure.

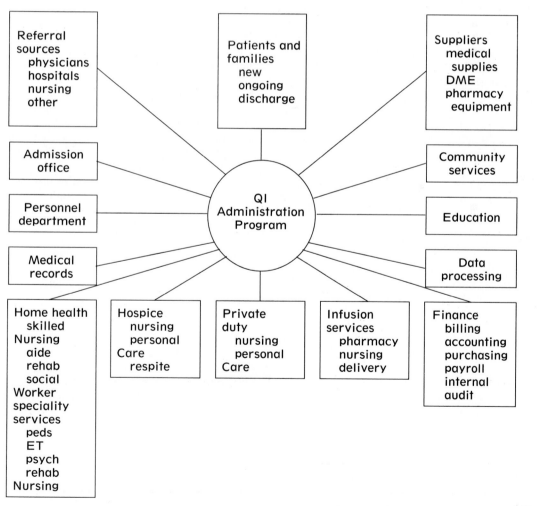

Figure 9-2 Contemporary QI program structure.

The Marker model

Carolyn Smith-Marker developed the Marker model to facilitate the development and implementation of standards that are useful in the QI program.[14] The Marker model reflects Donabedian's framework of structure, process and outcome standards of care.[5]

Structure standards define how a system operates. They *encompass all aspects of the* home health system except the process of giving care and the desired outcomes. They define optimal conditions that support staff function, agency operation, and patient care. *Expressed as policy, structure standards have legal, regulatory, and professional implications.* Because of this, Medicare regulations and state licensure requirements form the basis for each home health agency's operational policies and procedures or structural standards.

Process standards define the actions, knowledge, and skills needed to provide quality patient care. These standards make up the bulk of any agency's set of standards because they cover such a wide range of nursing activities and patient care. They can be directed toward the home health nurse, another discipline, or the patient. Process standards may assume many different forms: job descriptions, performance standards, procedures, protocols, guidelines, and patient standards of care.

Outcome standards specify the end to be achieved. These standards define the benefit from the service or care received.[19] The home health nurse and other disciplines use outcome standards as short-term and long-term goals in the patient care plan. (See Chapter 4 for information about developing outcomes of care.)

In the Marker model, *structure* defines home health agency organization including staff qualifications, *processes* defines policies and procedures for appropriate service delivery, and *outcomes* identifies the expected patient service results.

QI PROGRAM COMPONENTS

The QI committee should identify what aspects of the home health agency's service is to be evaluated. The Joint Commission on the Accreditation of Healthcare Organizations (JCAHO) refers to these categories as "important aspects of (patient) care."[7,9] Key patient services, as well as regulatory issues, help determine and prioritize the important aspects of patient care. For example, patient satisfaction should always be an important aspect of care. In a customer-driven business such as home health, patient satisfaction with the delivery of home health services is always an expected outcome. A key element in obtaining JCAHO accreditation is to provide evidence of patient satisfaction with both skilled (RN, PT, OT, ST, MSW) and nonskilled (aide, homemaker) services.[9]

To get started the QI committee should select two or three areas that are significant and feasible to examine. Important aspects of care can be ranked according to high-volume service needs, high-risk patients, or intrinsically problem-prone areas in order to help the committee discuss their options and develop a plan of action (Table 9-2).

MEASURING QUALITY
Indicators

Indicators serve as signals of potential or actual problems or barriers to the delivery of quality patient care. They do this by *quantifying* and

Table 9-2 Identification of important aspects of care grid

Important aspect of care	High-volume	High-risk	Problem-prone
Physician satisfaction	Yes	Potential	Potential
Infection control	No	Yes	Yes
Service delivery	No	Yes	Potential
High-tech services	Yes	No	No
Typical home health			
Complication and/or complaint resolution	No	Potential	Yes
Risk management (for example, incidents)	No	Yes	Yes

qualifying patient care events identified as important aspects of care. *Quantifying* means counting the number of events compared to all events. This is best presented in a ratio:[10]

$$\frac{\text{Number of patients for whom a}}{\text{specified event occurs}}$$
$$\frac{}{\substack{\text{Number of patients experiencing condition or} \\ \text{procedure that indicator is measuring}}}$$

For example:

$$\frac{\substack{\text{Number of patients with hematomas} \\ \text{following venipuncture}}}{\text{Number of patients receiving venipuncture}}$$

Qualifying refers to the quality and appropriateness of the event. Quality indicators may measure efficacy, appropriateness, availability, timeliness, effectiveness, continuity, safety, efficiency, respect, and caring. For example:

$$\frac{\text{Number of patients involved in their own care decisions}}{\text{Number of all active patients}}$$

Indicators are categorized by the type and seriousness of the event they measure.[8,10,19]

Structure indicators measure whether or not agency policies are followed. For example, if the important aspect of care is timeliness and the agency policy states all patients are evaluated for admission within 24 hours of referral, the structure indicator may read:

$$\frac{\text{Number of patients evaluated within 24 hrs}}{\text{Number of patients admitted}}$$

This would be further categorized as a rate-based, desirable indicator.

Process indicators measure specific processes or steps critical to quality patient care. For example, the agency may define wound care management techniques or treatment in a standard of care based on the wound description. A rate-based, desirable process indicator may read:

$$\frac{\substack{\text{Number of wound-care patients} \\ \text{with management techniques}}}{\text{Number of wound-care patients}}$$

Outcome indicators measure what happens or does not happen after something is or is not done. For example, the agency may evaluate goal achievement based on the patient care plan. With effective-

ness as the important aspect of care, the rate-based, desired outcome indicator may read:

$$\frac{\text{Number of patients reaching stated goals}}{\text{Number of active patients}}$$

Desirable outcome indicators are expected to improve or be maintained. Unexpected or undesirable outcomes may include worsening of a condition, a new complication, rehospitalization, unexpected death.

To keep the QI program manageable, the selection of quality indicators should be based on the home health agency's services that have the greatest impact on care. When selecting the events or indicators, consider the following:[23]

1. Include large numbers of patients (for example, wound-care patients).
2. Include indicators that entail a high degree of risk for patients or produce problems for patients or staff (for example, acquired infections).
3. Involve low-volume but complex services, (for example, infusion therapy).

Patient satisfaction is a desired outcome in all home health services. As such it should be included in these three activities, and defined separately to gauge overall home health agency performance.

Involving patients is very helpful when the QI committee is defining and measuring patient satisfaction.[2,12,16,20] It is important to recognize that, when asked what is important regarding their health care needs, patients' perceptions may differ greatly from those of the agency.[20] To summarize, patient care standards define *quality* while quality indicators measure and monitor *quality.*

Threshold parameters or ranges

Indicators may be measured against threshold parameters (ranges) or finite numbers. Ranges allow for natural variances in the performance of the patient care standard. The range is determined by calculating a standard deviation for the sample used and determining an acceptable and safe deviation from the standard. The range may also be set by the committee members based on their knowledge, experience, and discussion of acceptable and unacceptable thresholds. Finite numbers give specific thresholds for the study group to achieve. When the number is less than 100% or more than 0% (depending on how the indicator is stated), variances are allowed as a rare occurrence.

Finite numbers are preferred because they are less ambiguous and keep the expectation simple and clear to the patient, nurse, and agency. For example, when monitoring staff availability as an important aspect of patient care, the indicator threshold may read 98% to 100%, or 100% of therapy cases opened within 2 days.

$$\frac{\text{Number of patients opened by PT within 2 days}}{\text{Number of patients with orders for PT services}}$$

Sentinel or undesirable indicators are always measured against finite thresholds because of their serious outcomes. For example, when monitoring **safety** as an important aspect of care, the outcome indicator threshold for patient falls may be 0%.

$$\frac{\text{Number of patient falls during}}{\text{direct patient contact (visit)}} \over \text{Number of patient contacts (visits)}$$

Safety of patient discharge should also be evaluated. This is especially important to do when the patient goals are not met and the patient is not being discharged to another health care delivery system. In addition, issues of patient safety are a prime consideration when working with a case management payment program with limited visits.

QI TOOLS

The following lists some scientific QI tools available to help the committee visualize a process, pinpoint problems, discover causes, and identify solutions:[8,18]

- Flowcharts or diagrams are excellent tools to use when reviewing the steps in a process. Self-stick notes are useful in developing and revising a flowchart because they can be moved quickly and the process steps are easily seen.
- Time plots and control charts are simple tools to plot points along a time line. Threshold parameters or numbers can be added to the chart to see if the values are above, below, within, or at the threshold parameter.

- Cause and effect or fish-bone diagrams are used to identify all the possible causes of a stated effect.
- Pareto charts are bar charts comparing two scales such as frequency vs cost.
- Scatter diagrams compare two variables such as time and frequency. The clustering of points shows the time the monitored event has the highest frequency.

The creation of charts has been made easier by computer spreadsheet and database software which allow data manipulation, make data display suggestions, compute complex formulas (such as standard deviations), and create charts with ease.

Analysis and evaluation

Once evaluation methods are identified, data is collected, analysis occurs, and evaluation follows. Effective groups for analysis are typically made up of five members plus a group leader.[18]

Variation and trending. Variation and trend reporting are two ways to analyze indicators not meeting threshold(s). Variation reporting is the variance from threshold for individual indicators on separate monitoring periods. Trend reporting is the threshold ratings from several monitoring periods plotted on a time graph.

These types of reports reveal the direction of trend lines as being stable, increasing, or decreasing. Trend lines are of special interest in evaluating care practices and identifying future program needs. For example, if pressure ulcers developed on patients during the course of services and the incidence was associated with bedbound or severely functionally limited patients, patient and nursing skin care practices may need to be altered to reduce the risk of pressure ulcer formation. As assessed by the home health nurse, such practices could be applied to all future patients who are at risk for pressure ulcer formation.

Analysis. The QI committee reviews the data; identifies the system, staff, or patient problem along with trends and variances; develops a corrective plan; and evaluates the indicator for improvement.[10]

Evaluation. To be effective, program evaluation must answer the following structure and process questions:

DEFINITIONS OF DIMENSIONS OF PERFORMANCE

Doing the right thing

- The **efficacy** of the procedure or treatment in relation to the patient's condition
- The degree to which the care or service for the patient has been shown to accomplish the desired or projected outcome(s)
- The **appropriateness** of a specific test, procedure, or service to meet the patient's needs
- The degree to which the care provided is relevant to the patient's clinical needs, given the current state of knowledge

Doing the right thing well

- The **availability** of a needed test, procedure, treatment, or service to the patient who needs it
- The degree to which appropriate care is available to meet the patient's needs
- The **timeliness** with which a needed test, procedure, treatment, or service is provided to the patient
- The degree to which the care is provided to the patient at the most beneficial or necessary time
- The **effectiveness** with which tests, procedures, treatments, and services are provided
- The degree to which the care is provided in the correct manner, given the current state of knowledge, to achieve the desired or projected outcome for the patient
- The **continuity** of the services provided over time to the patient with respect to other services, clinicians, and providers
- The degree to which the care of the patient is coordinated among services, among organizations, and across time
- The **safety** of the patient (and others) to whom the services are provided
- The degree to which the risk of an intervention and risk in the care environment are reduced for the patient and others, including the staff members
- The **efficiency** with which services are provided
- The relationship between the outcomes (results of care) and the resources used to deliver patient care
- The **respect and caring** with which services are provided
- The degree to which the patient or a designee is involved in his or her own care decisions and to which those providing services do so with sensitivity and respect for the patient's needs, expectations, and individual differences

Source: Joint Commission on Accreditation of Healthcare Organizations: *1995 Accreditation manual for home care,* vol 1, standards, Oakbrook Terrace, Ill, 1994, The Commission. Reprinted with permission.

- Was the care delivered according to agency policies and procedures? (*Structure*)
- Was the care delivered as ordered? (*Process*)

Program evaluation must also answer the following outcome-related questions:

- Was the delivered care *appropriate* to the patient need?
- Was the delivered care *effective* based on expected patient response and outcome?
- Was the delivered care *efficient* according to parameters defined by the agency, clinical path, or national statistics?

JCAHO offers clear definitions of QI terms that may be included in your agency's QI program. (See the box titled Definitions of Dimensions of Performance.)

COST VERSUS BENEFIT

Today health care consumers and payers want the best quality care for the lowest cost. This has created dramatic changes in the health care delivery system. Now cost accounting methods must give not only overall costs by expense categories but also costs by specific patient service or condition type. This emphasis on costing services is being led by managed care providers who are gatekeeping

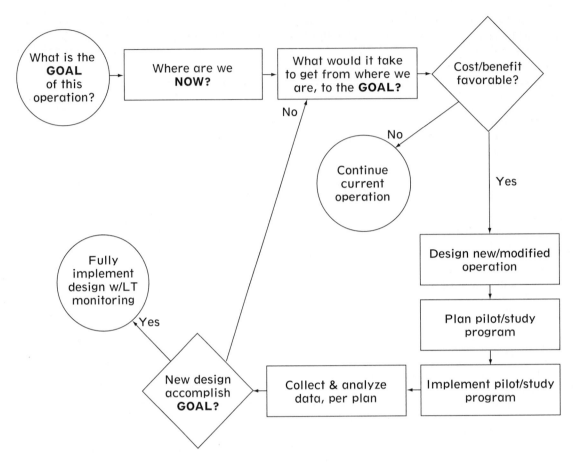

Figure 9-3 DHHS organizational performance improvement process. (Courtesy Deaconness Home Health Services, St Louis, Mo.)

home health and other health care services. Home health staff must be able to look at the mix and cost of services they provide and, based on the achieved patient outcomes, maintain or improve their competitive place in the home health market.

Never before have two opposing groups needed each other more: administration and staff. Both have much to offer the other in improving agency systems and practices in order to achieve better patient outcomes. In the past, administration may

have focused on costs while staff focused on quality. The QI committee now serves as a melting pot for both focuses to be addressed.

Paying more or less for a product does not always mean the product is better or worse. The same may be said of a service such as home health care. By defining and measuring important aspects of patient care, the QI committee and agency staff become aware of the cost of quality care. When alternatives or revisions are needed, the cost benefits of the change must be analyzed for more informed decision making. Acknowledging the importance of the budget, tempered by a concern for quality patient care, is the heart of an effective QI program. (See Figure 9-3 for an illustration of the cost performance process.)

FUTURE PERSPECTIVES

The momentum for quality outcome indicators and their acceptance is growing.[23] JCAHO has developed and is testing home health infusion indicators and will score them nationally in 1996.[7]

The Community Health Accreditation Program (CHAP)"In Search of Excellence in Home Care" project, funded by the W. K. Kellogg Foundation, is currently (1) defining quality outcomes using consumer input, (2) developing a system to assess quality using these outcomes, and (3) incorporating the process into CHAP's accreditation process. The home health quality management plan includes 11 quality pulse points divided into the consumer, clinical, and organizational categories. The six consumer pulse points are consumer, empowerment, caregiver relationship, knowledge/information needs, family support, and consumer expectations. The two clinical pulse points are functional ability and physiological functioning. The four organizational pulse points are team building, commitment to quality, coordination of care, and financial viability.[15]

A study conducted by the Center for Health Policy Research and the Center for Health Services Research at the University of Colorado Health Sciences Center has published a set of quality indicator groups (QUIGs) to measure changes in health status, in specific conditions, at various points of time.[13,19] The principal investigator is Peter W. Shaughnessy. Patient data from 49 home health agencies were used to define and measure patient care outcomes. The study population was 3,427 patients including 729 non-Medicare patients. Funded by the Health Care Financing Administration (HCFA), the outcome measurement system proposed in the study is expected to be the focus of the Medicare survey process. Figure 9-4 and Appendix 9-1 list the acute and chronic conditions which have identified indicators, examples of the conditions, and an example of the outcome measures.[19]

The QI paradigm will continue to influence home health nursing in the years to come. Why?

- It provides the basis for the most extensive definition, evaluation, and advancement of home health nursing practice today.
- It offers a model for continual improvement which has application in everything the home health nurse does both professionally and personally.
- It expands home health nursing teams to a multidiscipline, multisystem (interdependent) team model for improving patient care systems and solving patient care problems. Just as no one piece is more important than the whole, home health nurses accomplish more working together than separately. As individuals we are limited by our knowledge and experience, together we expand our limits to that of the group.[3]

SUMMARY

However quality is defined and measured, every home health patient wants it and every agency wants to deliver it.[2] The direction of home health quality and performance improvement programs is clear: every home health agency activity should be directed toward achieving the best possible care for each patient.[1]

In the final analysis, the quality of patient care is only as good as the involvement and commitment of the home health agency to achieve that quality. The extent to which agency operations provide quality patient care will depend on the support of the agency leaders and active involvement of the agency staff with the commitment of home health nurses in defining the QI process. Home health nurses are needed to keep quality patient care the focus of all agency operations and to promote professional standards of practice.

Self-directed home health nurses ultimately **have** the power to effect improvements in the delivery of services and to participate in other QI functions. This promotes nurses' autonomy and responsibility for meeting the health care needs of the public today and tomorrow. For it is recognized that"no one owns healing" and those who evaluate the performance of a profession control it.

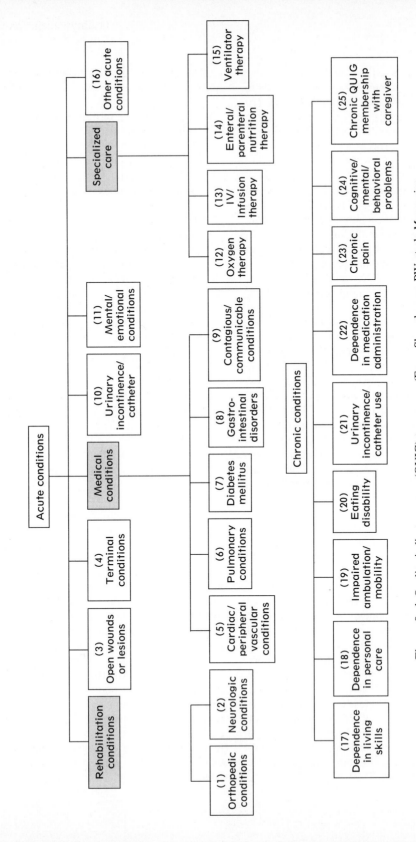

Figure 9-4 Quality indicator group (QUIG) taxonomy. (From Shaughnessy PW et al: *Measuring outcomes of home health care*, Denver, 1994, Center for Health Policy Research, University of Colorado Health Sciences Center.)

REFERENCES

1. Berhang-Doggett J, Lowenstein A: Quality assurance: achieving compliance with home care regulations, *Caring* 10:37-43, 1991.
2. Brook R Ellwood P, Berwick D: Assessing quality of care: three different approaches, *Bus Health* August:27-42, 1990.
3. Covey SR: *The 7 habits of highly effective people: powerful lessons in personal change,* New York, 1990, Simon & Schuster.
4. Dienemann J: *C Q I: continuous quality improvement in nursing,* Washington, DC, 1992, American Nurses Publishing.
5. Donabedian A: *Explorations in quality assessment and monitoring, vol 2, The definition of quality and approaches to its assessment,* Ann Arbor, Mich, 1980, Health Administration Press.
6. Hawk AB, Miyamuara JB: Quality improvement: how does it differ from quality assurance? *Hawaii Med J* 52(2):34, 36-37, 1993.
7. Joint Commission on Accreditation of Healthcare Organizations: *Primer on indicator development and application: measuring quality in health care,* Oakbrook Terrace, Ill, 1990, The Commission.
8. Joint Commission on Accreditation of Healthcare Organizations: *Quality improvement in home care,* Oakbrook Terrace, Ill, 1993, The Commission.
9. Joint Commission on Accreditation of Healthcare Organizations: *1995 Accreditation manual for home care,* volume 1, standards, Oakbrook Terrace, Ill, 1994, The Joint Commission.
10. Katz J, Green E: *Managing quality: a guide to monitoring and evaluating nursing services,* St Louis, 1992, Mosby.
11. Kramer AM, Shaughnessy PW, Bauman MK, Crisler KS: Assessing and assuring the quality of home health care: a conceptual framework, *Milbank* 68(3):413-443, 1990.
12. Largen CW: Bringing quality to the customer: a new paradigm for quality managers, *J Nurs Care Qual* 8(2):81-84, 1994.
13. Mann L: HCFA-sponsored study to yield outcome measures, *Home Health Line* 191(31):7, 1993.
14. Marker C: *Nursing standards* (audiocassette), Baltimore, 1985, Resource Applications.
15. Peters DA: A new look for quality in home care, *JONA* 22(11):21-26, 1992.
16. Riley PA, Fortinsky RH, Coburn AF: Developing consumer-centered quality assurance strategies for home care, *J Case Man* 1(2):39–48, 1992.
17. Saba VK: Diagnoses and interventions, *Caring* 3:50-57, 1992.
18. Scholtes PR: *The team handbook: how to use teams to improve quality,* Madison, Wis, 1988, Joiner Associates.
19. Shaughnessy PW et al: *Measuring outcomes of home health care,* Denver, 1994, Center for Health Policy Research, University of Colorado Health Sciences Center.
20. Smit J, Spoelstra S: Do patients and nurses agree? *Caring* 10:34-36, 1991.
21. Swanson JE, Albrecht M: *Community health nursing: promoting the health of aggregates,* Philadelphia, 1993, W B Saunders.
22. Wagner DM: QA in home care: the staff nurse's challenge, *JHQ* 14(2):30-32, 1992.
23. Wagner DM: Quality indicators: an approach to quality improvement in home healthcare, *JHQ* 14(3):8-10, 1992.
24. Zlotnick C, Decker R: Home visiting outcomes and quality of life measures, *J Community Health Nurs* 8(4):207-214, 1991.

Appendix 9-1

Quality Indicator Groups

QUALITY INDICATOR GROUPS (QUIGs) WITH EXAMPLES OF SELECTED CONDITIONS[11]

Acute conditions

QUIG no	Description of QUIGs and examples
1	Acute orthopedic conditions (e.g., fracture, amputation, joint replacement, DJD)
2	Acute neurologic conditions (e.g., CVA, multiple sclerosis, head injury)
3	Open wounds or lesions (e.g., pressure ulcers, surgical wounds, stasis ulcers)
4	Terminal conditions (e.g., palliative care for malignant neoplasms, advanced cardiopulmonary disease, end-stage AIDS)
5	Acute cardiac/peripheral vascular conditions (e.g., CHF, angina, coronary artery disease, hypertension, myocardial infarction)
6	Acute pulmonary conditions (e.g., COPD, pneumonia, pulmonary edema)
7	Diabetes mellitus*
8	Acute gastrointestinal disorders (e.g., gastric ulcer, diverticulitis, constipation with changing treatment approaches, ostomies, liver disease)
9	Contagious/communicable conditions (e.g., hepatitis, tuberculosis, AIDS, salmonella)
10	Acute urinary incontinence/catheter*
11	Acute mental/emotional conditions (e.g., anxiety disorder, depression, bipolar disorder)
12	Oxygen therapy*
13	IV/infusion therapy*
14	Enteral/parenteral nutrition therapy (e.g., TPN, gastrostomy/jejunostomy feeding)
15	Ventilator therapy*
16	Other acute conditions*

Chronic conditions

QUIG no	Description of QUIGs and examples
17	Dependence in living skills (e.g., meal preparation, housekeeping, laundry)
18	Dependence in personal care (e.g., bathing, dressing, grooming)
19	Impaired ambulation/mobility (e.g., ambulation, transferring, toileting)
20	Eating disability*
21	Urinary incontinence/catheter use*
22	Dependence in medication administration*
23	Chronic pain*
24	Chronic cognitive/mental/behavioral problems (e.g., Alzheimer's, confusion, agitation, chronic brain syndrome)
25	Chronic QUIG membership with caregiver*

*An example is not given since the QUIG name is sufficient to define the condition(s) included.
Source: Center for Health Policy and Services Research, Denver.

ILLUSTRATIVE GLOBAL AND FOCUSED OUTCOME MEASURES[11]

Outcome measures for all QUIGs (Global measures)

End-result outcomes and utilization outcomes

Functional outcome measures
   Improvement in ambulation
   Stabilization in ambulation
   Improvement in management of oral medications
   Improvement in patient/caregiver ability to manage equipment
Utilization outcome measures
   Acute hospitalization

Intermediate-result outcomes

Family/caregiver strain outcome measures
   Improvement in perceived ability to manage demands
   Stabilization in perceived ability to manage demands

Outcome measures for QUIG 5: acute cardiac/peripheral vascular conditions (focused measures)

End-result outcomes and utilization outcomes

Functional outcome measures
   Improvement in management of oral medications
Health status outcome measures
   Improvement in dyspnea
   Stabilization in weight
   Improvement in activity level
Utilization outcome measures
   Nonemergent MD/outpatient care for cardiac problems/medication side effects
   Emergent care in hospital, ER, or MD office for cardiac problem

Intermediate-result outcomes

Knowledge/skill compliance outcome measures
   Improvement in knowledge of contraindications to cardiac glycoside medication
   Stabilization in compliance with cardiac glycoside medications
   Stabilization in compliance with diuretics
   Improvement in knowledge of signs/symptoms to report

Outcome measures for QUIG 1: acute orthopedic conditions (focused measures)

End-result outcomes and utilization outcomes

Functional outcome measures
   Improvement in ambulation
   Stabilization in transferring
Health status outcome measures
   Improvement in pain
   Stabilization in pressure sores
Utilization outcome measures
   Emergent/urgent care (i.e., hospitalization, emergency room/clinic/office visit) resulting from fall
Acute care hospitalization

Source: Center for Health Policy and Services Research, Denver.

Continued

ILLUSTRATIVE GLOBAL AND FOCUSED OUTCOME MEASURES—cont'd

Intermediate-result outcomes

Family/caregiver strain outcome measures
  Improvement in perceived ability to manage demands
  Stabilization in perceived ability to manage demands
Knowledge/skill/compliance outcome measures
  Improvement in ambulation/walking/exercise program

Outcome measures for QUIG 24: chronic cognitive/mental/behavioral problems (focused measures)

End-result outcomes and utilization outcomes

Functional outcome measures
  Stabilization in communication ability
  Stabilization in socialization activities
  Stabilization in use of telephone
Health status outcome measures
  Stabilization in depression
  Stabilization in frequency of confusion
  Stabilization in frequency of behavioral problems
Unmet need outcome measures
  Improvement in unmet need for supervision

Intermediate-result outcomes

Knowledge/skill/compliance outcome measures
  Improvement in knowledge of safety
  Improvement in knowledge of medications
  Compliance with medications

PART

Clinical Application

10 The Patient with Chronic Obstructive Pulmonary Disease

Robyn Rice

Breathing, like the beating of our hearts, is largely taken for granted. Consider for a moment what life would be like if the simple act of breathing became an everyday struggle to survive. Picture the changes in our lives if we could not even walk from the kitchen table into the bathroom without becoming short of breath. These scenarios are real experiences and concerns of patients with chronic obstructive pulmonary disease (COPD).

COPD describes a group of diseases manifested by obstruction of the small airways within the lungs. Such diseases include chronic bronchitis, asthmatic bronchitis, and pulmonary emphysema.[11,32,38,40]

Chronic bronchitis is a clinical disorder caused by inflamed and edematous bronchial mucosa. Excessive mucus production results, producing a chronic, productive cough (minimum duration of 3 months per year for at least 2 successive years).[40]

Asthma is caused by bronchospasm and subsequent hypersecretion of mucus into the airways. Patients with asthma experience severe attacks of wheezing and coughing. Allergies, exertion, changes in temperature or environment, and emotional factors can trigger an asthmatic attack.[25] Childhood asthma is usually attributed to allergies and may dissipate as the child grows older.[31] Adult asthma, however, is associated with COPD. In adults with asthma, scarred and hypertrophied lung tissue resulting from repeated allergy attacks gives rise to asthmatic bronchitis.[31,40]

Emphysema is a pathological disorder characterized by destruction of lung tissue and overinflation of the small airways. Patients with emphysema develop structural defects in the lungs that hamper exhalation. Collapse of airways and subsequent air trapping prevent these patients from exhaling the "old" air and inhaling fresh, oxygenated air.[11,31,38]

COPD is a progressive, debilitating disease for which, at present, there is no cure.[11,26] At the time of initial diagnosis, usually some degree of irreversible damage to the lungs is already present.[31]

Symptoms of COPD may begin with a chronic, productive cough, repeated "chest" colds, and dyspnea or "shortness of breath" upon exertion.[39] The underlying problem of all COPD patients is a decrease of air flow in and out of the lungs.[21,22] Hypoventilation, shunting, diffusion impairment, and—most commonly—ventilation-perfusion abnormalities contribute to hypoxemia and the severe dyspnea experienced by this group.[40]

Advanced stages of COPD are characterized by a decline in mental and physical functioning, decreased activity levels, heart failure, and recurrent pulmonary infections.[26] Pulmonary infections can precipitate acute respiratory failure and are a frequent cause of repeated hospitalizations.

The purpose of this chapter is to review what is known about COPD to assist home health nurses in developing a plan of care for these patients. Patient education emphasizing home pulmonary rehabilitation and ongoing biopsychological interventions recommended in this chapter can be used to (1) prevent exacerbations of disease, (2) promote self-care management for patients and their families, and (3) offer patients with COPD respite from the enormous financial and emotional stressors associated with hospitalization. It is likely that home health nurses will visit many patients with COPD because of the large number of reported cases in the United States.

EPIDEMIOLOGY

Nearly 26 million Americans are now living with chronic lung disease.[2] As of 1994 the American Lung Association reported the incidence of chronic bronchitis to be estimated at 12.5 million, emphysema at 16.5 million, and asthma at 11.7 million. The estimated number of COPD sufferers has risen 41.5% since 1982.[2]

In 1994 the costs of respiratory diseases in the United States were estimated at $26.8 billion in direct costs, plus indirect costs of more than $29.5 billion—a total of $56.3 billion dollars.[2] These costs include lost earnings, hospital expenses, and disability payments. For example, people with asthma will experience well over a million days of restricted activity annually, and nearly 20% of them suffer self-care deficits with activities of daily living.[2]

The reported incidence of COPD is higher in urban areas and within lower socioeconomic classes.[2] Initial diagnosis is usually made between 30 and 50 years of age, and the course of the disease progresses for 25 to 30 years from origination to death.[11,28] COPD is more prevalent in men than in women and in smokers than in nonsmokers.[2,28] COPD is one of the primary chronic conditions afflicting the U.S. population and is now the fourth leading cause of death in the United States.[2] The most common causes of COPD-related deaths are respiratory insufficiency, pneumonia, and cor pulmonale.[26]

ETIOLOGY AND PATHOPHYSIOLOGY

Understanding the basics of alveolar gas exchange in relation to the structure of the lungs provides a framework for understanding the causes and effects of COPD. (See the box on page 159.)

Causes of COPD that determine specific disease manifestations are interrelated. They include smoking, environmental factors, and familial or hereditary factors.[2,4,35]

Smoking

Cigarette smoking is primarily responsible for nearly all COPD deaths.[2] Smoking destroys cilia lining the airways and represses the formation of alpha-antitrypsin (see the chapter section on Familial Factors). Excessive mucus production results when particles and irritants, previously cleared by the cilia, collect in the airways and cause inflammation and edema. A chronic cough develops. This further stimulates hypertrophy and hypersecretion of mucosal glands, which are characteristic of chronic bronchitis.

Ideally a sterile area, the lungs accumulate mucus and debris from continued smoking and become a breeding ground for infection.[6,24] Additionally, smoking encourages further migration of inflammatory cells into the lungs, which intensifies tissue irritation and edema. These repeated infections cause more damage, eventually destroying the smaller air passages and narrowing the larger ones.

Problems with airflow and hypersecretion of mucus create additional complications. For example, when oxygen does not reach the capillary network within the alveoli, the amount of oxygen in the blood decreases. In response, pulmonary vessels constrict. As a result, some areas of the lung will be well ventilated but have almost no blood flow while other areas may have good blood flow but no ventilation. This phenomenon, referred to as ventilation-perfusion imbalance, is common in chronic bronchitis and is related to obstruction of airways, poor ventilation of alveoli, and constriction of pulmonary vessels.[30,40] The net effect is low arterial oxygen content (hypoxemia) and increased concentrations of arterial carbon dioxide (hypercapnia).[38] As a consequence of vessel constriction, pulmonary hypertension develops. The heart must work harder to circulate blood through these narrowed vessels. In response to a magnified cardiac workload, the right ventricle thickens and enlarges. Right-sided failure, or cor pulmonale, can develop; and left-sided failure may follow.[40]

An increase in the production of red blood cells, or polycythemia, related to hypoxemia may also occur as a consequence of COPD.[26] Initially the increase in the number of oxygen-carrying red blood cells is helpful in compensating for hypoxemia. However, when the hematocrit exceeds 50%, blood viscosity increases so much that the blood actually clogs the vessels, which can lead to heart failure.[26]

Additional effects of hypoxemia result in a decreased blood flow to the kidneys. The glomerular filtration rate declines, and conservation of sodium occurs.[26,40] This promotes fluid retention and exacerbates heart failure.

THE PHYSIOLOGICAL RELATIONSHIP BETWEEN THE LUNGS AND COPD[26,39,40]

As air is inhaled, it moves through the upper airways where it is warmed, cleaned, and moisturized. Air then descends through the large and smaller airways and onward into the alveoli.

Cilia covered by a thin mucus layer (secreted by bronchial glands and goblet cells) line the epithelial airways. Cilia beat in a rhythmic, upward movement that impels the mucus layer toward the mouth and clears the lungs of debris left unfiltered by the upper airways. If mucus becomes too thick or if the amount is excessive, the cleaning action of the cilia is retarded. A cough is elicited in response to irritants or when the capability of the mucociliary system is overwhelmed. A chronic cough, however, is not a "normal" lung defense mechanism and suggests destruction of the mucociliary system.

Inflated with air, the alveoli become the final pathway for diffusion of oxygen and carbon dioxide. A fine capillary network from the pulmonary vessels brings blood to the membranes of the alveoli. Across these membrane surfaces, oxygen attaches and is transported in combination with hemoglobin (a component of red blood cells) to tissue capillaries where it is absorbed by tissues. Concurrently, as a by-product of metabolism, carbon dioxide moves out of the cells and eventually diffuses across pulmonary capillary membranes into the alveoli for exhalation.

During exhalation, elastic recoil and structural support of the airways force air out of the alveoli in preparation for inspiration. Elastic recoil is the tendency of the lung to return to its resting volume. A hallmark of COPD is the destruction of the mucociliary clearance system and the structural support and elastic recoil of the lungs. Consequently, arterial oxygen falls (hypoxemia) while arterial carbon dioxide increases (hypercapnia), giving rise to further sequelae of COPD.

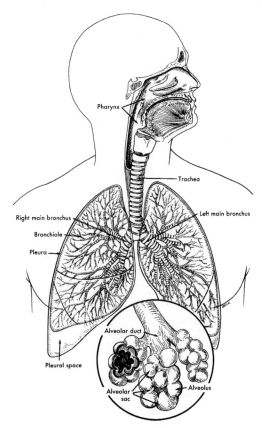

Artwork from Thibodeau, *Anthony's textbook of anatomy and physiology,* 1987.

Environmental factors

Occupation, air pollution, and allergens can influence the development of COPD. Exposure to substances such as molds, fungi, nitrogen or sulfur gases, asbestos, animal hair, hairsprays, and household pollutants may trigger asthmatic attacks.[11,39] During acute attacks, spastic contractions of the airways make breathing difficult and creates an overwhelming feeling of suffocation. An increase in mucosal goblet cells, thickening and hypertrophy of airways, and copious, thick mucus secretions are typical of chronic asthmatic bronchitis.[40]

Familial factors

Many diseases, including those of the respiratory system, tend to run in families. Genetic predisposition, as well as household habits passed from one generation to the next, can affect disease manifestation. For this reason, taking a health history is important.

Although emphysema is primarily associated with smoking, it may also result from an inherited deficiency of alpha-antitrypsin (AAT). AAT is a nonspecific, antiproteolytic enzyme. It normally represses the release of proteases, which are enzymes that can disintegrate and lyse lung tissue.[2,40] Proteases are released by blood leukocytes, alveolar macrophage, and bacteria as part of the inflammatory response. If unchecked, proteases destroy the structural elastin of lung tissue, and functional elastic recoil of the smaller airways is lost. Enlargement of air passages distal to the terminal bronchioles develops. Upon loss of elastic recoil, airways tend to collapse with exhalation. Overinflation and air trapping may cause the already distended alveolar walls to rupture. Large pockets filled with stagnant air called bullae may form. As the functional number of alveoli declines, dyspnea increases.[38,40] Therapy by replacement of AAT is now available.

In summary, patients with COPD frequently have elements of chronic bronchitis, pulmonary emphysema, and asthma in the pathogenesis of their disease. The predominant manifestation is shortness of breath, which becomes a primary focus of treatment.

HOME OXYGEN THERAPY

Many studies have documented the benefits of low-flow continuous or as needed (prn) oxygen therapy for patients with COPD.[9,11,15,33] A general improvement of primary organ function, along with increased mobility and cognitive processes such as abstraction and memory, is associated with low-flow oxygen administration to COPD patients. Additionally, reduced mortality rates are noted in these study groups. Cardiac output, hemoglobin concentration, and the partial pressure of arterial oxygen saturation (PAO_2) primarily determine oxygen transport, tissue perfusion, and the need for oxygen therapy. Generally speaking a patient whose PAO_2 is less than 55 mmHg on room air will require oxygen.

Oxygen flow is usually ordered at 2 to 3 L/min. When carbon dioxide levels remain chronically high, as with COPD, the body relies on low oxygen levels, or the hypoxic drive, as a stimulus for breathing. Although not all COPD patients are carbon dioxide retainers, the administration of oxygen at levels greater than 3 L/min may suppress the hypoxic drive in these patients and lead to respiratory arrest. Signs and symptoms of carbon dioxide narcosis include confusion, lethargy, and a patient who cannot be aroused. Home health nurses should stop the oxygen administration if inappropriately high oxygen levels occur and should alert the physician as soon as possible. If tampering with the flow rate is suspected, the home medical equipment (HME) vendor can be asked to put a lock on the flow meter.

Home oxygen therapy is expensive, but Medicare reimbursement can be obtained for eligible patients. Medicare guidelines specified on the Health Care Financing Administration's (HCFA) form 484 (Certificate of Medical Necessity or CMN) outlining the appropriateness of oxygen therapy include the following:[6,26,34,35]

1. A PAO_2 56 to 59 mmHg (or O_2 saturation to 89% on room air by ear oximetry); and
2. Evidence for end organ damage to include a diagnosis of COPD, cor pulmonale suggested by congestive heart failure, ECG evidence of heart disease, persistent erythrocytosis (a hematocrit of 57% or more), impairment of cognitive function, and dependent edema.

A written order for home oxygen therapy by the patient's physician is necessary for Medicare reimbursement. The prescription should provide a specific patient diagnosis indicative of end organ damage, specific laboratory evidence of hypoxemia, and should include flow rate and oxygen concentration, frequency of use, and duration of need. The prescription should be updated each certification period or for the duration of use since Medicare will not accept a lifetime prescription.

The usual goal of treatment is an oxygen saturation of 90% to 93%.[19,34] Patients should be taught that although oxygen is not addictive, it is a prescribed drug and should be respected as such. It is important to explain to COPD patients that oxygen should be used when needed but only at the prescribed amount because with certain patients high flow rates can lead to respiratory arrest. Patients receiving home oxygen therapy should be instructed that although oxygen does not burn, it is combustible. Contact with a spark or flame is to be avoided because this can cause an explosion. Oxygen should be kept at least 10 feet away from any potential explosive hazard such as smoking, gas burners, or electrical appliances.[26] Patients should notify the local fire department that they have oxygen equipment in the home.

Oxygen equipment in the home

Tanks, liquid oxygen and concentrators, are the oxygen systems most frequently used at home.[19,26] Cost, duration, ease of use, system portability, and individual patient needs influence the selection of the system.

Medicare uses a fixed reimbursement schedule based on market pricing rather than the type of system or actual volume of oxygen used. As a result, HME vendors who accept Medicare provide home oxygen at a fixed rate, regardless of the home system used. This policy has encouraged the use of oxygen-conserving devices but has priced liquid oxygen and related equipment (an inherently more expensive, yet portable, system that is ideal for numerous home care patients) beyond the resources of many patients.[19]

The operation, maintenance, and cleaning of oxygen systems and related equipment should be a routine part of patient education. This training is usually initiated by the HME vendor's respiratory therapist as part of discharge planning and is reinforced by the home health nurse.

High-pressure cylinders. Compressed gas is usually stored in small cylinders, green E tanks, or larger H cylinders. These tanks do not "vent" so oxygen is not lost. Cylinders and tanks are the most economical oxygen system for patients requiring low-flow or prn use. The cylinder or tank should be chained or supported in a cylinder cart or base and routinely fitted with pressure-relief devices that allow gas to escape if a sudden increase in pressure (such as that caused by exposure to heat) should occur. Patients should be instructed not to place or store their oxygen cylinders or tanks near radiators, steam pipes, or heat ducts in their homes.

The capacity of the cylinders is small, and prolonged use away from the larger tanks is very limited.[19] Frequent replacement and limited portability of the heavy tanks are among their disadvantages.[26]

Liquid oxygen. A liquid-state system uses low temperature rather than pressure to contain the oxygen. As a result, 1 L of liquid oxygen is equivalent to 861 L of compressed gas.[19] This makes for a lightweight system that greatly enhances patient mobility.

Liquid oxygen is stored in stainless steel, canister-type bottles. These canisters should be stored in well ventilated areas. Portable units can be filled from a reservoir tank kept at home. Fewer deliveries are required because these reservoirs hold twice as much as a gas cylinder.[19,26] Small and lightweight, liquid oxygen is the system of choice for high-volume users who desire a very portable system.[39]

Disadvantages include cost (because the gas will vent when not in use) and the potential for thermal burns when refilling canisters.[26] Liquid oxygen may be unavailable in many rural areas.

Concentrators. Oxygen concentrators draw air through a special filter that removes nitrogen, water vapor, and hydrocarbons to "concentrate" oxygen from room air.[26] Electrically powered concentrators are the most economical form of continuous oxygen use; they are easy to use and require fewer deliveries.[19,39]

However, concentrators are not always an appropriate oxygen source. They are not designed to provide high oxygen concentrations (>90% at flow rates >4 L/min), nor are they suitable for systems that require high flow pressures, such as the Venturi mask.[19,26,39]

Concentrators are, however, frequently used for home mechanical ventilation. Although the concentrator is the most cost-effective system at present for continuous oxygen therapy, patients can expect its operation to increase their electric bill about $30 to $40/month.[19,26]

Disadvantages include noise (depending on the model), immobility, and routine replacement of filters.[26,39] In addition, all concentrators require a power source (a portable backup tank should be installed along with the concentrator in case of machine or power failure).[26]

Oxygen enricher. Similar to an oxygen concentrator, an oxygen enricher uses a permeable membrane to separate and concentrate oxygen molecules. The net result is a constant 40% oxygen concentration at all flow rates.[9,26] Enrichers are less commonly used than oxygen concentrators but continue to be refined and will probably become more popular. Some patients may prefer high air flows to relieve their sense of suffocation. The oxygen enricher can provide maximal flow rates without a corresponding increase in oxygen concentration.[26] Additionally, the membrane of the oxygen enricher allows water vapor to pass, so there is no need for a humidifier.

Ancillary equipment and techniques

The nasal cannula, the Venturi mask, and more recently, transtracheal therapy are prominent methods of oxygen administration in the home.[16,26,37] The nasal cannula, by far the most popular, provides flows of 1 to 6 L/min with an oxygen concentration of 24% to 45%.[39] Venturi masks provide more controlled oxygen concentrations from 35% to 45% with flows of 4 to 6 L/min.[39]

To reduce the amount of oxygen that is wasted with use of the nasal cannula, reservoir nasal cannulas are becoming more popular in home care. A reservoir nasal cannula stores oxygen in a 20-ml collapsing chamber during exhalation. This allows the patient to use lower flow rates than would otherwise be needed. Reservoir cannulas at a flow rate of .5 L/min provide saturation equivalent to that of continuous flow at 2 L/min.[19] One of the cheapest oxygen-conserving devices now available, reservoir nasal cannulas retail for about $20 and require replacement monthly.[19]

Many patients wearing nasal cannulas complain about irritation from plastic prongs in the nose or soreness where the tubing rests on the ears. Alternate styles for the nasal cannula can be recommended by the HME vendor to promote patient comfort. Cotton balls placed over the ears, or a number of home improvisational techniques can alleviate pressure and soreness.[36] If sores should develop in the nose from tubing irritation, instruct patients to rub vitamin E and *not* a petroleum product (such as Vaseline) over the area.

Transtracheal oxygen therapy. Transtracheal oxygen therapy (TTOT) is a newer method of oxygen delivery. TTOT is accomplished by administration of oxygen directly into the trachea via a SCOOP catheter held in place by a bead chain necklace. Advantages of TTOT include a cost savings of 50% to 60% for the same flow provided by nasal cannulas, improved appearance, and increased patient mobility.[37]

Disadvantages include catheter dislodgment, tenderness, and a potential for subcutaneous emphysema around the catheter site. In addition, a mucus plug may form at the opening of the catheter, causing a potentially fatal obstruction.[19] To prevent this complication, the patient should be well hydrated; mucolytic agents may be used. Patients with TTOT should be taught to recognize the signs of mucus deposition—unexplained dyspnea, back pressure resulting in pop-off of the humidifier, persistent cough, etc—and to irrigate the catheter or cough the mucus out if they notice these signs.[19,37]

SCOOP catheters should be cleaned at least daily to prevent infection and should be replaced every 3 months. Cleaning requirements should be reviewed with the supplier. If the catheter accidentally comes out and the patient is unable to reinsert it, the patient should be instructed to loosely cover the insertion site with a lint-free gauze pad, put on the nasal cannula, and notify the physician.

AEROSOL THERAPY

Although aerosol treatments are ordered by the physician, home health nurses should monitor patients' abilities to administer medication, as well as the therapeutic effects of medications. Sterile normal saline is frequently used with aerosol therapy and can be made in the home. (See the box on page 163 for instructions.) Microscopic drop-

HOMEMADE STERILE NORMAL SALINE[36]

1. Add ¼ teaspoon of noniodized table salt to 1 cup of tapwater in a small clean glass jar with a screw-on lid.
2. Loosely place the lid on the jar.
3. Place the jar in a saucepan of water (water level in the saucepan should be three-fourths the height of the jar).
4. Cover the top of the saucepan.
5. Put the saucepan on the stove and boil the water for about 25 minutes.
6. Remove the saucepan from the stove and cool the solution. Remove the jar and tighten the lid.
7. If rapid cooling is desired, place the hot saucepan in another pan that contains water and ice cubes. Take care that the ice water does not flood over the rim of the saucepan and thereby contaminate the sterile saline. Do not place the hot glass jar directly in ice water as the glass may crack.
8. Store saline solution in the refrigerator. Important: Make fresh solution every week. Discard any solution that has become discolored or cloudy.

INHALER ADMINISTRATION[36]

Open mouth technique
1. Shake the inhaler canister 15 to 20 times.
2. Remove the protective cap.
3. Inhale a deep, slow breath and then exhale completely.
4. Open your mouth *wide*.
5. Hold the inhaler canister 1 to 1½ inches from your lips.
6. Hold your breath for as long as is comfortable.
7. Exhale slowly through pursed lips.
8. As prescribed by your physician, wait 1 minute between puffs and then repeat steps 1 through 7.

Inspirease technique
1. Take a slow breath in and exhale completely.
2. Insert the inhaler canister in the mouthpiece.
3. Make sure the bag is connected to the mouthpiece.
4. Shake the inhaler canister 15 to 20 times.
5. Insert the mouthpiece between teeth, and close lips.
6. Gently compress the inhaler canister.
7. Take three to four deep and slow breaths from the bag. *Do not* make the inspirease whistle. Hold your breath as long as is comfortable between breaths to allow the medicine to deposit in the lungs.

lets of medication can be inhaled by intermittent positive pressure breathing (IPPB), by compressor nebulizer, or by a cartridge inhaler.

IPPB therapy

Prescribed IPPB treatments should be given before meals. When ready to begin treatments, patients should be instructed to sit upright in a comfortable position.[36] After the machine is turned on, a mist forms at the mouthpiece. Patients then close their lips around the mouthpiece and breathe slowly, letting the machine fill their lungs.[36] To conserve the medicine, the machine should be turned off if any interruption (coughing) occurs and used until all the medicine is gone (10 to 20 minutes).[36,39]

Routine administration of IPPB therapy is generally becoming less popular in home care today. It is usually used as a last resort for patients who cannot inhale deeply. IPPB may induce pneumothorax in patients with emphysema. Generated pressures may also reduce cardiac output since increased intrathoracic pressures diminish venous return to the heart. Hyperventilation and infection from contaminated equipment are additional complications associated with IPPB.[26,39]

Compression nebulizers

Compression nebulizers require that the patient be able to take a deep, slow breath and cough effectively.[26,39] They are similar in operation to IPPB. Two basic types of nebulizers are currently available, a continuous mode and one operated by a finger valve.

Cartridge inhalers

Very popular in home care, cartridge inhalers are handheld, pocket-sized, metered-dose inhalers. Each inhaler contains approximately 200 puffs. An empty cartridge will float, whereas one that is half empty will partially submerge in water. (See the box titled Inhaler Administration.) Spacers used in the inspirease technique, are helpful for those patients who lack coordination for the open mouth technique of administration.[35]

INFECTION CONTROL

All home respiratory equipment should be routinely cleaned to prevent potential infection. Soap and water are effective for cleaning equipment such as nasal cannulas, masks, tubing, the cap and mouthpiece of cartridge inhalers, and humidifiers. Home respiratory equipment is then usually soaked in a white vinegar/water (1:3 cups) solution for 20 minutes, thoroughly rinsed with warm running water, and allowed to air dry.[36]

Surfaces of all equipment should routinely be wiped with a disinfectant. For most equipment, cleaning should be done daily or at least 2 to 3 times per week. Cleaning of equipment is also recommended after each IPPB or aerosol treatment.[36] After being cleaned, humidifiers should be refilled with fresh distilled water to prevent bacterial growth. All equipment should be dry when stored. Cleaning recommendations from the HME vendor and product manufacturer should be reviewed. (For a more detailed discussion of infection control principles, see Chapter 5.)

HOME CARE APPLICATION

Providing home care for patients with COPD is not an easy task. COPD patients and their families are frequently overwhelmed by the physical and psychological complexities of a progressively debilitating disease.

Planning visits

Within the Medicare system, the nurse cannot make a home visit just because the patient has chronic COPD. (Refer to Chapter 4 for Medicare guidelines for reimbursement of home health services.) However, services *are* usually reimbursable when the following are documented:

- Need for procedural services (chest physiotherapy)
- Unstable vital signs
- Unstable cardiopulmonary status (sudden weight gain or edema, syncope, lung congestion)
- Pulmonary infection (changes in the color or amount of sputum; elevated temperature)
- Need for patient/caregiver education (e.g., medications, diet, activity, procedural care)

- Any coexisting medical problems that require the services of a skilled nurse or therapist

In addition, the home health nurse must be alert to problems that may emerge as the patient/caregiver assumes responsibilities for care. As described in this section, issues involving patient/caregiver self-care management, home air quality, psychosocial concerns, and pulmonary rehabilitation will certainly be a focus of care.

Developing the plan of care

The plan of care and visit frequency will depend on the home health nurse's assessment of patient/caregiver needs. (See the box below and on page 165.) Patient care should be directed toward the following goals:

- Relief of physical symptoms
- Relief of psychosocial symptoms; anxiety, depression
- Patient education regarding self-care management of COPD and disease process; financial considerations including billing and reimbursement issues; home "survival needs"
- Increased independence and activity tolerance; general physical reconditioning

 PRIMARY NURSING DIAGNOSES/ PATIENT PROBLEMS

Ineffective breathing pattern.
Ineffective airway clearance
- Knowledge deficit; disease process and risk complications, medications including home oxygen therapy, operation of home medical equipment, procedural care, diet, pulmonary rehabilitation, infection control, socioeconomic resources, available community services, etc.
- Altered nutrition, less than body requirements
- Activity intolerance: ___ Ambulation, ___ ADLs, ___ Other *(Specify)*
- Self-care deficit: ___ ADLs, ___ Feeding, ___Toileting, ___Other *(Specify)*
- Risk for pulmonary infection
- Ineffective individual coping
- Hopelessness
- Altered sexuality patterns

**PRIMARY THEMES
OF PATIENT EDUCATION**

- COPD: signs and symptoms of disease process to report to the case manager and physician
- When to call 911
- Pulmonary infection: recognition and treatment
- Breathing techniques to conserve energy
- Postural drainage to clear mucus secretion
- Home oxygen therapy: operation and maintenance of equipment
- Medications: purpose, action, dosage, side effects, and methods of administration
- Diet
- Energy conservation
- Positive coping strategies to use when living with a chronic disease
- Adaptations to promote positive sexual relationship with significant other
- Socioeconomic resources
- Community services available for people with COPD

- Prevention of exacerbation of COPD and subsequent hospital readmission
- Improved quality of life
- Increased knowledge of disease process with appropriate interventions, community resources

A multidisciplinary approach is a must for patients with COPD. The pulmonary rehabilitation home program will involve nursing (includes use of the home health aide and/or homemaker services), rehabilitation services, respiratory therapists, nutritional therapists, and possibly the services of the social worker in assisting the patient to achieve his or her best level of functioning. The home care team should coordinate activities to assist the patient to build strength and endurance, clear excess mucus secretions, and overcome fears of dyspnea.[19]

Physical assessment

Clinical manifestation of COPD is similar to that for congestive heart failure (CHF). In addition, many ventilator-dependent patients have a diagnosis of COPD. (See Chapters 11 and 12.)

General. Patients with chronic bronchitis are stocky, typically cyanotic, and bloated as a result of heart failure. This group is sometimes referred to as "blue bloaters." Patients with emphysema often have barrel-shaped chests and ruddy complexions resulting from constant lung inflation and secondary polycythemia.[17] They are sometimes referred to as "pink puffers." Many COPD patients will show signs and symptoms of both chronic bronchitis and emphysema.

Observe patients' outward appearance in terms of dress and personal hygiene. Patients with COPD may not dress or bathe because the effort required to do so increases shortness of breath. Be aware that complaints of extreme fatigue, shortness of breath, sudden disorientation, or belligerency may be signs of hypoxemia and impending respiratory failure.[39]

Assess the patient's activity tolerance. Does shortness of breath occur at rest? Does it occur after 5 minutes of conversation or with 10 to 30 feet of ambulation? Use a rating scale to have patients identify how they describe their shortness of breath on a scale of 0 to 10. This is especially useful in caring for patients with changes in the treatment regimen as a means to evaluate the effectiveness of nebulizers, oxygen therapy, and steroids.

Obtain a health history to identify factors that may contribute to COPD such as smoking, occupation, and environmental or familial considerations. Does the patient look well nourished, overweight, or underweight? Does the patient look rested? Many patients with COPD are afraid to sleep for fear they will stop breathing. Some patients may do a lot of pointing and speak in short, abrupt phrases because they are short of breath.

Cardiopulmonary. Inspect the chest, noting size and shape. A barrel-shaped chest with an increased anteroposterior diameter (1:1) results from chronic hyperinflation of the lungs. An irregular heart rate, clubbing of the fingers, jugular venous distension, dependent edema, and oliguria are some of the clinical manifestations of hypoxemia and pulmonary hypertension. Limited bilateral excursion of the diaphragm and a decreased area of cardiac dullness, along with faint heart sounds, may be detected as a result of hyperinflation of the lungs.

Auscultate the lungs for abnormal or adventitious lung sounds. Specific abnormal lung sounds include the following:

- Wheezes (continuous whistling noises due to narrowed airways)
- Crackles (discontinuous popping sounds associated with the movement of fluid in the airways; crackles may be described as fine, medium, or coarse)
- Rubs (coarse scraping or grating noises resulting from the rubbing of inflamed pleura)

If patients cough, ask them how often they cough and at what times of the day. Ask if the cough is productive or nonproductive of mucus. If productive, ask about the consistency, color, and amount of mucus. If possible, inspect the mucus when it is coughed up. A green or yellowish color is characteristic of a pulmonary infection.[43]

The physician should be notified of any changes in the patient's baseline status. An awareness of complications from COPD or coexisting health problems—including diabetes, poor nutrition, depression, pump failure, and hypertension—should be a routine component of patient assessment.[28]

Medications

Patients with COPD are frequently on multiple medications. Primary medications used to treat COPD are oxygen, bronchodilator, corticosteroids, and antibiotics.[29,31,39]

Oxygen. Oxygen is usually administered at 1 to 3 L/min by nasal cannula. (See previous discussion of oxygen therapy including home safety precautions.)

Bronchodilator. Bronchodilators (beta-agonists and methylxanthines) relax smooth muscle around the bronchial tubes. They are usually inhaled or administered orally.

Beta-agonist inhalers include isoproterenol (Isuprel), isoetharine (Bronkosol), metaproterenol (Alupent), and albuterol (Proventil).[35] They are administered via metered-dose inhaler. Recommended dosage is 1 to 2 puffs every 3 to 4 hours.[35] Excessive use may increase tolerance. Side effects include increased heart rate, muscle tremors, and palpitations.[29]

Although not classified as a bronchodilator, cromolyn sodium acts prophylactically to prevent anaphylactic reactions. It is used with asthmatics and should be administered before possible contact with an asthmatic agent. Cromolyn sodium may be administered at 2 to 4 puffs, 4 times daily by metered-dose inhaler.[29,40]

Methylxanthines (theophylline) are not as effective as inhalers but do improve diaphragmatic contractility and act as a mild diuretic.[3] Optimal benefits occur with plasma levels of theophylline between 10 and 20 mg/ml.[3] Be aware of signs of theophylline toxicity to include anorexia, nausea, headache, tremors, and cardiac dysrhythmia.

Corticosteroids. Corticosteroids decrease inflammation and mucus secretion. Their onset of action is delayed compared with that of inhalers (bronchodilator). If using both, the bronchodilator should be administered first.[1,39] If prolonged steroid therapy is considered, a preliminary tuberculin test is recommended.[39]

A trial of 40 mg of prednisone per day is typically started over a 2-week period.[29] If the patient responds, the drug should be administered at the lowest effective dose. When being discontinued, steroids should be tapered off slowly.[1] Side effects include weight gain, cataracts, glucose intolerance, edema, hypokalemia, and a "moon face."[1,29]

Antibiotics. Antibiotics should be administered when sputum becomes purulent. *Haemophilus* influenzae and *Streptococcus* pneumoniae are the organisms most commonly isolated from the sputum of COPD patients.[31,43] Treatment for 7 to 10 days with tetracycline, penicillin, ampicillin, or trimethoprim-sulfamethoxazole is typically used.[43] Be aware that many antibiotics have drug and food interactions that require the patient to take the drug 1 hour before or 3 hours after eating or taking the antacid.[43] Emphasize the importance of completing antibiotic therapy for effectiveness even if the patient feels better.

Other. Be aware that the major side effect of a number of antianxiety medications is respiratory depression. Antidepressants, narcotics, analgesics, and sedatives should be used sparingly for the same reasons. Tricyclics widely used for older depressed patients include nortriptyline (Aventyl) and desipramine (Norpramine).[14]

Activities of daily living

In planning care, it will be important to determine what activities the patient can perform. Self-care activities include cooking, cleaning, laundry, shopping, etc. Can the patient move around in the home? Consider a referral to rehabilitation services for problems identified in this area. A request for home health aide services to assist the patient with ADL care may be needed.

Nutrition

Nutritional support will be an important part of nursing care because many patients with COPD are malnourished.[41,42] Be aware that malnutrition is associated with decreased ventilatory muscle strength, endurance, and force of contraction.[41,42] Good nutrition will restore these functions.

A high fat, low cholesterol diet to maintain an adequate weight is recommended.[41,42] Carbohydrate metabolism creates increased blood levels of carbon dioxide as a by-product. Because carbon dioxide is excreted primarily by the lungs, calories from fat and protein sources rather than carbohydrates are preferred for carbon dioxide retainers.[41,42] Liquid drinks that contain a relatively low percentage of carbohydrates are frequently used as a dietary supplement for COPD patients. Note that total parenteral nutrition (TPN) products and many nutritional supplements have a high carbohydrate content and therefore may produce shortness of breath in patients with COPD.[39]

The registered dietitian can be asked to review appropriate food choices and eating patterns. A high calorie diet with multiple small meals is frequently recommended, although diet may vary according to specific patient needs and concurrent diagnoses.[24,25,39] Frequent small feedings avoid problems with gastric distension that pushes against the diaphragm, making it more difficult to breathe.[24,25,39] Small meals eaten frequently also require less energy for metabolism than do large meals.

Gas-forming foods such as beans, brussels sprouts, and cabbage should be avoided.[24,25] Patients may wish to refrain from drinking milk because it thickens mucus. Alcohol depresses respiration and should be discouraged. Since caffeine is a stimulant, coffee, tea, and sodas should be avoided by patients in danger of heart failure.

Unless contraindicated, encourage the patient to drink 6 to 8 glasses of water a day to thin mucus secretions and promote hydration.[24,25]

If the patient is using steroids, a monitored regimen of oral calcium and vitamin D may be recommended to prevent osteoporosis.[29] Frequent oral hygiene improves the sense of taste. To conserve energy, encourage patients to use their oxygen equipment when they eat, if possible.

Home air quality

Instruct patients to avoid respiratory irritants such as smoke-filled rooms, animal hair, feather pillows, sudden changes in room temperature, pollen, or aerosol sprays.[2,36] Air-conditioning should be used in hot weather. Recommend that a humidifier be used, if possible, to keep airways from drying out, particularly in dry climates or during the winter when heated air is dry. Tell patients to stay indoors on days when pollen counts are high or air quality is poor. Recommend that scarves or masks be worn over the face during cold weather to prevent bronchospasm.

Psychosocial considerations

Patients with COPD are often depressed, lonely, and socially isolated.[14] The role losses associated with COPD are greater than those of other illnesses and contribute to the depression.[14] Shortness of breath and easy fatigability are primary factors. It may be necessary to alter the home environment to prevent patient isolation. Encourage patients to have their bedroom on the main floor with easy access to the bathroom and kitchen.

As the spouse assumes the family roles that the patient with COPD is no longer able to perform, the spouse is also placed under severe stress. Family conflicts may arise as a result of role changes and redefinition of lifestyles, or they may be caused by financial strain arising from the impact of a chronic disease. Likewise the spouse and family may absorb some of the patient's overwhelming sense of deprivation and loss.[8]

Dyspnea causes many patients with COPD to withdraw from day-to-day activities and hobbies. In addition, patients with COPD have been shown to have higher levels of anxiety during times of high dyspnea as compared to periods of low dyspnea.[10,13] Research indicates that effective treatment strategies include pharmacological therapy including tricyclic antidepressants, exercise, individual and family therapy, and family interventions.[6,4,12,13,18] It is important to facilitate positive coping by encouraging patient/family communication and by being attentive to behaviors that stress household relationships.

The frustrations and anxiety of air hunger should be reviewed with families to promote their understanding of patients' labile emotional states and sudden outbursts of anger. However, manipulative behaviors by patients are not acceptable. When coping with patient discomfort or distress, families should be instructed to remain calm and encourage patients to control their breathing, use their inhaler, put on their oxygen, and sit still until breath is regained.[4,6,18,21] Also, it may be necessary to remind caregivers "not to do everything for the patient" in balancing household support with the patient's best interests, which is to promote activity.

Refer patients to social services for assistance with financial planning. Instruct patients in stress reduction and relaxation techniques such as visual imagery. Support groups like the Better Breathers Club can help patients and their families explore activities that can be done together such as walking, reading, or driving.

Sexual counseling. Sex is an important aspect of life for all people, including those with COPD.[23] Sexual dysfunction often parallels the course of lung disease.[10] Loss of touch or fear of intimacy may increase feelings of anger and isolation. The fear of dyspnea and fatigue may limit participation in sexual activities.[23] The subject may be broached with a simple question such as, "Are problems with your breathing affecting your sex life?" If the patient and/or spouse wishes to discuss the subject, the home health nurse can suggest measures such as the following that may make breathing easier:[7]

- Have sex in a familiar environment with a room temperature controlled at 68° to 72° F and 40% humidity to promote comfort.
- Use the inhaler before sex or keep the metered-dose inhaler by the bedside for quick relief if shortness of breath occurs.
- Use oxygen via nasal cannula during sex.
- Try positions that do not require the patient to support all the body weight. Lying side by side, lying with the non-COPD partner on top, or using an armless chair with the non-COPD partner on top may alleviate patient dyspnea.

- Encourage patients and their spouses to take rest periods during sex as needed. Sometimes simply hugging can provide the greatest intimacy of all.

Patient education

Home management of COPD is complex. There is much patients and their families can learn to better their lives.[5] Patient education regarding home "survival needs" should be a priority of health teaching. As described in Chapter 12, survival needs include information about procedural care, medications, operation of equipment, what to do in emergencies, when to call the physician, etc. Never forget to ask patients what they perceive their immediate learning needs to be.[27]

Teach patients the early signs of respiratory infection (such as fever, increased sputum, color changes in sputum, extreme shortness of breath, or lung congestion) and stress the importance of starting antibiotic therapy promptly. Patients should know that a sudden weight gain (greater than 2 lb in 1 day) should be reported to the physician as a possible sign of heart failure.[36]

Patients with COPD often complain of lack of sleep related to shortness of breath. Teach them that pillows or a foam wedge obtained from the HME vendor can ease the effort of breathing and may encourage rest. Instruct them to keep medicines, clothes, tissues, personal articles, and the telephone by the bedside for convenience and ease of use.

Morning is typically a very difficult time for patients with COPD because mucus has accumulated in the lungs throughout the night.[18] The day is begun by coughing and expectoration of mucus, which can be exhausting. Instruct patients to use their inhaler in the morning to ease breathing and to wear their oxygen equipment when needed.

Encourage patients to use their oxygen equipment with extension tubing when bathing. Patients should be told to shower with warm water because extremes of temperature increase energy consumption. Bath blankets and robes help prevent chilling when drying. Shoes of the slip-on variety and shirts, dresses, and trousers with Velcro fasteners ease dressing.[24,25,39]

Emphasize the importance of cessation of smoking. In empowering patients to make healthy choices, make them aware of the hazards of

---

TIPS FOR ENERGY CONSERVATION FOR THE PATIENT IN THE HOME SETTING[36]

If you have COPD, save your energy for daily activities. Avoid rushing. A slow, steady rate of work with frequent rest periods is best. Never work so long or hard that you feel very weak, tired, or short of breath. High-energy tasks never should be done back-to-back. Use pursed-lip or diaphragmatic breathing as you do your work so your energy will not be wasted. Take your inhaler or use your oxygen as prescribed and needed. Remember, one of the best ways to conserve your energy is to assign priorities and preplan your day.

Ways to conserve energy

1. Plan rest periods of at least 5 to 15 minutes between activities.
2. Ensure adequate room ventilation and a comfortable temperature. Excessive heat, cold, or humidity may cause shortness of breath. Avoid places with dirty air such as dusty or smoke-filled rooms. Avoid animal hair, scented soaps, colognes, powders, cleaners, aerosol sprays, glues, or paints if they cause problems with your breathing.
3. When possible, sit while performing activities such as bathing, brushing teeth, or washing dishes. Avoid unnecessary walking or standing. Try to push or slide objects rather than lifting them (use a portable cart).
4. Ask family or friends to help with heavy work as needed. Delegate particularly strenuous chores such as mowing the lawn or vacuuming the carpet to other family members as needed.
5. Let dishes air dry instead of toweling them dry.
6. Space personal activities such as shaving, bathing, and washing hair over several hours or days.
7. Take a quick shower if the moisture in the air makes it difficult to breathe. Turn on tepid water and wet yourself. Turn off the water and soap yourself all over. Turn the water back on to rinse. Immediately towel dry to prevent shivering.
8. Wear loose-fitting clothes with elastic waistbands or Velcro fasteners and front closures. Wear shoes that are easy to slip on such as loafers or thongs.
9. To stand, first take several slow, deep breaths. Then, while breathing out through pursed lips, stand up.
10. To climb stairs, first breathe in deeply through your nose while standing. Next, exhale through pursed lips as you climb a couple of stairs. Stop, rest, and breathe deeply and slowly. Continue climbing two or three steps *while you exhale.* Stand still when inhaling. Hold onto the stair rails whenever possible for extra support.
11. Always remember to exhale when lifting or pushing heavy objects or when performing the action part of any activity.

---

smoking. According to the American Lung Association, an estimated 419,000 people die every year of smoking-related diseases.[2]

As discussed in the remainder of the chapter, techniques to increase strength, clear excess mucus secretions, and conserve energy will be a focus of patient education.

PULMONARY REHABILITATION

Pulmonary rehabilitation involves breathing retraining and chest physiotherapy. The goal of pulmonary rehabilitation is to improve the patient's breathing and oxygenation. This is accomplished by strengthening muscles, learning proper breathing patterns, and using effective mucus expectoration and clearance methods.

The physical therapist will develop a home exercise program helpful in building the patient's strength and endurance. In developing the plan of care, physical therapy will focus on functional loss. For example, if the patient is unable to walk, ambulation will be a priority of training.

An occupational therapist may be utilized to teach COPD patients to perform the activities of daily living (ADL) in a way that conserves their energy. Patients should learn to plan their day so that activities are coordinated with rest periods in order to prevent shortness of breath. Expending energy wisely reduces the effort of breathing. (See the box above for tips on how patients at home can conserve their energy.)

Specific techniques

Breathing techniques. There are a number of breathing techniques useful for COPD patients. Pursed-lip and diaphragmatic breathing are

---

BREATHING TECHNIQUES[36]

Controlled breathing exercises help get the maximum amount of air in and out of the lungs with the least amount of effort. These exercises should be practiced every day so that they become a natural way of breathing.

Pursed-lip breathing

Relax. Breathe in slowly. Purse lips into a whistling position and exhale slowly and evenly. Exhalation should be 2 to 3 times longer than inhalation. Count 1-2-3 for inhalation and 5-6-7-8-9 for exhalation.

Diaphragmatic breathing

Sit down. Relax your abdominal muscles with inhalation. This moves the diaphragm down. Tense the abdomen with exhalation. This helps push the diaphragm up. Place your hand over the abdomen just below your breastbone. Your hand will move as you breathe. With correct diaphragmatic breathing, your hand will move out as you inhale and move in as you exhale.

---

commonly taught. (See the box titled Breathing Techniques.) Consider hooking the patient up to a pulse oximeter during breathing exercises as a means of biofeedback.

Pursed-lip breathing helps keep the airways open, thus improving oxygenation. In diaphragmatic breathing, patients use their diaphragms for respiration instead of accessory muscles of the chest and neck. This promotes a more normal breathing pattern and reduces the work of breathing. Patients learn to exhale as they work since exhalation requires less effort than inhaling.[4,17,39]

Chest physiotherapy consists of procedures that cause postural drainage and clear the lungs of mucus. In addition, patients are taught to clear secretions from the lungs with effective breathing techniques such as the huff cough and the cascade cough. (Appendix 10-1 describes chest physiotherapy frequently used in the home.)

SUMMARY

Breathing affects every aspect of life. A simple and largely automatic process, breathing may become a daily struggle for people with COPD. Anger,

depression, and withdrawal are the understandable consequences of a lifestyle restricted by the effort of breathing.

A multidisciplinary approach to treating COPD is especially important for these patients because of their special diet, exercise, educational, and psychosocial needs. As case managers, home health nurses are in an excellent position to refer patients to various agency services. Networking with other disciplines strengthens the plan of care. COPD is a chronic, but not hopeless, disorder. With successful home management, men and women with COPD can resume optimal participation in life activities.

REFERENCES

1. Alberts W, Corrigan K: Corticosteroid therapy for chronic obstructive pulmonary disease, *Postgrad Med* 81(5):33, 1987.
2. American Lung Association: *Lung disease data-1994,* New York, 1994, The Association.
3. Aubier MA, Roussos C: Effect of theophylline on respiratory muscle function, *Chest* 86(2):91-97, 1985.
4. Brown S: Helping your COPD patient improve exercise capacity, *J Resp Dis* 7(5):40, 1986.
5. Brundage D, Swearengen P, and Johnsie W: Self-care instruction for patients with COPD, *Rehabil Nurs*, 18(5):321-325, 1993.
6. Carroll P: Good nursing gets COPD patients out of hospitals, *RN* 7:10, 1989.
7. Curgian L, Gronkiewicz M: Enhancing sexual performance in COPD, *Nurs Pract* 13(2):24, 1988.
8. Diethorn M: Preventions of sensory deprivation for the COPD victim's spouse, *Nurs Clin* 1:32, 1985.
9. Flenley D: Long-term home oxygen therapy, *Chest* 87(1):46, 1985.
10. Fletcher E, Martin R: Sexual dysfunction and erectile impotence in chronic obstructive pulmonary disease, *Chest* 81(4):21, 1982.
11. Francis P: Chronic obstructive lung disease and acute respiratory failure, *Postgrad Med* 79(1):64, 1986.
12. Gift A, Austin D: The effects of a program of systematic movement on COPD patients, *Rehabil Nurs* 17(1):8-10, 1992.
13. Gift A, Moore T, Soeken K: Relaxation to reduce dyspnea and anxiety in COPD patients, *Nurs Res* 41(4):242-246, 1992.
14. Gift G, McCrone S: Depression in patients with COPD, *Heart and Lung* 22(4):289-296, 1994.
15. Goldstein R: Effect of supplemental nocturnal oxygen on gas exchange in patients with severe obstructive lung disease, *N Engl J Med* 310(7):9, 1984.
16. Grandstrom D, Wierzbicki L: A better way to deliver long-term oxygen therapy, *RN* 9:7, 1989.
17. Hahn K: Slow-teaching the COPD patient, *Nursing 87* 17(4):10, 1987.

18. Heaton R et al: Psychologic effects of continuous and nocturnal oxygen therapy in hypoxemic chronic obstructive pulmonary disease, *Arch Intern Med* 143:1941, 1983.

19. Hodgkin JE et al: Your role in COPD home care, *Patient Care* 3:147-172, 1992.

20. Hoffman L, Mazzocco M, Roth J: Fine tuning your chest p.t., *Am J Nurs* 87(12):50, 1987.

21. Kohlman-Carrieri V, Janson-Bjerklie S: Strategies patients use to manage the sensation of dyspnea, *West J Nurs Res* 8(3):44, 1986.

22. Kohlman-Carrieri V, Murdaugh C, Janson-Bjerklie S: A framework for assessing pulmonary disease categories, *Focus Crit Care* 11(2):135, 1984.

23. Levine S, Stern R: Sexual function in cystic fibrosis, *Chest* 81(4):10, 1982.

24. Logan-Davis A: Managing the patient with advanced chronic obstructive pulmonary disease, part 1, *Hosp Med* 22(1):32, 1986.

25. Logan-Davis A: Managing the patient with advanced chronic obstructive pulmonary disease, part 2, *Hosp Med* 22(2):54, 1986.

26. Lucas J et al: *Home respiratory care,* Norwalk, Conn, 1988, Appleton & Lange.

27. McBride S: Patients with chronic obstructive pulmonary disease: their beliefs about measures that increase activity tolerance, *Rehabil Nurs* 19(1):37-41, 1994.

28. McDonald G: Long-term oxygen therapy delivery systems, *Resp Care* 28(7):43, 1983.

29. Mengert T, Albert R: Pulmonary therapeutics. In Larson E and Ramsey P, editors: *Med Ther,* Philadelphia, 1989, WB Saunders.

30. Mims B: The risks of oxygen therapy, *RN* 7:34, 1987.

31. Mitchell R, Petty T: Chronic obstructive pulmonary disease. In Mitchell R, Petty T, Schwartz J, editors: *Synopsis of clinical pulmonary disease,* ed 4, St Louis, 1989, Mosby.

32. National Institutes of Health: *Chronic obstructive pulmonary disease,* Pub No 83-2020, Washington, DC, 1983, US Department of Health and Human Services.

33. Nocturnal Oxygen Therapy Trial Group: Continuous or nocturnal oxygen therapy in hypoxemic chronic obstructive lung disease, *Ann Intern Med* 93(391):42, 1980.

34. Openbrier D, Hoffman L, Wesmiller S: Home oxygen therapy: evaluation and prescription, *Am J Nurs* 88(2):14, 1988.

35. Owens GR: New concepts in bronchodilator therapy, *AFP Practical Ther* 33(1):218-229, 1986.

36. Rice R: *Manual of home health nursing procedures,* St Louis, 1995, Mosby.

37. Spofford B et al: Transtracheal oxygen therapy. A guide for the respiratory therapist, *Resp Care* 32:345-352, 1987.

38. Traver G: Ineffective airway clearance: physiology and clinical application, *Dimens Crit Care Nurs* 4(4):44, 1985.

39. Vogt-Yanta M, Dettenmeier P: Pulmonary disease. In Martinson I and Widmer A, editors: *Home health care nursing,* Philadelphia, 1989, WB Saunders.

40. West J: *Pulmonary pathophysiology,* ed 4, Baltimore, 1992, Williams & Wilkins.

41. Wilson DO, Rogers RM, Hoffman RM: State of the art; nutrition and chronic lung disease, *Am Rev Respir Dis* 132:1347-1365, 1985.

42. Wilson DO, Rogers RM, Openbrier D: Nutritional aspects of chronic obstructive disease, *Clin Chest Med* 7(4):643-656, 1986.

43. Yoshikawa TT: Antibiotic treatment of lung infections, *Resp Ther* 6:26-28, 71-73, 1986.

Appendix 10-1

Chest Physiotherapy at Home[36]

Maneuvers used to assist in the removal of secretions:

Percussion is performed by clapping the cupped hand on the chest wall over the area of lung to be drained. Rhythmic clapping increases vibrations that stimulate the movement of secretions and helps clear secretions sticking to the bronchial walls. The hand is cupped to create a cushion of air against the chest wall. (See Figure 10-1.) Raise hands 3 to 4 inches above the chest wall and alternately clap lungs to vibrate secretions. Clapping should be vigorous but not painful.

Vibration is used to stimulate the flow of secretions into the larger airways where they can be removed by coughing. To accomplish this technique, the home health nurse's hand should be pressed firmly over the area of the chest wall to be vibrated. The muscles of the home health nurse's upper arm and shoulder are tensed (isometric contractions) to produce fine tremors on the chest wall as the patient exhales. Vibration is done with the flattened, not the cupped, hand.

Deep breathing by the patient assists in the movement of secretions and may stimulate coughing. A deep rapid inhalation followed by a slow, prolonged expiration may move secretions into larger airways for removal by coughing. Encourage deep breathing during chest physiotherapy.

Productive coughing is enhanced by placing the patient in a sitting position, leaning forward. Encourage coughing after chest physiotherapy.
a. Cascade cough: Have the patient take a deep slow inhalation, then cough 2 to 3 times in a row at the end of the breath to move secretions to larger airways.
b. Huff cough: Have the patient take a deep breath and make a "huff" sound when exhaling instead of the usual cough.

Postural drainage uses specific positions to let the force of gravity assist in removing lung secretions. A physician's order must be obtained before the home health nurse can carry out this procedure. There are six basic drainage positions commonly used in home care. Each is specific for major areas of the bronchopulmonary segments. Drainage positions should be maintained for 10 to 15 minutes each. During this time, alternate 2 to 3 minutes of percussion with 10 to 12 vibrations. These exercises should be performed before breakfast and at bedtime or prn. **Administer the inhaler before postural drainage.**

Primary drainage positions commonly used at home: Use a sturdy ironing board and a couch or other sturdy object of appropriate height to achieve the tilt of the Trendelenburg position. Place the narrow end of the board on the couch. Adjust the angle of the board to about 30 degrees. Brace the end of the board to prevent slipping. Pillows placed under the patient's hips/torso can also be used to achieve correct positioning (hips/torso should be elevated 12 to 20 inches to facilitate proper drainage). Exercises should be done to drain the lower bases of the lung first and proceed to the upper bases. (See Figure 10-2.)

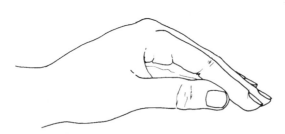

Figure 10-1 Cupped hand. (From Wade JF: *Comprehensive respiratory care: physiology and technique,* ed 3, St Louis, 1982, Mosby.)

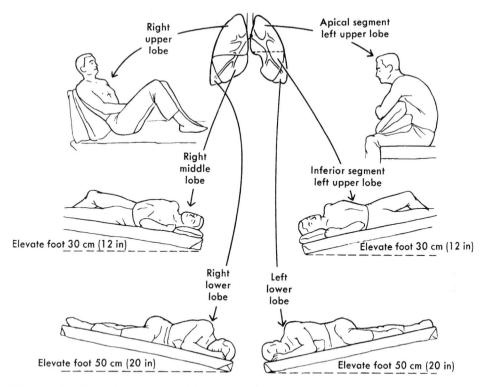

Figure 10-2 Postural drainage positions frequently used in home care. (From Phipps WJ, Cassmeyer VL, Sands JK, Lehman MK: *Medical-surgical nursing: concepts and clinical practice,* ed 5, St Louis, 1995, Mosby.)

1. To drain base of left lung (left lower lobe): Have patient well turned into right side-lying position. Percuss and vibrate over lower rib area.
2. To drain base of right lung (right lower lobe): Have patient well turned into left side-lying position. Percuss and vibrate over lower rib area.
3. To drain right middle lobe: Have patient in left side-lying position with right side of body supported. Percuss and vibrate over midchest/nipple area.
4. To drain left middle lobe: Position patient as in step 3, but in right side-lying position. Percuss and vibrate over midchest/nipple area.
5. To drain anterior upper lobes: Have patient sit up and lean back. Percuss and vibrate over collarbone/shoulder area.
6. To drain posterior upper lobes: Have patient sit up and then lean forward over a pillow. Percuss and vibrate over shoulder area.

When performing chest physiotherapy, have a cup or basin and paper tissue available for draining mucus. Offer mouthwash and assist with oral care as needed following postural drainage. Encourage patients to rest after the procedure. Note: Observe for potential contraindications of the Trendelenburg position, such as abdominal distension or irregular heart rate. If any of these conditions exist, check with the physician before positioning the patient.

11 The Patient with Congestive Heart Failure

Robyn Rice and *Troy McMullin*

Congestive heart failure (CHF) occurs when the heart is no longer able to pump and circulate blood effectively. The resulting circulatory overload or congestion is accompanied by clinical symptoms related to fluid pooling in body tissue. Long-term pharmacologic therapy, functional disability, and frequent rehospitalizations associated with this syndrome, pose severe financial and emotional stress for patients and their families.[4]

CHF may be acute or chronic and is associated with a poor prognosis.[1] For example, of newly diagnosed cases in Rochester, Minnesota, in 1981, survival following diagnosis was 80% at 3 months, 66% at 1 year, and 30% at 8 years.[9] In 1990, CHF was the underlying cause of death for about 38,000 persons; approximately 92% were among persons 65 years of age or over.[4] Increases in CHF death rates from 1980 to 1990 are attributed to a growing elderly population and longer survival of persons with hypertension or cardiac disease who subsequently develop CHF at an older age.[4]

An estimated 2 to 3 million Americans have CHF, and many are treated in their homes.[1,11] Patient assessment and education regarding precipitating factors of CHF with recommendations for lifestyle changes to control hypertension and reduce the incidence of myocardial infarction are primary focuses of this chapter.

PATHOPHYSIOLOGY

An understanding of the pathophysiology of CHF provides a framework for intervention and treatment and is based on two key concepts:[14]

1. The relationship among stroke volume, heart rate, and cardiac output
2. The heart as a two-system pump

The relationship among stroke volume, heart rate, and cardiac output must be considered when describing mechanical and physical factors that determine cardiac workload and the circulation of blood.

Stroke volume

Stroke volume represents the amount of blood pumped into the circulatory system by each myocardial contraction (normally, 60 to 130 ml of blood are ejected with each contraction). The following forces determine stroke volume:

Preload. This refers to filling pressures or the amount of blood in the left ventricle at the end of diastole, just before systole (ejection). It is also referred to as left ventricular end-diastolic pressure (LVEDP). In a normally functioning heart, an increase in preload is matched by an increase in the amount of blood pumped out of the ventricles and into the circulatory system. This phenomenon is referred to as Frank Starling's Law, which says that up to a point, increases in ventricular blood volume parallel the strength and force of contractions as the ventricle is stimulated to eject additional volume. However, in patients with CHF, sustained increases in preload lead to signs of clinical deterioration as overstretching and overworking of the myocardial muscle cause the heart to be unable to pump even moderate amounts of blood. Preload is the major determinant of myocardial oxygen consumption.[12]

Afterload. This refers to pressures in the aorta and peripheral vascular system that the heart must pump against to eject blood out of the ventricle. It is a function of both arterial pressure and left ventricular size. Any increases in vascular pressure or resistance will increase ventricular contractility as the heart attempts to maintain stroke volume and heart rate. Hypertension is one of the major factors that increase afterload.

Contractility. This refers to the strength and force of the mechanical pumping action of the heart. Increases in contractility are associated with a reduction in afterload.

Heart rate

Heart rate determines the timing and pattern of myocardial contractions and is controlled by specialized conduction cells of the heart and the autonomic nervous system.[13] Normally, increases or decreases in heart rate serve as compensatory mechanisms for variations in physical activity, emotional state, blood composition, and fluid balance. However, an irregular or abnormally slow heart rate impairs blood circulation and tissue oxygenation just as an extremely rapid heart rate shortens ventricular filling time and produces a smaller circulating blood volume. Therefore, inappropriate extremes of heart rate (lower than 50 beats/min or higher than 120 beats/min) may produce clinical signs and symptoms associated with oxygen deprivation and hypoxemia.

Cardiac output

Cardiac output describes the amount of blood pumped by the left ventricle per minute. A normal cardiac output is about 4 to 8 L/min. The relationship among cardiac output, stroke volume, and heart rate is expressed by the following equation:

$$\text{cardiac output} = \text{stroke volume} \times \text{heart rate.}$$

When stroke volume or heart rate declines, cardiac output also decreases. As cardiac output falls, so does blood pressure. If left untreated, the patient may progress to a state of cardiogenic shock. In addition, limited increases in stroke volume and heart rate cause increases in cardiac output. However, overloading the ventricle with too much fluid in patients with CHF may only serve to aggravate failure because the pumping ability of the heart cannot manage sustained increases in workload.

In maintaining fluid balance, the heart essentially functions as two pumps that are regulated by the left and right ventricles. Any damage to the heart can result in reduced pumping ability of either or both ventricles.

Left-sided failure refers to backward failure in which blood is not pumped into the arterial system and instead backs up into the pulmonary vessels and lungs. Of note, pulmonary vascular congestion and edema are the dominant clinical features of left-sided CHF. CHF rarely remains one-sided.

Right-sided failure results from disease primarily affecting the right heart. Right-sided failure most often follows left-sided failure and occurs when venous blood is unable to be pumped into the pulmonary circuit where carbon dioxide is exchanged for oxygen. Venous blood subsequently backs up into the systemic circulation, enhancing cardiac anoxia and failure. Systemic edema and circulatory congestion are the dominant clinical features of right-sided CHF.[9,10]

Left- and right-sided CHF are interrelated, and both result in an insufficient cardiac output. Compensatory mechanisms of the body functioning to offset a low cardiac output and restore volume may only aggravate fluid overload and pump failure. For example, as the anterior pituitary gland reflexively senses a decrease in blood pressure, the adrenal cortex is stimulated to secrete mineral corticoids, causing sodium and chloride retention.[11,12] This electrolyte retention can increase fluid volume and place additional stress on the heart. Also, in response to a decrease in blood pressure, the posterior pituitary releases antidiuretic hormone (ADH). ADH causes the kidneys to conserve fluid and intensifies circulatory congestion.

In summary, the causes of CHF are related to an inadequate tissue perfusion and are associated with the following clinical disorders:[2,9,11]

1. An increase in afterload (hypertension)
2. An increase in preload (circulatory overload)
3. A decrease in preload (hypovolemia, sepsis)
4. Impaired heart rate and contractility (electrolyte imbalance, myocardial infarction, pacemaker failure, coronary artery disease, congenital heart disease, valvular heart disease, cardiomyopathy)

All four may result in decreased cardiac output.

The home setting presents another variable for home health nurses when assessing and caring for patients with CHF. External and environmental factors will certainly influence the physiological response and clinical manifestations of a weakened heart and must be considered when developing the plan of care.

HOME CARE APPLICATION

Patients typically seen in home care are those with unstable CHF;[7] acute exacerbations will require hospitalization. Observation and assessment of the patient's condition regarding abnormal or fluctuating vital signs, weight changes, edema, respiratory changes, medication compliance, and dietary habits are the basis for home visits.

Planning visits

Home health nurses usually see patients with CHF 2-4 × wk depending on patient acuity, the patient's support systems, and teaching needs. Daily visits may be necessary if the patient has a new medication regimen, new diet, or changes in oxygen therapy. Visit frequency and the plan of care is based on the nurse's ongoing physical assessment and identification of patient health care needs.

Physical assessment

When evaluating decompensation (failure of the heart to maintain adequate circulation), compare any variations in the physical assessment with the patient's baseline status and vital signs. Always assess mentation and affect because confusion, combativeness, or unusual expressions of anger may be a sign of oxygen deprivation and hypoxemia. Ask patients if they have experienced fatigue, weakness, shortness of breath, or dizziness; these may be signs of pump failure.

Cardiac. Auscultate heart sounds for rate, rhythm, and intensity. Extra heart sounds such as an S_3 caused by turbulent blood flow within a weakened and damaged ventricle are characteristic of left ventricular failure in adults.[11,12] Assess for tachycardias or dysrhythmias when recording the apical-radial pulse and check blood pressure. A rapid or irregular heart rate may indicate an inadequate cardiac output.

Palpate the point of maximal impulse (PMI). Normally, the PMI is palpated at the fifth left intercostal space (5th LICS) at the midclavicular line. The PMI represents the contraction of the ventricle as it pushes upward against the chest wall.[3] With left ventricular failure, the PMI is displaced to the left. With right-sided failure, the PMI shifts to the right of the 5th LICS.

Patients with CHF may exhibit pulsus alternans, which is an alternation of strong and weak pulse amplitudes, frequently accompanied by alternating loud and soft heart sounds.[3] Pulsus alternans is common with left-sided failure and is best palpated in the radial or femoral arteries. Evaluate all peripheral pulses, noting rate, amplitude, and quality. Patients with CHF may have diminished or faint pulses due to poor circulation.

Inspect patients for signs of jugular venous distension (JVD), which is characteristic of right-sided failure. To evaluate for the presence of JVD, have patients sit in the bed with the head elevated at a 30-degree angle. Neck veins are considered abnormally distended when distension of the jugular veins can be measured at a horizontal line more than 3 cm above the sternal angle. JVD is a sign of elevated central venous pressure and fluid retention.[3]

Determine whether patients have a positive hepatojugular reflex, which is symptomatic of hepatic congestion and elevated central venous pressure. Have patients lie down, and exert firm pressure over the right upper quadrant of the abdomen while observing the neck veins. Patients are positive for a hepatojugular reflex if an increase of more than 1 cm is visible in neck veins as pressure is applied over the liver. A positive hepatojugular reflex is characteristic of right-sided CHF.[3]

Pulmonary. In left ventricular failure, blood backs up into the pulmonary circuit, causing fluid to diffuse into the alveoli and creating adventitious lung sounds. If left untreated, pulmonary congestion may progress to pulmonary edema, which presents with cyanosis, noisy respirations, and frothy pink sputum. Assess oxygenation status with arterial blood gas or by pulse oximetry. Be aware that the patients with CHF are at risk for hypoxemia and hypercapnia.

Evaluate for a cough. Is the cough dry or productive of sputum (phlegm)? Ask the patient, "How much do you think you cough up within 24 hours? A teaspoon, a tablespoon, a cup, or what?" Of note, purulent sputum has a green or yellowish color. Be aware that a cough is an important symptom of left-sided heart failure.[3]

Auscultate the lungs for crackles and wheezes. These occur when air moves into the fluid-filled alveoli and are characteristic of left-sided failure.[3] Patients also may have coarse gurgles that clear with coughing. Note the use of accessory muscles (such as the diaphragm and sternomastoids) and the respiratory rate in assessing the degree of failure. Normal resting respiratory rates in adults are about 8 to 16 breaths/min. Assess for breathing patterns associated with left ventricular failure such as the following:[3]

- Dyspnea with activity: shortness of breath that occurs with an increase in physical activity (exertional dyspnea). Ask patients to identify activities that cause shortness of breath, and ask them what they do to alleviate shortness of breath. Ask patients to ambulate to determine if shortness of breath occurs with activity.
- Orthopnea: shortness of breath that occurs when patients lie down, causing excess fluid within the vessels to move into the alveoli. To assess orthopnea, have the patient lie down. Next, raise the patient's legs and observe for orthopnea. In evaluating the severity of orthopnea, ask if the patient uses extra pillows at night to make breathing easier and, if so, how many.
- Paroxysmal nocturnal dyspnea: shortness of breath that occurs suddenly, waking patients up. Associated with sudden fluid shifts, paroxysmal nocturnal dyspnea may be accompanied by nightmares that cause patients to complain of feeling anxious and frightened.

Skin. The skin and hair can show signs of cardiac failure. The color of the skin and paleness of mucous membranes may indicate poor circulation. Of note, patients with CHF often have skin that is dusky, cool, and dry. Hair may be coarse and brittle with partial loss present.

Nail beds may show signs of poor capillary refill. Capillary refill can be evaluated by depressing the nail bed of a finger until the skin blanches. Release pressure and observe the length of time it takes for the patient's normal color to return. Return of color to the nail bed that takes longer than 3 seconds is considered abnormal and a sign of poor circulation.[3]

Clubbing of nail beds indicative of poor peripheral circulation may also be present. The angle

between the normal fingernail and nail base is approximately 160 degrees. The nail base feels firm to palpation. In late stages of clubbing (associated with hypoxia), the base of the nail is visibly swollen and the angle between nail and nail base is greater than 180 degrees.

Fluid/electrolyte and blood chemistries. On each visit measure the circumference of the ankle, dorsum, and calf of both legs to objectively evaluate dependent and peripheral edema, which are characteristic of right-sided failure. Pitting edema may or may not be present; it is evidenced by a depression left in the swollen extremity when compression is removed.

Observe for weight gain by weighing patients on the same scale and at the same time on each visit. A weight gain of 3 to 4 lb in 1 week or 2 lb in 1 day is an indicator of decompensation or problems in lifestyle habits.

Laboratory work should be obtained to assess fluid and electrolyte imbalance, which can cause problems with heart rate and contractility. Blood chemistries should be checked every other week, particularly if the patient is on intravenous furosemide (Lasix). Verify the frequency of laboratory work with the physician. Table 11-1 lists normal ranges of blood chemistries. Observe for signs and symptoms of hypokalemia, hyperkalemia, hyponatremia, and hypochloremia which may result from medication and fluid retention (Table 11-2).

Gastrointestinal. Note patient complaints of nausea, vomiting, or diarrhea. These symptoms are related to congestion of the gastrointestinal tract and typify right-sided heart failure. Abdominal distension or ascites can be evaluated by measuring abdominal girth.

Table 11-1 Blood chemistries pertinent to congestive heart failure

Measurement	Normal ranges
Potassium (K)	3.5-5.0 mEq/L
Sodium (Na)	135-145 mEq/L
Chloride (Cl)	95-106 mEq/L
Calcium (Ca)	8.5-10.0 mg/dl
Magnesium (Mg)	1.5-2.0 mEq/L
Blood urea nitrogen (BUN)	8-21 mg/dl
Creatinine	0.3-1.2 mg/dl

Table 11-2 Signs and symptoms of primary fluid and electrolyte imbalances associated with congestive heart failure[2,13]

Imbalance	Signs and symptoms
Electrolyte	
Hypokalemia	Generalized weakness and fatigue, irregular heart rate, hypotension, nausea, vomiting, apathy, coma
Hyperkalemia	Muscle twitching, musculoskeletal weakness, oliguria, nausea, diarrhea, abdominal distension
Hyponatremia	Thirst, decreased skin turgor, anorexia, nausea, vomiting, headaches, restlessness, apprehension
Hypochloremia	Hyperexcitability of nervous system and muscles, shallow breathing, hypotension, tetany
Fluid	
Hypovolemia	Weight loss, hypotension, oliguria, poor skin turgor, skin that is cool and dry, thirst
Hypervolemia	Puffy eyelids, peripheral and dependent edema, ascites, pulmonary edema, wheezes in lungs, sudden weight gain

Assess for ascites by having the patient lie down. Place the palm of one hand against the side of the patient's abdomen, and tap the opposite side of the abdomen with the other hand. A wave of fluid shifting across the abdomen indicates ascites.

In right-sided CHF, fluid backs up into the hepatic system, causing liver failure. This is associated with a rise in BUN and creatinine levels and jaundice. Palpate for an enlarged liver. Normally the liver should not be felt below the ribs after expiration.[3]

Renal. CHF affects all body organs, including the kidneys. A decline in cardiac output is accompanied by a decrease in the glomerular filtration rate. The kidneys respond by conserving fluid, and reduced urine output results. The minimal 24-hr urine output for adults is about 750 ml. The urine of CHF patients is often dark amber in color with a high specific gravity (>1.030).[4] Assess for proteinuria and glucosuria as BUN and creatinine rise with a decreased glomerular filtration rate. Be aware that the patient is at risk for metabolic acidosis or alkalosis with a decline in cardiac output.

Evidence of cardiac decompensation can be identified by a meticulous physical assessment. Any variation from the patient's baseline status should immediately be reported to the physician. Signs and symptoms of pulmonary edema and changes in level of consciousness warrant prompt medical attention. Under such circumstances home

health nurses should place the patient in a high Fowler's position, administer oxygen, and stay with the patient, fostering a calm environment, until emergency medical services arrive.

Developing the plan of care

The box below lists primary nursing diagnoses for patients with CHF. Medical treatment and nursing interventions for patients with CHF should be directed toward the following:[2,5,8,12]

- Reduced cardiac workload and enhanced performance
- Fluid management
- Reduced metabolic demands
- Stabilization of CHF at home through patient education regarding precipitating factors of cardiac failure: knowledge of medications, diet, activity regimen, etc.

Medications. A variety of medications are prescribed for patients with CHF. These medications are used to reduce afterload and/or preload and to increase contractility in an effort to improve cardiac output and restore fluid balance (Figure 11-1). Table 11-3 lists medications commonly used to treat CHF in the home.

Diuretic therapy remains a traditional treatment of CHF, and a diuretic may be the only medication required in mild failure. Diuretics reduce preload, and this reduction is usually accompanied by a

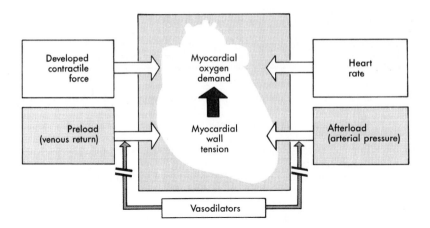

Figure 11-1 Mechanism of vasodilator action in the therapy of chronic congestive heart failure. (From Brody TM, Larner J, Minneman KP, Neu HC: *Human pharmacology: molecular to clinical,* ed 2, St Louis, 1994, Mosby.)

decrease in the patient's weight. Side effects of diuretic therapy include hypokalemia, hyponatremia, hypochloremia, and hypovolemia (Table 11-2). A record of the patient's weight helps assess the effects of the diuretic. Also, measurement of serum electrolytes is important because electrolyte imbalances may predispose patients to an irregular heart rate and sudden cardiac death.[8,11]

Thiazide diuretics are initially used in cases of mild failure. A potassium-sparing diuretic used in combination with a thiazide or loop diuretic is appropriate for patients who are taking digitalis and who are prone to hypokalemia.

Cardiac glycosides such as digoxin enhance cardiac performance by improving contractility. Electrolyte imbalances such as hypercalcemia, hypokalemia, and hypomagnesemia precipitate digoxin toxicity, as does compromised renal function. Clinical manifestations of digoxin toxicity include an irregular heart rate along with complaints of nausea, vomiting, and confusion in the elderly. Digoxin levels should be periodically monitored in patients with CHF; therapeutic levels range from 0.8 to 2 mg/ml.

Although not common in home care, intravenous dobutamine and dopamine may be administered via cassette to patients with CHF. Many of these patients are candidates for heart transplants. Dobutamine stimulates beta-adrenoreceptors and improves contractility of the heart. Depending on dose and concentration, dopamine can improve renal blood flow or cause peripheral vasoconstriction and increased myocardial contractility.

Venodilator therapy reduces preload. Venodilators such as nitrates increase venous capacity, redirecting blood flow from the pulmonary vasculature into the systemic vessels.[8]

Arterial dilators or vasodilators reduce systemic vascular resistance and afterload, resulting in reduced force against which the heart must pump to circulate blood. Arterial dilators such as hydralazine or captopril are frequently used in the treatment of hypertensive or valvular disorders that reduce cardiac output. As a vasodilator, nitrates play a major role in alleviating pain associated with angina.

Other medications administered to patients with CHF include potassium supplements, antiarrhythmics to control irregularities of heart rate, and anticoagulants to prevent thrombus formation. Reglan may be helpful with complaints of nausea.

Supplemental oxygen should be available as required and is usually administered via a nasal cannula. Flows greater than 2 to 3 L/min should be avoided in patients with an additional diagnosis of chronic obstructive pulmonary disease because high flows with these patients may remove the respiratory stimulus to breathe. (See Chapter 10.)

Diet. Diet is a primary component in the treatment of CHF. Sodium and fluid restrictions alone may be sufficient to control mild fluid retention. If

Table 11-3 Medications commonly used to treat CHF in the home

Medication	Dose/route	Side effects
Reduce afterload		
Angiotensin converting ***enzyme inhibitors***[a]		
benazepril (Lotensin)	20-40 mg PO qd	chronic cough, hyperkalemia, renal dysfunction
captopril (Capoten)[b]	50-100 mg PO tid	chronic cough, hyperkalemia, renal dysfunction, neutropenia
enalapril (Vasotec)[b]	5-20 mg PO bid	chronic cough, hyperkalemia, renal dysfunction, neutropenia
fosinopril (Monopril)	20-40 mg PO qd	chronic cough, hyperkalemia, renal dysfunction
lisinopril (Prinivil, Zestril)[b]	20-40 mg PO qd	chronic cough, hyperkalemia, renal dysfunction, neutropenia
quinapril (Accupril)[b]	10-20 mg PO bid	chronic cough, hyperkalemia, renal dysfunction, neutropenia
ramapril (Altace)	5-20 mg PO qd	chronic cough, hyperkalemia, renal dysfunction
Direct vasodilators		
hydralazine (Apresoline)	50-100 mg PO tid	hypotension, reflex tachycardia, headache, lupus, erythematosus
Reduce preload		
Loop diuretics		
bumetenide (Bumex)[b]	1-2 mg PO qd	hypocalcemia, hypokalemia, hypomagnesemia, hyponatremia
ethacrynic acid (Edecrin)[b]	50-100 mg PO qd	hypocalcemia, hypokalemia, hypomagnesemia, hyponatremia
furosemide (Lasix)[b]	40-80 mg PO qd	hypocalcemia, hypokalemia, hypomagnesemia, hyponatremia
torsemide (Demadex)[b]	10-20 mg PO qd	hypocalcemia, hypokalemia, hypomagnesemia, hyponatremia
Nitrates		
isosorbide dinitrate (Isordil, Sorbitrate)	10-40 mg PO tid	headache, dizziness, postural hypotension
isosorbide mononitrate (ISMO, Monoket)	10-20 mg PO bid	headache, dizziness, postural hypotension
nitroglycerin (Nitro-Bid, Nitrong)	2.5-9 mg PO tid	headache, dizziness, postural hypotension
nitroglycerin transdermal (Deponit, Nitro-Dur)	2.5-10 mg TOP qd	headache, dizziness, postural hypotension
pentaerythritol tetranitrate (Peritrate)	10-40 mg PO tid	headache, dizziness, postural hypotension
Improve contractility		
Cardiac glycosides		
digoxin (Lanoxin)[b]	0.125-0.25 mg PO qd	cardiac arrhythmias, nausea, vomiting, confusion, visual changes

[a]Mixed afterload and preload reduction
[b]FDA approved for the treatment of CHF

PRIMARY NURSING DIAGNOSES/ PATIENT PROBLEMS

- Decreased cardiac output
- Fluid volume excess
- Knowledge deficit; disease process and risk complications, medications, operation of home medical equipment, procedural care, diet, activity, socioeconomic resources, available community services, etc.
- Activity intolerance: ___ Ambulation, ___ ADLs, ___Other*(Specify)*
- Self-care deficit: ___ ADLs, ___ Feeding, ___Toileting, ___Other*(Specify)*
- Ineffective individual coping
- Potential for noncompliance with the therapeutic regimen

PRIMARY THEMES OF PATIENT EDUCATION

- Congestive heart failure: signs and symptoms of disease process to report to the case manager and physician
- When to call 911
- Anginal pain: recognition and treatment
- Medications: purpose, action, dosage, side effects, and methods of administration
- Diet: caloric, fluid, and sodium restriction to prevent fluid overload
- Activity: exercise and rest program
- Home oxygen therapy: operation and maintenance of equipment
- Positive coping mechanisms to use when living with a chronic disease
- Importance of following the medical regimen in order to prevent exacerbation of CHF
- Socioeconomic resources
- Community services available for people with CHF

possible, refer the patient to the registered dietitian for assistance with meal planning and specific dietary instructions. The registered dietitian can provide information about alternative ways to season and cook foods. Patients may wish to use the services of Meals-on-Wheels.

Sodium intake is usually limited to 2 to 4 g of salt daily, depending on the severity of fluid retention. Also, these patients are generally limited to 1 to 1.5 L of fluid per day. To evaluate diet and response to medication, have patients keep a record of their daily intake and output as well as a log documenting diet recall. (See Chapter 25 (hospice) for managing complaints of nausea.)

Activity. Physical activity should be planned to prevent exhaustion and should be determined by the patient's general condition. Identify those household tasks that cause exhaustion or shortness of breath, and devise strategies to reduce cardiac workload. For example, frequent rest periods before and after activities, or using oxygen while doing chores may reduce fatigue. As available, make a referral to social services for instruction in progressive relaxation techniques and guided imagery to assist patients in coping with the stress and anxiety associated with illness and subsequent changes in lifestyle.

Patient education. Patient education is a cornerstone of any plan of care. (See the box titled Primary Themes of Patient Education.) This is particularly true for patients with CHF because

lifestyle and habits strongly influence the stabilization of a weakened heart. In a 1994 study by Hagenhoff, patients with CHF ranked medication as the most important category of information to learn followed by anatomy/physiology and then, risk factors for exacerbation of CHF.[6]

The disease process and pathophysiology of CHF should be explained in such a way that patients understand the importance of taking prescribed medication and following dietary restrictions to prevent fluid retention. For example, patients should be able to name foods high in salt and should eliminate items such as potato chips, canned meats, and beer from their diet. Instruct patients to determine sodium content by reading food labels.

Avoidance of dusty and humid environments will make breathing easier for patients with CHF. Because smoking increases the demands on the heart, patients should be encouraged to stop. Using extra pillows or a foam wedge (available from the HME vendor) under the head at night can ease breathing and promote rest. If patients should suddenly become short of breath, instruct them to use their oxygen and sit up with their legs and arms in a dependent position to decrease preload and increase oxygenation.

Instruct patients to weigh themselves at the same time each day using the same scale. They should notify the physician's office if more than 2 lb are gained in 1 day. Patients who are recording intake and output can measure their fluids in standard household measuring cups. Calibrated plastic liners that fit inside the toilet to collect and measure urine can be purchased at most medical supply centers.

When evaluating patients, home health nurses may see signs of noncompliance or confusion with medication. When this occurs the purpose, action, and side effects of *all* medications should be reviewed with the patient. Using charts, coordinating medications with meals, using medication boxes or placing the week's supply of medications in separate envelopes marked for each day and stored in a shoebox for convenience may help remind patients to take their medications. As appropriate, patients should be provided instructions for home oxygen therapy. (See Chapter 10.) Patients should understand why it is important to take a potassium supplement if they are taking Lasix and should know the signs and symptoms of hypokalemia. They should be instructed to use their nitroglycerin tablets at the onset of anginal pain. Patients on digoxin should be shown how to take their own pulse. If their pulse is lower than 60 beats/min or higher than 110 beats/min, patients should consult with their physician before taking their digoxin. If on warfarin (Coumadin) or anticoagulant therapy, patients should be instructed to avoid over-the-counter medications high in vitamin K and to report signs of inappropriate bleeding (nosebleeds, red or black stools, spontaneous bruising) to the physician.

Home health nurses can use patient education to heighten patient awareness and assist with the stabilization of patients' cardiac status by reviewing conditions or situations that place extra workload on the heart, such as obesity, anemia, infection, or stress. Strategies related to these conditions should be incorporated into the plan of care. For example, instruct patients to avoid or limit physical activities that are excessively fatiguing. Patients with CHF should be aware of signs and symptoms of progressing failure such as clothes or belts suddenly becoming tight, increases in weight or fatigue, chest pain, unusual congestion of the lungs, and increased frequency of shortness of breath or coughing. They should also receive instruction regarding when to seek immediate medical attention.

SUMMARY

The treatment of CHF is aimed at reducing cardiac workload and fluid retention, improving oxygenation, and decreasing patient anxiety associated with changes in lifestyle. To live at home with CHF and prevent rehospitalizations, patients must learn to accept their disease and cope with necessary changes of habits in a positive manner. These adjustments may be particularly difficult for patients with CHF because periods of illness are interspersed with frequent periods of wellness. As patients begin to feel better, the temptation to return to old habits is great and may precipitate fluid retention. Home health nurses can provide patients with scientific explanations of the disease process as well as psychological support to foster a sense of responsibility for self-care and positive coping mechanisms. This is important, as it is recognized that no plan of care or medicine can take the place of concern for one's own health.

REFERENCES

1. American Heart Association: *Heart and stroke facts-1991,* Dallas, 1991, National Center.
2. Armstrong PW, Moe GW: Medical advances in the treatment of congestive heart failure, *Circulation* 88:2941-2952, 1993.
3. Bates B: *A guide to physical examination and history taking,* ed 6, Philadelphia, 1995, JB Lippincott.
4. Center for Disease Control: Mortality from congestive heart failure-United States, *MMWR* 43(5):77-81, 1993.
5. Dolan M: *Community and home health care plans,* Springhouse, Pa, 1990, Springhouse.
6. Hagenhoff B et al: Patient education needs as reported by congestive heart failure patients and their nurses, *J Adv Nurs* 19:685-690, 1994.
7. Health Care Financing Administration: Pub No 11 -Thru T273, Rev 3/95, Washington, DC, 1995, US Department of Health and Human Services.
8. Medical Economics Co: *Physician's desk reference,* Oradell, NJ, 1995, Medical Economics.
9. Rodeheffer RJ et al: The incidence and prevalence of congestive heart failure in Rochester, Minnesota, *Mayo Clin Proc* 68:1143-1150, 1993.
10. Ryan M: Stopping CHF while there's still time, *RN* 49(8):28-33, 1986.
11. Schocken DD et al: Prevalence and mortality of congestive heart failure in the United States, *J Am Coll Cardiol* 20:301-306, 1992.
12. Stanley M: Helping an elderly patient live with CHF, *RN* 49(9):35, 1986.
13. Thompson M et al: *Mosby's clinical nursing,* St Louis, 1993, Mosby.
14. Van Parys E: Assessing the failing state of the heart, *Nursing 87* 17(2):42, 1987.

12 The Ventilator-Dependent Patient

Robyn Rice

Clinical applications of advances in medical technology continue to have favorable influences on home health care. Patients with debilitating respiratory disease and/or respiratory insufficiency who were previously maintained in intensive care units or chronic care facilities, are now being discharged on home mechanical ventilation. Initially used as a lifesaving procedure, mechanical ventilation has evolved into either a life-support or augmenting procedure for patients unable to be "weaned," or taken off the ventilator;[25,39] hence the term *ventilator-dependent patient.* Once stabilized on ventilatory support, these patients continue to require varying degrees of caregiver help with their needs.

Ensuring safe and competent care for these technology dependent patients at home presents many challenges for the home health agency. With the assistance of home health nurses and the multidisciplinary team, ventilator-dependent patients and their families can return home and begin to rebuild their lives and renew relationships. Reasons for home treatment and the philosophies of home mechanical ventilation are well documented in the literature.[20,28,31,42]

One argument for home mechanical ventilation is that it improves the quality and length of life. Patients who return to their homes can benefit from nurturing environments that relieve the psychological and physiological stressors of hospitalization.[7] Independence and socialization are promoted as patients resume interactions with family and friends in the community and, frequently, in the workplace or school setting.[32] Additionally, cognitive and psychosocial development advances when ventilator-dependent children leave the restrictive hospital environment and experience the world around them.[1,17]

As mental health is optimized, physical health often follows.[7] The home affords ventilator-dependent patients a sense of privacy and allows them to resume normal sleeping and eating patterns. Physiological well-being is further enhanced as these patients are removed from potential sources of nosocomial, or hospital-acquired, infections that can be fatal.

Another factor that supports home treatment is the cost reduction. Home care for mechanical ventilation is much less costly than hospital care.[11,24,29] This is of special importance to patients and their families whose finances and insurance resources have been exhausted by the enormous costs of prolonged hospitalization. Estimates for the ventilator, oxygen, and adjunct equipment necessary for home discharge are cited as 10% to 25% of the costs for the same care in the hospital.[28] Other surveys cite an estimated 77% cost reduction for home mechanical ventilation in comparison with hospitalization.[37] Sivak et al.[39] surveyed costs of home care for 10 ventilator-dependent patients for a 38-month period and estimated the savings from the use of home care (as opposed to hospitalization) at $2.8 million. Monthly home care costs for mechanical ventilation may vary from $500 to $6,000,[37,39] whereas acute care costs can exceed $30,000 per month.[31]

Documented disadvantages of home mechanical ventilation include family stress related to long-term patient physical care needs, special transportation needs, lack of equipment support, and costs not covered by third-party payers including supplies and utility bills.[43] Changes in employment

185

status of caregivers (with a subsequent loss of income) due to caregiving responsibilities for disabled patients are not uncommon.[44] Advantages must be carefully weighed against disadvantages when considering home mechanical ventilation. These patients typically require a great deal of support in order to successfully make the transition from the hospital to the home setting. Before patients are allowed to go home on mechanical ventilation, safety factors (including a home environmental assessment) must also be considered. Most important, to qualify for home discharge, ventilator-dependent patients must be physiologically stable. Their caregivers must be *willing* and *able* to accept the sometimes awesome responsibility of self-care management at home.[28,29,42]

With these stipulations in mind, the home health nurse caring for ventilator-dependent patients gives attention to the following:

- Reinforcing self-care management with patient/caregiver education; identifying patient/caregiver needs as a part of discharge planning and continued service
- Patient assessment and procedural skills
- Socioenvironmental assessment to ensure cost-effective and safe patient care
- Assessment of the ventilator and the availability and functioning of related supplies and equipment to maintain the patient's well-being

The following sections of this chapter focus on the clinical management of ventilator-dependent patients in the home setting.

PATHOPHYSIOLOGY

The concepts underlying mechanical ventilation relate to respiration and the mechanics of breathing. The lungs assist cellular metabolism by providing body tissues with oxygen while removing carbon dioxide. The respiratory centers in the brain (pons and medulla) control involuntary respiratory function, and the cerebral hemispheres are responsible for voluntary respiration. Breathing is primarily an automatic process regulated by arterial blood levels of oxygen and carbon dioxide, expressed as the partial pressure of arterial oxygen (PAO_2) and the partial pressure of arterial carbon dioxide ($PACO_2$).[10,27] (See the box titled Normal Arterial Blood Gas Values.)

NORMAL ARTERIAL BLOOD GAS VALUES

- pH 7.35-7.45 (expression of hydrogen ion concentration, measures acidity of the blood)
- $PACO_2$ 35-45 mm Hg (partial pressure of carbon dioxide)
- PAO_2 60-100 mm Hg (partial pressure of oxygen)
- HCO_3 22-26 mEq/L (amount of bicarbonate dissolved in the blood)
- SAO_2 95% to 100% (oxygen saturation; if PAO_2 is between 60 and 95 mm Hg, SAO_2 should be greater than 90% with a normal pH, temperature, etc.)

Rhythmic patterns of breathing vary according to tissue oxygen needs and metabolic demands of the body. For example, breathing is slower during sleep and relaxed states and is faster with activity or any condition that increases metabolism. Concurrently, certain pulmonary, neurologic, disease, or drug-induced states may inappropriately speed or slow respiration.

The process of breathing involves two phases: (1) ventilation which consists of inspiration-expiration (the movement of air between the environment and alveoli) and (2) respiration, the gaseous exchange of oxygen and carbon dioxide between alveoli and blood circulating through the lungs and other body tissue.[4,21] The actual mechanics of ventilation occur because of pressure differences between the lungs (intrathoracic pressure) and the external environment (atmospheric pressure).[21] Contraction of the respiratory muscles and descent of the diaphragm, associated with inhalation, decrease intrathoracic pressure in relation to atmospheric pressure. This causes air to flow from the environment (high pressure) into the lungs (low pressure). At the end of inspiration, as respiratory muscles relax with exhalation, the diaphragm rises to its resting position, increasing intrathoracic pressure in relation to atmospheric pressure. This causes air to flow passively from the lungs into the environment.

Bronchitis or emphysema, bronchopulmonary dysplasia, cystic fibrosis or kyphoscoliosis (structural defects), poliomyelitis, muscular dystrophy, obstructive sleep apnea, central apnea, and trauma (neuromuscular origins) are conditions known to predispose certain patients to respiratory failure or insufficiency.[4,8,20] Whatever the cause, patients require ventilatory support when respiration is insufficient to meet the demands of metabolism.[26]

Specific equipment used to assist respiration depends on individual patient needs to balance ventilatory effort (the need for tissue oxygenation) with metabolic demands (the need to eliminate carbon dioxide as a by-product of metabolism) and to conserve respiratory muscles by preventing the fatigue of breathing.[21] Therefore equipment for ventilatory support may be used continuously or intermittently (e.g., during the day or night).

PRINCIPAL EQUIPMENT USED FOR HOME RESPIRATORY SUPPORT

Devices used to assist respiration and ventilatory effort in the home may be classified as positive pressure ventilators for invasive or noninvasive support or as negative pressure ventilators for noninvasive support, and are frequently accompanied by a variety of supplies needed to sustain home mechanical ventilation.

Ventilator-dependent patients are often advised to rent equipment. Most HME vendors rent ventilators for a monthly fee. As a part of the equipment rental package, HME vendors typically provide 24-hour service for equipment malfunction, deliver medical supplies such as tracheostomy tubes and suctioning equipment, and provide educational resources. Medicare presently pays 80% of the rental cost for most home mechanical ventilation equipment if the need is well documented and is supported by a physician's order.[15] Medicare also reimburses for home health nurse visits if the need for a skilled service (for example, monthly tracheostomy tube changes) is documented and the service is ordered by a physician.[15] When considering equipment, clarify cost and medical insurance reimbursement issues with the patient/caregiver.

Positive pressure ventilators

With positive pressure mechanical ventilation, air is forced into the lungs by application of positive pressure to the airway.[10,24,26] In other words, positive pressure ventilation is accomplished by pushing air into the chest. At the end of inspiration, positive pressure to the airway is removed and the diaphragm passively descends, allowing for exhalation. The exception is application of positive end-expiratory pressure (PEEP) with positive pressure ventilation. PEEP maintains positive pressure at the end of exhalation to keep alveoli open and improve oxygenation and ventilatory function.[31] PEEP is becoming more commonly prescribed for use in the home setting. However, PEEP usually requires more complex monitoring and equipment because it may be associated with an increased incidence of hypotension and trauma to the lungs.[28]

Mechanical ventilators are classified according to how the inspiratory phase ends[10]: (1) volume-cycled—a preset volume ends inspiration, (2) pressure-cycled—a preset pressure attainment ends inspiration, (3) flow-cycled—the decrease in patient inspiratory flow requirement ends inspiration, and (4) time-cycled—a preset time interval ends inspiration.

Piston-driven volume-cycled ventilators are commonly used in home care today because they easily compensate for changes in lung compliance and resistance.[24,28] Many of the current models are microprocessor controlled, which augments the device's precision in delivering consistent breathing patterns. Easy to use and lightweight, these ventilators are readily transported under wheelchairs and require a minimum level of preventive maintenance to ensure long-term, safe operation. Examples of volume-cycled positive pressure ventilators seen in home care today include the LP6PLUS and LP10 (Aequitron Medical, Inc.), the PLV100 and 102 (Life Care), and the Bear 33 (Bear Medical Ventilator). Although these ventilators differ in size and design, many have basic features that are quite similar (see Appendixes 12-1 and 12-2).

Invasive support. Frequently, positive pressure ventilators in the home setting are used with patients who cannot maintain ventilation for any length of time and who often require continuous mechanical ventilation.[28] Under these circumstances a backup respiratory support system must be placed in the home in the form of a self-inflating manual ventilator (AMBU bag) and a second ventilator to ensure patient safety and adequate ventilation.[19]

Noninvasive support. Patients whose conditions or disease do not require continous support can frequently be ventilated via a mouthpiece, oral/nasal mask, nasal mask adaptor or pneumobelt in place of a tracheostomy tube. This noninvasive delivery by the volume ventilator meets the needs of patients who typically have neuromuscular dysfunction or early stage respiratory insufficiency-type diseases who cannot maintain a normal PO_2 or PCO_2 with only spontaneous respirations. Augmenting their spontaneous breathing (respite ventilation), which generally occurs at night, allows the patient daytime freedom.

Negative pressure noninvasive support. Another form of noninvasive ventilatory support in the home may be accomplished with negative pressure ventilators, or rocking beds, or by use of continuous positive airway pressure (CPAP), or by use of a bi-level pressure device (BiPAP).[19] This equipment also does not require a tracheostomy and is typically used with patients who have neuromuscular dysfunction and require ventilatory support at night or periodically during the day.[19] Home health nurses should consult the respiratory therapist from the patient's HME vendor with any questions or concerns regarding the operation and use of this equipment.

Oxygen therapy

Supplemental oxygen may not be necessary for ventilator-dependent patients who need assistance with breathing but do not require additional oxygen to maintain an appropriate PAO_2. As a general guideline, supplemental oxygen should be added to the ventilator circuit to maintain a PAO_2 at or above 60 mm Hg.[20,21] Oxygen concentrators are frequently used as the primary source of supplemental oxygen for ventilator-dependent patients. An oxygen cylinder and regulator are usual backup reserves and improve patient mobility when traveling. Liquid oxygen systems are an alternative for those patients who consume high liter flows of oxygen and are also ambulatory (e.g., students with bronchopulmonary dysplasia). (Review Chapter 10 for further information on home oxygen therapy.)

Adjunct equipment

Additional ancillary equipment and supplies used for home mechanical ventilation are listed in the box on p. 189. Their use varies with patient needs. The HME vendor will deliver requested supplies on a monthly basis or as needed.

Tracheostomy tubes. Tracheostomy tubes are artificial airways made of silver, stainless steel, and plastic or other synthetic materials (see Figure 12-1, A-H). Costs for tracheostomy tubes range from \$14 to \$100.[24] Many are reusable. Oxygen and communication needs, as well as comfort level, are critical determinants when selecting a tracheostomy tube to meet specific patient requirements.

Tracheostomy tubes may be cuffed or uncuffed. A cuffless tracheostomy tube or fenestrated tracheostomy tube (which has an opening in the outer cannula above the cuff) allows the patient to talk as air moves upward and over the vocal cords. Patients who require continuous ventilation, for whom aspiration may be a problem, generally benefit from the Bivona FOME-CUF tracheostomy tube or one of the high-volume, low-pressure cuffed tracheostomy tubes made by Shiley/Portex.[31,35] The cuffs on these types of tracheostomy tubes prevent occlusion of tracheal capillary blood flow, which can cause tissue necrosis. Pediatric tracheostomy tubes are usually uncuffed.

A tracheostomy tube is basically composed of three parts: the outer cannula, the inner cannula, and the obturator. The outer cannula is the main part of the tracheostomy tube and essentially holds the stoma open while the tube is fitted into the tracheostomy and downward into the trachea. The outer cannula is held in place with tracheostomy ties or a Velcro collar (Figure 12-2).

Tracheostomy ties are recommended to secure the tracheostomy tube in pediatric or highly mobile patients because Velcro ties can pop open. Tracheostomy ties should be secured by a double knot at the side of the neck with room for only one finger to slip between the ties and the patient's neck. Change tracheostomy ties daily to prevent irritation to the neck.

The inner cannula fits inside the outer cannula and locks into place. The inner cannula is easily removed from the outer cannula. To prevent buildup of secretions, the inner cannula should be removed and cleaned at least daily. Be aware that not all tracheostomy tubes have inner cannulas.

The obturator is a stylet with a smooth, rounded end that fits inside the outer cannula and is used to insert the outer cannula. The tip of the obturator extends beyond the end of the outer cannula and is designed to protect the tracheostomy from damage during insertion of the outer cannula. The obturator completely occludes the airway when in place.

PRINCIPAL EQUIPMENT AND SUPPLIES USED FOR HOME MECHANICAL VENTILATION[19,24,48]

A. Primary ventilator
1. Ventilator circuits
2. Ventilator filters
3. Heated humidifier or cascade
   a. Sterile or distilled water (optional), or tap water boiled for 15 minutes
   b. Condensation drainage bags
   c. Heat and moisture exchangers (optional)
4. External 12-volt battery with power cord
5. Volume bag (optional)
6. Disinfectant

B. Secondary ventilator
1. Identical backup ventilator (optional)
2. AMBU bag (manual resuscitator)

C. Oxygen and related supplies
1. Oxygen source (optional): oxygen concentrator with backup compressed gas cylinder (tank)
2. Oxygen connecting tubing: pressure-compensated flowmeters are recommended with the use of 50 feet of connecting tubing
3. Air compressor and aerosol tubing for nebulizer treatments (optional)

D. Tracheostomy equipment and related supplies
1. Extra tracheostomy tube(s)—keep a tube 1 size smaller in home
2. Dressings (absorbent and lint-free)
3. Extra tracheostomy tube ties, Velcro collar, or twill tape
4. Water-soluble lubricant
5. Syringes
6. Sterile and nonsterile gloves
7. Cotton swabs
8. Stoma ointment (as prescribed by physician)
9. Sterile unit-dose and bottled normal saline (optional)—-may use tap water to rinse suction catheter *after* suctioning is completed
10. Hydrogen peroxide
11. Suction machine
    a. Extra collection bottles
    b. Suction catheters (Yankauer catheter—optional)
    c. Extension tubing

E. Home medical equipment
1. Hospital bed (optional)
2. Patient communication aid
3. As needed, equipment to assist with patient bowel/bladder management and personal care
4. Wheelchair/walker/cane

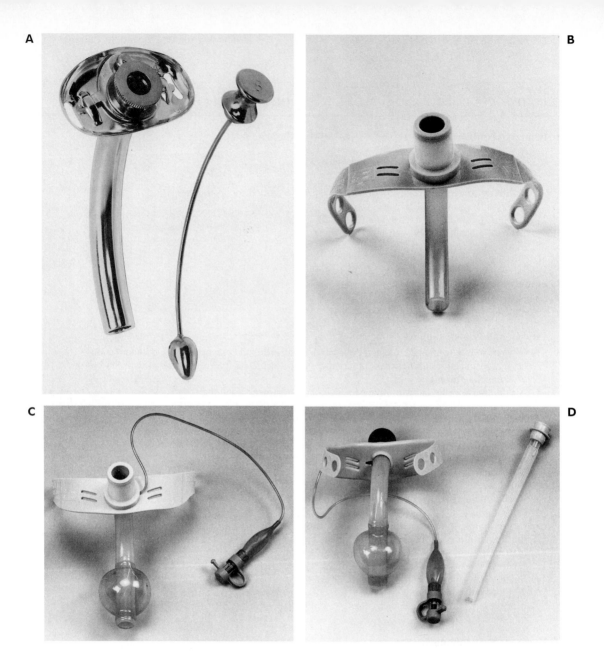

Figure 12-1 A, Silver tracheostomy tube and obturator. (Photo courtesy Pilling Co, Fort Washington, Pa.) **B,** Cuffless tracheostomy tube. (Photo courtesy Concord/Portex, Inc, Keene, NH.) **C,** Cuffed tracheostomy tube: anterior view. (Photo courtesy Concord/Portex, Inc, Keene, NH.) **D,** Cuffed tracheostomy tube: posterior view and inner cannula. (Photo courtesy Concord/Portex, Inc, Keene, NH.) **E,** Cuffed fenestrated tracheostomy tube, inner cannula, and obturator. (Photo courtesy Pfizer/Shiley, Inc, Irvine, Calif.) **F,** Neonatal and pediatric tracheostomy tubes and obturators. (Photo courtesy Pfizer/Shiley, Inc, Irvine, Calif.) **G,** FOME-CUF tracheostomy tube. (Photo courtesy Bivona, Inc, Gary, Ind.) **H,** DPRV tracheostomy tube, inner cannula, and obturators. (Photo courtesy Pfizer/Shiley, Inc, Irvine, Calif.)

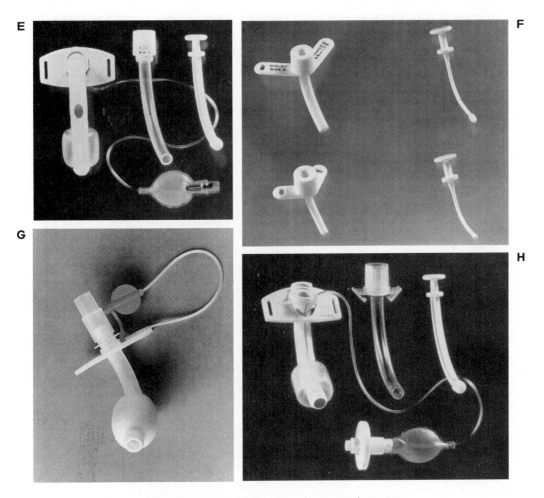

Figure 12-1, cont'd. For legend see opposite page.

Therefore it is *essential* to remove the obturator as soon as the outer cannula is inserted.

Communication devices. There are numerous communication devices currently available. These include reusable tracheostomy speaking valves that direct exhaled air upward over the vocal cords, an electronic larynx held by hand against the outside of the neck, electronic resonators that are activated by a small tube placed in the mouth and do not require functional upper extremities, typewriters, keyboards, computer terminals, and simple pen and paper. All of these devices encourage ventilator-dependent patients to communicate their needs and feelings.[25,28] More specialized equipment may be either rented or purchased from the HME vendor.

HOME DISCHARGE PLANNING

Predischarge planning should begin at least 2 weeks before discharge. The HME vendor and professional staff from the hospital usually provide initial patient and caregiver instruction sessions regarding

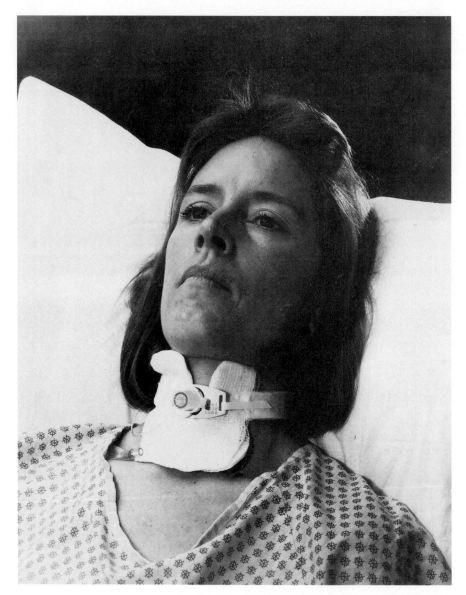

Figure 12-2 Using a Velcro collar to secure the tracheostomy tube. (Photo courtesy Dale Medical Products, Inc.)

ventilator management and related care to ensure a safe transition from hospital to home.[25,28]

The home health nurse, home health aide, clinical nurse specialist, respiratory therapist or designated home care coordinator, and physician (the multidisciplinary team) should attend as many of these patient instruction sessions as possible. Do-

ing so enables them to later reinforce previous instruction and also helps to identify any potential problem areas or special patient/caregiver concerns that should be addressed before discharge. It also provides home health personnel with realistic goals in developing the plan of care for these patients. For example, prior to discharge the home health nurse should establish who will be responsible for changing the outer cannula of the patient's tracheostomy tube and frequency of changes. Any concerns with this procedure should be brought up at this time.

An environmental evaluation of household structural needs and considerations, before patient discharge, further ensures a safe and practical return to the home.[29] For example, patients' rooms should have appropriate electrical outlets for the ventilator and related equipment, and afford easy access to the bathroom and kitchen. If the patient uses a wheelchair; widened doors, walkways, and ramps may need to be installed. The bathroom may need to be modified or have special equipment installed for patient use and convenience. A working telephone, running water, and adequate heating and air-conditioning are other household features that support discharging ventilator-dependent patients to their homes. The local electric company should be notified of the patient's electrically powered life-support equipment. These patients are usually placed on a priority list for service. These patients would certainly be priority clientle in the home health agency's disaster plan.

Patient/caregiver needs to consider prior to discharge

Smith, Findeis, and Thomas report that caregivers' most immediate self-perceived needs are to learn essential survival knowledge and skills of home ventilator management such as handling equipment, techniques for suctioning and tracheostomy care, and correct responses to emergency situations.[9,41,46] In planning for discharge, understanding everyday patient care needs appears to be more essential information for caregivers as opposed to pathophysiologic content.[40] Patient perceptions of immediate discharge planning needs commonly reflect those of caregivers; physical care and safety needs appear to overshadow knowledge of lung disease.[47] In addition, knowledge of financial and other matters including insurance coverage, how to fill out forms, money for supplies, utility bills, oxygen equipment, and transportation to the physician appear to be primary concerns of patients/caregivers and should be addressed as a part of discharge planning.[46]

Ideally, patients/caregivers should be able to administer the majority of required procedural care

with little intervention from professional staff before patient discharge (Figure 12-3). This capability helps to reduce patient/caregiver anxiety caused by separation from continuous hospital support.[40]

HOME CARE APPLICATION

Home health agencies should regard patients discharged to the home setting on ventilators as being at high risk for potential problems with equipment and complications with care. The following conditions of acceptance should be considered as policy when admitting ventilator-dependent patients to home health agency services:

- A working telephone in the home
- An HME vendor on call 24 hours a day, 7 days a week, for equipment malfunction and support
- An alternate ventilatory support system and (as appropriate) an additional oxygen source in the home
- A patient support system; (caregivers) *willing* and *able* to assist with patient care

These conditions of acceptance support patient safety and ensure that home health nurses have reasonable resources to work with.

Visit frequency

The HME vendor installs equipment and plays a major role in establishing the ventilator-dependent patient at home. The home health nurse should make an initial co-visit with the respiratory therapist from the HME vendor to review equipment and to mutually decide learning needs and outcomes of care with the patient/caregiver.

For the first week the home health nurse often makes daily visits to assess the patient's cardiopulmonary status and patient/caregiver progress with procedural aspects of care. The frequency of visits after this period depends on patient needs. During the first 2 weeks, 24-hour private duty care may be requested because this is a very anxious time for patients/caregivers who are developing independence from the hospital setting. As the ventilator-dependent patient and the caregivers settle into their routine and become comfortable with equipment and related care needs, visit frequency typically is decreased to monthly visits for procedural requirements such as tracheostomy tube

Patient's Name:_____ Caregiver's Name:_____

	Met	Not Met

1. Verbalize phone numbers to post by ventilator:
   - Home health agency
   - Home medical equipment (HME) company   _____   _____
   - Physician   _____   _____
   - 911/Local emergency room   _____   _____
   - Local power company (notify the power company
     that the patient is ventilator-dependent and
     request priority service)   _____   _____
   - Fire department   _____   _____
2. Demonstrate operation of ventilator
   (See manufacturer's manual, equipment varies):
   A. Identify parts of the tubing circuit
      - inspiratory and expiratory tubing   _____   _____
      - patient pressure tubing and port
        on rear panel of ventilator   _____   _____
      - exhalation valve tubing and port
        on rear panel of ventilator   _____   _____
      - exhalation valve   _____   _____
      - trach adapter   _____   _____
      - air inlet on rear panel of ventilator   _____   _____
      - DC power hookup   _____   _____
   B. Identify location and demonstrate replacement of fuse   _____   _____
   C. Check/adjust ventilator setting as ordered
      - mode   _____   _____
      - rate   _____   _____
      - inspiratory time   _____   _____
      - flow   _____   _____
      - high-pressure alarm   _____   _____
      - low-pressure alarm   _____   _____
      - PEEP/CPA   _____   _____
   D. Verbalize/demonstrate cleaning, storage and/or
      replacement of equipment   _____   _____
   E. Verbalize/demonstrate how to troubleshoot alarms   _____   _____
3. Verbalize/demonstrate what to do in case
   there is a power or equipment failure:
   - Manual resuscitation of the patient   _____   _____
   - Use of backup home ventilator, if available   _____   _____
   - Call and notify the power company   _____   _____
   - Call the respiratory therapist, from
     the HME company, for assistance   _____   _____
   - Call the home health agency for assistance   _____   _____
   - Consider 911 for emergency situations   _____   _____
4. Verbalize/demonstrate tracheostomy care (refer
   to manufacturer guidelines as tracheostomy
   tubes vary in use/cleaning):
   - Changing the tracheostomy tube   _____   _____
   - Cleaning the tracheostomy site
     and changing ties   _____   _____
   - Suctioning the patient   _____   _____
   - Cleaning and storage of equipment   _____   _____

Comments:

_____Passed   _____Needs to repeat

Professional's Signature:_____ Date:_____

Figure 12-3 Discharge patient/caregiver checklist for home mechanical ventilation.

changes and prn need. Visits by the respiratory therapist from the HME vendor essentially follow the same pattern as home health nurse visits, eventually occurring monthly to evaluate the patient, deliver supplies, and check equipment.[21]

Developing the plan of care and patient education

Although the respiratory therapists from the HME vendor are routinely responsible for instructing patients and caregivers in procedural aspects of care, home health nurses should reinforce instructions and evaluate compliance with teaching during their visits. The ventilator-dependent patient's care can be complicated and requires sound thinking. An important part of the home health nurse's role in patient/caregiver education is to provide a basis for sound decision making and to foster a sense of competency and good judgment. (See the boxes titled Primary Nursing Diagnoses and Primary Themes of Patient Education.)

The HME vendor typically leaves a patient care manual outlining equipment management and procedural aspects of care in the patient's home. The home health nurse should review this manual as an additional resource for patient education.

When developing a plan of care, no matter how much equipment surrounds the ventilator-dependent patient, home health nurses should never let technology take precedence over basic physical and psychological assessment of the patient. In other words, pay attention to the patient *before* paying attention to the machines.

A holistic assessment of ventilator-dependent patients should include the following:

- Baseline vital signs and cardiopulmonary status as a standard for future evaluation
- Physiological factors that relate disease process and issues involving ventilator dependence
- Patient/caregiver educational needs (includes physical aspects of self-care management as well as ongoing issues with finances and insurance)
- Psychosocial concerns related to ventilator dependence and caregiving
- Spiritual concerns and needs
- Availability of community resources to facilitate self-care management

PRIMARY NURSING DIAGNOSES/ PATIENT PROBLEMS

- Impaired verbal communication
  Ineffective breathing pattern
- Fluid volume overload
- Risk for infection: respiratory
- Knowledge deficit: disease process and risk complications, socioeconomic resources, troubleshooting and operation of equipment, procedural care, medications, diet, infection control, available community services, etc.
- Altered nutrition: potential for less than body requirements
- Activity intolerance:___ Ambulation, ___ ADLs, ___Other *(Specify)*
- Self-care deficit:___ ADLs, ___Grooming, ___Toileting, ___Other *(Specify)*
- Risk for pain: stress ulcers
- Risk for injury: tracheostomal trauma
- Risk for impaired skin integrity
- Body image disturbance
- Risk for loneliness
- Powerlessness
- Spiritual distress
- Ineffective individual coping
- Risk for caregiver role strain
- Ineffective family coping

Physical assessment of primary complications and nursing management

When conducting the physical assessment, home health nurses should observe for the following complications associated with ventilator dependence.[45]

Ineffective breathing pattern. **Assess** for over- or underventilation as related to inadequate ventilator settings or trauma to lung tissue (for example, as a result of positive pressure from the ventilator producing a rupture in alveolar or pulmonary structures, such as a pneumothorax). Primary signs and symptoms of respiratory distress are patient complaints of unrelieved shortness of breath, a change in the patient's level of consciousness or mentation (the patient may suddenly become combative), and changes in baseline vital signs or skin color. Assess for leaks or cracks in the ventilator circuit tubing which may cause suspected hypoxia.

**PRIMARY THEMES
OF PATIENT EDUCATION**

- The use of alternative speech methods
- Disease process: signs and symptoms to report to the case manager and physician
- When to call 911
- Socioeconomic resources
- What to do in case of equipment or power failure (manual resuscitation of the patient, who to call, etc.)
- Operation and maintenance of equipment
- Procedural care
- Medications
- Diet
- Positive coping strategies to use when living with a chronic illness (positive lifestyle adaptations to school, work, the home milieu, or family role changes)
- Strategies to promote patient ties to religion, family, friends, and community
- Caregiver/family respite alternatives
- Community services available for ventilator-dependent patients and their caregivers/families

Assess for mucus plugs or for very thick tracheal secretions, particularly in children. Mucus plugs can block the airway and cause respiratory distress. Very thick secretions or yellow/green secretion may indicate either insufficient humidity or a possible infection.[14]

Interventions include reporting signs and symptoms of respiratory distress to the physician. Duct tape can be temporarily used to seal circuit air leaks until tubing is replaced. As appropriate, recommend that patients go to a hospital emergency department for further evaluation and administer supplemental oxygen until emergency medical services arrive. Techniques for CPR should be reviewed with caregivers during the first home visit.

A source of humidity is essential for routine tracheostomy care because the tube bypasses the nose and mouth, which normally humidify inspired air. A tracheostomy collar, vaporizer, room humidifier, or in-line ventilator humidifier can be used to prevent the drying of secretions and formation of mucus plugs.[22]

Risk for infection: Respiratory. **Assess** for an elevated temperature, increased heart rate, or changes in the color, consistency, and amount of mucus produced. Be aware that infection in these patients can arise from many different sources including the environment; evaluate accordingly.

Interventions include reporting an elevated temperature to the physician, who may request a sputum specimen for laboratory evaluation. The patient/caregiver should be instructed to routinely initiate antibiotic therapy at the first signs of respiratory infection.[35] Teach infection control procedures to ventilator-dependent patients and their caregivers, focusing on handwashing and proper techniques for draining tubing, and cleaning humidifiers and related equipment.

Fluid volume overload. **Auscultate** the lungs for increased wheezes, increased lung sounds, or deviations from baseline status. Palpate extremities for edema, and if possible, weigh the patient to evaluate fluid overload. In ventilator dependence, edema originates from the following:[28]

- Heart failure
- Hypoalbuminemia
- Unchanged body position; dependent edema (poor venous return)
- Rebreathing moisture that is normally lost with exhalation (The ventilator-dependent patient may gain as much as 300 to 500 ml of extra water within 24 hours.)
- Positive pressure ventilation (Increases in intrathoracic pressure cause decreased venous return to the heart. This produces a low cardiac output, resulting in a backup of fluid in the extremities. Additionally, a low cardiac output stimulates ADH production, which conserves fluid in response to the body's false assumption of a dehydrated or hypovolemic state.)
- Renal failure as a consequence of congestive heart failure (CHF) or related disease process

Interventions include diuretics as part of the medication regimen to treat fluid overload. In addition, blood should be drawn for evaluation of electrolytes (particularly sodium and potassium levels because ventilator-dependent patients are prone to hyponatremia and hypokalemia) as well as for BUN and creatinine levels to evaluate renal function.[17,18] Dependent edema can be managed by encouraging mobility and periodically elevating extremities. Chest physiotherapy is helpful to clear the airway of excess secretions. (See Chapters 10 and 11.)

Altered nutrition: Less than body requirements. **Assess** patients for inappropriate weight loss. Malnutrition is frequently associated with COPD and is caused by poor intake, infection, and increased work of breathing.[30]

Interventions include recommending a diet in which half the patient's caloric requirements are met by a fat source (this limits CO_2 production and excess ventilatory demands).[5] As possible, initiate a referral to the dietitian for further evaluation. Patients with malnutrition may require enteral feedings or parenteral alimentation.

Pain: Stress ulcers. **Assess** patient complaints of nausea, abdominal pain, and vomiting. Assess for black, tarry stools which usually indicate an upper GI bleed. Bright red blood in the stool usually indicates lower GI bleeding. Be aware that ventilator-dependent patients are prone to stress ulcers and gastrointestinal hemorrhage.

Interventions include antacid therapy. Stools should be tested for occult blood when possible. Request ventilator-dependent patients to report blood in their stool or abdominal discomfort to their nurse or physician. Consult with the physican regarding treatment for pain control because some medications may exacerbate gastrointestinal hemorrhaging.

Risk for injury: Tracheostomal trauma. **Assess** for signs and symptoms of bleeding from the stoma. Tracheostomal trauma can be caused by the following:

- Too vigorous suctioning
- Overinflation of the tracheostomy tube cuff
- Strictures and adhesions of tissue to the tracheostomy tube

Interventions include teaching the patient and caregiver techniques of tracheostomy care. Tracheostomy tubes should be routinely changed to prevent adhesions and should never be forced into the patient's neck.

Risk for impaired skin integrity. **Assess** for signs/symptoms of skin breakdown caused by immobility or incontinence. Ventilator-dependent patients may become afraid to move from their beds for fear of losing their breath or disrupting the ventilator. This can progress to an essentially bedridden state, although it should be noted that many ventilator patients are not bedbound.

Interventions include obtaining a hospital bed for the patient. This will ease the patient's ability to make transfers. Some patients may require wheelchairs, walkers, or a hoyer lift to improve mobility. Consider a referral to rehabilitation services for a home exercise program to promote mobility. (Review wound care in Chapter 13 and incontinence management in Chapter 15.) Consider utilizing the services of the social worker or psychiatric home health nurse for support with patient stress management.

Medication regimen and procedural care

Medications and treatments for ventilator-dependent patients are similar to those for patients with COPD. (See Chapter 10.) Bronchodilators, diuretics, steroids, electrolyte supplements, cardiotonic medication, and chest physiotherapy are used to enhance respiration and to control edema.[17,24] In addition, ventilator-dependent patients are occasionally given antibiotics because they are susceptible to pulmonary infections.

Tracheostomy tube care. Tracheostomy tube changes are a primary skilled service provided by home health nurses for uncomplicated ventilator-dependent patients. Because of potential problems with bleeding and unknown patient response, the first outer cannula exchange should be done by the patient's physician in the medical office or hospital.

The patient's tracheostomy tube should be changed at least monthly to reduce the incidence of infection and esophageal strictures.[35] Infants and children will require more frequent outer cannula changes as related to growth and development factors. For complicated cases, a joint visit by two home health nurses may be required for this procedure. Changing the tracheostomy tube in a calm, reassuring, and expedient manner is important because any interruption of the airway can be a frightening and anxious experience for patients and their caregivers.

Tracheostomy tube changes are frequently done with the patient supine. A towel is placed between the shoulder blades to expose the stoma. Although this is a traditional position and useful with infants and children, many adult patients may tolerate this procedure best when sitting up. An upright position may give patients some feeling of control during the procedure and decrease the risk for aspiration and a choking sensation. In addition, instructing the patient to look upward and swallow during the procedure opens the airway to a correct anatomical position for tube insertion and may facilitate insertion.[35] This may also provide a mental focus that distracts the patient from some of the anxiety caused by the procedure and decrease the risk of aspiration.

If possible, caregivers should be taught the fundamentals of changing the tracheostomy tube and encouraged to assist the home health nurse with this procedure. If the tube should become dislodged in the middle of the night or when the patient is away from home, the family is then prepared to handle the situation—without emergency intervention from the ambulance service—until evaluation by the physician or home health nurse is possible.

If the tracheostomy tube accidentally comes out and the caregivers cannot reinsert it or reinsert a tracheostomy tube one size smaller, they should be advised to make a tight seal over the patient's stoma with their hand and manually ventilate the patient with the AMBU bag via a face mask until the nurse, the respiratory therapist from the HME vendor, or the emergency medical service arrives to provide assistance.

The inner cannula should be cleaned and replaced at least daily. Some inner cannulas are disposable for one time use only. If reusable, extra outer and inner cannulas may be cleaned with soap and water, rinsed with tap water, air dried, and stored in plastic bags.[24] A 50% hydrogen peroxide solution followed by a tap water rinse may help remove crusted material on the tracheostomy tube. Pipe cleaners or small brushes can be used to clean the inside of the tracheostomy tube.

Metal tracheostomy tubes may be washed with soap and water, boiled for 5 minutes, and then air dried for storage. Do not use hydrogen peroxide with metal tracheostomy tubes because it will corrode the metal.[24]

Tracheostomy tube cuff management. A tracheostomy cuff is useful for precise oxygen and air volume administration. Additionally, a tracheostomy cuff minimizes aspiration in patients with poor ability to swallow. A standard Luer syringe is used to inject air into the cuff via the pilot balloon for most cuffed tracheostomy tubes. An exception is the FOME-CUF tracheostomy tube, which requires a 60-ml syringe to deflate the cuff before insertion and upon removal.

Cuffed tracheostomy tubes should be periodically deflated to prevent tissue damage and promote communication.[35] The syringe should be inserted into the Luer valve and air should be withdrawn until resistance is felt. When the cuff is deflated, the pilot balloon becomes flat.

Cuff inflation varies according to patient comfort levels and with the minimal amount of air required to seal the tracheostomy. The minimal leak technique is commonly used to reduce the incidence of tracheostomal wall necrosis. As the ventilator gives the patient a breath, the cuff is slowly inflated until it presses against the tracheostomal wall and prevents auscultated air leaks when the patient inhales and exhales. Air is then withdrawn from the cuff until a small air leak is auscultated the next time the ventilator gives a breath. Usually 5 cc's of air are required to achieve a minimal occluding volume.[24] The Bivona FOME-CUF is designed to passively inflate until it meets the tracheal wall, providing good occlusion with minimal pressure against the tracheal wall.[3]

Stoma care. The stoma should be cared for daily and as needed. When making a visit, home health nurses inspect the skin surrounding the tracheostomy for signs of redness or infection and report findings to the physician as appropriate. The stoma should be gently cleaned with soap and water. Avoid the use of hydrogen peroxide and Betadine, if possible, as they may enhance skin breakdown.[23] After cleaning, apply an absorbent, lint-free dressing around the stoma.

Suctioning. Suctioning should be done whenever the patient's secretions build up in the airway and before and after the tracheostomy tube is changed. Although home health nurses should perform all procedures in as aseptic a manner as possible, in most cases suctioning, like stoma care and routine inner cannula changes, can be done by caregivers using clean technique.[12] Instruct caregivers to irrigate suction catheters with distilled or tap water and store them in a clean paper towel between uses. Suction catheters should be discarded

---

PROBLEM SOLVING HOME MECHANICAL VENTILATOR ALARMS[10,24]

Low-pressure alarms

1. Check the circuit for leaks; change circuit tubing as needed.
2. Check the tracheostomy cuff for a leak; inflate per comfort level.
3. Check exhaled air with volume bag. If range is unacceptable, call HME vendor. Manually ventilate the patient with the AMBU until the respiratory therapist from the HME vendor arrives.

Alarms as patient experiences cardiopulmonary distress

1. Take vital signs.
2. If unsure whether patient is getting sufficient oxygen, disconnect from the ventilator and ventilate the patient with the AMBU bag.
3. As time allows, suction and administer bronchodilator treatment.
4. Alert the physician. Stay with the patient until the emergency medical service arrives.
5. Administer cardiopulmonary resuscitation as appropriate.

High-pressure alarms

1. Suction; use saline to thin mucus plugs.
2. Check tubing for obstructions or collapse. Change circuit tubing as needed.
3. Drain excess water in tubing into drainage receptacle.
4. Administer bronchodilator treatment as ordered.

Note: These are general guidelines. Specific interventions should be based upon individual patient assessment and circumstance, as well as home health agency policy and procedures.

within 24 hours, or they may be cleaned with a 50% hydrogen peroxide solution and then boiled in water for 10 minutes, air dried, and stored in a new plastic bag for reuse.[36] The suction canister should be emptied and cleaned daily with soap and hot water. Suction tubing should also be cleaned daily with soap and hot water per home health agency policy or per HME vendor guidelines.[12]

Ventilator assessment

The home health nurse should become familiar with the ventilator dials and settings as well as circuit maintenance and proper responses to equipment alarms. See the box above for troubleshooting guidelines. Ventilator settings are primarily determined by patient comfort levels.[28] Ventilator assessment should become a routine part of the home health nurse's visit. (See Appendix 12-3.)

Infection control

Typically, ventilator setups (tubing) and the humidifier should be changed 2 or 3 times a week or per HME vendor guidelines for disinfection.[24] Tubing and the humidifier reservoir may be washed in soapy water, soaked in a 1:3 white vinegar/tap water solution for 15 to 20 minutes, and then rinsed thoroughly with tap water and air dried.[24,36] When

tubing is dry, it can then be stored in a new plastic bag. The exterior of the ventilator should be cleaned with a common disinfectant. (Review Chapter 5 for infection control guidelines.)

Psychosocial and spiritual assessment

Psychosocial and spiritual needs related to ventilator dependence are well documented.[6,7,16,17] Depression, fear, and a profound sense of loss are common feelings experienced by ventilator-dependent patients.[35] These feelings can be caused by a restrictive lifestyle, problems with communication and finances, and a high dependency upon others for basic needs.[13]

Fear is usually related to equipment malfunction and the possibility of not being able to breathe.[7] Patients with these fears often become very fixated on their immediate surroundings and the length of their tubing. These fixations can progress to complete activity intolerance and magnify problems caused by immobility.

Encourage patient mobility. Most wheelchairs can be set up with a ventilator attached to the back. Additionally, disposable heat and moisture exchangers can be added to the patient circuit so cumbersome humidifiers are not needed when traveling.[24]

Fear of equipment and alarms can be managed by patient education. Review the use of alternate ventilatory support systems and help the patient and caregiver identify circumstances when the HME vendor and home health agency should be called. The family may wish to tape the telephone number of the HME vendor on top of the ventilator, along with their physician's number, the home health agency's number, and the local emergency service's number.

Communication should be encouraged. Most ventilator-dependent patients are quite capable of directing their own care. In the home setting this can restore a sense of control and self-esteem. Home health nurses or speech therapists may help the patient choose a communication system that is easy to use and fits within the household budget.

When assessing the integrity of the patient's support system, be aware of problems that can result from constant care needs. Caregivers may become stressed when coping with continuous patient demands.[40,46,47] In addition, preexisting conflicts that may have temporarily abated with acute illness may resurface when the patient comes home. The impact of illness and the finality of ventilator dependence may not be experienced by patients and their caregivers until they are home where lost routines and changes in role and body image are poignantly felt.[7]

Caring, listening, being available to encourage communication, and providing information and support as needed are probably the best ways to assess and promote the integrity of the household as well as the intactness of the family system. Once a feeling is expressed and a problem verbalized, it can then be dealt with realistically as a part of interpersonal relationships. As mentioned earlier, a referral to the psychiatric home health nurse, social worker, the patient's religious leader, or respite services may be necessary to alleviate acute patient and caregiver stress.

PEDIATRIC ISSUES

Pediatric tracheostomy tubes less than a size 4 are usually cuffless and do not have an inner cannula. These tubes should be changed at least 1 to 2 times a week.[24] Parents with infants should be taught that if the tracheostomy tube accidentally comes out and they cannot reinsert it, they should try to reinsert a tracheostomy tube one size smaller.[2] If

this tube cannot be inserted, a suction catheter can be placed in the stoma, and breaths given through the catheter. When the infant relaxes, instruct parents to attempt to reinsert the tracheostomy tube.[14] If problems persist, EMS should be contacted immediately and the infant transported to the hospital.

The use of a positive pressure volume ventilator has become common practice for ventilating pediatric home care patients. This type of ventilator provides cardiopulmonary support through the delivery of a preset volume at a guaranteed minimum rate and is protected from barotrauma by a high-pressure cycle control.[48] However, the ventilator configuration is commonly modified to accommodate the pediatric patient's small lung capacity and variable leak. (Note: The cuffless tracheostomy tubes that are traditionally used for the pediatric population allow variable leaks.) Two types of modifications commonly used are (1) pressure limiting of the volume to preset levels for the duration of the inspiratory phase to prevent lung injury and to promote adequate oxygenation, and (2) supplying a continuous gas flow to ease the work of spontaneous respirations.

Caregivers should pay special attention in cleaning and handling equipment because children and infants are frequently subject to respiratory infections and other infectious disease related to their young age and immature immune systems. Diet and exercise are essential features of care to increase strength, endurance, and growth. Communication development is a concern for children with tracheostomies. However, extensive cooing and babbling does not appear necessary for later speech development.[38] Sibling adjustment and family coping with long-term ventilatory care will need to be evaluated. Quint (1990) reports that the family's ability to cope with the many needs of the ventilator-dependent child may decline with a longer duration of home ventilatory care.[34]

Coming home to a familiar, busy, and interesting environment will have special importance for pediatric patients, for whom growth and development are essential tasks. There should be an emphasis upon feeding and oral stimulation in the plan of care. The use of rehabilitation services is highly recommended. Seek additional resources when caring for pediatric ventilator-dependent patients; their needs are quite different from adults.

SUMMARY

The technical focus of this chapter highlights issues involving safe and competent management of ventilator-dependent patients in the home setting. This is not to say that home health nurses should let technology and procedural requirements dominate the plan of care. A humanistic and sensitive approach to patient care is the basic foundation of all nursing practice. When working with equipment, never forget to look at the patient; a grimace or a smile can say a lot.

Home mechanical ventilation can offer ventilator-dependent patients much richer and more fulfilling lives than the institutional setting of the hospital.[6] The home environment affords patients the noises, sights, and smells of life and living where relationships and friendships begin anew. Sitting on the porch on a warm summer's day, shopping at the mall, visiting friends, going to church, or returning to work or school restores a sense of self for ventilator-dependent patients and offers hope for tomorrow. This is the ideal, and with proper encouragement from home health nurses, it is certainly possible.[8,25,42]

As with most things, however, a darker side exists. Home health nurses may work with patients who have essentially become part of the bed, neither moving nor talking, as if in a comatose state.[33] As one family asked, "When is Dad going to die? When we brought him home, they said he wouldn't last long and that was 4 years ago."

Home health nurses should always assess the intactness of the family as caregivers as well as the biopsychosocial integrity of the patient. When the patient is without purposeful thought or function and is merely being aerated by the ventilator, the family as the patient's support system *will* show signs of disintegration. In addition, the literature supports a decline in the caregiver's/family's ability to cope with a longer duration of home ventilatory care.[9,34,40,46] In these circumstances, home care of ventilator-dependent patients becomes more complex and confronts highly sensitive issues.[33] Home health nurses can best meet these challenges by encouraging communication between the household and the patient's physician. If the patient can no longer be cared for at home, other choices (including placement in an extended care facility) should be discussed.[32]

At its best, home mechanical ventilation allows ventilator-dependent patients a rewarding life in a loving environment. At its worst, home mechanical ventilation becomes nothing more than the beeps and hisses of machines. It is critical that home health nurses recognize the vast difference between the two and intervene as is best for both patients and their families.

REFERENCES

1. Aday LU et al: *Pediatric home care: results of a national evaluation of programs for ventilator-assisted children,* Chicago, 1988, Pluribus Press.
2. Beard B, Monaco F: Tracheostomy discontinuation-impact of tube selection on resistance during tube occlusion, *Resp Care* 38(3):267-270, 1993.
3. Brackney S: Personal communication, Spring 1995.
4. Braun N: Intermittent mechanical ventilation, *Clin Chest Med* 9(1):153, 1988.
5. Cane R, Green S: Nutritional support of the ventilator-dependent patient, *Nutr Support Serv* 1:51, 1985.
6. Charles R: Coping with life on a portable ventilator, *Home Health Care Nurs* 3:27, 1985.
7. Clark K: Psychosocial aspects of prolonged ventilator dependency, *Resp Care* 31(4):329, 1986.
8. Elpern E et al: Long-term outcomes for elderly survivors of prolonged ventilator assistance, *Chest* 96(5):1120, 1989.
9. Findeis A et al: Caring for individuals using home ventilators: an appraisal by family caregivers, *Rehabil Nurs* 19(1):6-11, 1994.
10. Fuch P: Understanding continuous mechanical ventilation, *Nursing 79* 9(12):26, 1979.
11. Gracey D et al: Financial implications of prolonged ventilator care under DRGs 474 and 475, *Chest* 96(1):193, 1989.
12. Harris R, Hyman R: Clean vs sterile tracheostomy care and level of pulmonary infection, *Nurs Res* 33(2):80, 1984.
13. Haynes N, Raine S, Rushing P: Discharging ICU ventilator-dependent patient to home healthcare, *Crit Care Nurs* 10(7):39-47, 1990.
14. Hazinski M: Pediatric home tracheostomy care: a parent's guide, *Pediatr Nurs* 12(1):41-49, 1986.
15. Health Care Financing Administration: *Health insurance manual,* Pub No 11, Rev 229, Washington, DC, 1990, US Department of Health and Human Services.
16. Hodgkin J: Non-ventilator aspects of care for ventilator-assisted patients, *Resp Care* 31(4):334, 1986.
17. Hughes C, Knapper J, Redder C: Caring for ventilator-dependent patients, *Caring* 1:41, 1985.
18. Irwin M, Openbrier D: A delicate balance—strategies for feeding ventilated COPD patients, *Am J Nurs* 3:274, 1985.
19. Kacmarek R, Spearman C: Equipment used for ventilatory support in the home, *Resp Care* 31(4):311, 1986.
20. Kopacz M, Muriarty-Wright R: Multidisciplinary approach for the patient on a home ventilator, *Heart and Lung* 13(3):255, 1984.
21. Kreit J, Eschenbacher W: The physiology of spontaneous and mechanical ventilation, *Clin Chest Med* 9(1):11, 1988.
22. Law J et al: Increased frequency of obstructive airway abnormalities with long-term tracheostomy, *Chest* 104:136-138, 1993.
23. Linneaweaver W et al: Topical antimicrobial activity. *Arch Surg* 120:257, 1985.

24. Lucas J et al: *Home respiratory care,* Norwalk, Conn, 1988, Appleton & Lange.
25. Make B: Long-term management of ventilator-assisted individuals: the Boston University experience, *Resp Care* 31(4):303, 1986.
26. Marini J: Mechanical ventilation: taking the work out of breathing, *Resp Care* 31(8):695, 1986.
27. Mayo J: A nurse's guide to mechanical ventilation, *RN* 8:18, 1987.
28. O'Donohue W et al: Long-term mechanical ventilation—guidelines for management in the home and at alternate community sites, *Chest* 90(1):15, 1986.
29. Pierson D, George R: Mechanical ventilation in the home: possibilities and prerequisites, *Resp Care* 31(4):266, 1986.
30. Pingleton S: Nutritional support in the mechanically-ventilated patient, *Clin Chest Med* 9(1):101, 1988.
31. Popovich J, McAvoy C, Doyle L: Home mechanical ventilation: how, when, and for whom? *J Resp Dis* 6:27, 1986.
32. Prentice W: Placement alternatives for long-term ventilator care, *Resp Care* 31(4):288, 1986.
33. Purtilo R: Ethical issues in the treatment of chronic ventilator-dependent patients, *Arch Phys Med Rehabil* 67(9):718, 1986.
34. Quint R et al: Home care for ventilator-dependent children. *AJDC* 144(9):1238-1241, 1990.
35. Rice R: *Working with ventilator-dependent patients: Case study analysis.* A presentation at the NACH Conference, 1990.
36. Rice R: *Manual of home health nursing procedures,* St Louis, 1995, Mosby.
37. Rosen R, Bone R: Economics of mechanical ventilation, *Clin Chest Med* 9(1):163, 1988.
38. Simon BM, Fowler SM, Handler SD: Communication development in young children with long-term tracheostomies. *Int J Pediatr Otohinolayngol* 6:37-50, 1983.
39. Sivak E et al: Home care ventilation: The Cleveland Clinic experience from 1977 to 1985, *Resp Care* 31(4):294, 1986.
40. Smith C, Parkhurst C, Pingleton S: Adaptation in families with a member requiring mechanical ventilation at home, *Heart and Lung* 20(4):349-356, 1991.
41. Smith C, Perkins S, Pingleton S: Caregiver learning needs and reactions to managing home mechanical ventilation, *Heart and Lung* 23(2):157-163, 1994.
42. Splaingard ML: Home positive-pressure ventilation—twenty years experience, *Chest* 84(4):376, 1983.
43. Splaingard ML et al: Home negative pressure ventilation: Report of 20 years experience in patients with neuromuscular disease, *Arch Phys Med Rehabil* 66:239-242, 1988.
44. Stone R, Short PF: The competing demands of employment and informal caregiving to the disabled, *Med Care* 28(6):513-526, 1990.
45. Strieter R, Lynch J: Complications in the ventilated patient, *Clin Chest Med* 9(1):127, 1988.
46. Thomas V et al: Caring for the person receiving ventilatory support at home: caregivers' needs and involvement, *Heart and Lung* 21(2):180-186, 1992.
47. Thompson C, Richmond M: Teaching home care for ventilator-dependent patients-the patient's perception, *Heart and Lung* 19(1):79-83, 1990.
48. Tures D: Personal communication, (respiratory therapist and certified respiratory therapy technician at Aequitron Medical, Inc, Minneapolis), Oct 1995.

Appendix 12-1

Typical Ventilator Circuit

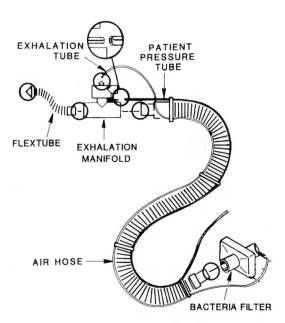

Figure A12-1 Drawing of a typical ventilator circuit. (Courtesy Aequitron, Inc, Minneapolis.)

Common Features of Home Mechanical Ventilators

A: Front panel (LP10 shown)

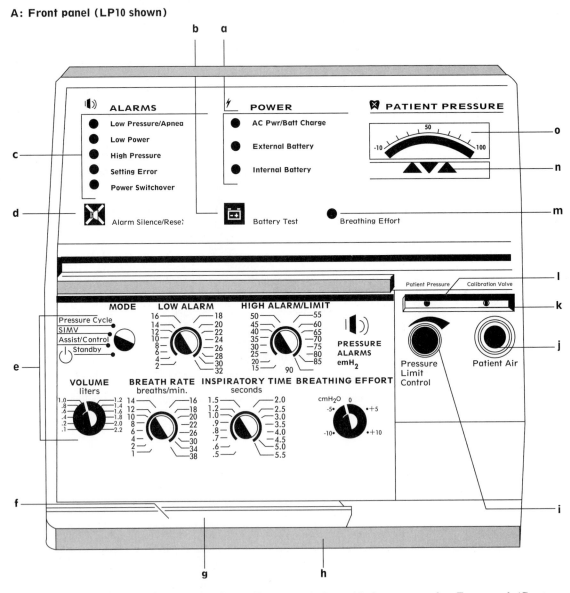

Figure A12-2a Example of a ventilator commonly used in home care today: Front panel. (Courtesy Aequitron, Inc, Minneapolis.)

a **Power source indicators.** Green light is on when AC power is in use and either battery is charging. Solid amber light is on when an external battery is providing power. Flashing amber light is on and audio signal every 5 minutes when internal battery is in use.

b **Battery test.** Press this button for a test of external/internal battery charge level (the ventilator must be operating on the battery being tested). Read results on battery condition scale of the **patient pressure** meter. Press in combination with **alarm silence/reset** for operating hours on machine. Read results on **patient pressure** meter and multiply the number indicated on the meter by 200.

c **Visual alarm indicators.** These **LEDs** identify alarm condition.

d **Alarm silence/reset button.** Push to test alarms. Push to silence any audible alarm (except setting error or apnea alarms) for 60 seconds. A silenced alarm will automatically reset when the condition is corrected.

e **Ventilator control knobs. Volume** and **breathing effort** controls are locking, skirted knobs; push in and turn to change setting.

f **Alarm reference guide.** Summary of alarm functions with suggestions for corrective action.

g **Control panel door.** Magnetically latched to protect controls.

h **Front carrying handle.**

i **Pressure limit control (LP10 only).** This control limits the patient pressure during an assisted or controlled breath. The pressure limit control knob has a locking outer ring; push the outer ring in and turn the small center knob to change settings.

j **Patient air port.** Standard 22-mm connection for patient air tube.

k **Exhalation valve port.** A connection for the exhalation valve tubing of the patient circuit.

l **Patient pressure port.** A connection for the proximal pressure line of the patient circuit. Connection and line are color coded with a black stripe.

m **Breathing effort.** Green light is activated by patient breathing effort. Breathing effort sensitivity is set by the **breathing effort** control knob.

n **Battery condition scale.** While pressing the **battery test** button, read the battery condition here.

o **Patient pressure meter.** Displays proximal pressure. Also displays battery charge level and machine hours of operation when appropriate buttons are pressed.

B: Operating controls

Warning | Periodically check the control panel to be sure that the controls are on the prescribed settings. The settings should not be changed without the order of a physician.

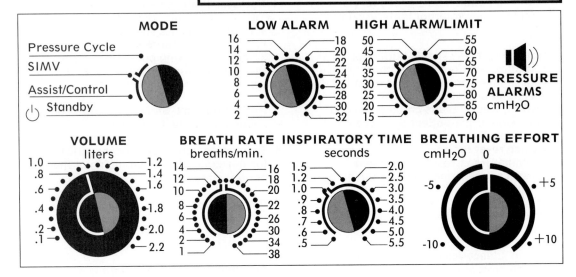

Mode control. Selects modes of operation.

Volume control. Sets the breath volume. Push in, then turn the knob to change the setting. When adjusted, the volume changes in 100-ml steps during each breath until the new volume is reached.

Breath rate control. Adjusts the number of breaths per minute.

Inspiratory time control. Adjusts delivery time for the breath.

Breathing effort control. Adjusts the patient effort needed to trigger a machine delivered breath. Push in, then turn to change the setting. When a breath is sensed, the **breathing effort** indicator lights.

Low alarm. Sets the low pressure limit. The low pressure alarm sounds if this limit is not reached for two consecutive breaths.

High alarm/limit. Sets the high pressure alarm or high pressure limit. The high pressure alarm sounds when the setting is exceeded (except in pressure limited mode). The alarm stops when the pressure drops to a lower level. Inspiration ends when the set point is reached.

Figure A12-2b Example of a ventilator commonly used in home care today: Operating controls. (Courtesy Aequitron, Inc, Minneapolis.)

C: Back panel

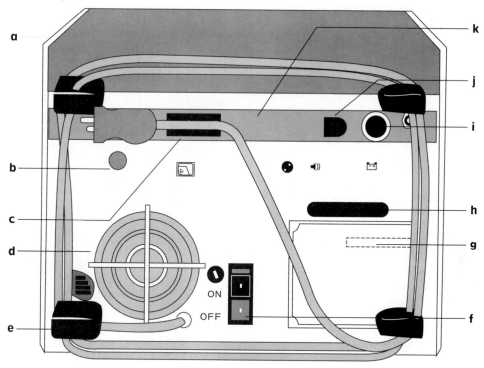

a Mounting rails. Connection for accessories.

b Vent. *Do not block.*

c AC plug holder.

d Inlet filter with screw-off cap. Patient air is drawn through this filter. Protects airflow and allows for easy filter change. *Do not block.*

e Cord wrap and rear feet.

f AC power switch/circuit breaker.

g Serial number plate.

h Communications port. Connection for optional printer.

i External 12VDC battery connection.

j Remote alarm connection.

k Rear carrying handle recess.

Figure A12-2c Example of a ventilator commonly used in home care today: Back panel. (Courtesy Aequitron, Inc, Minneapolis.)

Home Ventilator Management

Purpose

1. To define the responsibilities of the home health nurse caring for the ventilator-dependent patient.
2. To provide guidelines for home ventilator management.
3. To maximize high-tech quality patient care in the home setting.

RELATED PROCEDURES:

Administration of Oxygen Therapy
Arterial Blood Gas Sampling-Specimen Collection
Chest Physiotherapy
Pulse Oximetry
Suctioning
Tracheostomy Care:Inner Cannula Care
Tracheostomy Care:Outer Cannula Exchanges

General Information

Defining the roles of the HME vendor respiratory therapist and the home health nurse regarding care of the ventilator patient in the home is the responsibility of the discharge planning team. Weeks prior to the patient's discharge, the patient's home care team including the caregiver should be given instructions about actual and potential patient care needs. Caregivers who are *willing* and *able* to assist with patient needs are necessary for home discharge.

The home health nurse is advised to review the patient care manual from the HME vendor, which should outline ventilator management in the home and serve as an additional instructional guide for the patient/caregiver. It is important to refer to individual manufacturers' recommendations to ensure safe and efficacious use of all equipment.

Although the respiratory therapists from the HME vendor are responsible for instructing the patient/caregiver in procedural aspects of care, home health nurses should reinforce instructions and **evaluate** compliance with the plan of care during visits.

Equipment

1. Ventilator ("2" ventilators are recommended for patients requiring 20 or more hours of ventilator support per day or patients who are ambulatory, i.e., students)
   a. Ventilator circuits, filters
   b. Heated humidifier or cascade
      i. Sterile or distilled water, tap water if boiled 15 minutes
      ii. Condensation drainage bags
      iii. Heat and moisture exchanger (optional)
   c. External 12-volt battery with power cord and charger
   d. Volume bag (optional)
   e. Disinfectant (See Infection Control) Chapter 5)
   f. Manual self-inflating resuscitation bag
2. Oxygen and related supplies
   a. Oxygen source (optional): oxygen concentrator with backup compressed gas cylinder (tank) or a liquid system with a portable cylinder
   b. Oxygen connecting tubing: pressure-compensated flowmeter is recommended with the use of 50 feet of connecting tubing
   c. Air compressor and tubing for aerosol treatments (optional)
3. Tracheostomy equipment and related supplies
4. Home medical equipment
   a. Hospital bed (optional)
   b. Patient communication aid
   c. As needed; equipment to assist with patient bowel/bladder management and personal care
   d. As needed; cane, walker, wheelchair

Procedure

1. Explain the procedure to the patient/caregiver.
2. Maintain a copy of the most recent plan of care to ensure that all orders are being implemented correctly. When faced with questions that fall outside of the established care plan,

contact the HME respiratory therapist and physician for answers. If available, consult with the pulmonary clinical nurse specialist or discharge planning coordinator from the referring hospital.

3. Perform physical assessment to include:
   a. Subjective assessment based on, but not limited to, patient/caregiver comments on shortness of breath, color change, mucus production, fever, and machine or equipment concerns.
   b. Objective assessment of physiological data, such as blood pressure, pulse, respiratory rate, breath sounds, and oxygen saturation.
   c. Assess for complications of ventilator dependence such as skin breakdown, infection, fluid/electrolyte imbalance, malnutrition, and depression.

4. Assess patient/caregiver ability to manage ventilator dependence at home, concerns regarding equipment, resources, psychosocial, spiritual and teaching needs etc.

5. Perform safety check of all equipment to include:
   a. Patient circuit:
      i. Drain all tubing of water. Excess water should be considered contaminated and disposed of accordingly.
      ii. Inspect the circuit for wear and cracks.
      iii. Check all connections for tightness.
      iv. Make sure tubing is routed to prevent excess water from draining into the patient's airway or back into the humidifier or ventilator.
   b. Inspect all equipment for proper function and wear, including battery level and operational hours of the ventilator.
   c. Confirm that equipment is being cleaned and changed as ordered or per manufacturer's recommendations.

6. Assess the mode of delivery:
   a. Control mode-delivers a preset tidal volume at a fixed rate. The patient cannot initiate breaths or change the ventilatory pattern.
   b. Assist control volume or rate (ACV)-allows patients to initiate breaths so they can breathe at a higher rate than the preset number of breaths per minute generated by the ventilator. Each breath is delivered at the same preset tidal volume.
   c. Intermittent mandatory ventilation (IMV)-delivers a preset number of mechanical breaths at a preset tidal volume, but also allows patients to breathe with no assistance (positive pressure) from the ventilator at their own tidal volume.
   d. Synchronized intermittent mandatory ventilation (SIMV) -the ventilator senses the patient's spontaneous breath and synchronizes the timed breath with the patient's breath. This reduces competition between machine-delivered and patient-spontaneous breaths.

7. Assess the breath rate (ventilator plus patient). Approximate range 1-38 breaths/min.

8. Assess the tidal volume (VT) that the ventilator is giving the patient. VT is 10-15 cc/kg. The dial setting of the tidal volume may be compared with results obtained by use of a volume bag.
   a. The HME vendor may provide a clear, plastic sleeve called a volume bag that is used to measure the VT. Attach the volume bag to the exhalation valve or gas collection head on the tubing. Count the number of breaths it takes to completely fill the bag. On the back of the volume bag, a diagram shows total number of breaths taken to fill the volume bag with corresponding tidal volume.
   b. Dial settings from the tidal volume should be similar to what is obtained with the volume bag measurement; if discrepancies are noted, inform the HME vendor's respiratory therapist for follow-up.

9. Assess low pressure alarm limit setting (when the pressure falls below the set rate, the alarm will sound. For example, if the patient becomes disconnected from the ventilator, the low pressure alarm will be triggered). Approximate range: 2-32 cm H_2O.

10. Assess high-pressure alarm limit setting (when the pressure rises above the set rate, the alarm will sound. For example, mucus plugs increase pressure, inhibiting the ventilator effort to deliver oxygen and triggering the high-pressure alarm). Approximate range: 15-90 cm H_2O.

11. Assess patient pressures by observing low and high limits as the patient breathes.

12. Assess the FIO_2 (fraction of inspired oxygen: room air is .21%) or amount of prescribed oxygen being delivered. Approximate range: 24 to 40%. $FIO_2 > .40\%$ is rarely used in home care.

13. Assess positive end-expiratory pressure (PEEP) if used. High levels of PEEP (>5 cm H_2O) may cause barotrauma.

14. Instruct the patient/caregiver to post the following phone numbers by the telephone: the HME vendor, the physician's number, the home health agency's number, local power/electricity service number, and local emergency service number for emergencies or problems with equipment. Help the patient/caregiver identify circumstances when emergency numbers should be called.

15. Notify the local power/emergency services of patient's home address and arrange for priority service.

16. Provide patient comfort measures.

Nursing considerations

Instruct the patient/caregiver in the use of alternate ventilatory support systems. Have them demonstrate the use of the manual self-inflating resuscitation bag.

Documentation guidelines

1. Documentation of home ventilator management on the visit report should include:

   a. Patient toleration of ventilator dependence, cardiopulmonary status along with any pertinent findings, teaching, intervention, or procedures implemented (for example, suctioning); any patient/caregiver concerns regarding home environment, equipment, resources, psychosocial needs, etc.

   b. Ventilator settings or any changes or pertinent findings-mode, breath rate, high- and low-pressure alarm limit settings, the patient's high- and low-pressure reading, TV, FIO_2, and PEEP (if used).

   c. Multidisciplinary services and care coordination (nutritional therapist, physical therapy, occupational therapy, speech therapy, social worker or psychiatric home health nurse, and home health aide may be involved).

   d. Infection control precautions/management.

2. Update the patient care plan.

From Rice R: *Manual of home health nursing procedures,* St Louis, 1995, Mosby.

13 The Patient with Chronic Wounds

Robyn Rice and *Laurel A. Wiersema*

As many as 500,000 to 1 million persons experience wounds each year in the United States.[2,3] The estimated cost of treating a wound varies from $1,000 to $25,000,[2,33,39] and the total cost of treating wounds in the United States is reported to be between $3 billion and $7 billion annually.[33,37,45] Clearly, wound care is big business.

Although there are a variety of different types of wounds, home health nurses commonly visit and plan care for those patients who have wounds that do not easily heal. These are referred to as chronic wounds. How do chronic wounds differ from acute wounds such as incisions? Chronic wounds tend to result from an underlying disease process such as vascular insufficiency as opposed to acute wounds which begin with a stab injury that disrupts vasculature, resulting in hemostasis and activation of the inflammatory response. Since the inflammatory response drives the wound-healing cascade, its absence or suppression may help explain delayed wound healing.[8]

Chronic wounds commonly seen in home care include pressure ulcers, arterial ulcers, diabetic ulcers, and venous stasis ulcers.[8,39] In a recent survey of one home care agency, patients with chronic wounds represented 42% of the open cases.[40] Indeed, home care may become the most cost-effective and patient-preferred way to manage these disorders, although there is a continuing need for research in this area.

The purpose of this chapter is to provide current information about wound healing to assist home health nurses in developing a plan of care for patients with chronic wounds.

ETIOLOGY AND PATHOPHYSIOLOGY OF CHRONIC WOUNDS

Cells join and network to form all body tissues, including the skin. The skin, which is composed of many different kinds of cells, provides support and protection for underlying structures. (See the box titled The Skin.)

The skin depends on adequate circulation to meet its metabolic needs. Blood transported by arteries and arterioles into capillary beds delivers the oxygen and nutrients that are vital for cellular growth and function. Deoxygenated blood containing toxic by-products of cellular metabolism moves out of the capillary beds and is transported away by venules and veins.

When circulation to the skin is insufficient or disrupted for significant periods of time, cells become essentially oxygen starved and die.[43] Cellular death and necrosis of the skin are manifested by *wounds,* areas of breakdown or lesions. The following etiologies of cellular necrosis and delayed wound healing are multifactorial but are primarily related to impaired circulation and a loss of skin integrity.[22,25]

Disease states. Certain diseases are related to circulatory impairment and tissue necrosis. For example, congestive heart failure and peripheral vascular disease contribute to edema and tissue ischemia. Diabetes mellitus, trauma, and neurologic or neoplastic disorders can produce losses in sensation and mobility that may cause tissue deterioration and delayed wound healing.

In addition, hyperglycemic-induced leukocyte dysfunction and valvular dysfunction predispose

THE SKIN

The skin is the largest organ of the body, comprising about 15% of the normal body weight.[8] An acid pH of 4.2 to 5.6 regulates and balances the skin's own natural flora of microorganisms. This flora is unique to each person and, under normal circumstances, serves as a complex line of defense against other potentially pathogenic microorganisms.

The skin is composed of three adjoining layers: the epidermis, the dermis, and the subcutaneous tissues. The outer layer of the skin, the epidermis, is about 0.04 mm thick and without blood supply.[8,18] The amount of melanin (a dark brown or black pigment) in the epidermis determines the color of the skin.[8,38]

The epidermis is composed of many layers. Of particular note are the horny layer (stratum corneum) and the basal layer. The basal layer (stratum germinativum) is the basement membrane of the epidermis and depends upon the underlying dermis for nutrition. Epithelial cells at the basement membrane of the epidermis slowly migrate to the outer surface of the skin, the stratum corneum. In this process, called *keratinization,* upwardly migrating epithelial cells lose their nuclei, becoming flat and densely packed. Keratinization occurs at a constant rate, ensuring that cells naturally sloughed off at the surface are regularly replaced. Dry and tough in character, the stratum corneum permits evaporation of water from the skin (insensible loss). The permeability of the stratum corneum allows for the delivery of topical medication into the underlying tissues and systems. Hair follicles, sebaceous glands, and sweat glands are a part of the epidermis and extend downward into the dermis.

The dermis is well supplied with blood and is about 0.5 mm thick. Containing blood vessels, nerve endings, lymphatics, and connective tissue, the dermis is elastic and hardy.[22] The major cell type of the dermis is the fibroblast, which is responsible for the production of collagen and elastin. Collagen gives the skin its tensile strength while elastin provides the skin with its elastic recoil. The dermis supports the epidermis and is composed of two layers, the papillary layer and the reticular layer. The dermis merges with the third layer of the skin, the subcutaneous tissues.

The subcutaneous layer, also referred to as the hypodermis, connects the dermis to underlying structures. It contains fat, connective tissue, and nerve endings in addition to blood and lymph vessels. The subcutaneous layer of the skin protects and insulates underlying structures from injury and also provides caloric reserves for the body.[8]

The function of the skin is to provide protection, thermoregulation, and sensation. All three layers of the skin play a role in wound healing. The epidermis is responsible for resurfacing of the wound; however, it is the dermis and subcutaneous tissues that regulate wound repair and tissue regeneration.[25,42]

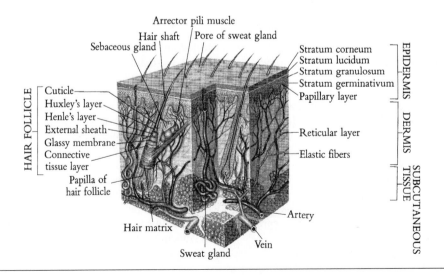

diabetics to infection and gangrene. This is why wound management of diabetics must include not only measures to maximize tissue perfusion, but also to *control blood glucose levels.*

Nutrition. Anemia and poor nutritional status affect the amount of oxygen and nutrients delivered to the cells and impair wound healing.[4,16,22] For example, vitamin C and iron are necessary for fibroblast proliferation and subsequent tissue granulation.[16,44] B complex vitamins, copper, and zinc are needed for collagen formation.[18] Furthermore, while undernourished patients with protein deficiencies may have defects in leukocyte (white blood cell) function, obese patients are especially hard to heal because of poor vascularization of fatty tissue. Additionally, hemoglobin levels below 12 g/100 ml slow healing because oxygen is required for collagen synthesis.[8,16]

Oxygen and nutrients are the building blocks of a healthy metabolism and tissue generation. In a study of 232 nursing home patients, Pinchcofsky-Devin and Kaminiski identified a positive correlation between the development of pressure ulcers and nutritional deficiencies.[37] Consequently a deficient caloric intake, especially a deficient protein intake, is associated with open and chronic, draining wounds.[4,16,37]

Wound contamination. Wound contamination due to moisture, incontinence and other sources of infection complicates and delays healing.[24] This can be related to inadequate skin care in which patient hygiene is neglected.

Chemical irritants. The presence of chemicals on the skin may cause damage and wound formation. For example, harsh solutions of povidone-iodine (Betadine), improper use of products (tape, skin sealants), and drainage of bodily fluids will erode the epidermis.[8]

Cognitive and behavioral status. Certain mental, cognitive, or behavioral states such as confusion, lack of education, or noncompliance with treatment may contribute to skin breakdown.[6] For example, smoking reduces the amount of oxygen delivered to cells for metabolic needs. In a study by Guralnik et al., smokers were shown to be 2.9 times more likely than nonsmokers to develop pressure sores.[16]

Medications. Medications have been shown to influence tissue destruction and repair.[24] For example, steroids delay wound healing.[34] Fibroblast production and tissue generation are slowed with topical administration of steroids onto the wound.[8] Systemic or topical administration of vitamin A can offset the antiinflammatory effects of steroids; however, vitamin A does not appear to speed wound repair in and of itself.[8,44]

Tranquilizers and analgesics can depress sensation and mobility, predisposing the patient to further tissue breakdown. Although topical antimicrobials can enhance healing of contaminated wounds, systemic antibiotics may have little effect on wound repair because of poor circulation and disbursement of medication.[24]

Mechanical forces. Among the primary causes of tissue destruction are prolonged pressure over weight-bearing bony prominences and external forces that interrupt or block circulation.[22] The internal capillary blood pressure, referred to as the capillary closing pressure, is estimated to be about 25 to 32 mmHg.[12,23] When external forces and prolonged pressure exceed capillary closing pressure, the vessels collapse and thrombose. They are then unable to assist in meeting the metabolic demands of tissue.[26] This results in ischemia and cellular death with subsequent tissue breakdown, the formation of the wound.

In addition to pressure, forces such as friction and shearing disrupt circulation and damage skin integrity. Abrasion and erosion of the epidermis occur when the skin rubs against another surface, causing friction. Such defects in the skin can become infected and promote ulcer formation. Sacral ulcers are largely attributed to the forces of shearing.[30] A common situation that results in shearing occurs when the patient sits with the head of the bed elevated, placing the majority of pressure on the sacral area.[8,12] As the patient slides down toward the foot of the bed, sacral skin sticks to the sheets and essentially remains in the same place. However, the deep, underlying tissue and muscle are pulled downward, resulting in stretching and tearing of integument and vessels. Consequently, ischemia and a shear ulcer with undermining usually develop. Improper techniques of turning and repositioning the patient also contribute to skin breakdown.[25,38]

Age. Age is a well cited factor in the formation of chronic wounds. A failing immune system and reduced mechanical strength of the skin (both associated with aging) place the elderly patient at risk for skin breakdown.[38] In addition, problems with circulation, diet, elimination, and mobility that are common in the elderly may complicate the course of wound healing.

CLASSIFICATION OF CHRONIC WOUNDS

Treatment of wounds rests on an understanding of the pathophysiology of tissue destruction and wound repair. For purposes of this chapter, chronic wounds are classified on the basis of etiology as pressure ulcers, venous ulcers, arterial ulcers, and diabetic ulcers.

Pressure ulcers

Pressure ulcers, also referred to as bedsores or decubitus ulcers, result from excessive, unrelieved pressure or from external forces such as shearing or friction. Pressure ulcers are likely to occur over weight-bearing, bony prominences or where the body is exposed to a firm, unyielding surface for varying lengths of time.[22,23] The patient's position determines the anatomic site at risk for ulceration. However, most pressure ulcers occur on the lower half of the body. The relationship among pressure, time, and body position appears to be a critical determinant in the formation of pressure ulcers.[22,23] Studies have shown that application of pressure to tissue in excess of 32 mmHg for 1 to 2 hours is sufficient to create pressure sores.[23,26]

Venous ulcers

Venous ulcers result from chronic venous insufficiency (a valvular defect) and are characteristically found on the lower extremities. Normally, venous flow is enhanced by exercise, during which contracting leg muscles create pressures that augment blood return to the heart. However, valvular incompetence and poor mobility predispose blood flow to back up into the venous system, leaking out of the capillaries and into tissue. Deprived of oxygen, this edematous tissue becomes necrotic and highly susceptible to ulcer formation.

Venous stasis ulcers are associated with firm but edematous extremities that often are stained reddish-brown. This is referred to as "hard" or brawny edema. Cellulitis may accompany these ulcers, which are characteristically shallow and have ragged, uneven edges with copious drainage. They may be painless to moderately painful.

There has been research into the role of fibrin cuffs in venous ulcer formation.[14,15] It has been postulated that fibrinogen, leaking into tissue as a result of incompetent valves, may accumulate around capillaries and form a fibrin cuff. These cuffs are believed to block the exchange of oxygen into the cell and prevent capillaries from dilating in response to increased metabolic demands of the tissue.[9] The role of fibrin cuffs in venous ulcer formation and treatment is still under investigation.

Arterial ulcers

Arterial ulcers develop as a result of a constricted or blocked artery. Blood flow to the cells is impaired, producing necrotic tissue or an ulcer. Arterial ulcers usually develop on the toes or heel of the foot.

The affected extremity is usually pale and hairless with a weak or questionable pulse that reflects an ischemic state. Typically a dry ulcer, the arterial ulcer has well defined edges and is deep with a necrotic and black wound base. Arterial ulcers are extremely painful.

Diabetic ulcers

Diabetics may exhibit an ulcer on the foot with both circulatory and neurological origins. Impaired circulation and neurological sensation occur as a result of a chronic hyperglycemic state. Ulcerations can also develop as a consequence of painless trauma in the presence of peripheral neuropathy.[8,26] Diabetic ulcers can appear similar to arterial ulcers. Diabetic ulcers may or may not be painful and are associated with osteomyelitis.

To summarize, when capillary blood flow to the skin is impaired, the cells become hypoxic and die. Tissue destruction and wound formation then occur. The patient's overall health and a number of other factors cited in this section will also reflect the course of skin breakdown and wound healing.

MECHANISMS OF WOUND HEALING

Wound healing is a very intricate and complex process that may be classified into three primary phases;[8,18,27] (1) the inflammatory phase, (2) the restoration phase, and (3) the remodeling phase. All three phases occur in sequence but may overlap. The duration of each phase varies with the extent of tissue damage and any concomitant disease state.

Inflammatory phase

In the inflammatory phase, initial tissue damage and bleeding cause vasoconstriction and the formation of a fibrin-platelet clot. Vasoconstriction lasts approximately 5 to 10 minutes. The injured tissue releases histamine and bradykinin, which cause capillary dilatation.[22] Intracellular fluid, proteins, and plasma components leak into the extracellular spaces, causing local increases in skin temperature, swelling, and redness (erythema).[22] This leakage creates a moist environment that attracts different kinds of leukocytes (white blood cells) to the injured area. The leukocytes then begin to debride and cleanse the wound by phagocytizing bacteria, dead cells, and necrotic debris, eventually becoming part of the wound exudate. Additionally, leukocytes stimulate healing. For example, macrophages, a type of leukocyte, not only clean up the wound but also release a protein that stimulates the formation of fibroblasts.[8,18] Fibroblasts, major components of the dermis, are responsible for collagen synthesis and connective tissue reconstruction which occur in the next phase.

Restoration phase

Wound repair in the restoration phase (sometimes referred to as the proliferative or fibroblastic phase) progresses at a rate dependent on the depth of the wound. If the wound is deep with significant loss of dermis and underlying tissue (full thickness wounds), angiogenesis (capillary growth) and granulation of lost tissue must precede the regeneration of the epidermis (epithelization). Superficial tissue loss (shallow or partial thickness wounds) may only need regeneration of the epidermis for repair.

In full thickness wounds, tissue regeneration begins with angiogenesis.[18] Angiogenesis, the formation and budding of new capillary beds that nourish cellular growth, is thought to be stimulated by macrophages and tissue hypoxia.[8,18]

During angiogenesis, the wound bed forms granulating tissue that is beefy red, highly vascular, and shiny in appearance. At this point, contraction of the wound bed may also occur, pulling the edges of the wound together and decreasing the area that needs to be filled by new tissue.

Epithelization takes place over a moist, vascular bed of tissue and often accompanies connective tissue repair of the dermis. The wound bed takes on a pink color, characteristic of the newly formed epithelial cells. Drawn to a moist substrate, epithelial cells migrate from the wound edges onto granulating tissue. Epithelial cells may also emerge from intact hair follicles, forming dots of pink tissue in the wound bed. These epithelial cells advance until they meet other epithelial cells. Once contact between epithelial cells is made, migration stops—a phenomenon referred to as *contact inhibition*. The defect in the skin is then closed.

Research has shown that a moist wound, free of contamination, promotes leukocyte migration and subsequent wound repair.[30,32,34,35] Dried, hard scabs and thick eschar have been shown to retard wound healing because epithelial cells must tunnel underneath the scab to close the wound.

Remodeling phase

During the remodeling phase, collagen (a fibrous protein that lends strength to all body tissues) is resynthesized and reorganized into increasingly tighter and stronger patterns. The collagen fibers are primarily remodeled by fibroblasts, forming the many layers of the epidermis and subsequent scar.

With the formation of the epidermis, the metabolic demands of the skin eventually slow down. When oxygen requirements lessen, capillary networks shrink and retreat, giving scars their characteristically white and bloodless appearance. Scars of full thickness or deep wounds are typically hairless because the hair follicles, a part of the epidermis, do not regenerate if destroyed. Scar tissue has about 80% of its previous strength and is very susceptible to recurrent tissue breakdown.[25]

The preceding review of the causes of tissue destruction and the mechanisms of wound repair leads to some general conclusions about treatment. Wound healing is enhanced by the following conditions:[13,31]

1. A moist wound environment
2. A wound bed free of necrotic tissue, eschar, and environmental contamination or infection
3. An adequate blood supply to meet metabolic demands for tissue generation
4. Sufficient oxygen and nutrition for cellular metabolism and tissue generation
5. Elimination of causative factors of skin breakdown

HOME CARE APPLICATION
Developing the plan of care

Several points should be considered when implementing wound care in the home. The patient and caregiver will have a very active role in wound care because the home health nurse's exposure to the wound will be periodic and intermittent. Therefore although the plan of care is guided by the physician, the home health nurse and the patient/caregiver must come to some agreement regarding its appropriateness. (See the box titled Primary Nursing Diagnoses/Patient Problems.) Even the best interventions are useless unless the patient and caregiver are willing and able to comply with specific wound care protocols and recommendations.

A patient referral to the registered dietitian may be helpful in reinforcing the importance of diet in wound healing. For example, patients with open and draining wounds may need to increase their caloric intake to as much as 3,000 to 4,000 calories/day with the recommended daily protein intake of approximately 2 g/kg.[4,16,37] A referral for home health aide services may be required for those patients who have limited functional ability and require assistance with ADLs. Consult with rehabilitation services to evaluate any problems with immobility or functional disability.

Wounds, like the patients who have them, are capable of dynamic changes. As the condition of the wound shifts, for better or worse, treatments and

planned visits should be adjusted accordingly. Documentation on the visit report should validate the visit frequency and subsequent need for treatment.

Visit frequency

The frequency of planned home visits is based on the assessment of patient/caregiver education needs, the condition of the wound, and related co-morbidities. Patients with complex, nonhealing wounds may require several certification periods of service before discharge is feasible.

In view of Medicare regulations for reimbursement, daily or b.i.d. visits of usually 1 or possibly 2 weeks may be done for infected, heavily draining, or complex wounds which are overwhelming for the patient/caregiver. Thereafter, visits to the home should decrease as the wound heals and the patient/caregiver becomes comfortable and adept in dressing changes. Eventually, the home health nurse would then visit the patient 1 or 2 times a week to evaluate the wound's progress toward healing and the patient's readiness for discharge.

Patient education

Self-care management of the wound is encouraged through patient/caregiver education. (See Chapter 6.) When devising the plan of care, initial assessment should determine whether the patient is able to learn wound care. If not, a designated caregiver or family member should be identified who is willing and able to assist with care plan implementation; this is the person who should observe initial dressing changes and learn the wound care regimen. (See the box titled Primary Themes of Patient Education.)

When teaching wound care in the home, it is important to be sure that the "why" and "how" aspects of care are understood. Consequently the patient/caregiver will require a great deal of instruction on wound assessment and when to call the physician and case manager regarding complications in care, dressing changes, proper use of any equipment, and lifestyle habits influencing wound repair and skin breakdown. Routine skin care will also be an important part of health teaching.

It may be worthwhile to write up guidelines for specific dressing changes and post them in a convenient place in the patient's home (such as on the refrigerator) as a way of ensuring that every-

---

PRIMARY NURSING DIAGNOSES/ PATIENT PROBLEMS

- Impaired skin integrity
- Pain
- High risk for infection
- Knowledge deficit; disease process and risk complications, medications, operation of home medical equipment, procedural care, diet, infection control, socioeconomic resources, available community services, etc.
- Altered nutrition, less than body requirements
- Body image disturbance
- Self-care deficit: _____ ADLs, _____ Feeding, _____ Toileting, _____ Other (Specify)

**PRIMARY THEMES
OF PATIENT EDUCATION**

- Wound assessment: when to call the case manager and physician
- When to call 911
- Medications: purpose, action, dosage, side effects, and methods of administration
- Use, operation, and maintenance of home medical equipment
- Dressing changes and related procedural care
- Diet
- Infection control
- Lifestyle habits that influence wound repair
- Socioeconomic resources
- Community services or alliances available for people with chronic and debilitating illness

one is correctly following treatment regimens. (See the box on p. 218 for sample guidelines.)

Infection control

Wound infection prolongs the inflammatory phase and delays healing. *Bacteroides* is the most common anaerobe with *Pseudomonas* and *Staphylococcus* being the most common aerobe cultured. A green color or fruity odor often indicates *Pseudomonas* while a fetid odor is often associated with an anaerobic infection. Assess the wound for infection and culture when appropriate.

When culturing the wound, gently cleanse with a physiological solution (such as normal saline) to remove debris before obtaining the culture. Using a swab, obtain the culture by moving across the wound bed using a zigzag motion (Figure 13-1). Consult with the physician; systemic antibiotics and/or topical antibacterials may be required.[41]

Home health nurses should perform dressing changes using an aseptic technique when possible. However, patients and their caregivers are usually taught clean technique. Of importance, the idea that infection slows healing should be explained to the patient/caregiver. Potential sources or circumstances promoting infection in the wound should be identified and discouraged. If the home is unclean or has dirt floors, ask the patient always to wear socks and shoes to protect the skin from germs. Medical supplies can be kept fairly clean if stored in a plastic trashbag.

Wound assessment and evaluation of healing

Although there is much information on wound management, nationally there is little agreement on uniform standards of evaluation. A variety of classification systems and measurement techniques exist in the literature. Prediction of wound development using the Norton or Braden scale is gaining recognition.[35] Classification methods to include staging and the Red, Yellow, Black system are popular. Photography, tracings, molds, and linear measurement techniques are also used.

Although it is recognized that trends among many practitioners are now focusing more on an objective assessment, staging of pressure sores or a decubitus wound continues to remain an acceptable method of classification. In the *Clinical Practice Guidelines on Pressure Ulcers in Adults: Prediction and Prevention* by the Agency for Health Care Policy and Research (AHCPR), staging of pressure ulcers reflects similar recommendations from the National Pressure Ulcer Advisory Panel (NPUAP) to include:[34]

- **Stage I:** Nonblanchable erythema of intact skin; the heralding lesion of skin ulceration. Note: Reactive hyperemia can normally be expected to be present for one half to three fourths as long as the pressure occluded blood flow to the area; it should not be confused with a stage I pressure ulcer.
- **Stage II:** Partial thickness skin loss involving epidermis and/or dermis. The ulcer is superficial and presents clinically as an abrasion, blister, or shallow crater. Painful.
- **Stage III:** Full thickness skin loss involving damage or necrosis of subcutaneous tissue that may extend down to, but not through, underlying fascia. The ulcer presents clinically as a deep crater with or without undermining of adjacent tissue. Undermining and copious drainage of exudates may be present; usually painless.
- **Stage IV:** Full thickness skin loss with extensive destruction, tissue necrosis or damage to muscle, bone, or supporting structures (for example, tendon or joint capsule). Copious drainage of exudates, undermining, and sinus tracts may be present; usually painless.

PATIENT/CAREGIVER EDUCATION GUIDELINES: WOUND CARE

1. Always wash your hands before and after changing your dressing because good handwashing will help keep your wound clean and prevent the spread of germs.
2. Keep all your medical supplies in a clean area; boxes of dressings, gloves, and other medical supplies may be stored in a clean plastic trashbag.
3. Discard wound care solutions after 1 week or sooner if you see particles forming in the container or if the solution changes color or becomes cloudy.
4. Notify the home health organization if you are running out of supplies.
5. Gather up your supplies. Prepare a plastic bag for disposal of dirty dressings and supplies.
6. Prepare your new dressing as your case manager has instructed you. All caregivers should wear gloves when assisting you with your dressing changes.
7. Carefully remove your old dressing and look at your wound. Any noticeable differences in size, color, or drainage should be reported to your case manager or home health aide at the next visit.
8. Apply your new dressing as the case manager has shown you. Follow the instructions below for specific steps to put on your new dressing. Your dressing should be changed according to schedule or if it comes off or becomes wet or moist. Seal and dispose of the bag in your family trash.
9. Call your case manager if you have an elevated temperature or problems with pus or excessive wound drainage or if swelling or pain occur with your wound.

SPECIFIC STEPS TO CLEAN YOUR WOUND AND CHANGE YOUR DRESSING:

Patient/caregiver signature: _____ Date: _____
Case manager signature: _____ Date: _____
Care path #: 1-Skin/Integumentary
White copy-patient's home record; Yellow copy-medical record
Copyright 1995; American Nursing Development, Maryville, Ill.

Be aware that staging has limitations which include (1) difficulties in staging pressure ulcers in patients with darkly pigmented skin, (2) difficulties in accurately staging the wound until the eschar has sloughed or the wound has been debrided, and (3) difficulties in problems with subjective interpretation among field staff when staging.

Wounds should be measured weekly by the case manager to ensure consistency in documentation. Irrigate the wound before assessing it to get an accurate measurement.

The visible portion of the wound may represent only a fraction of actual tissue necrosis (undermining).[12] Therefore when assessing depth and size of the wound, explore the wound base with a sterile swab for signs of undermining or sinus tract formation.

Skin assessment and measurement of wounds should include the size and extent of the wound along with any potential areas of breakdown. Black patients may not show typical reddened areas over affected tissue; however, heat and

Start

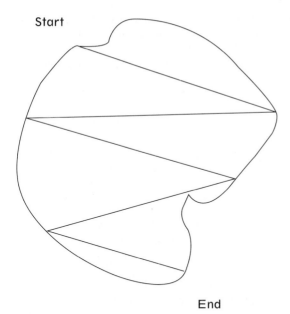

End

Figure 13-1 Using a zigzag method to culture the wound.

swelling can easily be palpated over tissue subjected to pressure. The authors recommend utilizing staging with a combination of descriptive wound assessment parameters to include the following:[34]

1. Measurements in centimeters
2. Anatomic location
3. Length, width, and depth of wound
4. Description of wound bed (color, appearance of tissue)
5. Presence/absence of undermining
6. Presence/absence of odor
7. Color and amount (small, moderate, large) of drainage
8. Wound stage according to AHCPR recommendations
9. Condition of surrounding skin
10. Associated risk factors predisposing patient to skin breakdown

Current trends in wound care

Wound care products. Many wound management products are noteworthy. As described earlier, leukocyte migration and epithelization are enhanced when a moist substrate is present. Current trends in many wound products suggest that use of a moist dressing to loosely fill dead space within the wound cavity fosters a healing environment, in addition to providing protection from contamination.[19,30] There is a vast array of wound care products on the market. Some of these products currently available are listed in Appendix 13-1.

Topical moisturizers, foams, transparent adhesive dressings, hydrocolloid dressings, and impregnated gauze dressings (to name a few) are now being used to moisturize the wound and protect it from secondary infections.[12,19,32] Occlusive dressings such as hydrocolloids should not be used on wounds with excessive purulence, deep sinus tracts, bone or tendon exposure, or in severely immunocompromised patients.[38] In these cases, a moist gauze dressing is recommended.[8,18]

Calcium alginate dressings are useful in controlling drainage.[5,41] Do not use calcium alginate dressings in wounds with minimal or no drainage because they will further dry out the wound bed.[5,41]

Research in chronic wound care is exploring the use of growth factors. Growth factors are small proteins, secreted as intercellular messengers, that regulate the growth of different cell types.[27] Addition of exogenous growth factors could be a new therapeutic approach to management of chronic nonhealing ulcers.

Cleansing and debridement. There also have been recent developments in wound cleansing and debriding. Along with the use of heat lamps, historically, wounds were essentially scrubbed out regardless of the appearance of the wound base. It is now known that just as the removal of eschar, pus, and exudate promotes healing, abrasive cleansing and irrigation of healthy, pink granulating tissue destroys the fibroblasts responsible for collagen synthesis.

Antiseptic solutions, such as Betadine and Dakin's, have been shown not only to kill bacteria but, in certain concentrations, to destroy fibroblasts and viable tissue.[28] The same holds true for aseptic solutions such as hydrogen peroxide. Therefore, physiological or detergent solutions (normal saline or water-based) are preferred as cleansers. If antiseptic or aseptic solutions are being used on infected wounds, apply a dilute concentration of 25% (one-fourth strength) or less.[28]

Plan cleansing and debriding treatments on the basis of wound bed assessment. Pink, healthy tissue may only require gentle irrigation with a physiological solution via a spray bottle.[10,11,12] Yellow, green, or black wound beds will require more vigorous debridement. Mechanical, chemical, or surgical means of debridement may be necessary.[10,12]

Mechanical debridement can be achieved by hydrotherapy (whirlpool or waterpick), normal saline wet-to-dry dressing changes, irrigation with a 35-ml syringe attached to an 18 or 19 gauge needle, or by gently cleansing the wound with soap and water.[10,34] If using home whirlpool therapy, the patient may wish to purchase a plastic trash can solely for whirlpool therapy. Bathtubs can be difficult for the elderly to move around in and often do not prevent oversplash of water created by the whirlpool. Instruct the patient/caregiver to clean the trash can after each use with a 10% bleach solution, rinse it out with tap water, and allow it to air dry. Emphasize that the trash can is to be used solely for the patient's whirlpool therapy.

Chemical debridement involves application of one of the numerous topical debriding agents now on the market. Topical debriding agents have enzymatic qualities that liquefy eschar, facilitating its removal.[10] Chemical debridement should be done by home health nurses and should be discontinued once eschar is removed. Product instructions must be followed carefully, avoiding application of the enzymatic compound to healthy tissue. When using a chemical debriding agent, consider encircling the wound with a hydrocolloid dressing during the procedure as an additional safety measure to prevent potential destruction of healthy tissue. Enzymatic preparations are not active in a dry environment and should not be used on dry eschar.[20] Crosshatch eschar with a scalpel and keep the wound surface moist.

When surgical debridement with a sharp instrument is needed for thick, black eschar, consult the physician.

Current trends in pressure management

Although the role of pressure in wound formation has been well described, pressure management continues to be redefined and improved.[3,7,38,46] Patients at risk for wound formation, as well as those with open wounds, should be placed on a regimen of skin care that controls exposure to forces of friction, shearing, and pressure. The use of elbow/heal protectors, socks, or a sheepskin may be helpful to relieve friction and prevent excessive pressure on soft tissues.[20] If pressure is not relieved, all other interventions are relatively ineffective.[29,47]

Minimize moisture from urine or stool, perspiration, or wound drainage to prevent chemical irritation. When moisture cannot be controlled, consider use of (1) pads or briefs that absorb urine and have a quick-drying surface that keeps moisture away from the skin, (2) a cream or ointment to protect the skin from urine, stool, or wound drainage, and (3) a rectal pouch to control incontinence of feces.

Emphasize proper seating position for bedbound or chairbound patients. In the presence or likelihood of skin breakdown on the ischia, sacrum, or coccyx, a correct upright sitting position is even more important to address. Sitting has many benefits (including improved breathing, circulation, mobility, and independence), which improve the healing process and overall health of the patient. (Refer to Chapter 16 for proper positioning techniques to seat chairbound patients.)

Wrinkle-free sheets, simple schedules for turning from side to back to side, and techniques of correct body positioning continue to be effective interventions in pressure management.[10] Placing the patient in a 30-degree oblique position almost totally prevents forces of shearing and can usually be done by family members using a couple of pillows.[6] Turning schedules should be individualized to meet the patient's needs or coordinated with care activities.[6] (See the box titled Recommendations for Pressure Ulcer Prevention in Adults.)

Not all patients have available caregivers to assist with a turning schedule or skin regimen. It may be necessary to recommend various types of medical equipment that can be purchased or rented from the home medical equipment (HME) vendor to prevent the deleterious effects of excessive pressure on soft tissue. At present, equipment recommended for pressure management is based on the degree of patient mobility and classified as either pressure reduction or pressure relief devices.[12,46]

Pressure reduction devices. Pressure reduction devices are recommended for patients who are able to assist with turning and have some degree

RECOMMENDATIONS FOR PRESSURE ULCER PREVENTION IN ADULTS

Skin care

1. All individuals at risk for pressure ulcers should have a systematic skin inspection daily.
2. Skin cleansing should occur at the time of soiling and at routine intervals.
3. Minimize environmental factors leading to skin drying such as low humidity (less than 40%) and exposure to cold. Dry skin should be treated with moisturizers.
4. Avoid massage over bony prominences.
5. Minimize skin exposure due to incontinence, perspiration, or wound drainage.
6. Minimize the forces of shearing and friction through proper positioning, transferring, and turning techniques. In addition, friction injuries may be reduced by the use of lubricants (such as cornstarch and creams), protective films (such as transparent film dressings and skin sealants), protective dressings (such as hydrocolloids), and protective padding.
7. Encourage good nutrition.
8. Consider rehabilitation referral for problems with immobility.

Mechanical loading and support surfaces

1. All individuals in bed who are assessed to be at risk for developing pressure ulcers should be repositioned at least every 2 hours if consistent with overall patient goals. Use a written turning schedule.
2. For individuals in bed, positioning devices such as pillows or foam wedges should be used to keep bony prominences (for example, knees or ankles) from direct contact with one another.
3. Individuals in bed who are completely immobile should have a care plan that includes the use of devices that totally relieve pressure on the heels. Do not use donut-type devices.
4. When the side-lying position is used in bed, avoid positioning directly on the trochanter.
5. Maintain the head of the bed at the lowest degree of elevation consistent with medical conditions and other restrictions. Limit the amount of time the head of the bed is elevated.
6. Use lifting devices such as a trapeze or bed linen to move (rather than drag) individuals in bed who cannot assist during transfers and position changes.
7. Any individual assessed to be at risk for developing pressure ulcers should be placed (when lying) on a pressure-reducing device, such as foam, static air, alternating air, gel, or water mattresses.
8. Any person at risk for developing a pressure ulcer should avoid uninterrupted sitting in a chair or wheelchair. The individual should be repositioned, shifting the points under pressure at least every hour or be put back to bed if consistent with overall patient management goals. Individuals who are able should be taught to shift weight every 15 minutes.
9. For chairbound individuals, the use of a pressure-reducing cushion is recommended. Do not use donut-type rings.
10. Positioning of chairbound individuals in chairs or wheelchairs should include consideration of postural alignment, distribution of weight, balance and stability, and pressure relief.

Source: Panel for the Prediction and Prevention of Pressure Ulcers in Adults: *Pressure ulcers in adults: prediction and prevention. Clinical practice guideline, No 3*, AHCPR Pub No 92-0047, Rockville, Md, 1992, Agency for Health Care Policy and Research, Public Health Service, US Department of Health and Human Services.

of mobility. Trapeze bars and side rails may also be used to aid in turning and moving. Pressure reduction devices do not consistently maintain pressure below capillary closing pressure but have been shown to be effective in preventing tissue necrosis with patients who are able to turn or move. This category includes water mattresses, gel pads, foam mattresses or pads, air support mattresses, and a variety of seated cushions.[29]

In recommending a cushion for the seated patient, correct wound care protocol dictates that the cushion should remove pressure from and ventilate the wound site. Therefore the ischials should be suspended in air, not encased in foam, gel, rubber, or vinyl. In addition, when considering what type of pressure reduction device to use, evaluate the appropriateness of the product as related to the patient's weight. For example, a high-density foam mattress may work well with a patient of normal weight but may be useless for an extremely obese patient. The HME vendor should be able to provide patient weight guidelines and product information. Avoid the use of donut rings; these generally do more harm than good.[34]

Pressure-relief devices. Pressure-relief devices are useful for patients with complete immobility and limited caregiver assistance.[3,29] Pressure-relief devices (for example, air fluidized therapy) maintain pressures below capillary closing pressures. The patient essentially floats on a fluid medium that distributes pressure evenly.[7] The patient's home must have appropriate electrical outlets and structural support because these beds are electric and may weigh 2,000 pounds or more.[1,47] Additional costs of these surfaces should also be a consideration because the continued use of electrical service will be realized in the patient's electric bill. Air flotation beds may render patient management at home easier for elderly caregivers who have difficulty meeting the demands of a frequent turning schedule, and may be more cost-effective in wound management for certain patients. Patients on air fluidized therapy should be well hydrated because this treatment can cause dehydration by increasing water loss through the skin and respiratory tissues.

Current philosophies of wound care blend the new with the old. Frequent position changes, use of medical equipment, application of cornstarch-based powder on the bed, use of transparent adhesive films or hydrocolloid dressings over areas at risk for breakdown, limiting the head of the bed position to 30 degrees to prevent shearing, incontinence management, and good nutrition all promote wound healing.[10,34,37] However, the question of what treatment is appropriate for what wound is necessary to consider.

Specific therapy: Matching wounds to treatments and products

Treatment for all types of wounds should be guided by three goals:[20]

1. Prevention of further tissue destruction by reducing or controlling predisposing etiologies of tissue destruction
2. Prevention of infection
3. Planning treatments as appropriate for (a) type of chronic wound (pressure, venous,

arterial, or surgical) and (b) condition and size of the wound (stage, amount of drainage, and related factors)

Recommendations for specific therapy of chronic wounds are as follows:[10,16,20,25]

Stage I: Nonblanchable erythema of intact skin

Interventions and specific treatment:

Prevention. Use pressure reduction techniques along with application of transparent adhesive films to protect "reddened" areas of skin at risk for breakdown. (See the box titled Application of Hydrocolloid Dressings and Transparent Adhesive Films.) Institute skin care regimen for stages I-IV. Condition is reversible with prompt intervention.

Stage II: Partial thickness wound

Interventions:

Cleansing/protection. Gently cleanse/irrigate pink wound bed with physiological or detergent solution. Application of a hydrocolloid dressing, transparent adhesive film, foam, topical moisturizer, or impregnated gauze dressing will maintain a moist environment for healing and protect the wound from environmental contamination.

Stage III: Full thickness wound: shallow

Interventions:

Disinfect/debride/absorb/protect. Filled with eschar, slough, and often copious exudate, these wounds may be infected. Use a physiological solution to cleanse and irrigate. A diluted concentration of an antiseptic or aseptic solution may be useful when working with infected wounds. Consult with the physician; antibiotic therapy—either systemic or topical (silver sulfadiazine cream)—may also be useful.[24]

Debride the wound as ordered by the physician. Eliminate dead space in the wound with an absorber (foam or granules) and cover with a protective dressing. Calcium alginate dressings may help control excessive drainage.[5]

Stage IV: Full thickness wound: Deep

Interventions:

Essentially same as for stage III. Avoid solitary use of transparent adhesive films or hydrocolloid dressings; these will not fill dead space.

APPLICATION OF HYDROCOLLOID DRESSINGS AND TRANSPARENT ADHESIVE FILMS

Purpose
- To promote wound healing
- To minimize pain and infection
- To protect the skin

General information

Hydrocolloid dressings and transparent adhesive films are useful to protect excoriated, reddened, or blistered areas of skin. They are used on partial thickness wounds. Transparent adhesive films are semipermeable dressings that are commonly used to protect skin against friction.

Equipment

1. Hydrocolloid dressing and transparent adhesive film (see Appendix 13-1, Wound Care Products)
2. Hypoallergenic tape
3. Plastic sheet or towel
4. Disposable nonsterile and sterile gloves, protective apron (See Infection Control, Chapter 5)

Procedure

1. Explain procedure to the patient/caregiver.
2. Assemble equipment in a convenient work area.
3. Assist the patient to a comfortable position to expose the wound. Place a plastic sheet or towel under the patient to prevent soiling of linen. Drape the patient for privacy.
4. Gently remove old tape and dressing. Assess the drainage on the old dressing; then discard in a plastic trashbag and secure.
5. Clean and irrigate the wound as prescribed by the physician. Clean from least contaminated area to the most contaminated area.
6. Inspect the wound, and evaluate it for healing.
7. Pat wound edges dry with a gauze pad, making sure surrounding skin is free of oily or greasy substances. Consider use of a skin prep to anchor the dressing.
8. Prepare dressing (hydrocolloid dressings and adhesive films are sterile and should be handled appropriately) in the following manner:
   a. Cut and prepare the dressing so that it covers a 1 1/2 inch margin of healthy skin.
   b. Carefully remove the paper backing from the dressing to prevent contamination of the sterile adhesive side.
9. Apply hydrocolloid dressing and adhesive film in the following manner:
   a. Gently *roll* the dressing over the wound (avoid stretching).
   b. Shape and mold the dressing into place, securing it around the wound edges; shape, mold, cut, and taper the dressing for hard to fit areas.
10. Secure the hydrocolloid dressing and adhesive film with hypoallergenic tape as needed.
11. Change the hydrocolloid dressing and transparent adhesive film about every 3 to 7 days or as required for leakage. (The hydrocolloid dressing may leave a gel residue in the wound bed; irrigate the wound with a normal saline solution; then apply a new dressing.)
12. Provide patient comfort measures.
13. Clean and replace equipment. Discard disposable items in a plastic trashbag and secure.

Nursing considerations

Perform wound care using sterile technique, unless ordered otherwise by the physician.
Instruct the patient/caregiver in the clean technique as approved by the physician.

Adapted from Rice R: *Manual of home health nursing procedures*, St. Louis, 1995, Mosby.   *Continued*

APPLICATION OF HYDROCOLLOID DRESSINGS AND TRANSPARENT ADHESIVE FILMS—cont'd

Documentation guidelines

Document the following on the visit report:

- The treatment and condition of the wound (each visit)
- Appearance of the wound bed (black, yellow, green, tan, red, or pink)
- Wound measurements (at least weekly), including the length, depth, and width of the wound in centimeters
- Depth and location of undermining in centimeters
- Inflammation or erythema of the skin around the wound
- Color, odor, and estimated amount of drainage
- Stage the wound weekly, and compare the progress with the goals of therapy
- Any patient/caregiver instructions on wound care and compliance with wound management; including ability to change dressings
- Other pertinent findings

Update the patient care plan.

Venous stasis ulcers. Treatment should control edema and promote healing. Underlying medical and nutritional disorders should be corrected. For example, congestive heart failure should be controlled to reduce lower extremity edema. If obesity is present, a weight reduction program should be initiated.

Periodically elevating the legs above the level of the heart with the use of compression therapy will control edema. Examples of compression therapy include compression stockings, elastic wraps, and the Unna boot. Instruct the patient to put compression stockings on before getting out of the bed in the morning. Compression stockings are to be worn all day. Elastic wraps or bandages should be placed on the leg when edema is minimal in order to maximize compression and venous return. Likewise, the application of the Unna boot is helpful to control edema. (See the box titled Application of an Unna Boot.)

A hydrocolloid dressing over the ulcer in combination with an impregnated gauze dressing or a hydrocolloid elastic bandage may also prevent edema and promote healing.[9,21] Calcium alginate dressings have been shown to be beneficial, because they pick up exudates and drainage yet maintain a moist environment for wounds that are at risk for maceration.[5,41] Follow suggested interventions for stage II wounds.

Arterial and diabetic ulcers. Arterial and diabetic ulcers are difficult to treat as related to their relatively ischemic state. Wound management should be directed toward the following:[8,26]

1. Avoiding excessive pressure to the area by total non–weight-bearing or corrective shoes/inserts
2. Cleansing/debriding the wound (consult with the physician regarding debriding agent; debridement is contraindicated in the presence of gangrene because removal of eschar results in an open wound with impaired blood flow and susceptibility to infection; in this case surgical intervention is recommended.)[8]
3. Preventing infection
4. Supporting the patient (encourage good nutrition, control edema, and control disease process-blood glucose and blood pressure)

Compression therapy is generally contraindicated in patients with an ischemic injury. Tight, restrictive clothing or ill-fitting shoes should be avoided.

As diabetics tend to lose sensation in the feet, improper weight distribution and subsequent tissue destruction may occur. Orthotics are specially fitted shoes designed to prevent such traumatic ulceration. In addition, total contact casts or below

APPLICATION OF AN UNNA BOOT

Purpose
- To promote healing of venous stasis ulcers and to minimize cellulitis
- To minimize pain and infection

General information
The Unna boot or medicated dressing is used to control edema and to promote healing of poorly vascularized areas of the leg and foot. The Unna boot is often used to treat venous stasis ulcers.

Equipment
1. Unna boot or medicated compression dressing (see Appendix 13-1, Wound Care Products)
2. Gauze or elastic bandage
3. Hypoallergenic tape
4. Plastic sheet or towel
5. Disposable nonsterile and sterile gloves, protective apron (see Infection Control, Chapter 5)

Procedure
1. Explain the procedure to the patient/caregiver.
2. Assemble the equipment at a convenient work area.
3. Assist the patient to a comfortable position to expose the lower leg. Place a plastic sheet or towel underneath the leg to prevent soiling the linen or the floor. Drape the patient for privacy.
4. Gently remove the old tape and dressing. Assess the drainage on the old dressing; then discard the dressing in a plastic trashbag.
5. Clean and irrigate the wound as ordered by the physician. Clean from the least contaminated area to the most contaminated area.
6. Inspect the wound and evaluate it for healing versus signs of infection.
7. Apply Unna boot by wrapping the dressing from above the toes to below the knee to control edema.
8. Cover the heel with oblique turns.
9. Make circular, figure-of-eight turns around the leg overlapping each turn by half the width of the medicated dressing.
10. Cover the entire area 2 to 3 times. Do not make reverse turns, because such turns cause unnecessary creases and pressure.
11. Cut and smooth the dressing to avoid creases or pleats.
12. Apply gauze or elastic bandage over the medicated dressing for support and to absorb copious drainage; then secure the gauze or elastic bandage with hypoallergenic tape.
13. Change the dressing 1 or 2 times a week. Remove the Unna boot in the following manner:
    a. Remove the elastic bandage or gauze wrap.
    b. Carefully cut and remove the dressing from the leg (soaking the dressing loose decreases the debriding effect).
14. Provide patient comfort measures.
15. Clean and replace the equipment. Discard disposable items in a plastic trashbag and secure.

Nursing considerations
Perform wound care using sterile technique, unless ordered otherwise by the physician.
Clean technique is often used with leg ulcers.

Adapted from Rice R: *Manual of home health nursing procedures,* St Louis, 1995, Mosby.   *Continued*

APPLICATION OF AN UNNA BOOT—cont'd

Documentation guidelines

Document the following on the visit report:

- The treatment and condition of the wound (each visit)
- Appearance of the wound bed (black, yellow, green, tan, red, or pink)
- Wound measurements (at least weekly), including the length, depth, and width of the wound in centimeters
- Depth and location of undermining in centimeters
- Inflammation or erythema of the skin around the wound
- Color, odor, and estimated amount of drainage
- Stage the wound weekly, and compare the progress with the goals of therapy
- Any patient/caregiver instructions on wound care and compliance with wound management; including ability to change dressings
- Other pertinent findings

Update the patient care plan.

---

the knee plaster casts with minimal padding over bony prominences may be used to reduce forces of shearing and pressure in noninfected ulcers.[26]

Trauma must be avoided. Activities will likely be limited for patients with peripheral vascular disease if the ulcer is to receive maximal perfusion. Patients with diabetes should never use hot water bottles or foot soaks to "warm up" the feet because as warmth increases the demand for blood. If neuropathy is present with arterial insufficiency and this increased demand for blood cannot be met, tissue injury results.[8] (Refer to Chapter 14; pay close attention to recommendations for diabetic foot care.) Utmost emphasis should be placed on teaching the patient to seek care for even the smallest wound.

The use of topical antibacterials and systemic antibiotics to treat an ischemic ulcer varies among practitioners. Although a topical antibacterial may help control infection, systemic antibiotics may not reach the wound bed because of poor circulation. Topical medications that contain steroids are not recommended because they trigger vasoconstriction.[8]

Patients with ischemic ulcers are at tremendous risk for gangrene and lower extremity amputation. Strict aseptic technique in dressing changes is advised and often difficult for the patient/caregiver to learn. Therefore the physician may order dressing changes to be done only by the home health

nurse until the wound is sufficiently healed to prevent the risk of gangrene.

Infected diabetic ulcers require immediate surgical excision of eschar and necrotic tissue. In addition, vascular surgery may be required when the blood flow is significantly impaired or treatment fails.

Documentation

Services planned and medical equipment and supplies ordered by the physician are the basis for Medicare reimbursement of wound care at home. Appropriate documentation of the patient's condition is crucial. Medicare views the following nursing skills as basic to wound care:[17]

1. Direct hands-on wound care treatment (procedural)
2. Skilled observation and assessment of the wound
3. Patient/caregiver education regarding treatment and interventions

On each visit, the home health nurse should document the treatment, and procedural care, and evaluate the wound for signs of healing versus infection. As discussed previously, measure and stage wounds weekly. Focus documentation of wound management on complicated procedural dressing changes, the need for patient education, and evaluation of wound healing along with any co-morbidity status that requires the services of the skilled nurse. Wound care is covered by Medicare as long as the need for skilled care and the need for treatment are clearly and precisely documented.[17] Despite everyone's best efforts, healing may not always occur, and the patient may require hospitalization for more intensive therapy.

SUMMARY

Home health nurses have a powerful influence over wound healing. Although the physician directs and guides the treatment, it is the home health nurse who orchestrates the plan of care. As case manager, the nurse's role is collaborative with patients, caregivers, and physicians. Changes in the plan of care rely heavily on nursing assessment and recommendations for treatment. It is not uncommon for patients and physicians to seek advice from the nurse regarding which products work best with different types of wounds, and when treatment should be modified.

Such a powerful voice must be informed. Home health nurses best meet this challenge by being knowledgeable about current trends and products for wound care and by being sensitive to the relationship between patient, wound, and home environment.

REFERENCES

1. Allman R et al: Air-fluidized beds or conventional therapy for pressure sores, *Ann Intern Med* 107:641, 1987.
2. Arjemi C: Statewide drive to eradicate decubitus ulcers launched in south Florida, *Fla Nurs News* 2:1, 1985.
3. Barnes S, Rutland B: Air-fluidized therapy as a cost-effective treatment for a "worst case" pressure necrosis, *J Enterostomal Ther* 13(1):27, 1986.
4. Bobel L: Nutritional implications in the patient with pressure sores, *Nurs Clin North Am* 22(2):379, 1987.
5. Bpharm T: Use of a calcium alginate dressing, *Pharm J* 8:188, 1985.
6. Braden B, Bryant R: Innovations to prevent and treat pressure ulcers, *Geriatr Nurs* 11(4):182, 1990.
7. Briston J, Goldfarb E, Green M: Clintron therapy: is it effective, *Am J Nurs* 8(2):120, 1987.
8. Bryant R: *Acute and chronic wounds. Wound repair.* St Louis, 1992, Mosby.
9. Convatec-Squibb: Wound healing: a delicate balance, *Adv Wound Healing* 5:9, 1989.
10. Cuzzell J: The new ryb color code, *Am J Nurs* 88(10):1342, 1988.
11. Diekmann J: Use of a dental irrigating device in the treatment of decubitus ulcers, *Nurs Res* 33(5):303, 1984.
12. Doughty D: Management of pressure sores, *J Enterostomal Ther* 15(1):39, 1988.
13. Doughty D: The process of wound healing: a nursing perspective, *Progressions* 2(1):10, 1990.
14. Excerpta Medica: *New insights into wound healing,* Princeton, 1988, Excerpta Medica.
15. Excerpta Medica, Cederholm-Williams, editors: *Fibrinolysis and angiogenesis in wound healing,* Proceedings of a symposium held Dec 4, 1987, Princeton, 1988, Excerpta Medica.
16. Guralnik J et al: Occurrence and predictors of pressure sores in the national health and nutrition examination survey follow up, *J Am Geriatr Soc* 36(9):807, 1988.
17. Health Care Financing Administration: *Home health insurance manual,* Pub No 11, Washington, DC, 1995, US Department of Health and Human Services.
18. Hess C: Wound care products: a directory, *Ostomy/Wound Management* 40(3): 70, 1994.
19. Hunt TK: The physiology of wound healing, *Ann Emerg Med,* 17(12):2-10, 1988.
20. Hutchinson J: Prevalence of wound infection under occlusive dressings: a collective survey of reported research, *Wounds* 1(2):123, 1989.
21. International Association for Enterostomal Therapy. *Standards of care for dermal wounds: pressure ulcers,* revised ed, Irvine, Calif, 1991, The Association.
22. Koone M, Burton C: Conservative management of long-standing venous stasis ulcer, *Wounds* 1(2):90, 1989.
23. Kosiak M: Etiology and pathology of ischemic ulcers, *Arch Phys Med* 40(1):63, 1959.
24. Kosiak M: Etiology of decubitus ulcers, *Arch Phys Med* 42(1):19, 1961.
25. Kucan J et al: Comparison of silver sulfadiazine, povidone-iodine and physiologic saline in the treatment of chronic pressure ulcers, *J Am Geriatr Soc* 19(5):232, 1981.
26. Kurzuk-Howald G, Simpson L, Palmieri A: Decubitus ulcer care: a comparative study, *West J Nurs Res* 7(1):58, 1985.
27. Laing P: Diabetic foot ulcers, *Am J Surg* 167(1A):31S-35S, 1994
28. Leigh R: Pressure ulcers: prevalence, etiology, and treatment modalities, *Am J Surg* 167(1A):25S-30S, 1994.
29. Linneaweaver W et al: Topical antimicrobial toxicity, *Arch Surg* 120:257, 1985.
30. Lovell H, Anderson C: Put your patient on the right bed, *RN* 53(5):66, 1990.
31. Madden M et al: Comparison of an occlusive and a semi-occlusive dressing and the effect of the wound exudate upon keratinocyte, *J Trauma* 29(77):924, 1989.
32. Margolin S et al: Management of radiation-induced moist skin desquamation using hydrocolloid dressing, *Cancer Nurs* 13(2):71, 1990.
33. The Medical Technology Forum: *Public policy implications related to use of the air-flotation bed treatment in the home setting,* Washington, DC, 1989, The Medical Technology and Practice Patterns Institute.
34. Mertz P: Occlusive wound dressings to prevent bacterial invasion and wound infection, *J Am Acad Dermatol* 12(4):662, 1985.
35. Murray S, Thompson R: We've organized our approach to pressure sores, *RN* 54(1):42, 1991.
36. Panel for the Prediction and Prevention of Pressure Ulcers in Adults: *Pressure ulcers in adults: prediction and prevention* (Clinical Practice Guideline No 3), 1992, Agency for

Health Care Policy and Research, Public Health Service, US Department of Health and Human Services.

37. Pinchcofsky-Devin G: Why won't this wound heal? *Ostomy/Wound Manage* 24:42, 1989.

38. Pinchcofsky-Devin G, Kaminiski M: Correlation of pressure sores and nutritional status, *J Am Geriatr Soc* 34(6):435, 1986.

39. Resnick B: Wound care for the elderly, *Geriatr Nurs*, 14(1):286-295, 1993.

40. Rice R: Wound prevalence and cost in home care: a survey of a community based home care agency-case study presentation. St Louis University, *Home Health Certification Exam Review Program*, St Louis, 1993.

41. Robson M et al: The efficacy of systemic antibiotics in the treatment of granulating wounds, *J Surg Res* 16:299, 1974.

42. Scurr JH, Wilson LA, Smith PD: A comparison of calcium alginate and hydrocolloid dressings in the management of chronic venous ulcers, *Wounds* 6(1):1-8, 1994.

43. Sebern M: Home-team strategies for treating pressure sores, *Nursing 87* 17(4):50, 1987.

44. Silane M, Oot-Giromini B: Systemic and other factors that affect wound healing. In Eaglstein W et al, editors: *New directions in wound healing,* Princeton, NJ, 1991, ER Squibb & Sons.

45. Stewart T: Materials, management and decubitus care, *J Healthcare Material Manage* 1:32, 1987.

46. Thomason S, Hawley G, Wurzel J: Specialty support surfaces: a cost containment perspective, *Decubitus* 6(6):32-40, 1993.

47. Ziegler-Cuzzell J, Willey T: Pressure relief perennials, *Am J Nurs* 87(9):1157, 1987.

Appendix 13-1

Wound Care Products

Product	Manufacturer	Comments
Physiological solutions		
Normal saline	Generic	Isotonic solutions used in wound irrigation and mechanical debridement, no chemical or antiseptic action.
Ringer's lactate	Generic	
Antiseptic solutions		
Acetic acid	Generic	Known to inhibit growth of *Pseudomonas aeruginosa, Trichomonas, and Candida.* Strong concentrations may destroy fibroblasts; dilute to <0.25%.
Alcohol/ethanol	Generic	Use only on iodine-sensitive patients.
Betadine	Generic	Can be absorbed through any body surface except adult intact skin. Dries skin. May destroy fibroblasts unless properly diluted to <1%.
Dakin's	Generic	Controls odor. May interfere with coagulation. Solution unstable; replace every 24 hours. Has been shown to adversely affect wound healing at strong concentrations; dilute to <0.5%.[47]
Domeboro (Burow's solution)	Miles Pharmaceuticals, Inc.	Antiinflamatory. Must be reconstituted. Stable for only 24 hours and should be refrigerated.
Hibiclens	Generic	Loses effectiveness when followed by soap rinse.
Isopropyl	Generic	Causes vasodilation below the skin; oozing from injection sites.

Please note: During 1995, Calgon Vestal was merged with ConvaTec. Products listed here with Calgon Vestal may in the future be found with ConvaTec.

Also, the Sween Corporation was recently purchased in 1995 by Coloplast. Products listed with Sween may in the future be found with Coloplast.

Continued

Product	Manufacturer	Comments
Aseptic solutions		
Hydrogen peroxide	Generic	Use only on wounds with necrotic debris. Can separate new epithelium from underlying tissue. Do not use in abdominal cavity as gas may invade capillaries and lymphatics. Slightly warms wound, enhancing vasodilation and decreasing inflammation. In strong concentrations, shown to destroy fibroblasts; dilute to <3%.
Zephiran	Generic	Inactivated by soaps; rinse wound thoroughly with normal saline before use. Reported to enhance growth of some *Pseudomonas* species; do not cover with occlusive dressings.
Detergent solutions		
Cara Klenz	Carrington Labs	Isotonic solutions used in wound irrigation and mechanical debridement. No antiseptic action.
Safclens	Calgon Vestal	
Constant-Clens	Sherwood Medical	
Biolex	C.R. Bard, Inc.	
Dermal Wound Cleanser	Smith & Nephew United, Inc.	
GENTELL PURELL	MKM Healthcare Carrington	
MICRO-KLENZ	Labs	
PURI-CLENS	Sween Corp.	
ROYL-DERM	Acme United Corp.	
SEA-CLENS	Sween Corp.	
Shur-Clens	Calgon Vestal	
ULTRA-KLENZ	Carrington Labs	
Cotton dressings (gauze)		
Fine-mesh gauze	Generic	About 41-47 thread count in a 4 × 4. Capillary beds rarely grow into the interstices of fine-mesh and are not damaged when the dressing is removed.
Wide-mesh gauze	Generic	About 30-39 thread count in a 4 × 4. Used in mechanical debridement, as coarse weave allows necrotic debris to adhere to dressing for removal.

Product	Manufacturer	Comments
Cotton dressings (impregnated)		
Adaptic	Johnson & Johnson	Drying out adversely affects wound healing.
Melolite	Smith-Nephew	
Mesalt	Scott Health Care	
Scarlet-Red		
Xeroform	Chesebrough Ponds, Inc.	
Vaseline gauze	Generic	
Aquaphor	Beiersdorf, Inc.	
Curity Oil		
Emulsion	Kendall	
Combination dressings		
Viasorb	Chesebrough Ponds, Inc.	Provide nonadherent, absorbent layer within a transparent membrane.
Polymem	Ferris Corp.	
Nu-Derm	Johnson & Johnson	
EXU-DRY	Exu-Dry Wound Care Products	
Leg ulcer wraps		
Unna boot (Dome-Paste)	Miles Pharmaceuticals, Inc.	Cotton mesh impregnated with zinc oxide, calamine (Unna boot), and gelatin. Dries to provide extremity with compression and support. No gaps should be left in bandage; otherwise edema will accumulate.
Viscopaste	Smith-Nephew	
Gelocast	Beiersdorf, Inc.	
Primer Flexible Unna Boot	Glenwood	
UNNA-FLEX	ConvaTec	
DuoDERM Adhesive	ConvaTec	Bandage systems used with a wound contact layer and compression to facilitate edema management.
Compression bandage	Smith & Nephew United, Inc.	
Profore		
Setopress	Acme United Corp.	Elastic bandage marked to facilitate application of correct pressure.
Exudate absorptive dressings		
Bard Absorption	Bard Home Health	Absorbs and picks up bacteria/exudates.
Debrisan	Johnson & Johnson	
DuoDerm Granules	ConvaTec	
DuoDerm Paste	ConvaTec	
Hydra-Gran	Baxter	
Hydron	Bioderm Sciences	
Algosteril	Johnson & Johnson	
Kaltostat	Calgon-Vestal-Merck	
Sorbsan	Dow Hickam	
AlgiDERM	ConvaTec	
Curasorb	Kendall	
DermaSORB	ConvaTec	
Wound Exudate Absorber	Hollister	
ChroniCure	Derma Sciences	May be used in conjunction with prescribed solution for copious draining wounds. Is not treatment of choice for wound management, as gauze may leave particles/fibers in the wound.
Medifil	BioCore, Inc.	
MULTIDEX	Lange Medical Products, Inc.	
Gauze	Generic	

Continued

Product	Manufacturer	Comments
Foam dressings		
Allevyn	Smith-Nephew	Avoid using in wounds with dry
Epi-Lock	Calgon Vestal	eschar.
Lyofoam	Acme United Corp.	
Primaderm	Absorbent Cotton Corp.	
Synthaderm	Calgon Vestal	
HYDRASORB	Calgon Vestal	
MITRAFLEX	Acme United Corp.	
Lyofoam "C"	Dow Hickam Corp.	
Flexzan		
Hydrocolloid dressings		
Comfeel Pressure Relief	Coloplast, Inc.	Dressing change required about every
Dressing	Coloplast, Inc.	4-7 days or prn for leakage. Rela-
Comfeel Ulcer Care Dressing	Beiersdorf, Inc.	tively impermeable to gas/vapor
Cutinova Hydro	ConvaTec	exchange. Use with caution in deep,
Duoderm/Duoderm	Baxter	full thickness wounds, as may foster
CGF	MKM Healthcare	anaerobic infection.
Hydrapad	Smith & Nephew United,	
DERMATELL	Inc.	
Replicare	Hollister	
Restore	Sween Corp.	
Sween-a-peel	3M Health Care	
Tegasorb	Sherwood Medical	
Ultec	Kendall	
Curaderm	Sween Corp.	
Triad		
Hydrogel dressings		
Intrasite gel	Smith-Nephew	Available in gel or sheet gel forms.
Vigilon	Bard Home Health	Normalize wound humidity. Sterile
Geliperm	E. Furgera & Co.	as packaged.
Nugel	Johnson & Johnson	
Elastogel	Southwest Technologies, Inc.	
Biolex	C.R. Bard, Inc.	
Carrasyn Gel	Carrington Labs	
Carrasyn V	Carrington Labs	
DuoDerm Hydroactive Gel	ConvaTec	
Gentell Hydrogel	MKM Healthcare	
Hypergel	Scott Health Care	
Iodosorb Gel	Occlassen Pharmaceuticals	
Normlgel	Scott Health Care	
Royl Derm	Acme United Corp.	
Wound'Dres	Sween Corp.	
Aquasorb	DeRoyal Industries	
ClearSite	NDM Wound Care	
Inerpan	Sherwood Medical	
Curagel	Kendall	

Product	Manufacturer	Comments
Hydrophilic powder dressings		
Chronicure	ABS LifeScience	Hydrophilic powder dressing which
Multidex	Lange Medical Products, Inc.	becomes a gel when contact is made with the wound surface.
Topical debriding agents		
Debrisan	Johnson & Johnson	Absorbs wound drainage, bacteria.
DuoDerm Paste	ConvaTec	Physiological debrider.
Elase	Parke-Davis	Indicated for slough/eschar.
Santyl	Knoll	Indicated for slough/eschar.
Silvadine Cream	Marion Labs	Physiological debrider with antimicrobial properties. Bacterial/fungicidal action maintained for about 12 hours. Change twice a day.
Travase	Flint Labs	Indicated for eschar. Moisten only with sterile water or saline. Not appropriate for pregnant women.
Panafil	Rystan	Indicated for removal of necrotic tissue.
Topical moisturizers		
Carrington Gel	Carrington Labs	These products are available in gel,
Dermagran	Dermasciences, Inc.	granulate, or sheet forms.
DuoDerm Paste	ConvaTec	
Geliperm Wet	E. Furgera & Co.	
Second Skin	Spence	
Transparent film (adhesive)		
Acuderm	Acme United Corp.	Semipermeable; dressing change required about every 4-7 days or prn.
Bio-Occlusive	Johnson & Johnson	May be used to protect skin against
Ensure	Deseret	friction.
Opraflex	Professional Medical Products	
Op-Site	Smith-Nephew	
Polyskin	Kendall	
Tegaderm	3-M	
Uniflex	Acme United Corp.	
Transparent film (nonadhesive)		
Omiderm	Jobst Dermatological Research Laboratories (D.R. Labs)	Cling to superficial open wounds without need of adhesive. Topicals may be applied to the dressing. Removal when falls off or by flushing with normal saline.

Continued

Product	Manufacturer	Comments
Miscellaneous (Traditional)		
Karaya	Generic	Absorbent, adhesive and hydrophilic properties; promotes moist wound bed.
Insulin	Generic	Enhances protein synthesis by skin. Observe for hypoglycemia and apply at meal times.
Stomahesive	ConvaTec	Useful in debriding thick, hard necrotic tissue.
Sugar	Generic	Hypertonic sugar solutions absorb moisture and debris, which may enhance wound healing. Use with caution; sugar may provide a medium for bacterial growth.
Granulex	Dow-Hickam	Softens and debrides eschar/slough; stimulates local vasodilatation.
Miscellaneous (Contemporary)		
Biobrane	Woodruff Labs, Inc.	Silicone membrane coated with collagen and hydrophilic peptide. Drying and sticking to wound bed may damage healthy tissue. Often used for burns.
Procurren	Curatec, Inc.	Platelet-derived formula containing growth factors to increase healing of severe/chronic wounds.

Diabetes is a disorder characterized by chronic hyperglycemia resulting from either an absolute or a relative deficiency of insulin secretion and/or action. The deficiency of insulin leads to marked abnormalities in carbohydrate, protein, and fat metabolism.[7] These disturbances are associated with the development of microvascular and macrovascular complications in persons with diabetes, including retinopathy, nephropathy, neuropathy, and cardiovascular[40] and peripheral vascular disease.[35] The prevalence of diabetes and its long-term complications result in high levels of morbidity and mortality, as well as tremendous personal, social, and economic costs to affected persons and society.[9,43]

Nearly 7 million people in the United States are known to have diabetes,[9] and probably an equal number have the disease but have not been diagnosed.[26] The prevalence of diabetes has been increasing (particularly in the older age groups) and is expected to continue to increase. The incidence is highest among women over age 64 and is increasing in this group. African Americans, Hispanics, and Native Americans are at increased risk for diabetes and its complications. The diabetes-related mortality rate varies by race and gender. Rates for black females are highest and are double those for white females; black males have the second highest mortality rate.[9]

Diabetes management and education are essential in reducing the incidence and severity of long-term complications.[4,6] Recent findings of the Diabetes Control and Complications Trial (DCCT) provide evidence that intensive therapy significantly delays the development and progression of retinopathy, nephropathy, and neuropathy in insulin-dependent diabetes mellitus.[19] The absence of known differences in the pathogenesis of complications in the two types of diabetes also suggests similar benefits of near normalization of blood glucose in non–insulin-dependent diabetes.[44]

Home health nurses encounter a wide variety of patients with diabetes and play a significant role in helping them to achieve improved glycemic control and effective self-management of their health care needs. Typical home care patients are older adults who may be in poor glycemic control and who may already have complications. This chapter focuses on adult home care patients. While some of the information also applies to patients who are children or adolescents, information addressing their specific needs is beyond the scope of this chapter.

PATHOPHYSIOLOGY AND CLASSIFICATION OF DIABETES

Diabetes is a heterogeneous syndrome with various forms having differing etiologies and clinical characteristics. The World Health Organization (WHO) clinical classification of diabetes mellitus includes four subgroups: insulin-independent diabetes mellitus (IDDM), non–insulin-dependent diabetes mellitus (NIDDM), malnutrition-related diabetes, and other types of diabetes associated with certain conditions and syndromes.[7] Because most home care patients with diabetes have either IDDM or NIDDM, this chapter focuses on these two types.

Insulin-dependent diabetes mellitus

IDDM is defined by the presence of hyperglycemia and classic symptoms such as polyuria, thirst, weight loss, and/or ketoacidosis and the necessity for insulin treatment. Persons with IDDM are dependent on insulin not only to control hyperglycemia and symptoms, but also to prevent ketoacidosis, diabetic coma, and death.[7]

The major defect in IDDM is the deficiency of insulin secretion resulting from autoimmune destruction of pancreatic beta cells.[7,20] The autoimmune response is thought to be triggered by environmental factors in genetically susceptible individuals, and has been associated with certain HLA types, the occurrence of viral infection, and the presence of islet cell antibodies.[7,20,33]

IDDM (formerly known as juvenile-onset diabetes and type I diabetes) is the most common form of diabetes in children and young adults.[7] Although the onset of IDDM occurs primarily among young individuals, with the major peak occurring between the ages of 11 and 14, IDDM may occur at any age. Symptoms often have an abrupt onset in children and a more insidious onset with increasing age. Girls often have monilial vaginitis.[33]

Non–insulin-dependent diabetes

NIDDM (formerly known as maturity-onset diabetes and type II diabetes) constitutes 85% or more of all cases of diabetes. NIDDM may present with classic symptoms without ketosis, but is often asymptomatic. Complications may be the first clinical indication of the disease. Insulin treatment may be needed to attain adequate blood glucose control, but is not necessary to maintain life or prevent spontaneous ketosis. Hyperglycemia in NIDDM is the consequence of abnormalities in insulin action, in insulin secretion, or both. NIDDM is also commonly associated with positive family history of the disease, obesity, and insulin resistance.[7]

During stress, such as infection, NIDDM may become transiently insulin-dependent. Adult-onset NIDDM progresses to IDDM at a rate of about 1% to 2% per year, even in those who attain and maintain ideal body weight.[16]

ACUTE COMPLICATIONS

Two hyperglycemic conditions, diabetic ketoacidosis and hyperosmolar nonketotic state, are associated with hospital admission and mortality in persons with diabetes.[30]

Diabetic ketoacidosis

Diabetic ketoacidosis (DKA) consists of the triad of hyperglycemia, ketosis, and acidemia. Insulin deficiency, elevated counterregulatory hormones,

and dehydration contribute to the development of DKA. Patients may become drowsy, stuporous, or comatose, with classical symptoms including polyuria, polydipsia, weight loss, vomiting, abdominal pain, Kussmaul respirations, dehydration, acetone odor on the breath, and signs of vascular shock. Precipitating factors include infection, intercurrent illness, and omission of or inadequate insulin therapy.[30]

Hyperglycemic hyperosmolar nonketotic state

Hyperglycemic hyperosmolar nonketotic state (HHNS) is defined by extreme hyperglycemia, increased serum osmolarity, and severe dehydration without significant ketosis or acidosis. Hyperglycemia is usually more severe ($>$600 mg/dl), dehydration is more pronounced, there is greater incidence of depressed sensorium, and the prognosis is poorer than in DKA. HHNS occurs more frequently in the elderly and in newly diagnosed diabetes and often has an insidious onset. Acute illness is the precipitating factor in many cases.[30]

Other common causes of DKA and HHNS are stress and ethanol abuse.[15] Treatment consists of fluid and electrolyte replacement and administration of insulin. Determination and elimination of precipitating factors is essential.[30]

Infection

Infection is the most common precipitating factor for diabetic ketoacidosis or coma, especially in the older person with newly diagnosed diabetes. The occurrence of infection complicates the management of diabetes. Whether the incidence of infection is higher in persons with diabetes remains debatable; however, those with diabetes appear to be at increased risk for infection at specific sites and due to certain organisms. Increased susceptibility to the following has been noted: urinary infection (in women only), complications of respiratory infection, bacterial infection of the skin or soft tissues (furuncles and carbuncles, infections of the extremities, necrotizing infections, postoperative wound infection), osteomyelitis, malignant external otitis, vaginitis or vulvitis, phycomycete infection, and periodontal infection. Poor metabolic control, vascular and neurologic abnormalities, and the increased performance of invasive medical procedures are associated with infection in diabetes.[36]

CHRONIC COMPLICATIONS

Long-term macrovascular and microvascular complications occur in both IDDM and NIDDM.[38]

Macrovascular disease

Macrovascular disease accounts for the majority of deaths in those with diabetes. Atherosclerosis involving the coronary, cerebrovascular, and peripheral vessels tends to occur prematurely and with greater severity in persons with diabetes than in the nondiabetic population.[10]

Cardiovascular disease. Persons with diabetes are twice as likely as nondiabetic individuals to die from coronary artery diseases. Since diabetes may be a significant independent risk factor for coronary disease, the importance of modifying other risk factors such as hypertension, hyperlipidemia, weight, and smoking is magnified.[48]

Cerebrovascular disease. Stroke occurs twice as frequently in the diabetic population. Hypertension is a major risk factor and should be adequately controlled.[37]

Peripheral vascular disease. Peripheral vascular disease, peripheral neuropathy, infections, and inadequate foot care increase the risk for lower extremity amputation in individuals with diabetes.[24] More in-hospital days are spent treating problems involving the lower extremities than any other complication of diabetes.[35]

Microvascular complications

Changes in the smaller vessels characterized by thickening of the capillary basement membrane associated with hyperglycemia lead to retinopathy, nephropathy, and neuropathy.[29]

Retinopathy. Diabetic retinopathy is a leading cause of blindness.[14] Retinopathy occurs frequently in both IDDM and NIDDM. The development is dependent on the duration of diabetes. Characteristic lesions include nonproliferative and proliferative retinopathy.[39]

Nephropathy. Nephropathy is a common complication of both IDDM and NIDDM,[51] and is the diabetes-specific complication associated with the greatest mortality.[39] Diabetic nephropathy is defined by persistent proteinuria in a patient with concomitant retinopathy and elevated blood pressure, in the absence of urinary tract infection, other renal disease, or heart failure.[51] Nephrotic syndrome develops, resulting in end-stage renal disease.[39]

Neuropathy. Distal symmetric sensorimotor neuropathy is the most common form of diabetic neuropathy. Loss of sensation and altered foot structure resulting from neuropathy lead to increased risk of foot trauma and diabetic ulcers.[39]

Autonomic neuropathy can affect cardiac function, bladder function, erectile function, and gastric or intestinal motility. Cardiac autonomic neuropathy may result in resting tachycardia and postural hypotension. Impotence is the most common clinical manifestation of autonomic neuropathy, affecting more than 50% of men with diabetes. Gastrointestinal effects include diarrhea and gastroparesis, which may not only cause symptoms but also alter the absorption of meals and impair glycemic control.[39]

HOME CARE APPLICATION

Specific goals of treatment in the home are to achieve normalization of blood glucose and prevent complications. Therapy for diabetes focuses on diet, exercise, and (for some patients) insulin or oral hypoglycemic agents. The emphasis of therapy varies according to the type of diabetes and the severity of the disease. For persons with IDDM, insulin therapy is essential for survival, but oral hypoglycemic agents are ineffective. Some of those with NIDDM may be treated with diet only, while others require insulin or oral hypoglycemic agents to control hyperglycemia. Nutritional management is a major priority for both types. Exercise is also an important factor in achieving metabolic balance.

The overall goal of home care is for patients and caregivers to acquire the knowledge and skills needed for accurate monitoring and effective self-management of diabetes and complications. This goal is achieved through assessment and education of the patient and caregiver.

Thorough diabetic assessment is essential regardless of the duration of diabetes. Assessment includes the interview integrated with the physical examination and evaluation of the patient's/caregiver's practices. A complete physical examination is usually performed, but only those areas related to diabetes will be presented here.

Physical assessment

General assessment. Check the patient's height and weight on the initial visit and the weight on each subsequent visit to assess nutritional status and hydration. Monitor blood pressure to assess for hypertension, which contributes to complications, and for postural hypotension which may result from autonomic neuropathy. Observe the skin for general hygiene and signs of infection. Check for heat intolerance and excessive sweating of the face and body, which may indicate autonomic dysfunction.[13]

Cerebrovascular. Check for symptoms of cerebrovascular disease, including intermittent dizziness, transient loss of vision, slurring of speech, and paresthesia or weakness of one arm or leg. Carotid bruits may be heard.[47]

Eyes/vision. Assess functional vision by noting whether the patient is able to do the following: (1) read printed materials, (2) compare blood or urine test strips with color chart accurately, and (3) draw up the dosage of insulin correctly. If vision is blurry, is this associated with hyperglycemia? Note any report of seeing "floaters" or "cobwebs," which may indicate retinal bleeding; or sudden, painless loss of vision, which may occur with a major retinal hemorrhage.[32] Refer patients to an ophthalmologist for evaluation if (1) blurry vision persists for more than 1 to 2 days and is not associated with a change in blood glucose, (2) sudden loss of vision in one or both eyes occurs, or (3) black spots, cobwebs, or flashing lights appear in the field of vision.[47]

Cardiovascular. Assess for typical symptoms of coronary heart disease such as chest pain, shortness of breath, or congestive heart failure. Since neuropathy may mask chest pain, myocardial infarction should be suspected in unexplained congestive heart failure or diabetic ketoacidosis.[4,7]

Gastrointestinal. Assess for symptoms of autonomic neuropathy. Anorexia, early satiety (a sense of fullness or bloating), and nausea after meals may indicate gastroparesis. Diarrhea that is nocturnal, is not accompanied by pain or cramps, is intermittent at first, and is associated with fecal incontinence may be related to autonomic neuropathy. Ask whether the patient is taking metoclopramide or other appropriate medications.[1,3]

Genitourinary/renal. Assess for neurogenic bladder, which is characterized by decreased urinary frequency, and urinary tract infection. Later, difficult or incomplete bladder emptying may occur. Test the urine for nitrite (which may indicate infection) and for protein (which may indicate nephropathy). In the elderly, the classic symptoms of urinary tract infection may be absent, with change in mental status being the only manifestation.[1,3]

With impotence, careful history and evaluation are essential to distinguish between psychogenic and organic erectile dysfunction. Organic impotence is gradual in onset and partner nonspecific. Early morning erection is absent. A referral to a physician may be needed to test for neurogenic impotence by monitoring nocturnal penile tumescence and rigidity.[1,3]

Lower extremities. Assess the feet for proper foot care. Guidelines appear in the Patient Education Guide. Check for signs and symptoms of peripheral vascular disease including intermittent claudication and decreased pulses in the lower extremities.[4,7] Typical symptoms of neuropathy include spontaneous uncomfortable sensations, contact paresthesias, impaired balance, diminished proprioception and position sense, absent or reduced vibratory sensation, numbness, and unnoticed injuries. An early sign is diminished deep tendon reflexes, especially of the Achilles tendon. Pain may be described as superficial or deep, burning, shooting, stabbing, aching, or tearing and is often more intense at night. The majority of patients report minimal or no symptoms, with deficits being noted on routine exam or because complications are present.[8]

With neuropathic ulcers, the foot is typically warm with easily palpable dorsalis pedis pulses. Note areas of local edema and warmth, which are at risk for tissue breakdown.[8]

Diabetes management and patient education

Each aspect of management should be reviewed to determine the plan of care and priorities. Patient education should be directed toward the knowledge and skills needed for competent self-management. (See the boxes titled Primary Nursing Diagnoses and Primary Themes of Patient Education.)

Insulin. Insulin is necessary for carbohydrate, protein, and fat metabolism.[2] Normally, the hormonal system is remarkably efficient in maintaining blood glucose within a narrow range despite alterations in periods of food intake and fasting.[27] The physiologic secretion of insulin to control blood glucose is timed precisely to meet the body's

---

PATIENT EDUCATION GUIDE: FOOT CARE[25]

The nurse should provide the patient with the following instructions:

Inspection

Look at your feet each day in a place with good light; use a mirror if you can't bend over to see the bottom of your feet.

Look for dry places and cracks in the skin, especially between the toes and around the heel; check for ingrown toenails, corns, calluses, discoloration, swelling, or sores.

If looking carefully at your feet is difficult for you, have a friend or family member help.

If corns, calluses, or other problems persist, see a foot doctor.

Bathing

Wash your feet daily in warm (not hot) water; always test the water temperature with your wrist or a bath thermometer to prevent burning yourself.

Do not soak your feet, because it will dry your skin.

Use a mild soap and rinse well; dry feet with a soft towel, making sure to dry between the toes.

To soften dry feet and keep the skin from cracking, use a cream or lotion such as Nivea, Eucerin, or Alpha Keri; do not put lotion between your toes.

If your feet sweat a lot, lightly dust with foot powder; wear cotton socks and change them several times a day.

Toenails

Trim your toenails only after bathing, when they are soft and easy to cut.

Always cut or file nails to follow the natural curve of your toe.

Avoid cutting nails shorter than the ends of your toes.

File sharp corners and rough edges of nails with an emery board so they do not cut the toes next to them.

Do not use sharp objects to poke or dig under the toenail or around the cuticle.

See a podiatrist for treatment of ingrown toenails and nails that are thick or tend to split when cut.

Corns and calluses

Control corn and callus buildup; after washing your feet, gently rub with a pumice stone.

Pad corns to reduce pressure.

Avoid using do-it-yourself corn or callus removers; they are caustic and may hurt healthy skin.

Never cut your corns and calluses with a razor blade; *no bathroom surgery*.

Socks

Wear clean, soft cotton or wool socks.

Socks should fit well and be free of seams and darns.

Never wear round garters or hose with elastic tops that might reduce the blood supply to your feet.

From Haire-Joshu DL: Nursing management of adults with disorders of the pancreas. In Beare PG, Myers JL, editors: *Principles and practice of adult health nursing,* St Louis, 1994, Mosby p. 1755.

Continued

---

needs. In persons with diabetes, insulin therapy attempts to duplicate this.[45]

Insulin regimens. Numerous patterns of insulin administration may be prescribed based on the needs of the individual. A commonly used regimen consists of two injections per day of an intermediate-acting insulin with the first dose given before breakfast and the second before supper or at bedtime. When the injection is given before meals,

regular insulin may be added when necessary to reduce postprandial hyperglycemia. More intensive regimens with multiple injections may be needed if the goal is to restore blood glucose levels to nondiabetic values throughout the day.[45]

Insulin preparations. Human insulin is manufactured by recombinant DNA technology, whereas animal insulin is made from beef or pork pancreas. Human insulin has a more rapid onset and shorter

---

PATIENT EDUCATION GUIDE: FOOT CARE—cont'd

Shoes

Always wear shoes or slippers to cover and protect your feet.

Wear shoes that fit well. Shoes that do not fit well can cause sores, blisters, and calluses, but shoes that feel good have room for all the toes to be in their natural place; avoid pointed shoes that pinch the toes. The top part of the shoe should be soft and pliable; the lining should not have ridges, wrinkles, or seams; the toe box should be round and high to allow space for toe deformities; you may need to see an orthotic specialist for special shoes or to have your shoes adapted to your feet.

When you buy shoes, make an outline of each foot from stiff paper to insert in shoes.

Before you put on your shoes, carefully check for stones or rough spots that might hurt your feet.

Improve your circulation

Try to quit smoking if you smoke.

Exercise every day; take a brisk daily walk for 1/2 to 1 hour; if you are not able to walk or move about easily, ask your nurse or doctor what types of exercises are best for you.

Avoid being in the cold for long periods; wear wool socks.

Treatment of injuries

Look at your feet if you stumble or bump a hard object.

If your foot is hurt, do not keep walking on it, since that can cause more damage.

Cuts and scratches should be treated right away; wash with soap and water and apply a mild antiseptic such as Bactine or Johnson & Johnson First Aid Cream; never use strong chemicals such as boric acid.

Notify physician or podiatrist of any blisters or sores on your feet.

---

duration of action. Beef insulin is more antigenic than pork or human insulin. Most patients currently beginning therapy are given human insulin. There is no reason for patients on animal insulin with good glycemic control and no adverse effects to change to human insulin.[45]

Insulin is available in short-, intermediate-, and long-acting forms. Short-acting insulins include regular ("R") and semilente. Intermediate-acting insulins are NPH and lente. Long-acting insulin is ultralente.[1] Action times for insulins are listed in Table 14-1 and shown in Figure 14-1.

Concentrations available in the United States are U-100 and U-500, with U-100 used most frequently and U-500 used only in rare cases of extreme insulin resistance.[45]

Storage and appearance. Insulin may be stored at room temperature for 6 to 8 weeks. Extreme temperatures should be avoided. Prefilled syringes should be kept in the refrigerator and used within 3 weeks.[45] Insulin should be at room temperature and inspected before use. Regular insulin should be clear and all other forms should be uniformly cloudy.[2]

PRIMARY NURSING DIAGNOSES/ PATIENT PROBLEMS

The following nursing diagnoses may be appropriate for the patient with diabetes mellitus:

- Knowledge deficit; diabetes care, prevention of complications
- Ineffective individual coping
- Alteration in nutrition, more than body requirements (if obese)
- Ineffective management of therapeutic regimen
- Risk for fluid volume deficit related to hyperglycemia
- Risk for injury related to neuropathy
- Risk for hypertension
- Risk for altered urinary elimination related to renal failure
- Activity limitation or intolerance related to diabetic complications

**PRIMARY THEMES
OF PATIENT EDUCATION**

- Diabetes self-care management
  Diet, importance of modifying fat
  Exercise
  Medication/insulin administration
  Blood glucose monitoring
  Foot care
  Sick day management
- Hypoglycemia: recognition and interventions
- Hyperglycemia: recognition and interventions
- Infection: recognition and interventions
- Importance of self-care management in prevention/reduction of complications

Mixing insulins. Mixtures of NPH and regular insulin can be used without any clinical difference in glycemic effect, compared with that produced by separate injection of each. Commercially available mixtures of NPH and regular insulin are available in a 70:30 ratio and a 50:50 ratio.[45] Premixed insulin is useful in patients with NIDDM who may not be able to master mixing of insulins.[11,45]

In mixtures of regular and lente, the binding of the regular insulin by the zinc is associated with blunting the effects of the regular insulin. When using mixtures of regular and lente, patients need to inject their insulin immediately after mixing in the syringe and keep their procedures for injection standardized.[45]

Syringes. Insulin syringes are available in 0.3-, 0.5-, and 1-ml capacity.[2] Syringes must match the concentration of the insulin being used (e.g., U-100 syringe for U-100 insulin).[45] Local guidelines for syringe disposal should be followed. Syringes which will not be reused should be placed in a punctureproof container for disposal.[2]

Syringe reuse. Syringes should never be shared with another person[2]; however, syringe reuse by an individual is safe and practical with certain precautions.[2,21] Syringes should be discarded when the needle becomes dull, is bent, or has touched any surface other than skin. Because of the increased risk of infection, those with poor personal hygiene, an acute concurrent illness, open wounds on the hands, or decreased resistance to infection should not reuse syringes. For reuse, the needle must be recapped after each use. To be capable of safely recapping a syringe for reuse, patients must have adequate vision, manual dexterity, and no obvious tremor. Skin around the injection sites should be inspected periodically for unusual redness or sign of infection.[2]

Injection sites. Insulin may be injected into the subcutaneous tissue of the upper arm, the anterior and lateral aspects of the thigh, the buttocks, and the abdomen (avoid a 2-inch radius around the umbilicus). Rotation of sites is important in pre-

Table 14-1 Insulin action curves

Insulin type	Onset (hours)	Peak (hours)	Usual effective duration (hours)	Usual maximum duration (hours)
Animal				
Regular	0.5-2.0	3-4	4-6	6-8
NPH	4-6	8-14	16-20	20-24
Lente	4-6	8-14	16-20	20-24
Ultralente	8-14	Minimal	24-36	24-36
Human				
Regular	0.5-1.0	2-3	3-6	4-6
NPH	2-4	4-10	1-16	14-18
Lente	3-4	4-12	12-18	16-20
Ultralente	6-10	?	18-20	20-30

Source: American Diabetes Association: Buyer's guide to diabetes products, *Diabetes Forecast* 46(10):52, 1993.

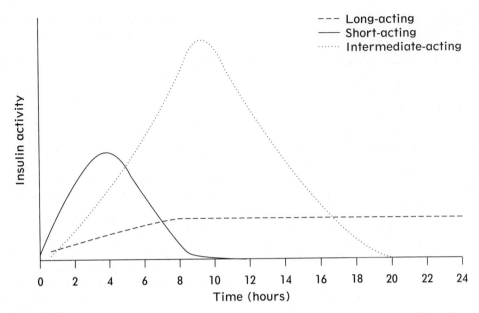

Figure 14-1 Insulin time action profiles: short- versus intermediate- versus long-acting. (From Haire-Joshu D: *Management of diabetes mellitus: perspectives of care across the life span,* St Louis, 1992, Mosby.)

venting lipohypertrophy or lipoatrophy. To obtain consistency in action of insulin, varying sites within the same anatomical region rather than between regions is recommended.[2] Using only abdominal sites may improve the consistency of insulin and glucose profiles in many cases.[45]

Absorption. Absorption of insulin may be affected by many factors. Speed of absorption varies with the site of injection, with the abdomen having the fastest rate of absorption, followed by the arms, thighs, and buttocks.[2] Insulin absorption may be increased by local application of heat, increase in room temperature, massaging the injection site, or exercising the injected limb. Injection depth affects insulin absorption, with intramuscular injection resulting in more rapid absorption than subcutaneous injection.[45]

Insulin administration. Home care nurses should observe the patient's/caregiver's techniques in preparing and injecting insulin. Patients with hyperglycemia without identifiable cause have been noted to be unaware of errors in their injection technique.

Several important deficits have been observed in patients' ability to measure and prepare insulin in a syringe. Inability to calculate total amount of regular and NPH insulin (due to difficulty with basic arithmetic involving addition), not rolling the NPH vial to mix it properly, not eliminating air bubbles from the syringe, and contaminating the regular insulin with the NPH insulin were noted. Factors associated with errors include age, arthritis of the hands, visual acuity, and education.[41]

Steps for preparation and injection of insulin are as follows:

1. Before each injection, the hands and the injection site should be clean.
2. For all insulin preparations except short-acting, gently rotate the vial in the palms of the hands (do not shake) to resuspend the insulin.
3. Draw up and inject an amount of air equal to the dose of insulin into the vial to avoid creating a vacuum. For a mixed dose, put sufficient air into both bottles.
4. Draw up the insulin. When mixing short-acting insulin with intermediate- or long-acting insulin, the clear short-acting insulin should be drawn into the syringe first.

5. Inspect the syringe for and eliminate air bubbles which could cause the injected dose to be decreased.
6. Lightly grasp a fold of skin and inject at a 90-degree angle. Thin individuals may need to inject at a 45-degree angle to avoid intramuscular injection.[2]

Prefilled insulin syringes. To promote independence in those who are capable of injecting insulin but are unable to draw it up, prefilled syringes may be appropriate. Home care nurses should use the following guidelines when using prefilled syringes:

1. Keep all prefilled single or mixed insulin syringes refrigerated and use within 21 days.
2. Never store syringes vertically with the needle down, as crystals may settle and clog the needle.
3. Instruct patients to resuspend the preparation before injection by rolling the syringe.
4. For consistent effect with mixtures of regular and lente or ultralente insulin, use only syringes that have been filled for at least 24 hours prior to injection. For example, on the day when the home health nurse visits and fills syringes, the patient should use a syringe filled on the previous visit, not a freshly mixed syringe.[5]

Assistive devices. Numerous devices designed to make giving an injection easier are available, including spring-loaded needle insertion aids, syringe magnifiers, dose gauges, needle guides, and vial stabilizers. These products may be especially helpful for people who are visually impaired or who have slight dexterity problems. Before a device is purchased, it should be tested by the user to determine whether it meets the individual's needs. One assistive device for those who are visually impaired is the Becton Dickinson Magni-Guide, which magnifies the entire length of the syringe and holds both the syringe and insulin vial, assisting the user to insert the needle into the vial properly.[1] A list and description of diabetes products that may assist persons to be independent in blood glucose monitoring and insulin administration, along with tips for teaching safe use and where the product may be obtained, is provided by Petzinger.[42]

Complications of insulin therapy. Hypoglycemia is by far the most frequent complication in patients treated with insulin.[45] Severe hypoglycemia may result in seizures, coma, long-term cognitive deficits, or death.[52]

As a general rule, hypoglycemia is defined as a blood glucose below 50 mg/dl.[17] In patients receiving insulin, hypoglycemia most often occurs because of a mismatch between the timing of insulin, meals, and exercise. Hypoglycemia may be caused by increased intensity or frequency of exercise, omission of meals, decreased caloric intake, weight loss, use of alcohol,[45] and sulfonylurea therapy.[17]

Symptoms of hypoglycemia vary and include sweating, trembling, weakness, visual disturbance, hunger, pounding heart, difficulty with speaking, tingling around the mouth, dizziness, headache, anxiety, nausea, difficulty concentrating, tiredness, drowsiness, and confusion.[28] Patients often have certain symptoms that are typical for them. Individuals and their significant others need to learn to recognize the symptoms of developing hypoglycemia that are most reliable for them.[12] Hypoglycemic unawareness (lack of classic symptoms) is common in those with IDDM, and increases their susceptibility to the adverse effects of hypoglycemia.[52]

Initial treatment of hypoglycemia for those who are able to swallow consists of consuming 15 g of carbohydrates such as orange juice (4 oz); sugar-containing cola (5 oz); honey, maple syrup, or corn syrup (1 tablespoon); candy (8 Lifesavers); sugar (4 teaspoons dissolved in water); cake icing (1 small tube); or glucose tablets or gel.[52] Monitor the patient's response, check the blood glucose, and follow with food to maintain the blood glucose.[17]

If the patient is unable to swallow, the nurse or caregiver should administer glucagon, 1.0 mg, intramuscularly or subcutaneously. After recovery from a hypoglycemic episode, every effort should be made to prevent recurrence by identifying the cause and correcting the treatment plan accordingly.[45] Assess the patient's/caregiver's knowledge of the causes, symptoms, and treatment of hypoglycemia and instruct as needed. Make sure the patient/caregiver understands the need to always carry a source of rapid-acting carbohydrate whenever leaving home.

Other complications of insulin therapy include lipoatrophy, lipohypertrophy, insulin edema, insulin antibody development, and insulin allergy.

Lipoatrophy, loss of fat at the injection site, is usually relieved by using purified insulin. In hypertrophy, the subcutaneous tissue becomes swollen or fibrous as a result of repeated injections at the same site, leading to poor or irregular absorption of insulin. Treatment consists of rotating injection sites.[45]

Insulin edema may result from marked improvement in blood glucose control. Swelling may occur in the feet and ankles or be generalized. The fluid retention is usually transient, but in rare cases may require treatment with a diuretic.[45]

Insulin allergies may be local or systemic, but they are infrequent as a result of the increased use of purified insulin. Local reactions range from small nodules to large, painful, pruritic erythematous areas.[45]

Oral hypoglycemic agents. Oral hypoglycemic agents, or sulfonylureas, are used in patients with NIDDM to stimulate the pancreatic beta cells to secrete insulin. Oral agents vary in their potency, rate of onset, and duration of action.[31] Characteristics of sulfonylureas are outlined in Table 14-2.

Hypoglycemia is the major adverse effect of sulfonylureas. Severe hypoglycemia is associated with the use of long-acting forms (such as glyburide and chlorpropamide); age (over 65); inadequate nutrition; intercurrent illness; chronic renal, hepatic or cardiovascular disease; and concomitant use of other drugs that cause hypoglycemia or potentiate sulfonylureas.[31]

Side effects other than hypoglycemia are infrequent and include nausea, vomiting, abdominal

Table 14-2 Characteristics of commonly used sulfonylurea drugs

Name of drug	Daily dose range (mg)	Duration of action (hr)
Tolbutamide	500-3000	6-12
Chlorpropamide	100-500	60
Tolazamide	100-1000	16-24
Acetohexamide	250-1500	12-18
Glipizide	2.5-40	15-24
Glyburide	1.25-20	24
Glyclazide	40-320	16-24

Adapted from: Lebovitz HE: Oral antidiabetic agents. In Kahn CR, Weir GC, editors: *Joslin's diabetes mellitus*, ed 13, Philadelphia, 1994, Lea & Febiger, p. 514.

discomfort, and skin rashes. Hematologic disorders and liver disease are rare. The use of chlorpropamide may result in water retention, hyponatremia, and alcohol-induced flushing.[31]

Have the patient/caregiver describe the action and side effects of the medication and how and when it is taken. Make sure the patient/caregiver understands the factors that may contribute to hypoglycemia.

Diet. Diet is regarded as both the cornerstone of treatment and the greatest challenge in diabetes management.[34] Although the dietitian ordinarily calculates the diet and develops the plan for diet management with input from the home care team, home health nurses have ongoing responsibility for instructing patients and assessing metabolic control. Nurses should be knowledgeable about the current dietary recommendations and rationale to assist the patient/caregiver in understanding this aspect of diabetes care.

Currently there is no one "diabetic" or "American Diabetes Association (ADA)" diet. The recommended diet is defined as a dietary prescription based on individual nutrition assessment and treatment goals.[3] General nutrition recommendations for people with diabetes, many of which are the same as for the general population, appear in Table 14-3.

For individuals using insulin therapy, it is important to eat at consistent times synchronized with the action times of the insulin preparation used. In NIDDM, emphasis is on achieving glucose, lipid, and blood pressure goals. Although weight loss is desirable, traditional dietary strategies have not been very effective in achieving long-term weight loss.[3]

In adults, a diet with adequate calories for maintaining or attaining reasonable body weight is recommended. Reasonable weight is the weight an individual and health care provider acknowledge as achievable and maintainable, both short- and long-term. This may not be the same as the desirable or ideal body weight.[3]

Improvement in food choices using nutritional guidelines such as *Dietary Guidelines for Americans*[49] and the *Food Guide Pyramid*[50] is an initial strategy. A nutritionally adequate meal plan with reduction of total fat, especially saturated fats, can be used. Mild to moderate weight loss (10 to 20 pounds) has been shown to improve diabetes

Table 14-3 Summary of nutrition recommendations

Calories	To achieve or maintain reasonable body weight
Protein	10%-20% of total calories
	10% with nephropathy
Fat and carbohydrate	80%-90% of total calories
Saturated fat	<10% of total calories
Cholesterol	≤300 mg/day
Fiber	25-35 g from a variety of sources
Sodium	≤3,000 mg/day
	≤2,400 mg/day with mild to moderate hypertension

Source: American Diabetes Association: Nutrition recommendations and principles for people with diabetes mellitus, *Diabetes Care* 17(5):519, 1994.

control, even if desirable body weight is not achieved. Weight loss is best attempted by a moderate decrease in calories (250 to 500 calories less than average daily intake) and an increase in caloric expenditure.[3]

Nonnutritive sweeteners (saccharin, aspartame, and acesulfame K) are safe to consume by all people with diabetes. Nutritive sweeteners (sucrose, fructose, corn syrup, fruit juice or fruit juice concentrate, honey, molasses, dextrose, maltose, sorbitol, mannitol, and xylitol) may be consumed when substituted for other carbohydrate foods, not simply added to the meal plan. Patients with dyslipidemia should avoid consuming large amounts of fructose. Excessive intake of sorbitol, xylitol, and mannitol may have a laxative effect.[3]

Precautions regarding alcohol use that apply to the general public also apply to people with diabetes. Alcohol in moderation will not ordinarily affect blood glucose levels when diabetes is well controlled. Because of the increased risk for hypoglycemia in those treated with insulin or sulfonylureas, if alcohol is consumed it should be ingested with a meal. Reduction or abstention from alcohol may be advisable for people with diabetes and other medical problems such as pancreatitis, dyslipidemia, or neuropathy. Calories

from alcohol need to be calculated as part of the total caloric intake, and substituted for fat exchanges or fat calories (1 alcoholic beverage = 2 fat exchanges).[3]

Diets should be individualized based on what patients are able and willing to do, their usual eating habits, and other lifestyle factors. Cultural, ethnic, and financial considerations are also very important.[3]

In the home, have the patient/caregiver record intake for 3 days, including the time, type, amount/portion size, and preparation (baked, fried, etc.). Observe the food available in the home. Is it consistent with the patient's needs? Ask the dietitian to review the diet record with the patient's diet prescription. Are there limitations due to inability to purchase, obtain, or prepare appropriate foods? If glycemic control is inadequate, consult with the dietitian to determine an appropriate plan for teaching and regimen adjustment.

Exercise. Many diabetic patients are homebound or unable to exercise because of complications. For those whose condition may improve or who have no contraindications for exercise, understanding the importance and effects of exercise is essential.

Benefits resulting from exercise include improvement in cardiovascular and pulmonary health, sense of well-being, and ability to cope with stress.[22] For NIDDM patients with insulin resistance, obesity, blood lipid abnormalities, and cardiovascular disease, the potential benefits of exercise are obvious and the risk of serious hypoglycemia relatively low. In patients with IDDM, the risk of serious hypoglycemia or worsened hyperglycemia and ketosis consequent to exercise merits caution. Attention must be given to balancing insulin, diet, and exercise so that the consequences of hypoglycemia do not outweigh the benefits of exercise.[23]

Before patients start an exercise program they should have a complete medical examination, including assessment of diabetic complications and blood glucose control. Exercise prescriptions must be individualized and should include the type, intensity, frequency, and duration of exercise.[22]

Assessment of glycemic control. Monitoring glycemic control is essential in assessing the need for adjustments in the therapeutic regimen and in evaluating diabetic control. In the home, glycemic control is evaluated by using devices for self-monitoring of blood glucose (SMBG) and by urine testing.

Blood glucose monitoring. SMBG is widely accepted as an important tool in diabetes management. SMBG in the home makes it possible to prevent many avoidable hospitalizations due to hypoglycemia and hyperglycemia, to evaluate the response to insulin replacement, to reveal the effects of overeating to those with NIDDM,[18] and to reinforce the benefits of exercise and medication.[11]

SMBG procedures involve obtaining a drop of capillary blood by fingerstick using a lancet, applying the blood to a reagent strip (or with some new meters to the glucose sensor), and reading the results at a specified time. Some strips can be read visually whereas others can only be read by meters. Accuracy of results depends upon following the manufacturer's instructions precisely.

Times and frequency of testing should be based on the individual's needs and goals. Until stabilized or with intensive therapy, many patients test 4 times a day: before each meal and at bedtime. Once a pattern is stabilized the frequency of testing may be decreased. The frequency of testing should be increased during illness. For patients who are not willing to or who cannot afford to test frequently, establishing a realistic schedule is important.

Blood glucose target goals are 80 to 120 mg/dl before meals and 100 to 140 mg/dl at bedtime. Individual glycemic target goals should be set based on the patient's ability to understand and carry out the treatment regimen, the risk for severe hypoglycemia, and other factors that may increase risk or decrease benefit.[4]

Assess the accuracy of SMBG by observing the patient's/caregiver's technique. Evaluate the present level of blood glucose control and teach the patient's/caregiver to do so by reviewing the patient's testing record. Ask the patient to state what glucose level is too high or too low and what action should be taken for each.

Glycosylated hemoglobin. Periodic measurement of glycosylated hemoglobin (Hb A_1 or Hb A_{1c}) is useful in patients with IDDM and NIDDM. The test provides an accurate estimation of the average blood glucose during the 6 to 8 weeks preceding the test.[11] Glycosylated hemoglobin should be performed at least quarterly in all insulin-treated patients and as frequently as necessary to assess achievement of glycemic goals in non–insulin-treated patients. The goal for hemoglobin A_{1c} is less than 7%.[4]

Urine testing. All patients should test their urine for ketones whenever blood glucose is consistently above 240 mg/dl, with acute illness, or symptomatic hyperglycemia.[45]

Urine testing for glucose has been replaced by blood glucose monitoring in many patients with diabetes. One limitation of urine testing is that in a patient with a high renal threshold for glucose, elevated blood glucose levels will not be reflected by urine testing. Hypoglycemia is not detected by urine testing. Because of its simplicity and low cost, urine glucose testing may be useful for those who are unable or unwilling to perform blood glucose monitoring.[45]

Although blood glucose testing is widely recommended, many patients still use home urine testing. In a study evaluating diabetic patients' home urine glucose testing technique, problems noted in performing urine testing included difficulty reading package insert instructions, inability to correctly read a clock, and waiting an incorrect amount of time before reading test results. Of the methods used, the largest number of errors occurred with Clinitest method.[46]

Urine testing products are sensitive to light, temperature extremes, and moisture. Patients and caregivers should follow manufacturer's instructions for storage, and keep tablets for urine testing out of the reach of children because they are poisonous.[1]

Hyperglycemia. Assess the patient's/caregiver's knowledge of the causes, symptoms, and treatment of hyperglycemia. Provide instructions regarding the importance of recognition and treatment of infection.

Sick-day management. Illness may disrupt the patient's diabetes management program. Since illness is often accompanied by hyperglycemia, the patient/caregiver needs to be instructed on the importance of continuing medication, maintaining adequate fluid and caloric intake on sick days, and seeking professional advice regarding temporary adjustment of the treatment program. Guidelines appear in the following Patient Education Guide box.

PATIENT EDUCATION GUIDE: "SICK-DAY" MANAGEMENT OF DIABETES MELLITUS

Sick means having fever, vomiting, nausea, diarrhea, or congestion. The nurse should provide the patient with the following instructions:

Insulin

If you take insulin shots, always take your insulin when you are sick, *even if you cannot eat your regular meals.* You may need extra insulin, for example:
1. If BG is 240-400 mg/dl add 2 to 4 units of regular insulin to the usual dose before meals and take the usual dose at bedtime.
2. If BG is 240-400 mg/dl and the urine is moderate to large for ketones, add 4 to 6 units of regular insulin to the usual dosage for *every* insulin dose until ketones are no longer moderate.

Medication

If you take a pill for diabetes, be sure to take it when you are sick. If vomiting, contact your physician or diabetes nurse educator.

Diet

If you are unable to eat your usual meals, try to drink fluids containing 10 g of carbohydrates every hour while awake. The following servings contain 10 g of carbohydrates:
  1/2 cup ginger ale (not diet)
  1/2 cup Coca-Cola (not diet)
  1/2 cup chicken soup with noodles
  3/4 cup chilled Gatorade
If you *are able to eat* usual meals, then drink 1/2 cup of calorie-free fluid every hour while awake. The following are calorie-free:
  Broth or bouillon
  Decaffeinated tea
  Sugar-free/caffeine-free soda, such as 7-Up or Sprite
  Water

Urine/blood testing

Check your urine for ketones/acetone and check your blood glucose level every 4 hours.
Seek professional advice if you have any of the following:
  Diarrhea or vomiting for more than 6 hours
  Moderate or large levels of ketones (++ or +++) in your urine even after two injections of regular insulin as
    instructed
  Your blood tests for glucose are over 400 or urine tests for glucose are 2% to 5% even after two injections
    of regular insulin as instructed

From Haire-Joshu DL: Nursing management of adults with disorders of the pancreas. In Beare PG, Myers JL, editors: *Principles and practice of adult health nursing,* St Louis 1994, Mosby, p 1742.

SUMMARY

Living with diabetes presents many challenges. Glycemic control may be difficult to achieve even in an ideal situation. Many home care patients have numerous barriers confronting them daily. Assessment of the individual's particular situation and practical, appropriate education and intervention are crucial in promoting adherence to the plan of care. The unique privilege of direct observation of the person's real-life situation may enhance the home health nurse's ability to tailor the treatment regimen to the individual's lifestyle. The mutual establishment of realistic goals and plans will demand the creativity of the home care nurse and the perseverance of the patient, but it is the best way to increase adherence and improve clinical outcomes.

REFERENCES

1. American Diabetes Association: 1994 Buyer's guide to diabetes products, *Diabetes Forecast* 46(10):50, 1993.
2. American Diabetes Association: Position statement: insulin administration, *Diabetes Care* 16(suppl 2):31, 1993.
3. American Diabetes Association: Nutrition recommendations and principles for people with diabetes mellitus, *Diabetes Care* 17(5):519, 1994.
4. American Diabetes Association: Standards of medical care for patients with diabetes mellitus, *Diabetes Care* 17(6): 616, 1994.
5. Anderson JH, Campbell RK: Mixing insulins in 1990, *Diabetes Educator* 16:380, 1990.
6. Beaser RS, Richardson DL, Hollerorth HJ: Education in the treatment of diabetes. In Kahn CR and Weir GC, editors: *Joslin's diabetes mellitus,* ed 13, Philadelphia, 1994, Lea & Febiger.
7. Bennett PH: Definition, diagnosis, and classification of diabetes mellitus and impaired glucose tolerance. In Kahn CR, Weir GC, editors: *Joslin's diabetes mellitus,* ed 13, Philadelphia, 1994, Lea & Febiger.
8. Broadstone VL et al: Diabetic peripheral neuropathy: sensorimotor neuropathy, *Diabetes Educator* 13(1):30, 1987.
9. Centers for Disease Control, Division of Diabetes Translation: *Diabetes surveillance 1980-1987,* Atlanta, 1990, US Department of Health and Human Services.
10. Chait A, Bierman EL: Pathogenesis of macrovascular disease in diabetes. In Kahn CR, Weir GC, editors: *Joslin's diabetes mellitus,* ed 13, Philadelphia, 1994, Lea & Febiger.
11. Cooppan R: General approach to the treatment of diabetes. In Kahn CR, Weir GC, editors: *Joslin's diabetes mellitus,* ed 13, Philadelphia, 1994, Lea & Febiger.
12. Cryer PE, Fisher JN, Shamoon H: Hypoglycemia, *Diabetes Care* 17(7):734, 1994.
13. Cyrus et al: Diabetic peripheral neuropathy: autonomic neuropathies, *Diabetes Educator* 13(2):11, 1987.
14. Dabbs CK, Meridith T: Diabetic eye disease. In Davidson JK, editor: *Clinical diabetes mellitus: a problem-oriented approach,* ed 2, New York, 1991, Thieme.
15. Davidson JK: Diabetic ketoacidosis and the hyperglycemic hyperosmolar state. In Davidson JK, editor: *Clinical diabetes mellitus: a problem-oriented approach,* ed 2, New York, 1991, Thieme.
16. Davidson JK: Diagnosis of diabetes mellitus. In Davidson JK, editor: *Clinical diabetes mellitus: a problem-oriented approach,* ed 2, New York, 1991, Thieme.
17. Davidson JK, Galloway JA, Chance RE: Insulin therapy. In Davidson JK, editor: *Clinical diabetes mellitus: a problem-oriented approach,* ed 2, New York, 1991, Thieme.
18. Davidson JK, Russo G: Monitoring of blood and urine glucose and ketone levels. In Davidson JK, editor: *Clinical diabetes mellitus: a problem-oriented approach,* ed 2, New York, 1991, Thieme.
19. Diabetes Control and Complications Trial Research Group: The effect of intensive treatment of diabetes on the development and progression of long-term complications in insulin-dependent diabetes mellitus. *NEJM* 329:977, 1993.
20. Eisenbarth GS, Ziegler AG, Colman PA: Pathogenesis of insulin-dependent (type I) diabetes mellitus. In Kahn CR,

Weir GC, editors: *Joslin's diabetes mellitus,* ed 13, Philadelphia, 1994, Lea & Febiger.
21. Fachnie JD, Whitehouse FW, McGrath Z: Reevaluation of single-use insulin syringes, *Diabetes Care* 11(10):817, 1988.
22. Giacca A, Vranic M, Davidson JK, Lickley HLA: Exercise and stress in diabetes mellitus. In Davidson JK, editor: *Clinical diabetes mellitus: a problem-oriented approach,* ed 2, New York, 1991, Thieme.
23. Goodyear LI, Smith RJ: Exercise and diabetes. In Kahn CR, Weir GC, editors: *Joslin's diabetes mellitus,* ed 13, Philadelphia, 1994, Lea & Febiger.
24. Habershaw G: Foot lesions in patients with diabetes: cause, prevention and treatment. In Kahn CR, Weir GC, editors: *Joslin's diabetes mellitus,* ed 13, Philadelphia, 1994, Lea & Febiger.
25. Haire-Joshu DL: Nursing management of adults with disorders of the pancreas. In Beare PG, Myers JL, editors: *Principles and practice of adult health nursing,* St Louis, 1994, Mosby.
26. Harris MI et al: Prevalence of diabetes and impaired glucose tolerance and plasma glucose levels in US population aged 20-74 years, *Diabetes* 36:523, 1987.
27. Henquin J: Cell biology of insulin secretion. In Kahn CR, Weir GC, editors: *Joslin's diabetes mellitus,* ed 13, Philadelphia, 1994, Lea & Febiger.
28. Hepburn DA: Symptoms of hypoglycemia. In Frier BM, Fisher BM, editors: *Hypoglycemia and diabetes,* London, 1993, Edward Arnold.
29. King GI, Banskota NK: Mechanisms of diabetic microvascular complications. In Kahn CR, Weir GC, editors: *Joslin's diabetes mellitus,* ed 13, Philadelphia, 1994, Lea & Febiger.
30. Kitabchi AE, Fisher JN, Murphy MB, Rumbak MJ: Diabetic ketoacidosis and the hyperglycemic hyperosmolar nonketotic state. In Kahn CR, Weir GC, editors: *Joslin's diabetes mellitus,* ed 13, Philadelphia, 1994, Lea & Febiger.
31. Lebovitz HE: Oral antidiabetic agents. In Kahn CR, Weir GC, editors: *Joslin's diabetes mellitus,* ed 13, Philadelphia, 1994, Lea & Febiger.
32. Lebovitz HE, editor: *Physician's guide to non-insulin dependent (type II) diabetes: diagnosis and treatment,* ed 2, Alexandria, Va, 1988, American Diabetes Association.
33. Lernmark A: Insulin-dependent diabetes mellitus. In Davidson JK, editor: *Clinical diabetes mellitus: a problem-oriented approach,* ed 2, New York, 1991, Thieme.
34. Lockwood D et al: The biggest problem in diabetes, *Diabetes Educator* 12(1):30, 1986.
35. Logerfo FW, Gibbons GW: Vascular disease of the lower extremities in diabetes mellitus: etiology and management. In Kahn CR, Weir GC, editors: *Joslin's diabetes mellitus,* ed 13, Philadelphia, 1994, Lea & Febiger.
36. McGowan JE: Infections in diabetes mellitus. In Davidson JK, editor: *Clinical diabetes mellitus: a problem-oriented approach,* ed 2, New York, 1991, Thieme.
37. McKenna MJ, Redmond JM, Whitehouse FW: Cerebrovascular diseases. In Davidson JK, editor: *Clinical diabetes mellitus: a problem-oriented approach,* ed 2, New York, 1991, Thieme.
38. Nathan DM: Long-term complications of diabetes mellitus, *NEJM* 328:1676, 1993.

39. Nathan DM: Relationship between metabolic control and long-term complications of diabetes. In Kahn CR, Weir GC, editors: *Joslin's diabetes mellitus,* ed 13, Philadelphia, 1994, Lea & Febiger.

40. Newman KD, Weaver MT: Insulin measurement and preparation among diabetic patients at a county hospital, *Nurs Pract* 19(3):44, 1994.

41. Perry A, Potter P: *Clinical nursing skills,* ed 3, St Louis, 1994, Mosby.

42. Petzinger RA: Diabetes aids and products for people with visual or physical impairment, *Diabetes Educator* 18:121, 1992.

43. Quickel KE: Economic and social costs of diabetes. In Kahn CR, Weir GC, editors: *Joslin's diabetes mellitus,* ed 13, Philadelphia, 1994, Lea & Febiger.

44. Rosenweig JL et al: Findings of the diabetes control and complications trial. In Kahn CR, Weir GC, editors: *Joslin's diabetes mellitus,* ed 13, Philadelphia, 1994, Lea & Febiger.

45. Rosenweig JL: Principles of insulin therapy. In Kahn CR, Weir GC, editors: *Joslin's diabetes mellitus,* ed 13, Philadelphia, 1994, Lea & Febiger.

46. Smolowitz JL, Zaldivar A: Evaluation of diabetic patients' home urine glucose testing technique and ability to interpret results, *Diabetes Educator* 18:207, 1992.

47. Sperling MA, editor: *Physician's guide to insulin-dependent (type I) diabetes: diagnosis and treatment,* Alexandria, Va, 1988, American Diabetes Association.

48. Steiner G: Hyperlipidemia and atherosclerotic cardiovascular disease. In Davidson JK, editor: *Clinical diabetes mellitus: a problem-oriented approach,* ed 2, New York, 1991, Thieme.

49. US Department of Agriculture, US Department of Health and Human Services: *Nutrition and your health: dietary guidelines for Americans,* ed 3, Hyattsville, Md, 1990, USDA's Human Nutrition Information Service.

50. US Department of Agriculture: *The food guide pyramid,* Hyattsville, Md, 1992, USDA's Human Nutrition Information Service.

51. Viberti G, Wiseman MJ, Pinto JR, Messent J: Diabetic nephropathy. In Kahn CR, Weir GC, editors: *Joslin's diabetes mellitus,* ed 13, Philadelphia, 1994, Lea & Febiger.

52. Widom B, Simonson DC: Latrogenic hypoglycemia. In Kahn CR, Weir GC, editors: *Joslin's diabetes mellitus,* ed 13, Philadelphia, 1994, Lea & Febiger.

15 The Patient with Bladder Dysfunction

Kathryn A. Houston

Bladder dysfunction resulting in altered urinary elimination is a clinical problem frequently encountered by home health nurses. Bladder dysfunction affects all age groups, is a major cause of disability and dependency, and is a source of significant stress for caregivers. Home health nurses play a vital role in helping patients and caregivers manage bladder dysfunction in the home. This chapter provides an overview of the pathophysiology and manifestations of bladder dysfunction and details nursing assessment and interventions for patients with urinary retention or urinary incontinence.

DEFINITION OF THE PROBLEM

Bladder dysfunction is a general term that refers to the failure of the bladder either to store urine or to empty urine properly.[24] Although the underlying causes of the problem vary, bladder dysfunction is manifested symptomatically as urinary retention, urinary incontinence, or both.

Urinary retention is defined as the inability to void and empty the bladder spontaneously.[56] *Urinary incontinence* is defined as the involuntary loss of urine in an amount or with a frequency sufficient to constitute a social or health problem.[26]

PREVALENCE

Urinary incontinence increases with age, is slightly more common in females, and is significantly more prevalent in persons with cognitive or functional impairments.[22,32] Although incontinence is most prevalent in long-term care settings,[9,39] a substantial proportion of the elderly population residing at home experiences urinary incontinence. Several studies have estimated the prevalence of urinary incontinence in the community-dwelling elderly population at approximately 30%.[14,22,23,53] The prevalence of incontinence in elderly persons cared for by family members has been reported to be as high as 53%.[37]

One survey of patients receiving home health services found that 22% of the sample were incontinent.[35] Most of the incontinent patients had mobility impairments (77%) or cognitive impairments (44%). Only 5% of those who were incontinent had received a formal evaluation of the problem. Management strategies to deal with incontinence most commonly consisted of the use of protective pads and garments (56%), a toileting schedule or habit retraining (38%), indwelling catheters or external collection devices (24%), and adaptive equipment (19%).

With rapid discharge of patients from acute care settings who have unresolved bladder dysfunction and with a growing amount of acute and long-term care being provided in the home, home health nurses will be increasingly involved with continence restoration and incontinence management.

PHYSIOLOGY OF THE LOWER URINARY TRACT

Bladder storage occurs under control of the sympathetic nervous system, whereas bladder emptying is a parasympathetic nervous system function. The sympathetic nervous system facilitates urine storage primarily by inhibiting the contractile effects of the parasympathetic system on the bladder. In addition, the sympathetic system is responsible for maintaining outlet resistance by stimulating alpha-adrenergic receptors in the bladder base and proximal urethra.[62]

Bladder function is regulated by means of an involuntary spinal cord reflex involving sacral spinal cord segments S2 to S4. As the bladder fills, stretch receptors located in the detrusor muscle are stimulated and carry impulses by way of parasympathetic nerves to the sacral spinal cord where these nerves synapse with motor fibers that innervate both the pelvic ganglia and bladder musculature. Stimulation of motor fibers results in detrusor contraction. This reflex can be voluntarily inhibited or facilitated through higher cerebral cortical control. Generally, between 150 and 350 ml of urine can be stored in the bladder before bladder pressure begins to increase and the initial urge to void is perceived. Normal bladder capacity is between 300 and 600 ml.[26]

ABNORMALITIES OF MICTURITION
The uninhibited neurogenic bladder

Damage to the brain stem or any portion of the spinal cord that interrupts the pathways transmitting inhibitory impulses to the bladder can result in an uninhibited neurogenic bladder. This condition is characterized by frequent, uncontrolled voiding that occurs whenever the micturition reflex is initiated. Conditions most commonly associated with this abnormality include cerebrovascular accidents, brain tumors or trauma, demyelinating disease such as multiple sclerosis, dementia, and Parkinson's disease.[5,51]

The atonic bladder

Lesions, damage, or deterioration of sensory or motor components of the sacral spinal cord can interfere with initiation or completion of the voiding reflex. The bladder fills to capacity, and urine leakage occurs as the bladder becomes overdistended. If sensory fibers are intact but motor nerves are involved, the individual is able to perceive bladder fullness but cannot voluntarily initiate voiding. If destruction of sensory nerve fibers is the cause of the atonic condition, stretch signals from the bladder cannot be transmitted and initiation of the micturition reflex is prevented. Common causes of an atonic bladder include infection, immobility, diabetes, pelvic surgery, medications, tumors, and injuries to the sacral region of the spinal cord (such as injuries that occur with vertebral compression fractures or trauma).

The automatic bladder (reflex bladder)

If the spinal cord is damaged above the level of the sacral region and anatomic components of the voiding reflex remain intact, reflex or automatic bladder dysfunction results. With this abnormality, voluntary inhibition of the micturition reflex is lost. The bladder can be emptied spontaneously, though, with elicitation of the micturition reflex by external cutaneous stimulation or other mechanisms. Reflex bladder is most commonly seen in individuals with upper motor neuron spinal cord injuries and multiple sclerosis.

EFFECTS OF AGING ON BLADDER FUNCTION

Although aging itself is not necessarily a cause of bladder dysfunction, certain anatomic and physiologic changes associated with aging can predispose elderly individuals to develop problems with urine storage and emptying.[49,52]

Degeneration and fibrosis of the bladder wall tissues result in a decline in bladder capacity as individuals age.[12,26,30] This reduction in bladder capacity may result in more frequent trips to the bathroom. In addition, the kidneys' ability to concentrate urine diminishes with age. Larger volumes of urine along with a smaller bladder capacity give rise to nocturia.

Changes in bladder contractility with advanced age can also alter bladder function. Decreased bladder contractility results in increased residual urine remaining in the bladder after voiding. Urinary residuals have been implicated as contributing to the higher prevalence of bacteriuria in the elderly population.[51] Detrusor instability associated with changes in the neuromuscular threshold to bladder stretch causes the prevalence of involuntary bladder contractions to increase with age. It has been estimated that approximately 15% of healthy elderly men and women have uninhibited bladder contractions in the absence of underlying pathology.[40]

In women the decline in estrogen production after menopause greatly reduces urethral resistance and urethral closure pressure. Urethral mucosal changes resulting from estrogen loss disrupt oxygenation, tissue integrity, and the normal flora predisposing the tissues to inflammatory and infectious states such as atrophic vaginitis and urethritis.[16] Childbirth, gynecologic surgery, and obesity further weaken the pelvic floor muscles, placing elderly women at greater risk for the development of stress incontinence.[54] In men prostatic hypertrophy can obstruct the bladder outlet, resulting in urinary retention or overflow incontinence.

The higher prevalence of cognitive dysfunction in older adults places them at greater risk for developing urinary incontinence. Dementias, depression, and delirium can interfere with the ability to recognize toileting needs and carry out the necessary psychomotor activities involved in toileting.

HOME CARE APPLICATION

Home health nurses caring for patients with bladder dysfunction must first assess the status of the patient. The information obtained is then used as a basis for initiating appropriate patient education and for choosing and implementing suitable interventions.

Health history and assessment

Despite the fact that many individuals with bladder dysfunction will benefit from assessment and treatment, studies indicate that a large proportion of them do not undergo any type of evaluation.[22,50] Patients are often embarrassed or reluctant to report bladder problems, and many older adults may consider loss of urine control part of the normal aging process. Therefore home health nurses should include an assessment of bladder function in the overall assessment of the patient.

Nursing assessment should be geared toward determining the cause of the bladder dysfunction so that potentially reversible factors can be corrected and management strategies appropriate for the particular condition can be instituted. A thorough assessment of bladder function should include a history, with emphasis on bladder habits and bowel function; a physical assessment including bedside urodynamic testing; functional, cognitive, and environmental evaluations; and collection of laboratory tests for further evaluation.

The history. Key aspects of the nursing history are summarized in the box that follows. Onset and duration of the problem, frequency of accidental urine loss, and volume of leakage should be ascertained. Characteristics that delineate the type of incontinence the individual may be having should be determined. For example, it is important to note whether urine loss is associated with a

---

ESSENTIAL ELEMENTS OF THE HISTORY: ONSET, DURATION, FREQUENCY OF SYMPTOMS
1. Volume of urine loss
2. Characteristics of bladder dysfunction: urgency, hesitancy, straining, dribbling, urine loss on exertion or with coughing, sneezing, or bending
3. Associated symptoms of bladder dysfunction: dysuria, frequency, nocturia, lack of sensation, vaginal discharge or itching, hematuria
4. Pattern of urine loss: times, activity at time of leakage, relationship to fluid or medication consumption
5. Past and current medical problems: neurologic disorders, diabetes, strokes, congestive heart failure, venous insufficiency
6. Past genitourinary/gynecologic history: childbirths, surgery, dilatations, radiation, recurrent urinary tract infections
7. Medications
8. Fluid intake: amount, type, times
9. Bowel habits: frequency, consistency

---

sudden sense of urgency or whether leakage occurs with exertional activities such as exercise, bending, coughing, or laughing. Hesitancy, straining to void, frequent dribbling, constant leakage of small amounts of urine, and a sensation of incomplete bladder emptying are symptoms of urinary retention. Associated symptoms such as burning on urination, frequency, urgency, hematuria, or fever may indicate a urinary tract infection, although these classic symptoms may be absent in elderly patients.[6] Vaginal discharge, itching, or dyspareunia are signs of atrophic vaginitis, which is often associated with stress incontinence.

The pattern of urine loss should be elicited. Morning incontinence may be related to daily use of a diuretic. Nocturia may be caused by the consumption of alcohol, caffeine, or other fluids near bedtime. Incontinence that occurs only when away from home might indicate a functional loss that results from the inability to find toileting facilities when needed.

Relevant medical history should be reviewed during the assessment because many medical problems can result in bladder dysfunction. Diabetic

Table 15-1 Medications that can potentially affect continence[26]

Type of medication	Potential effects on continence
Diuretics	Polyuria, frequency, urgency
Anticholinergics	Urinary retention, overflow incontinence, impaction
Psychotropics	
Antidepressants	Anticholinergic actions, sedation
Antipsychotics	Anticholinergic actions, sedation, rigidity, immobility
Sedatives and hypnotics	Sedation, delirium, fecal impaction
Narcotic analgesics	Urinary retention, fecal impaction, sedation, delirium
Alpha-adrenergic blockers	Urethral relaxation
Alpha-adrenergic agonists	Urinary retention
Beta-adrenergic agonists	Urinary retention
Calcium channel blockers	Urinary retention
Alcohol	Polyuria, frequency, urgency, sedation, delirium, immobility

patients may experience incontinence as a result of polyuria associated with elevated blood sugar levels or because of diabetic neuropathy rendering the bladder hypotonic. Neurologic disorders such as strokes, Parkinson's disease, dementia, and multiple sclerosis are frequently associated with detrusor instability, which when coupled with the functional disabilities of these medical conditions can result in urinary incontinence.[67] Patients with congestive heart failure or venous insufficiency may experience frequency, urgency, and nocturia as a result of postural diuresis associated with assuming a horizontal position.[36]

Past genitourinary and gynecologic history in females should ascertain the number of vaginal births, bladder or abdominal surgeries, and urethral dilatations. In males, prostate surgery and radiation therapy are important to note. In both men and women the frequency of urinary tract infections should be determined because recurrent infections may necessitate referral to a urologist.

A careful review of medications the patient is taking should be conducted, since many medications can alter bladder function (Table 15-1).

Assessing fluid intake is another important aspect of the patient's history. Amount, type, and times of fluid consumption should be determined. Fluid consumed close to bedtime may contribute to nocturia or nighttime incontinence. Beverages containing alcohol, caffeine, or aspartame (Nutrasweet) can cause urinary frequency and urgency and often have prolonged effects on elderly individuals.

Assessment of bladder habits. Description of the patient's bladder habits is also useful in determining appropriate nursing interventions. A bladder record (Figure 15-1) is a good way to establish the patient's bladder habits and pattern of incontinence.[1,55] The bladder record can be kept by the patient, family, or formal caregiver. The patient is checked for wetness every 2 hours for several days, and a log is filled out describing the times and volumes of successful voids, incontinent episodes, and fluid intake.[19,25] The bladder record not only helps assess the type and pattern of accidental urine loss, but it also is used to establish behavioral interventions and protocols for managing incontinence.

BLADDER RECORD

Name_____Date_____

Time	Amount Urinated in Toilet	Urine Leakage Small Amount	Urine Leakage Large Amount	Activity when Leakage Occurred	Leakage of Stool	Fluid Intake
8:00 am	ml					
9:00 am	ml					
10:00 am	ml					
11:00 am	ml					
12:00 pm	ml					
1:00 pm	ml					
2:00 pm	ml					
3:00 pm	ml					
4:00 pm	ml					
5:00 pm	ml					
6:00 pm	ml					
7:00 pm	ml					
8:00 pm	ml					
9:00 pm	ml					
10:00 pm	ml					
11:00 pm	ml					
12:00 am	ml					
1:00 am	ml					
2:00 am	ml					
3:00 am	ml					
4:00 am	ml					
5:00 am	ml					
6:00 am	ml					
7:00 am	ml					

Figure 15-1 Sample bladder record.

Assessment of bowel function. Constipation may be a major factor contributing to incontinence because stool mass in the rectum obstructs the bladder outlet. In addition, fecal incontinence may coexist with urinary incontinence and often will improve with use of the same treatment modalities employed to manage bladder problems.

Patients and caregivers should be questioned to determine the frequency and consistency of bowel movements; when the last bowel movement occurred; whether or not patients have problems with constipation, fecal incontinence, or impactions; what types of foods are eaten; how much fluid is consumed on a daily basis; and whether laxatives are used and if so how often.

Physical assessment. The physical assessment of incontinent patients should include neurologic, abdominal, pelvic, and rectal examinations. A brief evaluation of cranial nerve responses, reflexes, muscle strength, and sensation to the lower extremities and perineal area should be conducted. Abnormalities such as focal and parkinsonian signs suggest that the bladder dysfunction has a neurologic component. Integrity of the sacral reflex arc can be determined by testing for the bulbocavernosus reflex. This is done by inserting a gloved finger into the patient's rectum. Gently stroking the glans penis in males and the skin near the clitoris in females should elicit an anal contraction if the reflex is present. Absence of the reflex does not always indicate pathology but can be helpful in further defining problems with neurologic innervation if focal findings are present.

The abdomen should be inspected for scars indicating previous abdominal surgeries and for distension. The abdomen should also be palpated to determine the presence of any masses, tenderness, or bladder distension.

The perineum should be examined for redness and skin breakdown. A simple pelvic examination involving inspection of the vaginal canal for atrophic vaginitis or infection and palpation for anatomic abnormalities and masses can be done in the home. During the rectal examination, the rectum should be checked for fecal impaction, masses, prostatic enlargement, and muscle tone. Having the patient squeeze the rectal muscles around the examiner's finger allows evaluation of sphincter tone.

Bedside urodynamic testing. Bedside urodynamic testing is a simple screening procedure to determine the cause of persistent urinary incontinence (i.e., urge, stress, or overflow). The procedure and its diagnostic usefulness are outlined in Table 15-2. Ouslander compared bedside with standard multichannel cystometry in 171 elderly incontinent patients.[42,43] Bedside testing was reported to have a 75% sensitivity and 79% specificity for detrusor instability. Diokno compared the provocative stress test (a component of bedside cystometry) with self-reported continence status and incontinence symptoms.[13] The estimated sensitivity of provocative stress testing was 39.5% with a specificity of 98.5%. Bedside urodynamic testing is neither sensitive nor specific for detrusor hyperactivity with impaired contractility or other forms of outlet obstruction.

Although multichannel synchronous pressure flow studies offer the most accurate method of evaluating bladder dysfunction, these studies are also more expensive, invasive, and time-consuming than bedside testing. Bedside testing, therefore, has value as an initial screening procedure to evaluate bladder dysfunction in the home setting.

Functional assessment. Because many patients suffer from impaired mobility, it is important for home health nurses to determine the extent to which functional disabilities contribute to urinary incontinence. An assessment of gait, balance, and transfer ability can ascertain whether bladder problems have a functional component. Patients should be observed as they rise from a bed or chair. Immediate standing balance, step symmetry, step continuity, speed, stability with movement, and appropriate or inappropriate use of assistive devices should be noted. If patients are confined to a bed or wheelchair, the ability to shift weight while sitting and lying should be assessed, since use of a urinal or bedpan will depend on the degree to which patients are able to maneuver themselves.

Assessment of cognitive function. Evaluating cognitive function is an important part of assessing patients with bladder dysfunction, since the nursing interventions chosen to treat the problem must be consistent with patients' abilities to learn, remember, and carry out instructions. There are standard forms available for assessing mental status. Multidisciplinary conferences with the mental health nurse may be helpful in obtaining and assessing this information.

Environmental assessment. Environmental factors that should be assessed include distance to the

Table 15-2 Bedside cystometry procedure

Procedure	Normal finding	Abnormal finding	Diagnostic usefulness
1. Have patient void. Then catheterize.	Catheter passes with ease.	Catheter is difficult to pass.	OVERFLOW INCONTINENCE from mechanical obstruction.
2. Measure postvoid residual urine.	Less than 100 ml PVR.	Greater than 100 ml PVR.	OVERFLOW INCONTINENCE secondary to retention.
3. Fill bladder slowly with sterile solution. Note volume when initial urge to void is sensed.	Initial urge to void generally sensed when bladder holds 250 ml to 300 ml.	Strong initial urge sensed at less than 200 ml.	URGE INCONTINENCE related to small bladder capacity.
4. Continue to fill bladder slowly until patient can hold no more.	Normal bladder capacity between 400 ml to 600 ml.	Patient unable to tolerate minimum of 400 ml.	URGE INCONTINENCE secondary to diminished bladder capacity.
5. Note any involuntary bladder contractions.	No contractions or leakage around catheter noted.	Retrograde movement of fluid into syringe. Leakage around catheter, patient expresses sense of urgency.	URGE INCONTINENCE related to uninhibited bladder contractions.
6. With bladder filled to capacity, remove catheter and have patient cough in supine and standing positions.	No leakage.	Leakage of fluid from bladder with stress maneuvers.	STRESS INCONTINENCE associated with pelvic muscle weakness.
7. Have patient empty bladder into measuring "HAT." Observe patient void.	Calculated postvoid residual less than 100 ml. Strong urine stream.	Calculated postvoid residual greater than 100 ml. Hesitancy, straining, intermittent stream present.	OVERFLOW INCONTINENCE secondary to an obstruction or atonic bladder.

toilet, toilet access, seat height, presence of safety or supportive devices, lighting, safety of floor surfaces, obstacles in the pathway to the bathroom, type of clothing and footwear worn by the patient, ability to manipulate clothing, accessibility of adaptive equipment, and availability of caregiver assistance.[33,36] Although not used commonly in the home setting, physical and chemical restraints should be recognized as environmental barriers that may interfere with the performance of toileting tasks.

Laboratory tests. Urinary tract infections can cause urinary incontinence and urinary retention.

This very treatable source of bladder dysfunction can be ruled out by laboratory evaluation. A postvoid catheterization should be performed on all incontinent patients to check for residual urine. A residual volume of 100 ml or greater indicates urinary retention. The urine sample that is collected should be sent to the laboratory for urinalysis and culture. A urine white blood cell count of 10 or greater is suggestive of a urinary tract infection.[6,67] The presence of red blood cells in the absence of pyuria or bacteriuria may indicate the need for a urologic evaluation to rule out tumors or calculi. Identification of the infecting organism by culture ensures the choice of appropriate antibiotic treatment.

Dipstick testing of urine is an acceptable screening technique of urinalysis. Urine that is dipstick positive for leukocytes, red blood cells, or nitrite is generally infected. Many physicians will initiate antibiotic therapy immediately based on dipstick findings alone.

Blood urea nitrogen (BUN) and serum creatinine, end products of metabolism, can be helpful in identifying renal failure. Urea nitrogen rises gradually during acute renal failure, and serum creatinine rises rapidly during chronic renal failure. The BUN may be elevated if the individual is dehydrated, febrile, or receiving increased proteins parenterally or in the diet.

Nursing management and patient education

The plan of care for patients with bladder dysfunction is based on assessment and subsequent determination of the cause of the problem. (See the box titled Primary Nursing Diagnoses/Patient Problems.) A variety of interventions are available for the management of urinary incontinence and retention. Therapies most appropriate for each type of bladder dysfunction are outlined in Table 15-3. Each management strategy is discussed in detail in the following sections.

PRIMARY NURSING DIAGNOSES/ PATIENT PROBLEMS

- Urinary elimination, alteration in pattern related to prostatic hypertrophy, retention, urethral sphincter weakness, infection, detrusor hyperreflexia, and functional impairment
- Bowel elimination, alteration in: constipation or fecal impaction related to immobility, decreased fluid intake, medication side effects, and decreased gastrointestinal motility
- Potential for urinary tract infection related to chronic indwelling catheter use
- Self-care deficit: toileting
- Potential for skin breakdown secondary to incontinence
- Self-concept/self-esteem alteration related to urinary incontinence

Interventions for patients with bladder dysfunction should be directed toward goals of care that are realistic and achievable, reflecting patients' and caregivers' physical, psychological, and intellectual capabilities. (See the box titled Primary Themes of Patient Education.)

Behavioral training procedures. Behavioral interventions aim to improve bladder function by providing a patient/caregiver-initiated stimulus and reinforcer to establish continent behavior.[8]

Pelvic floor exercises. Pelvic floor (Kegel) exercises are used to treat stress incontinence in men and women with intact cognitive function. These exercises involve repetitive contraction and relaxation of the periurethral muscles to help strengthen them so that tighter urethral closure can be achieved. (See the box titled Kegel Exercises for a description of the technique.) Success rates of 70% or more have been reported with the use of Kegel exercises.[21,63] Although the optimal number and frequency of pelvic floor exercises required to achieve urine control have not been established,[64] several training times per day are generally suggested.[25] Anywhere from 6 to 12 weeks of continued exercise will be necessary before patients begin to see results. Ongoing exercise to maintain muscle tone will be necessary once the desired results are achieved. Having patients perform these exercises during a digital rectal or vaginal exam provides feedback to ensure that the correct muscles are being tightened. Instruct patients to practice starting and stopping the flow of urine when voiding to become familiar with the muscles that need to be targeted. Once learned, these exercises should be practiced frequently. Patient motivation and compliance are essential for the success of this treatment.

Bladder retraining. Bladder retraining involves progressive lengthening or shortening of toileting intervals to correct the negative habit of frequent voiding or waiting too long to void. This improves the patient's ability to suppress the urgency caused by bladder instability. Bladder retraining incorporates adjunctive techniques such as triggering and emptying techniques, intermittent catheterization, and the use of a bladder record to identify a voiding schedule and adjust the amount and timing of fluid intake.

Bladder retraining is applicable to patients with a neurogenic bladder or patients who have had an

Table 15-3 Types, causes, and treatments of persistent urinary incontinence

Classification	Definition	Characteristics	Causes	Treatment options
Stress	Loss of urine with intraabdominal pressure	Small-volume urine loss Common in women Urine loss with coughing, laughing, bending, lifting, sneezing, or when standing up	Pelvic muscle relaxation secondary to decreased estrogen production, childbirth(s), trauma, surgery, and obesity Damage to urethral sphincter from surgery, radiation treatment, or trauma	Pelvic floor exercises Suspension surgery Artificial urinary sphincter Alpha-adrenergic agonist Estrogen replacement Electrical stimulation Vaginal pessary Penile clamp Biofeedback
Urge	Sudden loss of urine associated with sense of urgency to void	Large-volume urine loss Loss of urine in any position Frequency Urgency Nocturia	Detrusor instability secondary to a neurologic condition or bladder irritation, e.g., infection, cancer, foreign body Idiopathic bladder instability	Anticholinergics, antispasmodics, or antibiotics Biofeedback Behavioral training procedures Electrical stimulation Surgical removal of irritating lesion
Reflex	Sudden urine loss when the spinal cord reflex arc is completed	Large-volume urine loss May or may not sense need to void	Spinal cord injury Multiple sclerosis	Cutaneous stimulation Credé maneuver Behavioral training Bladder relaxants
Overflow	Leakage of urine from an overdistended bladder secondary to mechanical obstruction of the urinary outlet or an atrophied state of the detrusor muscle	Frequent or continuous dripping of urine Urine loss in small volumes Hesitancy or straining to void Diminished urine stream	Bladder outlet obstruction due to enlarged prostate, urethral stricture, cancer, pelvic prolapse Atonic detrusor muscle due to medications or neurologic involvement, e.g., diabetes, multiple sclerosis, or trauma	Surgery to relieve obstruction Intermittent catheterization Cholinergic Temporary use of indwelling catheter
Functional	Urinary leakage associated with inability to toilet because of cognitive impairment, physical disability, psychological unwillingness, or environmental barriers	Large-volume urine loss Normal muscle and sphincter function Voiding at inappropriate times	Impaired mental status as with dementia, head injury, depression, psychosis Physical disabilities that slow down or impair motor function, e.g., arthritis, strokes, Parkinson's disease Unfamiliar environment Environmental barriers such as restraints, distance to the toilet	Habit training Scheduled training Adaptive equipment Absorbent pads and pants Environmental manipulation

PRIMARY THEMES OF PATIENT EDUCATION

- Complications from disease process; when to call the physician and case manager
- Catheter management
- Medications: purpose, action, dosage, side effects, and methods of administration
- Urinary tract and bladder infection: recognition and treatment
- Diet: fluid intake (volume, types, scheduling); dietary measures for managing constipation
- Infection control
- Skin care
- Toileting schedules

KEGEL EXERCISES

Kegel exercises are a technique used to strengthen the pelvic floor muscles to prevent loss or leakage of urine that can occur when these muscles are weak. Here's how you do Kegel exercises:

- Sit or stand. Without tensing the muscles of your legs, buttocks, or abdomen, imagine that you are trying to control the passing of urine by squeezing the muscles of the vagina together. Hold one hand on your stomach to make sure the abdominal muscles are not moving as you slowly squeeze the sides of the vagina together.
- As you do this, the ring of muscles around the rectum will also squeeze together. This is normal.
- Practice squeezing the vagina together, counting to three as you squeeze tightly. Give one last extra squeeze on the count of four, and then relax the muscle for three counts.
- Do a series of 10 exercises 4 times per day. Count one, two, three, extra squeeze, relax. Two, two, three, extra squeeze, relax. Three, two, three, extra squeeze, relax, and so on up to a total of 10 Kegel exercises.
- Good times to practice Kegel exercises are in the morning before getting up, in the evening at bedtime, and during the day when you go to the bathroom. When you are passing urine, practice stopping the urine flow and then restarting it again.

It is important to do your Kegel exercises daily. It will take about 6 to 8 weeks of *daily* exercising before you begin to notice any results.

indwelling catheter.[19] Adequate cognitive function, mobility, and motivation are necessary for bladder retraining to be successful.

Scheduled toileting. Scheduled toileting, or prompted voiding, assists patients to void at fixed intervals, usually every 2 hours during the day and every 4 hours at night. The goals of scheduled toileting are to prevent incontinent episodes and to help the patient establish bladder control. Prompted voiding therapy has been found to decrease incontinent episodes in patients with significant cognitive and physical dysfunction.[11] Because this intervention is caregiver dependent, its potential success relies heavily on the availability and motivation of caregivers to implement the procedure. Scheduled toileting is useful for managing urge and functional incontinence.

Habit training. Habit training, as opposed to scheduled toileting, consists of a flexible toileting schedule based on the patient's pattern of incontinence. Positive reinforcement for continent behaviors is an important component of habit training. The goal of habit training is to avoid incontinent episodes while gradually increasing the voiding interval to approximate a normal voiding pattern of every 3 to 4 hours. Generally, adjustment in the timing and volume of fluid intake is necessary to achieve the desired goal. Habit training can be used to manage functional and urge incontinence but is largely caregiver dependent.

Credé maneuver. In the Credé maneuver, bladder emptying is aided by manually exerting pressure over the lower abdomen to express urine. This method can be used for patients with urinary retention secondary to a neurogenic bladder or with reflex incontinence. It should not be performed if an abdominal mass or aneurysm is present. Patients should be instructed to sit upright on the toilet and place hands flat—one on top of the other—on the abdomen just below the umbilicus. They should press down firmly toward the perineum 6 or 7 times until urine starts flowing. Once the urine stream begins, they should maintain light pressure until it stops. After relaxing for 2 minutes the maneuver should be repeated until urine can no longer be expressed.

Catheters and catheter care

Several types of catheters and catheterization procedures are used in the home setting to manage urinary incontinence. These include indwelling catheters, intermittent catheterization, and external catheters or collection devices. Indications and nursing management practices for each type of catheter or catheterization procedure are discussed in the following sections.

Indwelling catheters. Chronic indwelling catheterization for the management of bladder dysfunction should not be regarded as a routine nursing intervention. It should be limited to the following situations: (1) when urinary retention is present and cannot be corrected either surgically or medically and intermittent catheterization is traumatic or impractical, (2) when skin wounds or pressure sores are present and need to be protected from urine contamination, (3) when patients are terminally ill or debilitated and bed or clothing changes are uncomfortable or disruptive, and (4) when it is the preference of patients or caregivers after all other treatments have failed.[26]

Both short- and long-term urethral catheterization are associated with a high risk of urinary tract infection.[48,57,60] Other complications include renal and bladder stones, hydronephrosis, bladder carcinoma, epididymitis, pyelonephritis, prostatic and urethral abscesses, and urethral fistulae.[57] Trauma, discomfort, leakage of urine, and encrustation causing blockage of the catheter lumen are problems that have been identified with chronic indwelling catheters.[46,47] For these reasons, catheters should be avoided unless absolutely necessary.

Selecting the catheter. Plastic and latex catheters are recommended for short-term use of 1 to 3 weeks.[46] Urethral pain and bladder spasms are more common with the less flexible plastic catheters, and a higher incidence of encrustation has been noted with latex catheters.[57] Silicone catheters should be used for long-term purposes, since lower incidences of encrustation and catheter bypassing (i.e., leakage of urine around the catheter) have been reported with their use.[27] Currently, silver-coated, antimicrobial, and lubricous-coated catheters are being evaluated to determine their safety and efficacy.[29]

Catheter size depends on the individual, how long the catheter will be in place, and the purpose for inserting the catheter. In general, a small catheter size is recommended because large-diameter catheters have been associated with more complications.[46] The catheter should be small enough to

pass with ease through the external meatus to ensure its passage through the rest of the urethra. A 14 to 16 French catheter is recommended in most instances. Catheter lumen sizes increase by 2 French increments. Each gradation of 2 French equals 0.33 mm. Two catheter lengths are currently available: the male length (41 cm) and the shorter female length (23 cm).

Balloon size is also a factor to consider in choosing a catheter. Urinary catheters come with balloon volumes of 5, 10, or 30 ml and can be inflated with water or air. The 30-ml balloon is often used after transurethral prostatectomy to prevent hemorrhage. Smaller balloon sizes of 5 or 10 ml should be used in most cases, since they take up less space, cause less mucosal irritation, and are less often associated with bladder spasms and bypassing of urine.[46]

Inserting the catheter. Using sterile technique, home health nurses should insert indwelling catheters according to policy and procedure guidelines of their agency. Resistance may be encountered during insertion when the catheter tip reaches the internal sphincter. Pausing for a few seconds to allow the sphincter to relax may help overcome this problem. Prostatic hypertrophy and urethral strictures cause greater resistance to catheter passage. Using a smaller lumen or a coudé catheter may make insertion easier. Force should never be used to overcome resistance, since edema or urethral perforation can occur. A physician should be notified if resistance continues and gentle manipulation of the catheter fails to allow insertion. With male patients, it is important to retract the foreskin back over the head of the penis once catheterization is completed.

The patient should not experience pain when the balloon is inflated. If pain occurs, the balloon is in the urethra instead of the bladder and needs to be advanced farther.

If the bladder has been distended with urine, it will need to be emptied slowly. Hypotension or bladder hemorrhage can occur if compressed bladder vessels are allowed to dilate too rapidly. Recommendations for bladder decompression are as follows:

1. Initially, remove no more than 800 ml of urine.
2. Clamp the catheter for 15 minutes.

3. Every 15 minutes unclamp the catheter and allow it to drain 100 ml.
4. Repeat this procedure until the bladder is empty.

Maintaining the catheter and drainage system. A closed catheter system should be the standard of care for patients requiring indwelling urethral catheters. However, even with a closed system, bacteriuria will occur. It is possible to delay the onset of bacteriuria with maintenance of a closed system.

The drainage system chosen should be suited to the patient's individual needs so that, once intact, disconnection of the system is unnecessary. For example, if the patient is fairly mobile, a leg bag can be used and a special drainage system can be connected to the distal part of the leg bag at night. In this manner, the closed system does not have to be interrupted to change drainage bags. The drainage system should also have a one-way valve between the bag and the catheter tubing to prevent reflux of urine back into the bladder. The collection bag should always be kept below the level of the patient's bladder.

The catheter should never be disconnected from the collection tubing to obtain urine samples. Aspiration of urine with a sterile needle and syringe from a port on the tubing for this purpose is the appropriate mechanism for obtaining a urine specimen.

Routine catheter care. Handwashing by the nurse, patient, or family caregiver before and after handling the catheter and drainage system is essential. Periurethral care includes cleansing the perineum with soap and water each day and after each bowel movement, using care to wipe from the urethra toward the anus. Application of antiseptic agents such as Betadine to the periurethral area has not been proven effective in reducing bacteriuria.[48] The catheter should always be secured to the upper thigh to help reduce movement in and out of the urethra, which can cause inflammation.

Changing the catheter. No data are available on how frequently catheters should be changed. Recommendations for frequency of catheter changes vary from every 4 weeks to only when obstruction or malfunction occurs.[48,55] The catheter material will partly determine how often it will require

changing. Wastling[59] suggests that silicone catheters can be left in place for up to 6 months. Kniep-Hardy et al.[27] recommend that all catheters be changed every 4 weeks unless problems necessitate changing more frequently. It is accepted that foley catheters should never be reused once they are removed.

Home health nurses should always use sterile technique when changing catheters because they might introduce microorganisms to which the patient has no resistance. Caregivers who learn to change the catheter may use clean technique. It has been reported that frail, debilitated, and elderly patients develop infections whether clean or sterile technique is used and that clean technique is easier and more practical for caregivers in the home setting.[27]

Bladder irrigation. The effectiveness of routine bladder irrigation in preventing infection and obstruction remains unclear. Evidence suggests that routine bladder irrigation does not prevent infection,[4] and both open and closed bladder irrigation methods have been reported to cause urinary tract infections.[18]

In the home, bladder irrigation is usually indicated for catheter obstruction or to instill medication. Bladder instillation is similar to intermittent bladder irrigation except that the catheter is clamped after the fluid is instilled to allow the solution to remain in the bladder for a specified time period. The flow rate of the irrigant must be controlled, and the patient must be observed closely for signs of bladder retention.

Solutions commonly used for bladder irrigation are sterile normal saline or sterile 0.25% acetic acid. Normal saline is isotonic and reduces the chance of hemolysis or fluid overload that can occur with the use of sterile water. Acetic acid acidifies the urine and prevents debris formation, which can lead to encrustation around the catheter tip.

Little evidence exists to support the efficacy of catheter clamping prior to discontinuation.[20,27,38,66] To remove an indwelling catheter, deflate the balloon by attaching a syringe to the balloon lumen and aspirating the fluid. The catheter is then withdrawn slowly. If the balloon does not deflate, the physician should be contacted immediately. Caregivers should be instructed to notify the home health agency of any problems with the indwelling catheter such as leakage, a lack of urine, patient complaints of abdominal pain or tenderness, change in urine color, or fever. They should be taught how to discontinue the catheter if problems arise during the night or when the home health nurse is not available. Simple instructions regarding discontinuation of the catheter may save an unnecessary and expensive trip to the emergency department. Ideally, home health agencies should have after-hours service managers taking calls to help patients and their caregivers troubleshoot problems with foley catheters or to help them make decisions regarding questionable situations.

Treating infections. Even with the use of aseptic technique, by the end of 30 days of catheterization, 78% to 95% of patients will be bacteriuric.[57] However, the majority of patients with long-term urethral catheters and bacteriuria are asymptomatic. Routine surveillance cultures are not necessary in the chronically catheterized patient. The use of antimicrobial agents for prophylaxis or treatment of asymptomatic bacteriuria is not recommended, since this practice may lead to the development of more resistant organisms and/or drug toxicity.[40,65]

Two thirds of febrile episodes in elderly, long-term catheterized patients are related to urinary tract infections.[58] Therefore temperatures of patients with indwelling catheters should be closely monitored. Mental status changes, diaphoresis, abdominal pain, tachycardia, hypotension, nausea and vomiting, and restless or agitated behaviors are other symptoms that may indicate the presence of a urinary tract infection or bacteremia. It is important to monitor the patient's response to antibiotics and correlate the laboratory sensitivity findings with the medical treatment because many strains of bacteria in long-term catheterized patients are resistant to commonly used antimicrobial agents. If symptomatic urinary tract infections recur frequently, patients should be referred to a urologist to rule out underlying pathology.

Encrustation and obstruction. Encrustation refers to accumulation of debris around the catheter tip that blocks the drainage holes. One way of preventing obstruction from encrustation is to change the catheter more frequently. In addition, maintaining an acidic urinary pH helps reduce encrustation. This can be achieved with dietary measures. Cranberry juice and an acid-ash diet

make the urine more acidic. It is recommended that the patient drink 5 to 8 oz of cranberry juice 3 times a day and incorporate meat, whole grains, eggs, prunes, and plums in the diet.[15]

Since encrustation occurs more frequently when the urine is concentrated,[27] patients should be encouraged to maintain a fluid intake of 2,000 to 3,000 ml per day. Adequate fluid intake will ensure a steady stream of urine in the catheter tubing, reducing the possibility of catheter obstruction.

Silicone catheters should be used whenever possible because this material is less susceptible to encrustation. Milking the catheter tubing several times a day can help maintain catheter patency. If the catheter does become obstructed, catheter replacement is recommended.

Leakage. Although leakage of urine around the catheter can occur if the catheter is obstructed, it may also occur if the patient is having bladder spasms. Bladder irritability and spasms may result from a variety of causes. Urinary tract infection, constipation or fecal impaction, bladder stones, or an oversized catheter balloon are possible sources of bladder irritability.

When leakage occurs, measures should be taken to alleviate the irritating condition. If such measures fail to maintain dryness, an antispasmodic agent such as oxybutynin (Ditropan) or flavoxate (Urispas) can be used to relax the bladder muscle.

Odor. Physical cleanliness is important in controlling urine odor. Perineal care with soap and water should be carried out daily. Odor from drainage bags and appliances is caused by bacteria, and reduction of bacterial growth in drainage bags has been found to eliminate odor.[10]

Drainage systems should be changed whenever the catheter is changed. Camasso[10] recommends adding 10 ml of sterile hydrogen peroxide through the drainage porthole each time the drainage bag is emptied. This allows maintenance of a closed system and reduces odor. Kniep-Hardy et al.[27] recommend deodorizing drainage bags by filling them with a solution of 2 parts vinegar to 3 parts water and soaking for 20 minutes. Because this method does not maintain a closed system, it is best used for cleansing external collection devices and associated drainage systems.

Intermittent catheterization. Intermittent catheterization is usually implemented in the home health setting for problems associated with persistent urinary retention. The goal of intermittent catheterization is to avoid high intraluminal pressure and overdistension, which decrease blood flow to the bladder muscle and make it susceptible to bacterial invasion. Intermittent catheterization should be performed frequently enough so that the bladder is not allowed to accumulate more than 500 ml of urine.[28]

Generally, clean technique is recommended when intermittent catheterization is done at home. Clean technique has not been found to significantly increase the overall incidence of urinary tract infections, and is reported to decrease the overall incidence of urinary tract complications.[3,31,45,60] Patients and caregivers should be taught to wash their hands before the procedure. Procedural guidelines outlined by agency protocols should be followed. After the procedure, the catheter should be washed with soap and water and allowed to dry thoroughly. Catheters can be stored or carried in plastic bags. They may be reused, but should be discarded when they begin to crack or develop an odor.

Suprapubic catheterization. A suprapubic catheter is inserted percutaneously through the abdominal wall into the bladder and is sometimes used after gynecologic and urologic surgery. As with indwelling urethral catheters, infection is a primary concern. Other complications of suprapubic catheters include cellulitis, leakage, hematoma near the insertion site, and obstruction.[57] These catheters are maintained much like an indwelling urethral catheter.

External catheters. External catheters and collection systems are used to manage rather than prevent or resolve the symptoms and problems associated with bladder dysfunction. These devices should be used only on patients who have not responded to other measures to correct problems with incontinence or on patients who are extremely physically dependent.

External catheters for men consist of either a penile funnel that is held to the pubic area by waist straps or a condom that is attached to the penis with adhesive and elastic straps. Condom catheters are the most common external device for men. Although many believe external catheters are quite safe, symptomatic urinary tract infections are more prevalent among men who wear condom catheters than among those who do not.[41,43,58] Complications of condom catheters include edema, skin

breakdown, penile constriction, penile ischemia, and urethral diverticula.[34,58]

The penis should be cleansed with soap and water and allowed to dry before application of an external device. For greater comfort and adherence, it may be necessary to shave the pubic hair. The condom should fit snugly but not tightly. If tissue swelling and color change occur, the condom is too tight and should be discontinued immediately. Condoms should be removed daily or every other day to wash and evaluate the skin.[7] Every 3 to 4 days the condom should be left off to allow the skin to be exposed for 24 hours. If skin irritation occurs, the condom should be removed until the area is completely healed.

If the penis is retracted, a condom catheter will not be useful. Special pouches, similar to ostomy bags, are available that fit over the penis and attach to the pubic area. These pouches need to be sized appropriately, and the pubic area must be shaved for them to fit properly. Their disadvantage is that the penis is not protected from urine contact.

External catheters for females are commercially available, but their safety and efficacy have not been established. Problems that have been encountered with the use of female external catheters include displacement, leakage, labial pressure sores, and erosion of soft tissues of the vulva.[44]

Environmental manipulation and supportive measures

Because many environmental factors can contribute to functional urine loss, adjustments in the environment may be necessary. These adjustments consist of removing environmental barriers or adding supportive devices.

Environmental barriers to toileting include such factors as inadequate lighting, distance to the toilet, clutter, the type of clothing the individual is wearing, and physical or chemical restraints. Bathroom lighting should be adequate at all times, especially at night. Night-lights in bathrooms not only help patients identify the location of the toilet but are also an important safety measure to prevent falls. Distance to the toilet should be no more than 30 to 40 feet from the living area.[7] Making toilet access easier by moving the bed or chair closer or by providing a toilet substitute may help the patient with impaired mobility maintain dryness. Walkways to the bathroom should be kept clean and clutter-free, and throw rugs on bathroom floors should be removed. Clothing must be non-constrictive and easy to remove. If buttons or zippers are difficult for the patient to manage, elastic-waisted pants or Velcro fasteners may be substituted. In some cases, underwear and stockings may need to be eliminated to allow independent toileting. Patients should always wear supportive, nonskid shoes or slippers when going to the bathroom. Physical restraints and pharmacologic agents that alter mental status should be avoided.

Supportive devices consist of mobility-enhancing adaptive equipment and toilet substitutes. Equipment to enhance mobility includes bathroom wall rails, toilet railings, canes, walkers, wheelchairs, electric chair raisers, trapeze bars, and elevated toilet seats. Toilet substitutes consist of bedside commodes, overtoilet chairs for transporting the patient to the toilet, bedpans, and urinals.

Absorbent pads and pants. Protective undergarments and pads are designed to absorb urine and provide a moisture barrier to protect clothing, bedding, and furniture. Absorbent products are either disposable or reusable and are the most widely used aid for managing urinary incontinence.[50] A catalogue of incontinence products can be obtained from an organization called Help for Incontinent People (PO Box 544, Union, South Carolina, 29379).

It is important that diapers and other absorbent products be prescribed only after a thorough evaluation of the bladder dysfunction. When used prematurely, these products simply obscure the problem.

Medication and fluid modification. Home health nurses can help patients modify medications and fluid intake to facilitate normal bladder function. Several types of medication can aggravate incontinence. Diuretics should be taken early in the morning to prevent patients from having to void frequently during the night. If the diuretic is being given for blood pressure maintenance but is considered a significant cause of incontinence, the nurse should discuss this problem with the physician. In many cases another antihypertensive agent can be prescribed in place of the diuretic. If the patient is receiving sedatives, tranquilizers, or narcotic analgesics, the nurse should be aware of the effects of these drugs on mentation. Caregivers

will need to be alerted to the fact that patients will need assistance to the bathroom or a reminder to toilet themselves. In some cases a voiding schedule will be necessary.

Oral fluid intake should be planned in conjunction with a toileting schedule. Voiding upon awakening, after meals, once between meals, and at bedtime is a schedule that works well, since most individuals drink the bulk of their fluids with meals. A daily fluid intake of 2,000 to 3,000 ml should be consumed between breakfast and supper with fluids limited to 150 ml after the evening meal. Consumption of alcohol and beverages containing caffeine (such as coffee, tea, and colas) should be avoided.

Cranberry juice. For many years, folk wisdom has suggested that cranberry juice can be used to prevent the occurrence of urinary tract infection. A recent study found that cranberry juice reduced bacteriuria and pyuria by 50% in elderly women who drank 300 ml daily over a 6-month period.[17] It is thought that cranberry juice somehow alters adherence of bacteria to the epithelial cells lining the mucosal surface of the urinary tract. Although additional research must be conducted, it does appear that cranberry juice may be clinically useful in the prevention and management of urinary tract infections.

Bowel management. Nursing measures to restore or maintain normal bowel function include (1) dietary modification, (2) increasing fluid intake, and (3) increasing the patient's level of activity. Adequate amounts of fluid and fiber, both of which are important in preventing constipation, are often lacking in the diets of homebound individuals. Between 4 and 6 g of fiber per day are recommended to facilitate normal bowel function.[2,7]

Increasing fluid intake to between 2,000 and 3,000 ml per day in the absence of cardiovascular disease, and to approximately 1,500 ml daily if the patient has a history of congestive heart failure, will help reduce the incidence of constipation. Popsicles or ice chips are helpful alternatives to water and juices. Intravenous fluids may be necessary to prevent dehydration and bowel complications in patients with nausea and vomiting.

Increasing the level of physical activity may be a seemingly impossible task for the debilitated homebound patient. However, even extremely frail individuals can benefit from the increased motion afforded by position changes (such as sitting in a chair) and by active or passive range of motion exercises. Wheelchair confined patients may receive motivation from music or exercise tapes, which are available through local libraries or specialty organizations such as the Arthritis Foundation.

Pharmacologic treatment

Drug therapy for bladder dysfunction can be implemented alone or in conjunction with other therapeutic modalities. The pharmacologic agents used most commonly are those that improve bladder emptying, decrease bladder hyperactivity, and increase or decrease resistance of the bladder outlet.[61] These drugs are summarized in Appendix 15-1.

SUMMARY

Home health nurses frequently care for patients with bladder dysfunction, a potentially debilitating condition that adversely affects the physical, psychological, and social well-being of patients and their families. Home health nurses can have a tremendous impact on patients' efforts to improve urinary control. Through assessment, planning, and implementation of strategies to achieve continence, home health nurses can significantly enhance patients' dignity and quality of life.

REFERENCES

1. Autry D, Lauzon F, Holliday P: The voiding record an aid in decreasing incontinence, *Geriatr Nurs* 5:22-25, 1984.
2. Behm RM: A special recipe to banish constipation, *Geriatr Nurs* 6:216-217, 1985.
3. Bennett CJ, Diokno AC: Clean intermittent self catheterization in the elderly, *Urology* 24:43-45, 1984.
4. Bergener S: Justification of closed intermittent urinary catheter irrigation/instillation: a review of current research and practice, *J Adv Nurs* 12:229-234, 1987.
5. Blaivis JG: Diagnostic evaluation of incontinence in patients with neurologic disease, *J Am Geriatr Soc* 38:306-310, 1990.
6. Brink CA: Evaluation of urinary incontinence, *Top Geriatr Rehabil* 3:21-29, 1988.
7. Brink CA, Wells TJ: Environmental support for geriatric incontinence, *Clin Geriatr Med* 2:829-840, 1986.
8. Burgio KL, Burgio LD: Behavior therapies for urinary incontinence in the elderly, *Clin Geriatr Med* 2:809-827, 1986.
9. Burgio LD, Jones LT, Engel BT: Studying incontinence in an urban nursing home, *J Gerontol Nurs* 14:40-45, 1988.
10. Camasso JA: Peroxide to prevent odor in drainage bags, *Geriatr Nurs* 5:284, 1985.
11. Creason NS, Grybowski JA, Burgener S et al: Prompted voiding therapy for urinary incontinence in aged female nursing home residents, *J Adv Nurs* 14:120-126, 1989.
12. Diokno AC: The cause of urinary incontinence, *Top Geriatr Rehabil* 3:13-19, 1988.
13. Diokno AC: Diagnostic categories of urinary incontinence and the role of urodynamic testing. *J Am Geriatr Soc* 38:300-305, 1990.
14. Diokno AC, Brock BM, Brown MB, Herzog AR: Prevalence of urinary incontinence and other urological symptoms in the noninstitutionalized elderly, *J Urol* 136:1022-1025, 1986.
15. Dolan M: *Community and home health care plans,* Philadelphia, 1990, Springhouse Corp.
16. Elia G, Bergman A: Estrogen effects on the urethra: beneficial effects in women with genuine stress incontinence, *Obstet Gynecol Surv* 48: 509-517, 1993.
17. Fleet JC: New support for a folk remedy: cranberry juice reduced bacteriuria and pyuria in elderly women. *Nutr Rev* 52:168-170, 1994.
18. Gilbert V, Gobbi M: Making sense of bladder irrigation, *Nurs Times* 85:40-42, 1989.
19. Greengold BA, Ouslander JG: Bladder retraining: program for elderly patients with post-indwelling catheterization, *J Gerontol Nurs* 12:31-35, 1986.
20. Gross JC: Bladder dysfunction after stroke: it's not always inevitable, *J Gerontol Nurs* 16:20-25, 1990.
21. Henderson JS: A pubococcygeal exercise program for simple urinary stress incontinence: applicability to the female client with multiple sclerosis, *J Neurosci Nurs* 20:185-188, 1988.
22. Herzog AR, Fultz NH: Urinary incontinence in the community: prevalence, consequences, management, and beliefs, *Top Geriatr Rehabil* 3:1-12, 1988.
23. Herzog AR, Fultz NH: Prevalence and incidence of urinary incontinence in community-dwelling populations, *J Am Geriatr Soc* 38:273-281, 1990.
24. Holland NJ, Levison PW, Madonna MG: Rehabilitation research: pathophysiology and management of neurogenic bladder in multiple sclerosis, *Rehabil Nurs* 10:31-33, 1985.
25. Jakovac-Smith DA: Continence restoration in the homebound patient, *Nurs Clin North Am* 23:207-218, 1988.
26. Kane RL, Ouslander JG, Abrass IB: *Essentials of clinical geriatrics,* ed 3, New York, 1993, McGraw-Hill.
27. Kniep-Hardy MJ, Votava K, Stubbings MJ: Managing indwelling catheters in the home, *Geriatr Nurs* 5:280-285, 1985.
28. Lewis NA: Nursing management of altered patterns of elimination, *J Home Health Care Pract* 1:35-42, 1988.
29. Liedberg H, Lundeberg T, Ekman P: Refinement in the coating of urethral catheters reduces the incidence of catheter-associated bacteriuria: an experimental and clinical study, *Europ Urol* 17:236-240, 1990.
30. Matteson MA, McConnell ES: *Gerontological nursing: concepts and practice,* Philadelphia, 1988, WB Saunders.
31. Maynard FM, Diokno AC: Urinary infection and complications during clean intermittent catheterization following spinal cord injury, *J Urol* 132:943-946, 1984.

32. McCormick KA, Burgio KL: Incontinence: an update on nursing care measures, *J Gerontol Nurs* 10:16-23, 1984.

33. McCormick KA, Scheve AS, Leahy E: Nursing management of urinary incontinence in geriatric inpatients, *Nurs Clin North Am* 23:231-263, 1988.

34. Melekos M, Asbach HW: Complications from urinary condom catheters, *Urology* 27:88, 1986.

35. Mohide EA, Pringle DM, Robertson D, Chambers LW: Prevalence of urinary incontinence in patients receiving home care services, *Can Med Assoc J* 139:953-956, 1988.

36. Morishita L: Nursing evaluation and treatment of geriatric outpatients with urinary incontinence, *Nurs Clin North Am* 23:189-206, 1988.

37. Noelker L: Incontinence in elderly cared for by family, *Gerontologist* 27:194-200, 1987.

38. Oberst MT, Graham D, Galler NL et al: Catheter management programs and postoperative urinary dysfunction, *Res Nurs Health* 4:175-181, 1981.

39. Ouslander JG: Urinary incontinence in nursing homes, *J Am Geriatr Soc* 38:289-291, 1990.

40. Ouslander JG, Elhilali MM: *The diagnosis and management of urinary incontinence,* New York, 1987, Clinical Medicine Research Institute.

41. Ouslander JG, Greengold B, Chen S: External catheter use and urinary tract infections among incontinent male nursing home patients, *J Am Geriatr Soc* 35:1063-1070, 1987.

42. Ouslander JG, Leach GE, Abelson S et al: Simple versus multichannel cystometry in the evaluation of bladder function in an incontinent geriatric population, *J Urol* 140:1382-1486, 1989.

43. Ouslander JG, Leach GE, Staskin DR: Simplified tests of lower urinary tract function in the evaluation of geriatric urinary incontinence, *J Am Geriatr Soc* 37:706-714, 1989.

44. Pieper B, Cleland V, Johnson DE, O'Reilly JL: Inventing urine incontinence devices for women, *Image* 21:205-209, 1989.

45. Plunkett JM, Braren V: Five-year experience with clean intermittent catheterization in children, *Urology* 20:128-130, 1982.

46. Roe BH: Aspects of catheter care, *Geriatr Nurs Home Care,* 6:21-23, 1987.

47. Roe BH, Brocklehurst JC: Study of patients with indwelling catheters, *J Adv Nurs* 12:713-718, 1987.

48. Schaeffer AJ: Catheter-associated bacteriuria, *Urol Clin North Am* 13:735-747, 1986.

49. Sier H, Ouslander JG, Orzeck S: Urinary incontinence among geriatric patients in an acute-care hospital, *JAMA* 257:1767-1771, 1987.

50. Starer P, Libow LS: Obscuring urinary incontinence: diapering the elderly, *J Am Geriatr Soc* 33:842-846, 1985.

51. Staskin DR: Age-related physiologic and pathologic changes affecting lower urinary tract function, *Clin Geriatr Med* 2:701-710, 1986.

52. Sullivan DH, Lindsay RW: Urinary incontinence in the geriatric population of an acute care hospital, *J Am Geriatr Soc* 32:646-650, 1984.

53. Teasdale TA, Taffet GE, Luchi RJ, Adam E: Urinary incontinence in a community-residing elderly population, *J Am Geriatr Soc* 36:600-606, 1988.

54. Turner SL, Plymat KR: As women age: perspectives on urinary incontinence, *Rehabil Nurs* 13:132-135, 1988.

55. Urinary Incontinence Guideline Panel: *Urinary incontinence in adults: clinical practice guidelines;* AHCPR Pub No 92-0038, Rockville, Md, 1992, Agency for Health Policy and Research, Public Health Service, US Department of Health and Human Services.

56. Voith AM: A conceptual framework for nursing diagnosis: alterations in urinary elimination, *Rehabil Nurs* 11:18-21, 1986.

57. Warren JW: Catheters and catheter care, *Clin Geriatr Med* 2:857-871, 1986.

58. Warren JW: Urine-collection devices for use in adults with urinary incontinence, *J Am Geriatr Soc* 38:364-367, 1990.

59. Wastling G: Long-term catheterization—a survey of home care, *Nurs Times* 79:29-32, 1983.

60. Webb RJ, Lawson AL, Neal DE: Clean intermittent self-catheterization in 172 adults, *Br J Urol* 65:20-23, 1990.

61. Wein AJ: Pharmacologic treatment of incontinence, *J Am Geriatr Soc* 38:317-325, 1990.

62. Wein AJ: Physiology of micturition, *Clin Geriatr Med* 2:689-699, 1986.

63. Wells TJ: Additional treatments for urinary incontinence, *Top Geriatr Rehabil* 3:48-57, 1988.

64. Wells TJ: Pelvic (floor) muscle exercise, *J Am Geriatr Soc* 38:333-337, 1990.

65. Whippo CC, Creason NS: Bacteriuria and urinary incontinence in aged female nursing home residents, *J Adv Nurs* 14:217-225, 1989.

66. Williamson ML: Reducing post-catheterization bladder dysfunction by reconditioning, *Nurs Res* 31:28-30, 1982.

67. Wyman JF: Nursing assessment of the incontinent geriatric outpatient population, *Nurs Clin North Am* 23:169-187, 1988.

Drugs Used to Treat Urinary Incontinence

Drug	Dosage	Mechanism of action	Type of incontinence	Adverse effects
Anticholinergic and antispasmodic agents				
Oxybutynin (Ditropan)	2.5-5 mg bid or tid	Increase bladder capacity; decrease involuntary contraction	Urge incontinence with detrusor instability	Dry mouth, blurred vision, constipation, delirium, elevated intraocular pressure, postural hypotension
Flavoxate (Urispas)	100-200 mg bid or tid	Increase bladder capacity; decrease involuntary contraction	Urge incontinence with detrusor instability	Above side effects plus cardiac conduction disturbances
Alpha-adrenergic agonists				
Pseudoephedrine (Sudafed)	15-30 mg bid or tid	Increase urethral smooth muscle contraction	Stress incontinence with sphincter weakness	Elevation of blood pressure, headaches, tachycardia
Phenylpropanolamine (Ornade)	75 mg bid or tid	Increase urethral smooth muscle contraction	Stress incontinence with sphincter weakness	Headaches, tachycardia, anorexia, elevation of blood pressure
Anticholinergic/ antispasmodic agents with alpha-adrenergic properties				
Imipramine (Tofranil)	10 mg tid	Decrease involuntary bladder contractions and increase urethral smooth muscle contraction	For mixed stress and urge incontinence	Postural hypotension, dry mouth, constipation, dizziness, blurred vision

*Cholinergics rarely used because efficacy controversial and side effect potential high.

Continued

Drug	Dosage	Mechanism of action	Type of incontinence	Adverse effects
Conjugated estrogens				
Premarin (oral)	0.625 mg qd	Strengthen periurethral tissues	Stress incontinence; urge incontinence associated with atrophic vaginitis	Elevation of blood pressure, breast tenderness, endometrial hyperplasia
Topical	0.5-1 g q hs			
Cholinergic agonists *				
Bethanechol (Urecholine)	10-30 mg tid	Stimulate bladder contraction	Overflow incontinence with atonic bladder	Bradycardia, hypotension, bronchoconstriction, dyspepsia
Alpha-adrenergic antagonists				
Terazosin (Hytrin)	1 mg qd up to 10 mg QD	Relax smooth muscle in bladder neck and prostate	Overflow incontinence associated with prostate enlargement	Postural hypotension, headaches, dizziness, syncope, tachycardia, palpitations
Doxazosin (Cardura)	Between 1 to 10 mg qd	Same as above	Same as above	Dizziness, headache, fatigue, tachycardia, edema
5-Alpha reductase inhibitor				
Finasteride (Proscar)	5 mg qd	Inhibits prostatic hyperplasia	Overflow incontinence associated with prostatic enlargement	Rash, breast tenderness, impotence

16 The Patient Receiving Rehabilitation Services

Robyn Rice and *Laurie Rappl*

Rehabilitation is an important and increasingly used service of the home health care industry. The availability of rehabilitation services has increased greatly over the past decade.[6] Rehabilitation as described in this chapter is a restorative process to help ill, physically impaired, or handicapped persons regain their maximum physical, mental, and vocational usefulness following disease or injury.[3,5,7]

The specific rehabilitation professionals referred to include physical therapists, occupational therapists, and speech language pathologists. Effective rehabilitation for patients with impaired mobility is an educational process involving the coordinated efforts of patients, caregivers, physicians, home health nurses, and various health specialists. The ultimate goal for patients with impaired mobility is to maximize their independence and daily functioning within their home environment.

As the average life expectancy for Americans increases, so does the incidence of illness, disease, and physical disability, resulting in an increased need for rehabilitation. In addition, since the onset of the prospective payment system, patients are being discharged from hospitals much sooner than in the past. When first seen at home, patients are frequently in the acute phase of their disease process or injury and often have received only initial instructions and an abbreviated version of the rehabilitation program.

Patients are frequently treated at home because of insurance coverage limitations for inpatient stay or a lack of available beds for admission into a rehabilitation unit or facility. Skills learned in a rehabilitation center may not apply to the patient's home setting, or may not be carried over by the patient into the home very easily. Oftentimes, a few visits by the

rehabilitation professional will accelerate the patient's ability to adapt skills to the home setting.

As is the case with any service related to home health care, financial coverage for rehabilitation services is provided by private, state, and federal government insurance programs. Patients receiving home care rehabilitation under their hospitalization Medicare benefit (Medicare Part A) must be homebound; that is, they must need the assistance of another person or device to leave their home.[4] This is not the case when receiving services billed under the supplemental medical insurance (Medicare Part B). Payment under Medicare Part B reimburses at a rate of 80% whereas reimbursement of 100% is provided under Medicare Part A.[4]

To receive the Medicare home care benefit, a patient must have a signed order from a physician for treatments and services to be rendered.[4] Rehabilitation treatments must require the skills of a professional physical therapist, occupational therapist, or speech and language pathologist.[4] The patient must have the expectation of improved physical mobility, or at least have a reasonable rehabilitation potential.[4] The exception to this requirement is for home visits to instruct and educate a caregiver regarding transfer and positioning techniques, range of motion exercises, and establishment of a home exercise program for patients with chronic disabilities or patients with no apparent rehabilitation potential.[4] Medicare will not, however, reimburse for maintenance therapy.[4]

INDICATIONS FOR REHABILITATION SERVICES

Nurses new to home care may experience difficulty in determining the appropriateness and need for rehabilitation services. This difficulty is largely due to a lack of working experience with patients who could benefit from physical, occupational, or speech therapy, and unfamiliarity with each discipline's area of expertise. Case management strategies for home health nurses would be to learn principles of rehabilitation therapy and build a collaborative practice with the home care team.

To ensure patients' maximal recovery or restoration of function, or to prevent further dysfunction, a multidisciplinary approach is essential. Open and ongoing communication among the nurse, the physician, and all rehabilitation professionals regarding the establishment of goals and the plan of care will result in an overall improvement in the quality of care. Likewise coordination of patient care with the home health aide and/or social services may be needed.

When establishing a plan of care for any patient, it is important that home health nurses take a holistic approach to assessing needs related to the patient's illness, injury, or disease process. These include, but are not limited to, physical, emotional, social, and economic needs.[3] The home health nurse will assume an important role in helping patients adjust to and accept alterations in body image secondary to disease or illness by addressing loss, anxiety, and depression.[2]

When home health nurses assess patients to determine the appropriateness of rehabilitation services, it is important that they assess patients' overall mobility levels and functional status. Asking seated patients if they have difficulty ambulating is frequently inconclusive. It is important to have patients demonstrate their abilities, rather than focusing on their subjective complaints of disability. By observing patients' abilities or assisting them to ambulate, home health nurses can quickly assess many areas of physical functioning and thus are able to determine the need for other services. For example, difficulty understanding or following commands may be indicative of speech or cognitive deficits. Prior to ambulating, patients must come to a standing position. When they are doing so, home health nurses can assess such things as balance and coordination deficits, the ability or inability to move forward and rise from a seated position, and the paralysis or dysfunction of any extremity. Patients may have an unawareness of body parts or a lack of perception or spatial orientation, making these tasks nearly impossible. Observing patients ambulate will help to determine their gait ability and possibly the need for additional equipment or gait devices. At this point, home health nurses can also identify those patients at risk for falls.

During the initial visit, the home health nurse should note if the patient has specific difficulties, such as maneuvering around the kitchen for meal preparation or cleanup, or using the bathroom facilities safely. Any details in these areas will assist the rehabilitation professional in determining if a referral is appropriate, and which discipline should be involved.

Equally important in determining the need for rehabilitation services is a knowledge and understanding of the patient's prior functional status. It is unlikely that patients with chronic disabilities who have not ambulated in several years will be appropriate candidates to receive physical therapy for gait training. It is also beneficial to investigate whether patients have previously received physical, occupational, or speech therapy for the same or similar conditions or problems and the degree of patient or caregiver compliance. It is also important to recognize that patients occasionally are not accepting of their disability or dysfunction and are therefore not amenable to receiving therapy services.

The majority of patients referred for rehabilitation services generally have a diagnosis that implies impairment of the neuromuscular and/or musculoskeletal systems. The box on p. 273 lists common conditions and diagnoses that may assist home health nurses to make appropriate referrals for specific rehabilitation services. Conditions and diagnoses must be acute or represent a recent exacerbation of a chronic disease. Patients who suffer from several of the conditions and diagnoses listed in the box may have multiple deficits and thus need services from any or all of the three rehabilitation disciplines (physical, occupational, or speech therapy).

Frequently, patients may appear to need skilled therapy because of weakness or impaired mobility. However, before making an interdisciplinary referral, home health nurses must consider the available reimbursement sources. Payment for rehabilitation services for patients experiencing weakness or immobility from prolonged hospitalization secondary to medical complications may be denied by Medicare. Fiscal intermediaries often view this as a weakness or temporary loss of function that will improve spontaneously and does not warrant the intervention of a skilled therapist. When assessing patients' needs for additional services, it is important that home health nurses not concentrate solely on the medical diagnosis, because the therapist treats loss of function and *not the specific disease or illness.*

COMMON CONDITIONS AND DIAGNOSES APPROPRIATE FOR HOME HEALTH REHABILITATION REFERRALS[4]

1. Patients who have sustained fractures or dislocations
2. Patients who have undergone orthopedic surgeries, including joint replacements or reconstructive surgeries
3. Patients suffering from degenerative joint or disc disease
4. Patients suffering from rheumatoid arthritis
5. Patients who have undergone amputations or require prosthetic training
6. Patients who have sustained burns with joint involvement or have physical impairment with an associated decrease in function
7. Patients who have suffered cerebral vascular accidents
8. Patients who have suffered head injuries or spinal cord injuries
9. Patients with multiple sclerosis
10. Patients with amyotrophic lateral sclerosis
11. Patients with Parkinson's disease
12. Patients with a decrease in function as a result of neuropathies and/or myopathies
13. Patients with chronic obstructive pulmonary disease who require postular drainage and teaching
14. Patients with cardiac impairment requiring cardiac rehabilitation
15. Patients with severe immobility as a result of any disease process requiring instruction to the caregiver in hoyer lift transfers or any assistive device
16. Patients suffering from newly diagnosed blindness
17. Patients with head/neck cancer resulting in partial or total laryngectomies or glossectomies
18. Patients whose underlying disease process, illness, or injury has resulted in dysphagia
19. Patients suffering from a hearing loss

Chapter 3 describes clinical indicators for a rehabilitation referral. In all phases of health care, as well as in the exploding home care arena, there is a severe shortage of qualified speech, occupational, and physical therapists. Often the home health nurse will have to fill the needs of the patient in the absence of a qualified therapist. Community resources may include the home medical supply dealer, representatives from manufacturers, and literature from journals. If a therapist is available, a consultation on an evaluation with instruction may be all that is necessary to maximally benefit the patient.

HOME CARE APPLICATION

Home health nurses can serve as an important link in the restoration of patients' function or in the prevention of further dysfunction. Their ability to assist patients with transfers, gait training, or range of motion exercise programs established by the rehabilitation professional hastens the recovery process. Spiritual and emotional support will also be needed by patients and their caregivers in adjusting to and accepting changes in body image resulting from disease and disability. (See the boxes titled Primary Nursing Diagnoses/Patient Problems and Primary Themes of Patient Education.)

Of note, when faced with the patient's many needs, caregivers may experience role strain and require respite services. Signs of caregiver role strain are discussed in Chapter 6. The home health aide and social worker may be of assistance in helping patients and their caregivers adjust and adapt to physical disability.

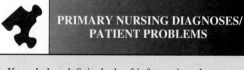

PRIMARY NURSING DIAGNOSES/ PATIENT PROBLEMS

- Knowledge deficit: lack of information about condition and care
- Activity intolerance: _____ Ambulation, _____ ADLs, _____ Other*(Specify)*
- Self-care deficit: ADLs, _____ Feeding, _____ Toileting, _____ Other *(Specify)*
- Body image disturbance
- Impaired physical mobility
- Risk for trauma
- Risk for caregiver role strain

PRIMARY THEMES OF PATIENT EDUCATION

- Disease process: when to call the case manager or physician
- When to call 911
- Medications: purpose, action, dosage, side effects, and methods of administration
- Body mechanics regarding lifting and transfers
- Gait training and strength endurance
- Range of motion exercises
- Operation and function of mobility aids (walkers, canes, crutches, or wheelchairs)
- Operation and function of home medical equipment and assistive devices (hospital beds, hoyer lifts, sliding boards, bedside commodes, bathtub seats, tub transfer benches, button hooks, dressing sticks, communication aids)
- ADL self-care management
- Home environmental safety
- Positive coping mechanisms to improve body image adaptation
- Socioeconomic resources
- Available community services for people experiencing stroke or problems with immobility
- Caregiver respite services

This section is primarily designed to provide home health nurses with a basic knowledge of techniques pertinent to rehabilitation. Working with patients experiencing loss and depression is discussed in Chapter 23. Many of the following techniques (such as body mechanics for moving and lifting, transfer training, gait training, and range of motion exercises) and assistive devices may be incorporated in the nursing care plan. Proper seating techniques are extremely important in order to prevent skin breakdown. (See Appendix 16-1, Seating Tips for the Chairbound Patient.)

Body mechanics/transfer training

An awareness and understanding of good body mechanics is essential for home health nurses to prevent injury to themselves and patients. By applying the principles of body mechanics when lifting or moving patients, home health nurses take advantage of the body parts best suited to lifting: the legs.[8] When moving or lifting a patient, it is important to maintain balance with the feet spread slightly apart to increase the base of support. The nurse's back should be kept in alignment, with the spine staying as erect as possible. When reaching over a patient in bed, it is beneficial to advance one foot forward and under the bed if possible, to allow the trunk to remain reasonably erect. Stooping or bending at the waist should be avoided. To prevent strain on the back muscles, it is important to squat, bending the hips and knees while keeping the back straight and in proper alignment. When returning to the standing position, the muscles in the legs should be allowed to do the actual lifting. Movements should be smooth and steady, never jerky or sudden. Turning while lifting should be accomplished by moving the feet rather than by twisting the trunk or waist.

When transferring the patient from a bed to a chair, it is important to place the bed at a moderate and comfortable height if possible. Place the chair parallel or at a slight angle to the bed, closest to the patient's uninvolved side if possible. Instruct the patient to assist with whatever movements he or she is capable of doing safely. Assist the patient to a sitting position on the edge of the bed; the patient's feet should be flat on the floor. If possible, have the patient push up with the hands on the bed while the nurse or therapist grasps around the waist or gait belt. Assist the patient to a standing position by straightening the patient's hips and knees. Block the patient's knees when paralysis or weakness exists.[8] Either turn slowly, sidestep, or pivot the patient one quarter turn until the backs of the legs rest against the chair. Have the patient reach for the arm of the chair, if able, to achieve a sitting position. This method of stand-pivot transfer is generally used with patients who can offer some assistance or who do not need transfers with the use of mechanical devices, such as hoyer lifts or sliding boards.

Range of motion exercises

The prevention of joint contractures and adhesions and the maintenance of joint mobility are essential aspects of any patient's care. These goals are accomplished through joint range of motion exercises, which can be performed by home health nurses and patients following instructions in basic range of motion techniques (Table 16-1 and Figure 16-1). Range of motion can be described in four ways:

Table 16-1 Range of motion exercises

Body part	Type of joint	Type of movement	Body part	Type of joint	Type of movement
Neck and cervical spine	Pivotal	Flexion: bring chin to rest on chest Extension: return head to erect position Hyperextension: bend head back as far as possible Lateral flexion: tilt head as far as possible toward each shoulder Rotation: turn head as far as possible to right and left			Internal rotation: with elbow flexed, rotate shoulder by moving arm until thumb is turned inward and toward back External rotation: with elbow flexed, move arm, until thumb is upward and lateral to head Circumduction: move arm in full circle. Circumduction is combination of all movements of ball-and-socket joint
Shoulder	Ball-and-socket	Flexion: raise arm from side position forward to position above head Extension: return arm to position at side of the body Hyperextension: move arm behind body, keeping elbow straight	Elbow	Hinge	Flexion: bend elbow so that lower arm moves toward its shoulder joint and hand is level with shoulder Extension: straighten elbow by lowering hand Hyperextension: bend lower arm back as far as possible
		Abduction: raise arm to side position above head with palm away from head Adduction: lower arm sideways and across body as far as possible	Forearm	Pivotal	Supination: turn lower arm and hand so that palm is up Pronation: turn lower arm so that palm is down
			Wrist	Condyloid	Flexion: move palm toward inner aspect of the forearm Extension: move fingers so that fingers, hands and forearm are in same plane

Continued

Table 16-1 Range of motion exercises—cont'd

Body part	Type of joint	Type of movement	Body part	Type of joint	Type of movement
		Hyperextension: bring dorsal surface of hand back as far as possible Lateral flexion: tilt head as far as possible toward each shoulder Rotation: turn head as far as possible to right and left	Hip	Ball-and-socket	Flexion: move leg forward and up Extension: move leg back beside other leg
Fingers	Condyloid hinge	Flexion: make fist Extension: straighten fingers Hyperextension: bend fingers back as far as possible			Hyperextension: move leg behind body
		Abduction: spread fingers apart Adduction: bring fingers together			Abduction: move leg laterally away from body Adduction: move leg back toward medial position and beyond if possible
Thumb	Saddle	Flexion: move thumb across palmar surface of hand Extension: move thumb straight away from hand Abduction: extend thumb laterally (usually done when placing fingers in abduction and adduction) Adduction: move thumb back toward hand Opposition: touch thumb to each finger of same hand			Internal rotation: turn foot and leg toward other leg External rotation: turn foot and leg away from other leg

Table 16-1 Range of motion exercises—cont'd

Body part	Type of joint	Type of movement	Body part	Type of joint	Type of movement
		Circumduction: move leg in circle			Inversion: turn sole of foot medially Eversion: turn sole of foot laterally
Knee	Hinge	Flexion: bring heel back toward back of thigh Extension: return heel to floor	Toes	Condyloid	Flexion: bring heel back toward back of thigh Extension: return heel to floor
					Abduction: spread toes apart Adduction: bring toes together
Ankle	Hinge	Dorsal flexion: move foot so that toes are pointed upward Plantar flexion: move foot so that toes are pointed downward			

Passive range of motion. This is range of motion in which patients offer no assistance. The movements are performed completely by another person.

Active-assistive range of motion. This is range of motion in which patients assist with the movements but still require assistance from another person.

Active range of motion. This is range of motion in which the patients perform all movements unassisted.

Resistive range of motion. This is range of motion in which movements are performed with weights or against physical resistance.

Caregiver education regarding range of motion exercises is important and should be done on an ongoing basis. This is especially true for patients who are bedridden, who are susceptible to skin breakdown, or who have an abnormality in muscle tone.

Gait training and mobility aids

Patients' abilities to function within the home are largely controlled by their gait ability or ability to manage a wheelchair. Gait safety is a primary concern with all patients. Older patients often have impaired vision, mild balance disturbances, or decreased sensation. Patients' lack of knowledge of safety measures frequently contributes to falls and further injury. All efforts should be taken to ensure maximal safety at home. Home health nurses can assist with this by reinforcing safety precautions

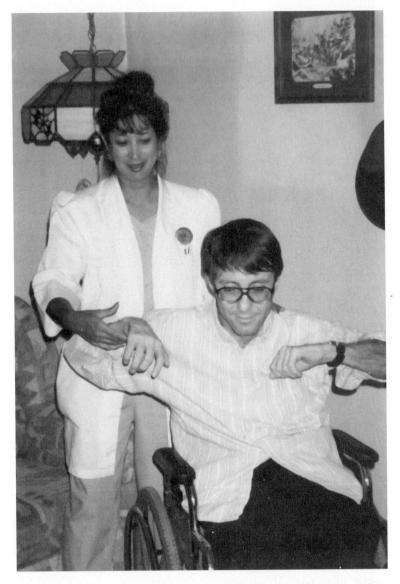

Figure 16-1 Home health nurse assisting with range of motion exercises. (Photo courtesy Home Health Department, Gila Regional Medical Center, Silver City, NM.)

and noting environmental hazards or barriers. Re-arranging furniture allows for ease of maneuverability. Removing throw rugs, telephone wires, and electric cords will contribute to increased safety within the home.

Frequently, patients live alone or with an elderly spouse or caregiver and are fearful of ambulating

in the absence of the nurse or physical therapist. Home health nurses can hasten the recovery process by assisting patients with their established gait programs. Patients may require standby assistance, verbal cueing, or gait devices when ambulating. There are numerous gait devices or mobility aids available. These include standard walkers, wheeled walkers, reciprocating walkers, hemi-walkers, standard canes, quad canes, standard crutches, and loft strand crutches.[1]

Walkers are generally used for patients who have lower extremity weight-bearing restrictions and whose balance or strength does not warrant the use of crutches. Walkers are used more often with the elderly, whereas crutches are commonly used with the younger population. Canes are frequently used for patients who have mild weakness or balance disturbances or for patients who have unilateral upper extremity limitation or absence of function and are unable to use devices requiring the use of both upper extremities. Wheelchairs may be the only means of locomotion throughout the house for some patients. Wheelchairs can be customized and adapted to the specific needs and requirements of each patient. Wheelchairs vary, ranging from standard wheelchairs to reclining wheelchairs, hemi-wheelchairs with one-arm drive, and electric wheelchairs. A variety of accessories and options are available.

Home medical equipment and assistive devices

Home medical equipment and assistive devices serve as an adjunct in the rehabilitation process for many patients. Hospital beds, overhead trapeze bars, and bed rails are used to assist patients' bed mobility and safety. Hoyer lifts and sliding boards ease the transferring of patients with impaired mobility. Raised toilet seats, toilet safety rails, bedside commodes, bathtub seats, tub transfer benches, tub safety rails, and grab bars all promote increased independence in performing such ADLs as toileting and bathing. Some of these items are shown in Appendix 16-2.

Self-help assistive devices used to facilitate independence with dressing, grooming, feeding, and cooking include long-handled reachers, sponges or shoe horns, stocking aids, button hooks, and dressing sticks. Universal cuffs are beneficial for patients who have a loss of motion or strength and need help holding objects when performing basic self-care activities. Built-up handles may be needed on eating and cooking utensils used by patients with diminished hand function or decreased coordination.

Patients with impaired communication or phonation may require augmentative communication devices, cassette talking tapes, or an electrolarynx.

With instruction and careful selection of the proper equipment and/or assistive device, patients have the potential to increase their independence and functional ability within the home. With knowledge of available equipment, home health nurses will have less difficulty in determining the need for physical therapy, occupational therapy, or speech pathology intervention.

SUMMARY

Through the collective efforts of home health nurses, rehabilitation professionals, and all involved caregivers, achieving the primary goal for any patient is possible. For patients requiring home health rehabilitation, that goal is to restore the maximum attainable level of functioning and independence. Likewise, by facilitating and understanding the grieving process, health caregivers can address the loss, anxiety, and depression that this group of patients may experience. Patients are encouraged to emphasize and utilize their assets, to become involved in activities of daily living, and to take pride in themselves and in the mastery of their accomplishments.[2]

With proper care and patient education, disabilities can be prevented from becoming handicaps. Consequently, team commitment and a knowledge of the care being delivered from each health professional is essential for the effective treatment of all patients receiving home rehabilitation services.

REFERENCES

1. Barnes MR, Crutchfield C: *The patient at home: a manual of exercise programs, self-help devices and home care procedures,* rev ed, Thorofare, NJ, 1984, Slack.
2. Drench M: Changes in body image secondary to disease and injury, *Rehabil Nurs* 19(1):31-35, 1994.
3. Guzelaydin SK: Treading the path of interdisciplinary boundaries: a community health care approach to rehabilitation services in the home, *J Home Health Care Pract* 4(4):24-30, 1992.
4. Health Care Financing Administration: *Health Insurance Manual,* Pub No 11 -Thru T273, Rev 3/95, Washington, DC, 1995, US Department of Health and Human Services.
5. Kauffman DD: Physical therapy interaction in the home, *Caring* 11(8):16-19, 1992.
6. Martinson IM, Widmer A: *Home health care nursing,* Philadelphia, 1989, WB Saunders.
7. Topp R, Mikesky A, Bawel K: Developing a strength training program for older adults: planning, programming, and potential outcomes, *Rehabil Nurs* 19(5):266-274, 1994.
8. William M, Worthingham C: *Therapeutic exercise for body alignment and function,* Philadelphia, 1957, WB Saunders.

Appendix 16-1

Seating Tips for the Chairbound Patient

The home care patient probably spends a majority of waking hours sitting up in some kind of chair: a wheelchair, a recliner, a couch, or a sofa. While assessing the patient and developing the plan of care, the home health nurse must address the position the patient is supported in when sitting. Proper positioning can reduce contracture formation and skeletal deformities, protect the skin from pressure ulcers, enhance internal organ functioning, improve patient comfort, and put the patient in as functional a position as possible to enhance independence in daily activities. It is healthy to sit correctly.

Standard living room furniture typically is made for generic comfort, and is not structured enough to provide positioning support for patients experiencing weakness, paralysis, or contractures. It will be easier to support patients in a more upright chair such as a wheelchair. Many patients have a tendency to sit in a slouched position with their hips placed forward on the seat, back curved, knees lower than the hips, and feet unsupported. Therefore in assisting patients to maintain an upright, neutral body position, the nurse must address patient seat, back, foot, and leg supports.

Seat. Begin by assessing the patient's sitting position by looking at the patient from the side. The keystone in proper positioning is pelvic control. The seat cushion should help hold the hips back on the seat as close to the backrest as the patient's body structure will allow. Securing the pelvis in this position will help the patient sit upright. This prevents a slouched position which is damaging to the patient's skin and uncomfortable over time. Use a cushion that cradles the ischials and blocks them from sliding forward on the seat.

Back. Back support must be addressed both for comfort, and to help keep the pelvis in a neutral position. If the back is allowed to slouch, the hips will tend to push forward away from the backrest, and the pelvic control gained by the seat cushion will be lost. Wheelchairs typically have a sling-type upholstery that encourages a slouched back position. Living room furniture occasionally provides back support. The home health nurse must ensure that the patient's back and lumbar (lower back) curves are supported as upright as the body allows. There is a wide variety of back cushions on the market, from small lumbar pillows to larger pieces that extend from the seat to the shoulders. Consult with the home medical supplier regarding cushion selection. The goal is to use the most economical piece that helps the patient maintain the most upright position the body structure will allow.

Feet. The patient's feet must be supported so that the weight of the legs does not drag the person forward out of position. Be sure that enough foot support is provided so that the knees and hips are on the same level; that is, the thigh is parallel to the floor. This can be accomplished in a wheelchair by raising the footrests, or in the living room by providing a stool of the proper height.

Legs. Now examine the patient from the front. The thighs should be aligned so that they are pointing straight ahead rather than rolling together or falling away from each other. Thigh supports may be needed to keep them properly aligned. Also, trunk support may be needed to help keep the patient from leaning heavily to one side.

Side and front assessment. Assess the patient from the side and front as follows:

1. Assess from the side
   a. Keep the pelvis as close to the backrest as possible by providing a seat cushion that keeps the ischials from sliding forward.
   b. Prevent a slouched back posture, and a pelvis that rolls backward by providing back support to maintain the natural lumbar curve.
   c. Bring the patient's knees to the same level as the hips by providing foot support.
2. Assess from the front
   a. Maintain the thighs in a flat, straight ahead position by providing support between or alongside the thighs if needed.
   b. Prevent leaning of the trunk to the side by providing side supports.

(Review Chapter 13 for recommendations for seating with skin breakdown.)

Appendix 16-2

Adaptive Equipment Commonly Used in the Home

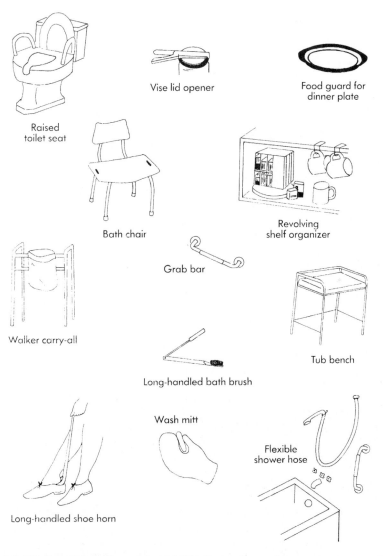

Raised toilet seat

Vise lid opener

Food guard for dinner plate

Bath chair

Revolving shelf organizer

Walker carry-all

Grab bar

Long-handled bath brush

Tub bench

Long-handled shoe horn

Wash mitt

Flexible shower hose

From Bronstein KS, Popovich J, Stewart-Amidei CM: *Promoting stroke recovery: a research based approach for nurses,* St Louis, 1991, Mosby.

17 The Patient Receiving Home Infusion Therapy

Lori B. Watkins and Robyn Rice

Home infusion therapy is no longer new to the home care industry. The first home intravenous (IV) therapy programs appeared with the advent of the prospective payment system in the 1970s.[1,11,15] In 1980 the home infusion industry consisted of a small, relatively underutilized service; by 1992 the total market was estimated to exceed $3 billion and growing.[15] Growth in the home infusion industry is influenced by several factors:[4,5,11]

Patient population. Patients discharged to the home now are often sicker than those who required home care in the past. As patient acuity levels rise, home health services such as home infusion therapies will expand to meet complex health care needs. Patients in home care now include cardiac, prenatal, and perinatal patients, as well as patients with infectious disease, all of whom require aggressive treatment.

Technology. Advances in technology have contributed to the safety and feasibility of home infusion therapy. Portable infusion pumps developed over the past 15 years are safer, more accurate, and easier to use. Patients no longer have to manipulate bulky and heavy equipment in their homes. A variety of flexible silicone catheters with longer dwell times have replaced large steel needles, improving the reliability and safety of home infusion therapy. For example, the refinement of the central venous catheter has made the infusion of vesicants and high-dextrose fluids safe in the home setting.

Cost. Home IV therapy costs substantially less than in-hospital therapy. Cost reductions of $2,370 to $3,665 per patient, per illness, have made home IV therapy an attractive option to both payers and patients.[1] The demand for cost-effective health care will continue to fuel a steady growth in the home infusion market.

Consumer awareness. As educated consumers, patients are taking a more active role in meeting their own health care needs. Many patients prefer to be treated at home, where they feel more in control of their body and the circumstances leading to recovery. In the fast-paced world of work, many people are reluctant to spend time away from careers and other obligations. Often, providing high-technology services at home allows patients and their families to participate in the recovery process with less disruption in their lifestyles.

Issues such as staffing, safety, patient education, availability of supplies, and clinical expertise to execute IV therapy services must be considered when implementing home infusion therapy. Home infusion therapy is *nursing-intensive* because coordination provided by trained nurses is vital to safely administer these therapies outside of the acute care setting. Services and products used include nursing care and pharmacy services, drugs, nutrients and solutions, supplies and specialized medical equipment, administration and support services, and quality improvement activities.[15]

The most common infusion therapies administered in the patient's home include antibiotic therapy, pain therapy, chemotherapy, parenteral nutrition, and enteral nutrition.[15] Home blood transfusion and other therapies described in this chapter are becoming more common. The purpose of this chapter is to present an overview of principles of home infusion management in order to prepare home health nurses to meet the complex needs of this patient population.

ADMINISTRATIVE ISSUES
Reimbursement

One of the key administrative issues in providing home infusion services is ensuring adequate reimbursement for services and supplies. Payment for home IV therapy services varies and should be researched thoroughly with each patient admission. Although services for IV therapy are covered, with the revocation of the Medicare Catastrophic Coverage Act of 1988, there is limited reimbursement for specific IV drugs under the Medicare program. Parenteral nutrition and a selected number of other drugs have coverage under Medicare Part B *if* they meet the appropriate clinical diagnosis and certain criteria requirements. Part B also provides limited reimbursement for supplies used in conjunction with skilled nursing visits and therapies as long as Medicare guidelines are met.[2,8] Medicaid, a state-administered health care plan, has requirements that vary from state to state.

Referrals and quality care

Once the patient population and potential needs are assessed, policies regarding admission and referrals should be developed by clinical and administrative managers. Most licensing bodies require procedures outlining specific patient admission criteria.

As part of quality control, trained personnel (usually nurses) should screen referrals for eligibility and appropriateness. Examples of criteria to be assessed for potential home infusion therapy include the patient's general health status as it relates to the appropriateness of home infusion therapy, patient and caretaker willingness and ability to assist with care, accessibility and licensure of the physician, and adequacy and safety of the home environment (including the availability of water, electricity, and telephone service).

It may be possible to correct any deficit(s) before providing home care services. However, referral sources should be informed of admission criteria to avoid confusion and inappropriate referrals.

Agency policies and procedures should be developed in accordance with local guidelines and standards of care. (See Chapter 9.) For instance, infusion therapy protocols can be developed from the national standards published by organizations such as the Intravenous Nurses Society (INS), the Oncology Nursing Society (ONS), and the American Society of Parenteral and Enteral Nutrition

(ASPEN). In addition, local hospitals and physicians may have specific requirements relating to home care that further ensure the delivery of quality patient care. For example, accreditation agencies, such as Joint Commission, now require the pharmacist to have a care plan for home IV therapy patients.[8] From a legal/ethical point of view, home health agency policy should provide field staff with clear guidelines to access top level agency administration if problems arise in the field (for example, inadequate response from on-call supervisory staff, or field staff requiring guidance in decision making for problematic situations).

The physician

The role of the physician should be clarified with staff when providing home infusion. Physicians, traditionally surgeons or gastroenterologists, have been solicited for their referrals by home infusion companies that provide parenteral nutrition therapy services. Recently, internal medicine specialists have proved to be a sound referral source. Once the referral is made, the physician acts as the medical case manager by ordering the plan of care and serving as consultant to the pharmacist and home health nurses.[2,12]

The home infusion department should also have a designated medical director to review the appropriateness of administering certain medications in the home. Many times the medical director will simply request clarification from the patient's physician as to how the infusion will be monitored (for example, therapeutic blood levels).

The nurse manager and staffing concerns

The role of the clinical nurse manager is one of coordinator and support person for patients and staff. Nurse managers need to be aware of the staff necessary to provide high-technology services. Nursing visits can range from 45 minutes for a follow-up visit to 4 hours for a blood transfusion. Taking into account the geographic size of the service area and the type of IV therapy to be provided, the nurse manager calculates the number of full-time equivalent (FTE) staff necessary. Many states and licensing bodies require that agencies provide 24-hour access to nursing care. Meeting such requirements may mean on-call services of a nurse and/or manager and the potential for visits after hours. Although 24-hour staffing may not be feasible or necessary, it should be noted that late discharges, total parenteral nutrition (TPN) setups, and instruction of caregivers most often occur after 5:00 PM. Early morning visits may be necessary for TPN disconnects, blood draws, and emergency IV restarts.

One staffing model used is coverage from 7:00 AM to 7:00 PM, using 8-hour staggered shifts. A 4-day workweek may make the unattractive shifts more acceptable.[3] A nursing supervisor should be on site as long as there are staff members in the field.

The issue of staff safety is of concern. The agency should have provisions to protect staff members making evening or night visits. Contracting with security services, "buddying-up" for visits in potentially dangerous areas, and providing adequate emergency communication systems (car phones, beepers, calling cards) are suggestions. Though some of these mechanisms can add to the cost per visit, they can be well worth their price in terms of staff satisfaction and safety.

The quality of the home health agency can be measured by the quality of its personnel. Another role of the nurse manager is to coordinate continuing education opportunities for the staff. A monthly scheduled in-service program to enhance clinical expertise may include such topics as infection control, new chemotherapeutic modalities, nutritional assessment, and stress management. Often professionals from local agencies are willing to provide such information.

HOME CARE APPLICATION

There are numerous reasons for the initiation of home infusion therapy. It is used to replace fluids and correct electrolyte imbalances in dehydrated patients; to replace fluids and electrolytes lost as a result of vomiting, diarrhea, suctioning, wound drainage, or blood loss; to provide caloric value for the malnourished or for those who cannot eat; and to administer IV medications such as antibiotics, chemotherapy, or blood products. Routes of administration most commonly used in home infusion therapy include the following:[15]

- Intravenous—into a vein
- Intramuscular—into the muscle
- Subcutaneous—under the skin
- Epidural—into the space just outside the dura, a membrane surrounding the spinal cord and brain

- Intrathecal—into the subarachnoid space that immediately surrounds the spinal cord
- Intraperitoneal—into the free space of the abdominal cavity
- Enteral—into the digestive system

Overview of intravenous fluids

Several different IV fluids are used in home care. Complications from these IV fluids may occur, and the home health nurse should be aware of their signs and symptoms.

The most commonly used IV fluid is **dextrose in water** (D_5W). D_5W is available in many concentrations and contains no sodium, potassium, or chloride. It is used for hydration, as a vehicle for administration of IV drugs, as a caloric source (when used in concentrations greater than 10%), and as a treatment for hypernatremia.[7,9] Possible complications from dextrose solutions include hyperglycemia with diabetic patients. A greater than 10% dextrose solution should always be infused through a central venous catheter because peripheral administration may cause thrombophlebitis.[9,14] Dehydration can occur through osmotic diuresis when dextrose is infused at a rate that exceeds the body's ability to metabolize the solution. (Glucose builds up in the blood stream and has a diuretic effect.) Prolonged infusions of dextrose can result in an imbalance of water in the extracellular fluid, thereby causing water intoxication. Hypokalemia can result from prolonged therapy with an electrolyte-free fluid.[10]

Normal saline (NS) is an isotonic solution that contains no calories. NS is used for treatment of sodium depletion, for extracellular fluid replacement, and as a vehicle for administration of blood transfusions.[7,9] Home health nurses should be aware that NS infusions may cause hypernatremia, acidosis, or circulatory overload.

Dextrose in sodium chloride solution (D_5NS) provides calories and sodium chloride, corrects moderate fluid loss, and promotes diuresis in dehydrated patients.[7,9]

Lactated Ringer's solution (LR) is an isotonic multiple electrolyte solution. LR is given to treat electrolyte imbalances and to replace fluid loss caused by vomiting, gastric suctioning, drainage, burns, or diarrhea.[7,9] Pulmonary edema or congestive heart failure can result from the sodium excess of LR.[7,9]

Peripheral and central line management

When initiating peripheral IV therapy, consider the size of the vein and the viscosity of the solution. Select the smallest gauge needle or catheter needed for the infusion. Upon selecting a site, consider the location and condition of the vein (Figure 17-1). Know the purpose of the infusion and the duration of the therapy. It is beneficial to know whether patients have previously received IV therapy and their tolerance to it.

Occasionally a patient may have poor peripheral venous access due to numerous IVs while hospitalized and therefore is not a candidate for long-term IV therapy. The administration of subcutaneous fluid or hypodermoclysis may serve as an alternate method of hydrating these patients.

A central venous catheter (CVC) is required for patients with a variety of medical conditions, including cancer and bowel disease. A CVC is generally a long silicone rubber catheter approximately 1/8 inch in diameter with a cuff to secure it in place once inserted. These catheters are used for long-term venous access and spare the patient repeated venipunctures. Common CVC catheters used in home care are subclavian catheters (e.g., Hohn catheter or Deseret triple lumen catheters), tunneled catheters (e.g., Hickman-Broviac catheters or Groshong catheters), implantable vascular access devices (IVAD) (e.g., Port-a-Cath), and peripheral venous access systems (e.g., PAS port or PICC line).[12]

The insertion of a CVC requires a minor operation, but the procedure should cause little discomfort. The patient is given a local anesthetic, and two small incisions are made: one directly above the collarbone and the second to the side of one of the breasts. After the incisions are made, the proximal end of the CVC is inserted into the superior vena cava leading into the heart's right atrium. The distal end of the CVC is placed beneath the skin and exited through the second incision. A cuff attached to the CVC, which lies beneath the skin inside the vein, prevents the catheter from migrating during daily activities or while being used.[4] The CVC may or may not be sutured at the exit site. The CVC is ready for use immediately after insertion. The patient may feel some discomfort at the incision sites for several days. (For recommended flushing of the CVC, see Appendix 17-1.)

Groshong catheter. The Groshong catheter has a patented 3-position valve near the closed tip, which opens outward during infusion and inward during blood withdrawal. The valve closes automatically when not in use because venous blood pressure is not great enough to spontaneously open the valve inward. If, for example, the catheter accidentally becomes disconnected from the infusion, the valve will automatically close and prevent air embolus.[9,12] This also prevents blood from backing up into the lumen and clotting the catheter. Because of this special valve, hepariniza-

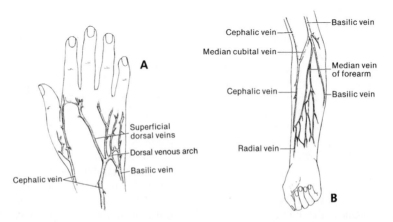

Figure 17-1 Venous anatomy. (From Perry AG, Potter PA: *Clinical nursing skills and techniques,* ed 3, St Louis, 1994, Mosby.)

tion and clamping of the Groshong are unnecessary. (For irrigation instructions, see Appendix 17-1.)

Implantable vascular access device. The subcutaneous or implantable vascular access device (IVAD) is also used for the delivery of medications, blood products, and nutritional fluids directly into the bloodstream. The terms *subcutaneous* and *implantable* refer to the fact that the device is placed in the subcutaneous layer beneath the patient's skin. The device, commonly referred to as a port, is visible as a raised area beneath the skin. Daily care is not required, and thus there is less disruption of the patient's normal activities.

The ports are made from special medical-grade materials designed for safe, long-term use in the body. The ports are small disks about 1 1/2 inches in diameter with a raised center or septum. The septum is made from a self-sealing rubber material. Ports may have a single or double septum. In the double-septum ports there is no communicating flow of fluid between ports. The noncoring needle is inserted into the septum for delivery of IV fluids. The IV fluid is carried from the port into the bloodstream through a small, flexible catheter. The port also provides a simple means for collecting blood samples.

The ports are inserted during a minor surgical operation that is usually performed with a local anesthetic. The physician places the port just beneath the skin and inserts the proximal end of the catheter into the vein selected for administration of the IV fluids. The port is frequently placed in the upper chest just below the collarbone, a position convenient for patient treatment.

Once the port is placed, it is ready for use. During the first few days after the insertion of the port, it is important for the patient to avoid heavy exertion. When the incision has healed, the patient may resume normal activities.

The port can be used in two ways. One method, referred to as a bolus injection, delivers the medication or IV fluid all at once with the special needle being left in place for only a short time. In the other method, referred to as continuous infusion, a sterile transparent dressing is placed over the needle and port to secure the needle. Extension tubing is attached to the needle with an injection cap on the distal end of the tubing. If the patient is receiving a continuous infusion or long-term daily IV therapy, the noncoring needle is changed once a week. A blood return should be confirmed each time the port is accessed or before an infusion is started. (For flushing procedure, see Appendix 17-1.)

PICC line. Current trends for venous access in the home setting favor a peripherally inserted central catheter, commonly referred to as a PICC line. A PICC line provides a peripherally inserted catheter into the median cephalic basilic, median cubital, or cephalic vein. It is used for venous access for intermediate-term (7 days) or longer (6 to 8 weeks) infusion therapies.[12] Final placement is in the upper arm (axillary vein) or the central venous corridor (subclavian vein or superior vena cava). Placement in the central venous corridor requires placement verified by a portable x-ray.

Only registered nurses certified in the insertion technique should place PICC lines.[2] Approval for insertion must be obtained from the physician, who indicates catheter dwell time and placement. PICC lines may be used for antibiotic, pain, hydration, and other selected therapies.[2,12]

Mechanical phlebitis may occur within 24 to 72 hours after insertion. Treatment involves application of moist heat 4 times a day and elevation of the arm. If phlebitis persists, consult the physician about possible removal of the PICC line. If catheter sepsis is suspected, the PICC line must be removed. Only a physician or a trained nurse may remove a PICC line.

Hemostats (or any clamp with teeth or sharp edges) should not be used on the PICC line. Blood pressure cuffs or tourniquets should not be placed on the arm where the line is inserted, and blood specimens should not routinely be obtained via a PICC line.

When providing central venous catheter or PICC line care, it is important to have a repair kit available in the home and/or establish at the time of admission which local emergency room can handle the repair of the line if necessary. These lines will crack and leak and can be repaired.

Dressing changes and catheter care. An IV gauze dressing should be changed at least 3 times a week. A transparent or occlusive IV dressing, commonly used with CVCs, should be changed 1 to 2 times a week.[7,12] Primary IV tubing should be changed every 48 hours in order to prevent infection.[12] Secondary tubing should be changed daily.[7,12] The IV catheter should be secured to the patient's arm or chest as appropriate and never allowed to hang loose. CVC injection caps should be changed once a week, or every 3 to 4 days if the CVC is used frequently.[7,12] In response to the OSHA bloodborne pathogen standard, many home health agencies have switched to needleless IV systems. (The reader is referred to individual manufacturer's guidelines for use and maintenance of needleless IV systems.) If used, needles inserted through the injection cap should be 1 inch or less in length. Injection caps should be changed weekly by the nurse.[7,12] Exit site IV catheter care includes cleansing the site with alcohol and Betadine.[7,12] Crusted drainage at the catheter exit site may be cleaned with hydrogen peroxide.

Other access methods for IV management used in home care

Continuous subcutaneous rather than intravenous infusion of narcotic therapy may be used for pain management. However, better results in pain management may be achieved using the intravenous route.

The **epidural** or **intrathecal space** may be also used for pain management. A minor surgical procedure is necessary to insert the catheter into the selected site. The catheter is then tunneled under the skin, where it is either connected to a subcutaneous implanted port or to an ambulatory infusion pump.[15]

Enteral access is used to administer nutrient solutions into the gastrointestinal tract. A gastrostomy tube is commonly used for long-term enteral therapy. A pump is recommended to ensure accurate flow rates.

Infusion device and pump management

The gravity drip system is the simplest system for home infusion therapy. The solution is hung on a pole above the patient, and the solution follows the forces of gravity. The rate of flow is typically managed by an in-line clamp that is adjusted to control a given rate of drops per minute as counted in the drip chamber. Because of an inherent inaccuracy and lack of alarm system to warn of blockage, this is not the ideal system for certain home infusion patients.[15]

Disposable elastomeric devices are pressurized pumps that consist of an elastic sphere containing

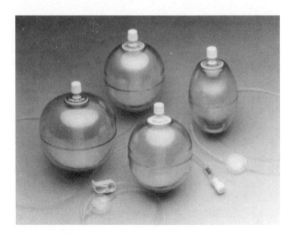

Figure 17-2 Elastomeric membrane pumps. (Courtesy Block Medical, Carlsbad, Calif.)

a small balloon, filled with the drug by the pharmacist (Figure 17-2). Once activated, the elastomeric membrane contracts, forcing the drug into the catheter and patient. The flow rate is usually accurate and the pump is easy to use. The primary disadvantage of this system is that because each dose requires a new device, it may not be cost-effective in the long run.

Many patients sent home from the hospital require IV antibiotic therapy, IV nutrition therapy, or IV pain control or cardiovascular medications. These can be administered through ambulatory infusion pumps, which are small, lightweight, and function on battery power, thus enabling the patient to move about freely. The pumps can be worn in a pouch carried over the shoulder or hooked to a belt. Attached to the pump is a reservoir that holds the necessary medication. The reservoir is usually connected to extension tubing, which is attached to a needle or catheter.[11]

Infusion pumps work in a variety of ways, depending on the patient's needs. The pumps deliver a constant rate of medication. Certain pumps are designed to deliver medication only when the patient activates a dose/rate button (for example, patient-controlled analgesia or PCA pump).

Complications of IV therapy

IV therapy is not without complications. A hematoma may develop at the insertion site, resulting in tenderness or bruising. It may be impossible to advance or flush the catheter. The vein may infiltrate or the needle or catheter may puncture through the vein wall at the time of insertion. When complications occur, nursing actions include removing the IV device, applying pressure and warm soaks to the affected area, and documenting assessment and interventions.[6,12] If resistance is met on venipuncture, do not try to advance the needle farther.

Infiltration of the IV occurs when the catheter becomes dislodged from or perforates the vein. The presenting symptoms of an infiltration are swelling and tenderness above the IV site, which may extend along the entire limb. There may be decreased skin temperature around the site. The backflow of blood may be absent, the flow rate may become slower or stop, or fluid may continue to infuse into tissue even if the vein is occluded. For infiltration of vesicant drugs, follow an established extravasation protocol, and document assessment and interventions. Infiltrations can be prevented by frequent assessment of the IV site, securing the IV site with an occlusive clear dressing or armboard, and not constricting the limb above the site with tape.

Phlebitis may occur when hypertonic or viscous medications and solutions are administered. Repeated use of the same vein, movement of the catheter in the vein, and use of a catheter too large or a flow rate too rapid for the size of the selected vein may also cause phlebitis.

Thrombophlebitis may occur if there is clotting at the tip of the catheter. The area proximal to the insertion site will become red, tender, and warm; the vein will be hard when palpated. There will be a decrease in IV flow rate, and the patient will experience increased pain or discomfort with the infusion. Prevention of phlebitis includes use of large or central veins for hypertonic solution, use of the smallest IV catheter to accommodate viscosity of fluid and size of vein, and regular IV site rotation every 3 days or as needed.

IV therapy can also produce site infection. Its presenting symptoms are redness, tenderness, swelling, and warmth at the insertion site, with a possible purulent exudate. Site infection may result from failure to maintain aseptic technique during insertion or site care. Site infection can also be caused by insertion of an IV catheter for longer than 3 days or by immunosuppression. The IV catheter should be removed if site infection is present. The home health nurse should obtain a culture of the catheter tip, notify the physician for follow-up, restart the IV at a different site, and document nursing assessment and interventions.[7,12] Site infections can be prevented by using aseptic technique during IV starts, dressing changes, and initiation of medications or solutions. Peripheral IV sites should be rotated at least every 3 days.[7,9,12]

Clotting of an IV site is another complication of IV therapy. It is likely to occur when the IV rate is too slow to maintain patency of the catheter or when a heparin lock solution is not routinely used to flush the catheter. The site may be clotted when the IV catheter does not flush easily, the IV flow rate is sluggish, or there is tenderness at the IV site. An attempt should be made to withdraw the clot with a syringe to clear the IV catheter.[7,12] If the clot cannot be withdrawn, the catheter should be removed and the IV restarted at another site.

As approved by the physician and per agency policy, heparinized saline or urokinase (a fibrinolytic agent) may be used to dissolve a clot which has formed in a CVC.[12] The fibrinolytic agent should be injected into the catheter and the catheter clamped. The home health nurse should wait for 10 minutes, unclamp the catheter and aspirate the clot. The procedure should be repeated with a 20-minute dwell time if the catheter remains clotted.[7,12] Then, the catheter should be irrigated with normal saline. Documentation should include the assessment and interventions. Flushing of the IV catheter routinely with a heparin lock solution and saline solution or maintaining a constant IV flow rate should prevent clotting of an IV site. Home health nurses should be aware that patient position may prevent CVC irrigation and blood sampling. Changing intrathoracic pressure may move the catheter tip away from the wall. This can be accomplished by having the patient breathe deeply or change positions such as turning to one side, lying flat, raising or lowering the arms, or by performing the Valsalva maneuver.[7,16]

Serious systemic complications of IV therapy include air embolism and circulatory overload. An air embolism may be caused by an empty solution container, IV tubing that has run dry or has not been properly purged or primed of air, or a disconnected IV.[7,16] Symptoms may include respiratory distress, a weak and thready pulse, hypotension, loss of consciousness, and diminished or absent breath sounds.

In the event of an air embolism, the IV infusion must be discontinued immediately. The patient should be turned onto the left side with the head down to allow the air to enter the right atrium and disperse through the pulmonary artery.[10] Oxygen should be administered, if available, and emergency services called as soon as possible. The physician should be immediately notified. Nursing assessment and interventions should be documented on the visit report. Prevention of an air embolism includes purging or priming the tubing of all air before initiating the infusion and securing all connections with tape.

Circulatory overload, another potential complication of IV therapy, is the result of miscalculation of the patient's fluid requirements or a "runaway" IV caused by a loosened roller clamp. The patients symptoms will include generalized discomfort, neck vein engorgement, hypertension, fluid-filled lungs, shortness of breath, and a fluid intake greater than fluid output. Nursing actions include decreasing the flow rate or stopping the infusion, elevating the patient's head, notifying the physician, and administering medications and oxygen as ordered. Document assessment and interventions. The patient may need to be seen by the physician for complications with infusion therapy.

Types of home infusion therapy

Antibiotic therapy. It is recommended that a CVC or PICC line be used for antibiotic therapy lasting longer than 3 weeks.[2] When possible, the patient should receive the initial intravenous dose of the antibiotic in a controlled environment (hospital, clinic, emergency department, or physician's office) to monitor for allergic or anaphylactic reactions. Intravenous home antibiotic therapy is usually administered 1 to 4 times a day depending on the drug and patient-specific factors such as disease severity.[15]

Most often gravity is used to infuse antibiotics. Many antibiotics are administered via pressurized devices that permit continuous infusion over 60 minutes. A pump is recommended for aminoglycoside or vancomycin infusions and for patients with fluid overload problems. IV tubing and needles

should be changed with each dose. Peripheral IV sites are rotated every 3 days or as needed.

Patients with diseases involving hepatic, renal, hematopoietic, cardiac, and pulmonary systems must be carefully evaluated for complications of infusion therapy. High doses of penicillin-related drugs can cause seizures and other central nervous system changes. Aminoglycosides and vancomycin require assessment for nephrotoxicity and ototoxicity. Any patient receiving long-term antibiotic therapy, especially an immunosuppressed patient, should be assessed frequently for signs and symptoms of superinfection with resistant organisms. In addition, home health nurses should be aware of appropriate laboratory tests when monitoring antibiotic administration. These tests are outlined in Table 17-1.

Chemotherapy. Qualified nursing personnel may administer oral, intramuscular, or subcutaneous chemotherapeutic agents. Approved chemotherapy for home administration should be listed according to agency policies and procedures and administered under the guidance of the medical director. It is recommended that only chemotherapy-certified nurses carry out home administration of intravenous push (IVP) or infusions of chemotherapeutic agents. Pregnant and lactating women are advised not to administer IV push chemotherapeutic agents.[11] IV push chemotherapeutic agents must be administered through the stopcock of a running IV. They should not be administered into the line containing solution with additives.

Patients should receive the first dose of chemotherapy in the hospital or physician's office.[2] It is recommended that intravenous infusions be administered only via central venous access devices, such as an implanted port or long-term tunneled silicone catheter.[11]

Extravasation kits should be available and must be taken to the patient's home along with written procedures for treating extravasation of vesicant chemotherapeutic agents. Chemotherapy spill kits should be provided by the home health agency for use in patients' homes in the event of a spill or leakage of the hazardous drug.

Before administering chemotherapeutic agents, home health nurses must be aware of certain baseline information.[2,11] In addition to a record of the patient's vital signs, they should know the

Table 17-1 Drug classification and suggested laboratory tests

Drug classification	Suggested test and frequency
Aminoglycosides	
Gentamicin	CBC, SMA6, peak and trough twice weekly
Amikacin	Audiogram if therapy greater than 2 weeks
Tobramycin	
Miscellaneous	
Vancomycin	CBC, SMA6, peak and trough weekly
Clindamycin	Audiogram weekly if therapy greater than 2 weeks
Beta-lactam cephalosporins	
Ancef	CBC, SMA6, SGOT weekly
Ceftriaxone	
Ceftazidime	
Penicillins	
Ampicillin	CBC, SMA6, SGOT weekly
Pen G	
Pen V	
Antifungals	
Amphotericin B	CBC, SMA6, Mg twice weekly,
Fluconazole	Fluids CBC, SMA6, SMA12 weekly
Sulfonamides	
Bactrim	CBC, SMA6 weekly
Antivirals	
Ganciclovir	CBC, SMA6 twice weekly
Acyclovir	
Foscavir	CBC, SMA6, Ca, Mg, Po_4 twice weekly fluids
Quinolones	
Ciprofloxacin	CBC, SMA6, SMA12 weekly
Colony stimulating factors	
GCSF (granulocyte colony stimulating factor)	CBC weekly
GMCSF (granulocyte macrophage colony stimulating factor)	
Erythropoietin	
Blood products	
Packed red blood cells	CBC, platelets before and after transfusion
Platelets	
Gammaglobulin	
Antineoplastics	
Refer to each antineoplastic drug to determine relevant clinical monitoring/observations.	CBC, SMA6, Ca, Mg before therapy

Continued

Table 17-1 Drug classification and suggested laboratory tests—cont'd

Drug classification	Suggested test and frequency
Diuretics	
Lasix	SMA6 weekly
	weight each SNV
Sympathomimetics	
Dobutamine	SMA6 and Mg weekly
	weight each SNV
Anticoagulants	
Heparin	CBC, protime weekly
Hydration	SMA6, Mg weekly
	weight each SNV

results of a complete blood count (including platelet) performed within 1 week of chemotherapy administration. (If white blood cells are >3,500 and/or the platelet count is <100,000, the patient's physician should be consulted.)

Home health nurses administering IV push chemotherapeutic agents must wear disposable protective gowns and sized sterile gloves during the procedure. When bubbles are removed from syringes or IV tubing, a sterile alcohol wipe should be placed carefully over the tip of the needle, syringe, or tubing in order to collect any of the drug that may be discharged. In case of skin contact with an antineoplastic drug product, the affected area should be washed thoroughly with soap and water. If the drug gets into the eyes, they should be flushed immediately with a copious amount of water.

Chemotherapeutic agents should be prepared for administration at a bathroom or kitchen counter on a plastic-backed field (a disposable diaper works well).[2,11,12] The area should be washed thoroughly before and after preparation with soap and water or 70% alcohol and allowed to dry. The work space should be free of food or other items that could become contaminated. Home health nurses should not mix chemotherapeutic agents. All chemotherapeutic agents should be prepared by a pharmacy. Any defective syringe or bag containing chemotherapy should be sent back to a pharmacy for safe disposal.

Home health personnel and caregivers should be cautioned to avoid skin contact with excreta of individuals treated with antineoplastic agents. Hands should be washed thoroughly and gloves worn when disposing of excreta. Institutional guidelines for the treatment of hazardous waste must be followed in disposing of excess portions of the agent or contaminated equipment:[2,11]

- Unused portions should not be disposed of down the drain or the toilet. (Contents should be left in the container and placed in a plastic "zipper" bag lined with paper towels.)
- Contaminated needles, IV bags, and syringes are disposed of intact to prevent aerosolization contamination. (These items should be placed in a container with a label specified for chemotherapy waste disposal.)

Pain management. Narcotics can be used for effective pain management to alleviate severe pain, decrease anxiety, and maximize the patient's best level of functioning. Cancer, neurologic, orthopedic, or certain AIDS-related diseases are conditions that may require pain management in the home.

Narcotics can be administered intravenously, intermuscularly, subcutaneously, intrathecally, or epidurally when the patient is no longer responsive to oral or rectal drug administration. Frequency and dosage of administration should depend on the patient's response to the medication.

Narcotics commonly infused in home care include morphine, hydromorphone, levorphanol, and methodone.[15] PCA pumps are often appropriate for use with narcotics.

Hemotransfusions. Blood transfusions are most frequently given to restore blood volume and blood components lost as a result of surgery, hemorrhage, or disease. Hemotransfusions maintain and promote the oxygen-carrying capacity of blood by supplying red cells, and supplement the coagulation properties of platelets. Red blood cells and blood components may be administered in the home by a qualified registered nurse in accordance with the standards of the American Association of Blood Banks.

A physician's order must be written for transfusion of blood or blood components. The order should state the type and amount of blood or component, the duration of the infusion, the date of the transfusion, and pretransfusion and post-transfusion blood work. The physician should be available for consultation by telephone throughout the time of blood or blood component administration in case complications arise. The following boxes list hemotransfusion criteria.

Informed consent must be obtained from patients receiving hemotransfusions prior to initiation of therapy. The physician is responsible for initial instructions related to the nature and purpose of the agent to be administered, the risks involved, and the alternatives available for treating the patient's condition. Home health nurses are responsible for reinforcing the physician's instructions, explaining the procedure to the patient, reviewing signs and symptoms of potential transfusion reactions (both immediate and delayed), and obtaining signatures on the consent form. (Blood for typing and crossmatching must be drawn and delivered to the blood bank 24 to 48 hours before the transfusion.)

Nurses administering hemotransfusion must bring an emergency drug kit to the home and keep it readily available during the entire length of the visit. Suggested contents of the drug kit are listed in the box on p. 294. For a patient with a history of allergic reaction, the physician may order premedication with an antihistamine prior to hemotransfusion and/or administration of a leukocyte-poor preparation. (The blood bank must be informed of leukocyte-poor needs at the time the request for blood is made.)

A patent IV must be established; 18 gauge or larger is ideal. The signs and symptoms of infusion reaction to observe for include chilling, fever, dyspnea, cyanosis, hives, headache, muscle ache, sharp pain in the lumbar area, a nonproductive cough, itching, vomiting, swelling, pain at the infusion site, dark urine, chest pain, flushing, shock, hypothermia or hyperthermia, hypotension, hypertension, and tachycardia. Reactions may occur immediately or 24 to 48 hours, 1 to 6 weeks (delayed hemolytic), or 1 to 6 months later (hepatitis, other viral infections).

Blood and blood components should not be piggybacked. Two successive units may be admin-

---

MEDICAL DIAGNOSES APPROPRIATE FOR IN-HOME TRANSFUSION[2]

1. Chronic gastrointestinal bleeding
2. Anemia in the presence of chronic renal disease
3. Anemia with bone marrow failure/transplant
4. Anemia associated with malignancy
5. Sickle cell anemia
6. Undiagnosed symptomatic anemia
7. Hemophilia
8. Thrombocytopenia due to bone marrow failure/transplant

REFERRAL CRITERIA FOR IN-HOME TRANSFUSIONS

The patient must:
1. Reside within the local community
2. Have physical limitations that render the patient homebound
3. Be alert, cooperative and able to respond to instructions
4. Have a medical condition that allows for safe transfusion therapy at home
5. Have available a responsible adult in the home during the procedure to witness verification checks and be available to call for help
6. Have adequate peripheral/central venous access as determined by a home health IV care nurse
7. Have a hemoglobin level of less than 10 g/100 ml (for red blood cell recipients)

EMERGENCY DRUG KIT CONTENTS

- One IV tubing (macrobore)
- 500 ml of 0.9% sodium chloride
- Two prefilled syringes of diphenhydramine hydrochloride, 25 mg each
- One 3-ml syringe with 25-gauge 5/8-inch needle
- One ampule of epinephrine, 1:10,000 (.1 mg/ml)
- Two ampules of epinephrine, 1:1,000 (1 mg/ml)
- Two 3-ml luer-lock syringes
- Two filter needles
- Two 23-gauge 1-inch needles
- Two 20-gauge 1-inch needles
- Povidone-iodine wipes
- Alcohol wipes
- One adult oral airway
- Index card for each allergic reaction procedure
- Two EDTA tubes
- One urine specimen cup
- One laboratory requisition
- Three labels

---

istered through one transfusion set by flushing with NS after each unit. An *exception* is a sepacell filter (for leukocyte-reduced blood), which may only be used for one unit. Infusion length is determined by the physician order and the patient's condition in accordance with the standards of the American Association of Blood Banks and the home health agency's policies.[2] One unit of packed red cells is usually transfused over 1 1/2 hours with a maximum time of 4 hours. A longer infusion time of 2 to 4 hours per unit is considered for the following:

- Infants
- Adults over age 60
- Patients with chronic anemia
- Patients with cardiopulmonary disease
- Debilitated patients
- Patients with a prior history of transfusion reaction

Enteral nutrition therapy. Enteral nutrition involves tube feeding into the patient's stomach or intestine. Such therapy is used for patients who are unable or unwilling to swallow or who can not otherwise ingest food or fluids by mouth, yet who have normally functioning lower gastrointestinal tract functions.[15]

Nasogastric tubes are preferred for short-term use whereas gastrostomy tubes are preferred for long-term use. Refer to manufacturer recommendations and agency policy for nasogastric and gastrostomy tube management. Complications may arise if the formula is not administered properly and may include aspiration, diarrhea, bloating, pneumonia, and possibly death.[12,15]

Routine monitoring for therapeutic effectiveness is also a part of enteral nutrition therapy. It is of extreme importance to instruct caregivers to sit the patient up at a minimum 45-degree angle during and for one hour after feedings to prevent aspiration.[12]

Total parenteral nutrition. TPN provides nutrition when the alimentary route cannot or should not be used (for example, for patients with malnutrition resulting from Crohn's disease, short-bowel syndrome, cancer, ulcerative colitis, and AIDS-related malnutrition).[15]

TPN fluids must be prepared in a pharmacy, and glucose concentrations greater than 10% should not be given peripherally.[10] Because of the high electrolyte and glucose concentrations and volumes used, the rate should not be increased or decreased dramatically because this can result in electrolyte imbalance, hyperglycemia, hypoglycemia, or fluid overload. An infusion pump is always used to ensure constant flow rates.

Administration of TPN requires a written physician order, which specifies the frequency of checks of vital signs and blood glucose. For patients with impaired renal function, serum chemistry panels are obtained and recorded weekly or as ordered. These are listed in Table 17-2.

The TPN solution must be refrigerated in the patient's home. The patient or caregiver must be instructed to remove the solution from the refrigerator to allow it to reach room temperature before infusion. Rapid infusion of a cold solution can cause shaking chills and lead to ventricular arrhythmias.[6] A 1.2-micron filter for lipid-containing TPN fluids is recommended, and strict aseptic tubing standards must be met. Needle changes are done every 24 hours.[2]

Blood samples should not be taken from the TPN line. An alternate intravenous route should be used for IV push medications and for intravenous piggybacks (IVPBs).

Other therapy. The following may also be administered in the home setting: hydration therapy,

Table 17-2 Serum chemistry and hematology panels[12]

Test	Normal adult range
Chemistry screens	
Serum sodium	136-145 mEq/L
Serum chloride	97-108 mEq/L
Plasma potassium	3.5-5.5 mEq/L
Serum creatinine	0.7-1.5 mg/dl
Serum urea nitrogen (BUN)	4-22 mg/dl
Serum uric acid	2.2-9.0 mg/dl
Serum total protein	6.0-8.2 g/dl
Serum albumin	3.5-5 g/dl
Serum total bilirubin	0.1-1.2 mg/dl
Serum cholesterol	150-270 mg/dl
Serum alkaline phosphatase	19-74 IU/L
Serum oxalic transaminase (SGOT)	0-41 IU/L
Serum glutamic lactic dehydrogenase (LDH)	60-220 IU/L
Serum calcium	9-10.5 mg/dl
Serum phosphorus	2.3-4.3 mg/dl
Serum carbon dioxide	23-30 mEq/L
Hematology screens	
Red blood cell	4,000,000-5,300,000/mm³
Hemoglobin	Male- 13-17 g/dl
	Female- 12-15 g/dl
Hematocrit	Male- 39%-51%
	Female- 36%-45%
White blood cells	4,000-10,000/mm³
Sedimentation rate	1-20 mm/hr
Platelet count	250,000-500,000/mm³

dobutamine or other inotropic agents to improve cardiac contractility for patients with severe congestive heart disease, tocolytic therapy (administration of terbutaline for the treatment of premature uterine contractions in high risk pregnancies), chelation (or iron overload) therapy for patients suffering from chronic iron overload conditions such as thalassemia, and growth hormone therapy. In addition, infusion therapies may include aerosolized pentamidine (or other medication by inhalation), hemodialysis, and hormonal treatments.

Stringent agency policies regarding admission, monitoring, and implementation of these therapies are highly recommended in order to ensure safe and efficacious patient care.

Developing the plan of care and patient education

Home infusion therapy patients typically are discharged from the hospital at higher acuity levels than the average home care patient. (See the box titled Primary Nursing Diagnoses/Patient Problems.) The delivery of services and supplies must be coordinated to ensure a safe transition from the hospital to the home.[15] As with any high-tech procedure in the home, feasibility of the service must be determined before admission. As described in the beginning of this chapter, the home milieu must be able to support IV therapy equipment and related services.

Although home infusion therapy is a very technical service, patient/caregiver requirements for self-care management are derived from a holistic needs assessment as described in Chapter 4. It should be emphasized that patient/caregiver education and active involvement is an essential component of successful home infusion therapy.

A major focus of service is to enable patients or caregivers to manage long-term home infusion safely with minimal intervention by home health nurses. Therefore the patient/caregiver *must* be able to demonstrate administration techniques, express a willingness to comply with techniques, understand the signs and symptoms of therapy complications, and be able to identify appropriate

PRIMARY NURSING DIAGNOSES/ PATIENT PROBLEMS

- Knowledge deficit; lack of information about home IV therapy and risk complications, medications, operation of home medical equipment, procedural care, diet, activity, socioeconomic resources, available community services, etc.
- Altered nutrition; less than body requirements
- Pain
- Risk for infection
- Activity intolerance:__Ambulation, __ADLs, __ Other *(Specify)*
- Self-care deficit:__ADLs, __Feeding,__Toileting, __ Other *(Specify)*

Table 17-3 Troubleshooting IV therapy in the home: Patient/caregiver education[2,5,6,7,11]

Complication	Action
Infusion slows or stops	Observe for swelling, pain, or hardness around needle/catheter site. If any of these are noted, stop the infusion and immediately notify the home health nurse and/or physician. If the above signs and symptoms are not present: 1. Check for twisted tubing or pressure on tubing. 2. See if the patient has moved or bent his or her arm. If so, return arm to original position. 3. If the flow rate remains slow or stopped, turn regulator off and contact the home health nurse.
Circulatory overload Occurs when patient has received too much fluid. Symptoms: Coughing, shortness of breath Increased respirations Headache, facial flushing Rapid pulse rate Dizziness	Stop the infusion and immediately call the home health nurse and/or physician. Call an ambulance directly if the situation is an emergency.
Air embolism Air gets into the blood stream. Symptoms: Extreme shortness of breath Anxiety Lips and nailbeds turn blue Rapid pulse rate Loss of consciousness	This is a medical *emergency.* Turn patient on left side with head down. *Immediately* call an ambulance. Stay with the patient.
Pyrogenic reaction May occur with exposure to contaminated equipment or solutions. Symptoms: Abrupt temperature, chills Complaints of backache, headache Nausea and vomiting Flushed face Dizziness	Discontinue IV therapy. Call home health nurse/notify physician. Stay with the patient until arrival of the home health nurse. (If symptoms are severe, take the patient to an emergency department.) Save the equipment/IV solution for laboratory analysis.
Severed catheter	Clamp the line and notify the home health nurse/physician.

Additional information can be obtained from the Family Service and Visiting Nurse Association, Alton, Ill.

**PRIMARY THEMES
OF PATIENT EDUCATION**

- Complications of IV therapy or disease process; recognition, treatment, when to call the case manager and physician
- When to call 911
- Medications: purpose, action, dosage, side effects, and methods of administration
- Administration and management of IV therapy
- Operation and maintenance of equipment
- Infection control
- Socioeconomic resources

interventions. (See the box titled Primary Themes of Patient Education.)

Patients and caregivers are taught how to initiate or discontinue the IV therapy, how to flush the catheter, and how to prepare IV fluids for administration. In addition, patients and caregivers are generally taught maintenance and operation of infusion pumps. This includes changing the battery, starting and stopping the pump, and responding appropriately to alarm signals. Finally, patients and caregivers must be taught how to deal with complications of IV therapy. Table 17-3 provides patient education guidelines for troubleshooting IV therapy in the home. In order to meet established outcomes of care, the plan of care is developed to reflect nursing assessments, actions, multidisciplinary collaboration, and ongoing monitoring and evaluation that includes physician and patient/caregiver involvement.[13]

SUMMARY

Medications previously administered in the hospital setting such as amphotericin B, dobutamine, heparin, Igg-globulin, ganciclovir, and pentamidine now are being administered in the home. As a result, home infusion therapy is possible only in conjunction with standards of nursing practice that stress the importance of staff expertise, systems coordination, and patient education emphasizing active involvement with therapies as fundamental to the plan of care. Such standards may be derived from guidelines published by the Centers for Disease Control (CDC) and the Intravenous Nurses Society (INS).

In conclusion, home IV therapy offers the promise of high-technology health care services in an environment that is safe, familiar, and cost-effective. With the information presented in this chapter, home health nurses can help to make the potential of home infusion therapy and quality patient care a reality.

REFERENCES

1. Appleby CR: For profits that are not humble, there's no place like the home-infusion market, *Healthweek* 3:18, 1990.
2. Barnes Home IV Care: *Clin policy proced man,* 1995.
3. Brown JM: Home care models for infusion therapy, *Caring* 1:24-27, 1990.
4. Davol: *Hickman subcutaneous port patient information,* Cranston, NJ, 1989, Davol.
5. The Family Services and Visiting Nurse Association of Alton, Ill: *Clinical policy and procedure manual,* 1995, The Association.
6. Handy CM: Home care of patients with technically complex nursing needs, *Nurs Clin North Am* 23(2):315-327, 1988.
7. Intravenous Nurse Society: *Revised intravenous nursing standards of practice,* Belmont, Mass, 1990, The Society.
8. The Joint Commission on Accreditation for Health Care: *1995 accreditation manual for home care, vol I and II,* Oakbrook Terrace, Ill, 1995.
9. Kentwich PF: *Intravenous medication care guides, intravenous therapy,* Boston, 1990, Jones & Bartlett Publishers.
10. O'Donnell KP: Physicians and home IV therapy: roles & risks, *Caring* 1:30-31, 1988.
11. Pharmacia Deltec: *A drug delivery system for the cancer patient,* St Paul, 1987, Pharmacia Deltec.
12. Rice R: Home IV therapy. In Rice R, editor: *The manual of home health nursing procedures,* St Louis, 1995, Mosby.
13. Treseler KM: *Clinical laboratory tests: significance and implications for nursing,* Englewood Cliffs, NJ, 1982, Prentice Hall.
14. Viall CD: Your complete guide to central venous catheters, *Nursing 90* 1:34-42, 1990.
15. Winter R, Parver A, Sansbury J: *Home infusion therapy: a service and demographic profile,* The National Alliance for Infusion Therapy, 1993, Philadelphia.
16. Wyeth-Ayerst Laboratories: *Proper care of the Hickman catheter,* Philadelphia, 1989, Wyeth-Ayerst Laboratories.

Appendix 17-1

Maintaining Patency of Peripheral and Central Access Devices

Access	Recommended flushing
PICC lines	Flush every 12 hr with a 2.5-ml heparin lock solution of 100 units per 1 ml of normal saline (NS).*
Peripheral lines	Flush every 24 hr with 2.0 ml of NS; follow with 1 ml of heparin lock solution to maintain patency of a heparin lock. Flush with 2.0 ml of NS before and after routine medication administration through a peripheral line.
Central venous catheter	
Hickman or Raaf	Flush each lumen every 24 hr with a 2-ml heparin lock solution.*
Groshong	Flushing of the Groshong depends on usage. Flush once per week with 5 ml of NS when CVC is not in use; flush with 20 ml of NS after blood sample withdrawal or if blood is observed in the catheter; flush with 30 ml of NS after TPN infusion and prior to blood sampling. Heparin is not used.
Subcutaneous or implantable ports	Flush after each treatment and once a month, between treatments with 5-10 ml of heparin lock solution. Be certain to flush both ports on a double-septum port.*

*The SASH method—saline flush, administer medication, saline flush, heparin flush—is used with the administration of medications.

18 The Patient with Neurologic Dysfunction

Ellen Barker

Individuals with a nervous system disorder must live not only with the effects of the disease, they also experience threats to their very existence in ways that are unlike any other type of illness. A neurologic disease may affect cognition (e.g., the ability to think, to learn, and to make judgments). In addition, it may affect the ability to move, ambulate, eat, eliminate, communicate, hear, and even breathe.

This chapter will focus on patients who have been diagnosed with one of the three most significant neurologic diseases home health nurses will encounter in the community: cerebrovascular accident (stroke), multiple sclerosis (MS), and dementia, specifically Alzheimer's dementia. While these diseases are the ones most frequently encountered, others may be seen that require similar care.

Nurses may feel that home management of patients with neurologic disorders is difficult and demanding; however, a basic review of pathophysiology and a summary of case management guidelines will enable the nurse to meet the needs of patients and families. Home health nurses will be personally and professionally rewarded as they strive to improve the quality of life for patients and provide dignity in the face of a neurologic illness. Expanded knowledge of the neurologic disease process, to include its progression and prognosis, is the foundation for providing high quality home care. Appropriate medication and treatment regimens tailored to the patient's needs in the home setting are necessary to ensure the best possible outcome, whether that be recovery or a peaceful and dignified death.

Family members of patients with neurologic deficits may feel particularly frustrated and stressed in their dual role as loved one and 24-hour caretaker. Extensive interaction with families is an integral part of the home nurse's responsibilities. The home health nurse may need to care for two patients in the home setting—the assigned patient and the spouse or loved one. Often the spouse or loved one is elderly and not in good health, which further complicates the home setting. Enormous support, teaching, and follow-up by the nurse are needed to ensure that family members also stay healthy, rested, and able to continue the important role of caretaker for the homebound patient with neurologic dysfunction. Ongoing family education and evaluation are an integral part of every home visit. (Refer to Chapter 6, which discusses working with families and caregivers.)

Patients and family members alike will benefit from the home health care nurse who is knowledgeable and competent, and who possesses a broad-based understanding of the neurologic disease.

CEREBROVASCULAR ACCIDENT (CVA)

Cerebrovascular disease or *stroke* is defined as an abnormal condition of the cerebral blood vessels characterized by an occlusion or hemorrhage that causes ischemia and damage to the brain tissue perfused by the involved vessel. This interruption in the blood supply to specific areas of the brain has been described in the past as "accidents of the vessels," hence the term *cerebrovascular accident* (CVA). Hippocrates provided the first description of stroke as far back as 460 to 370 BC. Despite the long history of this serious and complex disease, it remains a primary cause of disability among adults and is the third leading cause of death in the United States after heart disease and cancer.[7]

Incidence

The National Stroke Association reports that 500,000 to 600,000 persons suffer a new or recurrent stroke each year, resulting in 150,000 deaths. Although stroke death rates are declining, the numbers of strokes may be increasing because of the growing elderly population where the incidence is higher. Men have a 25% increased risk of stroke because of high rates of hypertension and poorer health risk habits. The risk of stroke among African Americans is twice that of the white population, primarily because of hypertension.[5]

Pathophysiology

There are four types of stroke syndromes: (1) transient ischemic attack (TIA) or temporary interruption of blood flow that lasts an average of 1 minute and no longer than 24 hours with no permanent damage (symptoms may include motor and sensory impairment, speech and visual impairment, and dysphasia), (2) reversible ischemic neurologic deficit (RIND), which lasts longer than 24 hours with no symptoms or neurologic deficits after 48 hours, (3) stroke in evolution, or progressing stroke, with increasing neurologic deficits lasting longer than 24 hours, and (4) completed stroke where the symptoms stabilize and the neurologic deficits cease to escalate.

Stroke is also divided into two groups or classifications: hemorrhagic and ischemic (or occlusive).

Hemorrhagic stroke. A cerebral hemorrhage can occur within the parenchymal or brain tissue as an intracerebral hemorrhage, or the bleed can be within the spaces surrounding the brain on its surface. For example, bleeding can occur from a subdural hemorrhage, under the dura and above the arachnoid membrane. The bleed can also result from a subarachnoid hemorrhage (SAH) where the bleeding is usually caused by an aneurysm or arteriovenous malformation (AVM). The subarachnoid space, which is between the arachnoid and pia, is the only "true space" over the brain and is filled with cerebrospinal fluid (CSF). The hemorrhage causes the CSF to become bloody as seen on lumbar puncture (LP). Vessels on the surface of the brain that rupture fill the spaces between the brain and the skull, exerting downward pressure on the surrounding brain tissue and resulting in increased intracranial pressure (ICP).

Aneurysms and AVMs are usually congenital and silent. There is no warning to herald the rupture. The sudden onset of a hemorrhagic stroke is dramatic as the blood enters the area surrounding the ruptured vessel. Headache, often described as "the worst headache of my life," invariably occurs as the blood products break down and irritate the meninges or brain tissue. Aneurysms can rupture at any time although it is more often a condition seen in healthy adults between 20 and 50 years of age.[1] After the initial rupture, the vessel constricts, a clot forms to seal the leak, and medical intervention is necessary to prevent a rebleed. Berry (saccular) aneurysms are the most common type. Giant, mycotic, and dissecting aneurysms are seen less frequently.

An SAH from a ruptured aneurysm may range from a small leak to a massive bleed, graded I through V. The symptoms from a grade I reflect only a minimal bleed with no deficits. When the hemorrhage is mild (grade II), the patient may develop a headache. Grade III, described as a moderate bleed, usually results in a change in the level of consciousness (LOC) with or without neurologic deficits. Grades IV or V produce life-threatening symptoms as a result of moderate to severe hemorrhage, and require intensive care and emergency measures.

When an intracerebral bleed is massive or near vital centers, the outcome can be fatal. This is considered "large vessel disease." If, however, the patient has had a long history of hypertension, the hemorrhage may occur in small penetrating vessels. This is called "small vessel disease," with a potentially more favorable outcome if detected and treated early.

Occlusive stroke. An occlusive or thrombotic stroke results when a cerebral vessel's circulation is decreased or completely obliterated by an infarct or stenosis. When an area of the brain has no blood supply, or too little blood supply, focal ischemia from low perfusion pressure will gradually cause symptoms. In a local process (e.g., atherosclerosis), fatty materials called plaque builds up in the inner lining of the artery, usually at the bifurcation in the common carotid. Over time, the plaque will enlarge and become irregular and pitted with ulcer craters that bleed or form clots. Platelets aggregate to the ulcer site, enlarging the clot, which eventually will completely fill the lumen of the vessel or break off. Clot fragments or plaque travel distally until they lodge in penetrating branches of vessels, obstructing blood flow and causing ischemia.

Local ischemia over time signals a compensatory response or collateral circulation that may delay stroke symptoms. When the collateral circulation fails or becomes inadequate to perfuse the brain, low perfusion will cause warning signals and symptoms of stroke.

In contrast to the slow progressive disease of thrombotic stroke, embolic strokes occur the instant a fragment or embolus that has traveled from another source (e.g., the diseased heart) enters the cerebral circulation. The blockage causes instant symptoms as the affected vessel becomes occluded. Cerebral edema accumulates around the lesion following the ischemia. The deficits correlate with the vascular territory involved.

Acute complications

The location of the affected blood vessel and the circumscribed cerebral area are dependent on the vessel's blood flow. The area deprived of blood will determine the stroke syndrome (Table 18-1). Damage will be measured by the amount of brain tissue deprived of oxygenated blood. Immediate signs and symptoms may include:

- Decreased LOC or coma
- Increased ICP
- Paralysis or decreased motor function
- Sensory loss
- Respiratory problems (e.g., atelectasis and pneumonia)
- Unstable vital signs
- Infection
- Aphasia
- Memory loss
- Dysarthria with impaired communications
- Dysphasia with the potential for choking and aspiration
- Impaired thought patterns
- Headache and/or pain
- Urinary tract infections

Treatment

In the acute phase, once neurodiagnostic studies are completed to determine whether the stroke is hemorrhagic or occlusive, measures are directed toward patient survival with appropriate interventions. The treatment is determined by the patient's age, state of health at the time of stroke, location and extent of the cerebral attack, and the degree of deficit that the patient has suffered. Surgery, angioplasty, or endoscopic procedures to obliterate an aneurysm may correct the hemorrhagic stroke.

Cerebral angioplasty, a newer experimental option available at some centers for "brain attacks" that have occurred within 6 to 8 hours, is showing great promise. A small dose of agents (e.g., urokinase) is injected in the cerebral vessel downstream from the clot via a small catheter threaded into the femoral artery to quickly dissolve the infarct and reopen the artery. Patients treated early with cerebral angioplasty may suffer less brain tissue death and therefore have a more rapid recovery with a much better chance for return of functions.

Surgery can also be an option for prevention of ischemia (e.g., carotid endarterectomy). Traditional modalities with pharmacologic treatment to prevent further thrombotic events include agents (e.g., anticoagulation and antiplatelet agents).

Once the patient has recovered from the acute event, rehabilitation and discharge planning are needed to prepare the patient for home recovery.

HOME CARE APPLICATION
Assessment

Patients recovering from a major stroke often require a multidisciplinary home health care team to regain activities of daily living (ADL) and instrumental activities of daily living (IADL). The nursing care is integrated with other health care professionals to meet patient goals for optimal outcome, with the nurse assuming the role as case manager or team leader. Helping the patient cope with the sequelae following the stroke, adjusting to the home environment, and gaining independence can be hampered by problems with immobility, musculoskeletal function, altered nutrition, altered elimination, skin integrity, and altered sensation. A combination of these problems creates a high risk for injury. Altered cognition compounds the patient's inability for self-care and patient teaching, especially if the patient has residual confusion following the stroke event.

Initial assessment focuses on a complete evaluation of the patient to plan functional restoration modalities or a death with dignity. (See the box

Table 18-1 Stroke syndromes secondary to occlusion or stenosis

Location / vessel	Area of brain infarcted	Signs and symptoms noted
Anterior and central circulation	NOTE: The internal carotid enters the Circle of Willis and supplies the lateral anterior and central portions of the cerebral hemispheres through the middle cerebral artery and the paramedial frontal lobe superior to the corpus callosum through the anterior cerebral artery; penetrating branches serve the deeper layers of the hemispheres.	
Internal carotid	If collateral circulation is intact, there is commonly no infarction; if infarcted, it is in the same area as the middle cerebral artery.	• Arterial pressure may be low in the retina. • Bruits over the internal carotid artery. • Possible retinal emboli. • History of TIAs. • Positive noninvasive studies.
Middle cerebral artery (MCA) (most common area); either stem or branches of MCA	Cortical motor area (face, arm, leg) and/or posterior limb, internal capsule, corona radiata.	• **Motor:** contralateral hemiparesis or hemiplegia, greater in face and arm than leg.
	Cortical sensory area (face, arm, leg) and/or posterior limb of internal capsule.	• **Sensation:** contralateral loss in same distribution as motor loss.
	Broca's area and deep fibers in the dominant hemisphere.	• **Speech:** expressive (motor) disorder with anomia (left hemisphere most commonly affected) with nonfluent aphasia and some comprehension defects.
	Broca's area and deep fibers in the nondominant hemisphere.	• **Speech:** dysarthria.
	Optic radiations deep in the temporal lobe.	• **Vision:** contralateral homonymous hemianopsia or quadrantanopsia.
	Location not known.	• **Motor:** mirror movements. • **Respirations:** Cheyne-Stokes respirations, contralateral hyperhidrosis, occasional mydriasis.
	Posterior limb or internal capsule and adjacent corona radiata.	• **Motor:** pure motor hemiplegia.
	Penetrating branches of MCA (lenticulostriate branches) into the basal nuclei.	• **Motor:** varying degrees of contralateral weakness of face, arm, or leg. • **Sensory:** little or no loss; if present, contralateral following the motor distribution. • **Speech:** transcortical sensory aphasia (communicating pathways are interrupted). • **Perception:** transient visual and sensory neglect on the left if a right lesion.

Modified from Adams RD, Victor M: *Principles of neurology,* ed 4, New York, 1989, McGraw-Hill; Bronstein KS, Popovich JM, Stewart-Amidei C: *Promoting stroke recovery: a research-based approach for nurses,* St Louis, 1991, Mosby; Kandel ER, Schwartz JH, Jessell TM: *Principles of neural science,* ed 3, New York, 1991, Elsevier; and Millikan CH, McDowell F, Easton JD: *Stroke,* Philadelphia, 1987, Lea & Febiger. In Barker E: *Neuroscience nursing,* St Louis, 1994, Mosby.

Table 18-1 Stroke syndromes secondary to occlusion or stenosis—cont'd

Location/vessel	Area of brain infarcted	Signs and symptoms noted
Anterior and central circulation—cont'd		
Anterior cerebral artery (ACA) (least common)	Proximal segment: corona radiata (rarely).	• **Motor:** when present, a mild contralateral hemiparesis, greater in leg; with bilateral occlusion of ACA, cerebral paraplegia in both legs can occur.
	Main stem (complete occlusion is uncommon, thus areas affected differ and collateral circulation may alleviate signs or symptoms); medial aspect of frontal lobes, caudate nucleus, and corpus callosum are supplied by the ACA.	• **Motor:** contralateral paralysis or paresis (greater in foot and thigh); mild upper extremity weakness. • **Sensory:** mild contralateral lower extremity deficiency with loss of vibratory and/or position sense, loss of two-point discrimination. • **Speech:** may have transcortical motor and sensory aphasia if left hemisphere.
Posterior circulation	NOTE: The posterior circulation includes the posterior cerebral artery, the vetebral arteries, and the basilar artery; the anatomic territory covered includes the posterior aspects of the hemispheres, the central areas of the thalamus and midbrain, and the brain stem; occlusion of the vessels is most commonly by emboli; effects of infarct in these vessels and their penetrating vessels can be specific or devastatingly global; many complex syndromes have been identified (see the original sources from which this table is compiled or basic neurology texts [e.g., Kandel] for detailed descriptions).	
Vetebral arteries	Medulla and spinal cord tracts, anterior spinal artery and penetrating branches (medial medullary syndrome).	• **Motor:** contralateral hemiparesis (face spared) and/or impaired contralateral proprioception; flaccid weakness or paralysis of the tongue and/or dysarthria.
Basilar artery (three sets of branches)	Midline structures of pons (paramedian branches); three general areas of infarction are common: (1) medial inferior pontine syndrome, (2) medial midpontine syndrome, and (3) medial superior pontine syndrome.	• **Motor:** contralateral hemiparesis or hemiplegia, ipsilateral lower motor neuron facial palsy, "locked-in syndrome". • **Sensory:** contralateral loss of vibratory sense, sense of position with dysmetria, loss of two-point discrimination, impaired rapid alternating movements. • **Visual:** inferior pontine: diplopia; impaired abduction of ipsilateral eye: internuclear ophthalmoplegia; medial superior: diplopia, internuclear ophthalmoplegia, skewed deviation.
	Corticospinal and corticobulbar tracts in pons, sensory tracts of medial and lateral lemnisci, vestibular nuclei, inferior and middle cerebellar peduncles, cranial nerve nuclei and/or fibers, cerebellar connections in tectum, descending sympathetic pathways, central brain stem, pontine tegmentum (vertebral basilar syndrome).	• **Motor:** upper motor neuron type of weakness: paralysis in combinations involving face, tongue, throat, and extremities; dysphagia, facial weakness, dysmetria, ataxia (either trunk or extremities), weak mastication muscles. • **Sensation:** combinations of impaired sensation (vibratory, two-point, position sense, pain, temperature), facial hypesthesia, anesthesia of cranial nerve V.

Continued

Table 18-1 Stroke syndromes secondary to occlusion or stenosis—cont'd

Location/vessel	Area of brain infarcted	Signs and symptoms noted
Posterior circulation—cont'd Posterior cerebral artery (PCA)	Central territory (thalamic area, dentothalamic tract, cerebral peduncle, red nucleus, subthalamic nucleus, and cranial nerve III).	• **Motor:** contralateral hemiplegia with possible dysmetria, dyskinesia, hemiballism or choreoathetosis, dystaxia, cerebellar ataxia, and tremor; contralateral upper motor neuron palsy; several syndromes are associated: (1) Weber: cranial nerve III palsy and contralateral hemiplegia; (2) thalamoperforate syndrome: superior, crossed cerebellar ataxia or inferior crossed cerebellar ataxia with cranial nerve III palsy (Claude syndrome), (3) decerebrate attacks. • **Sensory:** contralateral sensory loss of all modalities without agraphia. • **Function:** prosopagnosia (inability to recognize familiar faces), topographic disorientation, memory deficits, alexia, inability to read, color anomia. • **Level of consciousness:** in bilateral PCA syndromes, coma with absent doll's eyes or loss of alertness may occur; if tegmentum of midbrain near hypothalamus and third ventricle is damaged, akinetic mutism may occur.
Small vessel disease	NOTE: Small penetrating vessels in brain parenchyma that supply areas near the basal ganglia are most vulnerable to infarction although any small vessels can occlude deep in the brain and cause injury, producing neurologic signs or symptoms; such infarcts are commonly called **lacunes** ("small pit or hollow"), a term that is changing in meaning. They can be caused by emboli but are most commonly associated with microatherosclerosis although they can be found in otherwise healthy people, those with concurrent therosclerosis, hypertension, and/or diabetes have a higher incidence of this type of infarct.	
	Internal capsule, most commonly.	• **Motor:** contralateral hemiparesis on a single side, with equal deficit in face, arm, and leg; often unaccompanied by detectable signs of sensory, visual, and speech loss, depending on location; old term is "pure motor stroke" although evidence suggests that other neurologic signs are present but overlooked because of low intensity.
	Thalamus, most commonly.	• **Sensory:** complete or partial loss in face, arm, trunk, and leg that appears exactly midline; may be accompanied by pain, hypesthesias, and uncomfortable sensations.

**PRIMARY NURSING DIAGNOSES/
PATIENT PROBLEMS**

Cerebrovascular accident (CVA)
- Impaired cognition
- Alterations in behavior
- Impaired physical mobility
- Altered nutrition, less than body requirements
- Incontinence
- Impaired skin integrity
- Altered sensory/perceptual status

**PRIMARY THEMES
OF PATIENT EDUCATION**

Cerebrovascular accident (CVA)
- Risk factors for stroke
- Signs and symptoms of stroke
- Aftercare from medical interventions and/or surgery
- Coping strategies
- Community reentry
- Management of neurologic deficits

titled Primary Nursing Diagnoses/Patient Problems.) This section will review how to preserve the patient's current neurologic status and/or help to restore the patient to the highest level of function. (See the box titled Primary Themes of Patient Education.)

Components of the neurologic assessment, to include cranial nerve assessment (Table 18-2), follow with interventions and expected patient outcomes. The nurse must maintain a high vigilance to detect a possible second stroke, complications related to the acute stroke, and side effects from medications, especially anticoagulants. Stroke risk factors to monitor for prevention of a recurrent stroke include:

- High blood pressure
- Heart disease
- High red cell count

- Cigarette smoking
- Alcohol consumption
- Obesity
- Cholesterol over 200
- Physical inactivity
- Diabetes mellitus (DM)
- Carotid bruit

Nursing interventions

Cognition, behavior and psychosocial. The nurse should determine the premorbid cognitive ability by reviewing the patient's history, interviewing family members, and reviewing the acute care record for results describing the location and degree of brain damage and neuropsychological reports. Initial and frequent serial testing are recommended using the Short Portable Mental Status Questionnaire (SPMSQ) (Figure 18-1) or Mini-Mental State Examination (Figure 18-2). Most stroke victims will regain the significant amount of lost functions within 1 to 2 years; however, individuals who receive consistent stimulation and rehabilitation may continue to recover smaller degrees of function up to 10 years. In working with patients who are cognitively impaired, effective therapy devices include items for a reminder of date, time, and orientation. For example, place the bed near a window to help the patient observe the changes of day and night, daily weather, and seasonal changes. Use verbal comments for emphasis.

Survivors of stroke may suffer from neurobehavioral deficits that range from an inability to adjust to the home environment to frank psychotic disorders. Interventions include first identifying the cause of the unwanted behavior, removing barriers that provoke it, and containing the behavior until it is no longer present. Medications that potentiate confusion should be eliminated or substituted. Pharmacologic or physical restraints should not be used if possible.[7]

A consistent routine, a calm approach combined with adequate periods of rest, and an environment with minimal noise and confusion are desirable. If depression, anxiety, and stress persist following discharge to home, consider a psychological referral to the psychiatric home health care nurse or social worker for early detection and treatment. Psychosocial concerns may be overwhelming for the patient, the family, and the caregivers.

Table 18-2 Cranial nerves

Cranial nerve	Origin and course	Function
I Olfactory Sensory	Mucosa of nasal cavity; only cranial nerve with cell body located in peripheral structure (nasal mucosa). Pass through cribriform plate of ethmoid bone and go on to olfactory bulbs at floor of frontal lobe. Final interpretation is in temporal lobe.	Smell. However, system is more than receptor/interpreter for odors; perception of smell also sensitizes other body systems and responses such as salivation, peristalsis, and even sexual stimulus. Loss of sense of smell is termed *anosmia.*
II Optic Sensory	Ganglion cells of retina converge on the optic disc and form optic nerve. Nerve fibers pass to optic chiasm, which is above pituitary gland. Some fibers decussate, others do not. The two tracts then go to the lateral geniculate body near the thalamus and then on to the end station for interpretation in the occipital lobe.	Vision.
III Oculomotor Motor	Originates in midbrain and emerges from brain stem at upper pons. Motor fibers to superior, medial, inferior recti, and inferior oblique for eye movement; levator muscle of the eyelid.	Extraocular movement of eyes. Raise eyelid.
Parasympathetic	Parasympathetic fibers to ciliary muscles and iris of eye.	Constrict pupil; changes shape of lens.
IV Trochlear Motor	Comes from lower midbrain area to innervate superior oblique eye muscle.	Allows eye to move down and inward.
V Trigeminal Sensory	Originates in fourth ventricle and emerges at lateral parts of pons. Has three branches to face: ophthalmic, maxillary, and mandibular.	*Ophthalmic branch:* Sensation to cornea, ciliary body, iris, lacrimal gland, conjunctiva, nasal mucosal membranes, eyelids, eyebrows, forehead, and nose. *Maxillary branch:* Sensation to skin of cheek, lower lid, side of nose and upper jaw, teeth, mucosa of mouth, sphenopolative-pterygoid region, and maxillary sinus. *Mandibular branch:* Sensation to skin of lower lip, chin, ear, mucous membrane, teeth of lower jaw and tongue.
Motor	Goes to temporalis, masseter, pterygoid gland, anterior part of digastric muscles (all for mastication), and the tensor tympani and tensor veli palatini muscles (clench jaws).	Muscles of chewing and mastication and opening jaw.

From Rudy E: *Advanced neurological and neurosurgical nursing,* St Louis, 1984, Mosby.

Table 18-2 Cranial nerves—cont'd

Cranial nerve	Origin and course	Function
VI Abducens		
Motor	Arises from a nucleus in pons to innervate lateral rectus eye muscle.	Allows eye to move outward.
VII Facial		
Sensory	Lower portion of pons goes to anterior two thirds of tongue and soft palate.	Taste anterior two thirds of tongue. Sensation to soft palate.
Motor	Pons to muscles of forehead, eyelids, cheeks, lips, ear, nose, and neck.	Movement of facial muscles to produce facial expressions, close eyes.
Parasympathetic	Pons to salivary gland and lacrimal glands.	Secretory for salivation and tears.
VIII Acoustic		
Sensory	*Cochlear division:* Originates in spinal ganglia of the cochlea, with peripheral fibers to the organ of Corti in the internal ear. Goes to pons, and impulses transmitted to the temporal lobe.	Hearing.
	Vestibular division: Originates in otolith organs of the semicircular canals in the inner ear and in the vestibular ganglion. Terminates in pons, with some fibers continuing to cerebellum. Only cranial nerve originating wholly within a bone, petrous portion of temporal bone.	Equilibrium.
IX Glossopharyngeal		
Sensory	Posterior one third of tongue for taste sensation and sensations from soft palate, tonsils, and opening to mouth in back of oral pharynx (fauces). Fibers go to medulla and then to the temporal lobe for taste and sensory cortex for other sensations.	Taste in posterior one third of tongue. Sensation in back of throat; stimulation elicits a gag reflex.
Motor	Medulla to constrictor muscles of pharynx and stylopharyngeal muscles.	Voluntary muscles for swallowing and phonation.
Parasympathetic	Medulla to parotid salivary gland via otic ganglia.	Secretory, salivary glands. Carotid reflex.
X Vagus		
Sensory	Sensory fibers in back of ear and posterior wall of external ear go to medulla oblongata and on to sensory cortex.	Sensation behind ear and part of external ear meatus.
Motor	Fibers go from medulla oblongata through jugular foramen with glossopharyngeal nerve and on to pharynx, larynx, esophagus, bronchi, lungs, heart, stomach, small intestines, liver, pancreas, kidneys.	Voluntary muscles for phonation and swallowing. Involuntary activity of visceral muscles of heart, lungs, and digestive tract.

Continued

Table 18-2 Cranial nerves—cont'd

Cranial nerve	Origin and course	Function
X Vagus—cont'd Parasympathetic	Medulla oblongata to larynx, trachea, lungs, aorta, esophagus, stomach, small intestines, and gallbladder.	Carotid reflex. Autonomic activity of respiratory tract, digestive tract including peristalsis and secretion from organs.
XI Spinal accessory Motor	This nerve has two roots, cranial and spinal. Cranial portion arises at several rootlets at side of medulla, runs below vagus, and is joined by spinal portion from motor cells in cervical cord. Some fibers go along with vagus nerve to supply motor impulse to pharynx, larynx, uvula, and palate. Major portion to sternomastoid and trapezius muscles, branches to cervical spinal nerves C2-C4.	Some fibers for swallowing and phonation. Turn head and shrug shoulders.
XII Hypoglossal Motor	Arises in medulla oblongata and goes to muscles of tongue.	Movement of tongue necessary for swallowing and phonation.

The return to a familiar world and the home setting may dramatically improve cognition. Old picture albums, newspapers, and favorite television and radio programs can be therapeutic and entertaining. A multidisciplinary team care plan should reflect a cognitive plan of care that becomes increasingly challenging and rewarding.

Medications. Patients may have received anticoagulants, such as heparin or warfarin sodium during their acute illness. Warfarin is a commonly prescribed anticoagulant for patients at discharge. The effects of warfarin are judged by prothrombin time (PT). The prescribed quantity may range from 1½ to 2½ times the baseline PT based on typical home dosage of 2 mg/day to 10 mg/day PO. Anticoagulation therapy will continue for as long as the patient is considered to be at risk. The nurse may be asked to collect weekly or biweekly blood work for PT values and to immediately report any abnormal values or adverse reactions.

Patients and family must be taught the risks of warfarin or antiplatelet (aspirin) therapy. The nurse will routinely assess for bleeding, evidenced by hematuria, hemoptysis, hematemesis, melena, bleeding gums, bruising of skin, or petechiae. Instructions for gentle toothbrushing, care when shaving, and prevention of nicks or skin cuts is emphasized.

Sensory status. Problems related to hemianopsia, field cuts, impaired depth perception, and unilateral neglect require that the patient be approached in a manner to avoid the "blind spots." Furniture in the home should be arranged appropriately and not moved about. Spatial disorders and impaired vision make it difficult for patients to be independent until they have readjusted to the home environment.

Patients with a parietal lesion of the nondominant side may experience a condition known as "neglect" and totally ignore the opposite side of the body. If asked to draw a picture of a clock, this patient will draw numbers only on one side of the clock's face. The neglected side needs to always be carefully protected. The patient can be re-

Short Portable Mental Status Questionnaire (SPMSQ)

Instructions: Ask questions 1-10 in this list and record all answers. Ask question 4a only if patient does not have a telephone. Record number of errors based on 10 questions.
Allow one more error if subject has had only a grade school education.
Allow one less error if subject has had education beyond high school.

+	−

1. What is the date today?_____
   Month   Day   Year

2. What day of the week is it?_____

3. What is the name of this place?_____

4. What is your telephone number?_____

4a. What is your street address?_____
   (Ask only if patient does not have a telephone)

5. How old are you?

6. When were you born?

7. Who is the President of the United States now?

8. Who was the President just before him?

9. What was your mother's maiden name?

10. Subtract 3 from 20 and keep subtracting 3 from each new number, all the way down.

_____ Total Number of Errors

0–2 Errors	*Intact intellectual functioning*
3–4 Errors	*Mild intellectual impairment*
5–7 Errors	*Moderate intellectual development*
8–10 Errors	*Severe intellectual impairment*

To be completed by interviewer

Patient's name: _____ Date:_____

Sex: 1. Male   Race: 1. White
      2. Female   2. Black
                         3. Other

Years of education:_____   1. Grade school
                                               2. High school
                                               3. Beyond high school

Interviewer's name:_____

Figure 18-1 Short Portable Mental Status Questionnaire (SPMSQ). (Modified from Pfeiffer E: *J Am Geriatr Soc* 23(10):433-441, 1975. In Barker E: *Neuroscience Nursing,* St Louis, 1994, Mosby.)

Mini-Mental State Examination

Maximum
Score   Score

Orientation

| 5 | ( ) | What is the (year) (season) (date) (day) (month)? |
| 5 | ( ) | Where we are: (state) (country) (town) (hospital) (floor)? |

Registration

| 3 | ( ) | Name three objects: 1 second to say each. Ask the patient all three after you have said them. Give 1 point for each correct answer. Then repeat them until he/she learns all three. Count trials and record. Trials |

Attention and Calculation

| 5 | ( ) | Serial 7s. 1 point for each correct. Stop after 5 answers. Alternatively, spell "world" backwards. |

Recall

| 3 | ( ) | Ask for the three objects repeated above. Give 1 point for each correct. |

Language

| 9 | ( ) | Give the name of objects: a pencil and a watch (2 points) |

Repeat the following "No ifs, ands, or buts." (1 point)
Follow a three-stage command:
  "Take a paper in your right hand, fold it in half, and put it on the floor." (3 points)
Read and obey the following:
  "Close your eyes" (1 point)
Write a sentence (1 point)
Copy design (1 point)
Total score
ASSESS level of consciousness along a continuum_____

Alert Drowsy Stupor Coma

Instructions for Administration of Mini-Mental State Examination

Orientation

(1) Ask for the date. Then ask specifically for parts omitted (e.g., "Can you also tell me what season it is ?"). One point for each correct.

(2) Ask in turn "Can you tell me the name of this hospital?" (e.g., town, country) 1 point for each correct.

Registration

Ask the patient if you may test his/her memory. Then say the names of three unrelated objects clearly and slowly, about 1 second for each. After you have said all three, ask him/her to repeat them. This first repetition determines his/her score (0-3), but keep saying them until he/she can repeat all three, up to six trials. If he/she does not eventually learn all three, recall cannot be meaningfully tested.

Attention and Calculation

Ask the patient to begin with 100 and count backward by 7. Stop after 5 subtractions (93, 86, 79, 72, 65).

Score the total number of correct answers.

If the patient cannot or will not perform this task, ask him/her to spell the word "world" backward. The score is the number of letters in correct order (e.g., dlrow = 5, dlrow = 3).

Recall

Ask the patient if he/she can recall the three words you previously asked him/her to remember. Score 0-3

Figure 18-2 Mini-Mental State Examination. (Modified from Folstein MF, Folstein SE, McHugh PR: *J Psychiatr Res* 12:189-198, 1975. In Barker E: *Neuroscience Nursing*, St Louis, 1994, Mosby.)

Language

Naming: Show the patient a wrist watch and ask him/her what it is. Repeat for pencil. Score 0-2.

Repetition: Ask the patient to repeat the sentence after you. Allow only one trial. Score 0 or 1.

Three-stage command: Give the patient a piece of plain blank paper and repeat the command. Score 1 point for each part correctly executed.

Reading: On a blank piece of paper print the sentence "Close your eyes" in letters large enough for the patient to see clearly. Ask him/her to read it and do what it says. Score 1 point only if he/she actually closes his/her eyes.

Writing: Give the patient a blank piece of paper and ask him/her to write a sentence for you. Do not dictate a sentence; it is to be written spontaneously. It must contain a subject and verb and be sensible. Correct grammar and punctuation are not necessary.

Copying: On a clean piece of paper, draw intersecting pentagons, each side about 1 inch and ask him/her to copy it exactly as it is. All 10 angles must be present, and 2 must intersect to score 1 point. Tremor and rotation are ignored.

Estimate the patient's level of sensorium along a continuum, from alert on the left to coma on the right.

Figure 18-2 Mini-Mental State Examination—cont'd

minded of the neglected side with visual attention and range of motion exercises to prevent injury and muscle wasting.

Pain in the affected limb may be one of the first signs of neural recovery. The repetitive exercises and physical therapy help to restore the lost neural circuitry and stimulate the neurons to rewire the damaged brain. Motor recovery follows sensory recovery. The healthy side may be stimulated to communicate with the damaged side. The nurse may observe that when the patient moves the unaffected arm, the opposite limb with the deficit also moves, but only slightly. These compensatory reactions should be recorded.

The OT and PT rehabilitation team's contribution is important to help the patient gain confidence and overcome sensory obstacles that interfere with autonomy and independence.

Language and communication. Left-sided stroke survivors may have receptive and expressive language deficits that impair meaningful communication. After discharge to home, patients' full awareness of their deficit may cause fear, anger, frustration, despair, hopelessness, and even rebellion as they develop nonverbal or healthy attempts to express themselves and make their needs known. It is therefore important to maintain the same caregivers who, over time, learn the meaning of damaged speech (much like a mother understands her baby's utterances). During this phase it is vital that the home health nurse address the

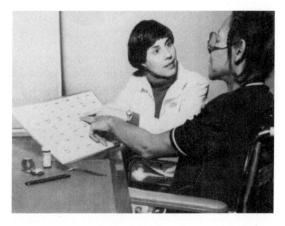

Figure 18-3 Using the Talking Pictures communication board. (Copyright Crestwood Company, Milwaukee, Wis. Used with permission.)

patient in a respectful way and refrain from using slang or babytalk communication.

Communication aids (e.g., Talking Pictures) for patients with communication difficulties following stroke augment and supplement communication and are useful for language therapy. Communication boards (Figure 18-3) may be the only means of communication for some patients after a stroke.

Physical mobility and musculoskeletal function. A rigidly adhered to routine of getting the patient out of bed (OOB), sitting in a specialized chair, and ambulating as soon as possible, is vital to the prevention of long-term complications of immobility and to achieve the expected outcome. Special equipment, the training of caretakers or volunteers, and a schedule for OOB activities are needed. The physical therapist (PT) and occupational therapist (OT) prescribe the type and amount of therapy with range of motion (ROM) exercises that can be passive or active. Exercises performed independently by the patient or by the family should be repeated up to eight or more times per day. As soon as the patient can ambulate, daily walks with measured distances are incorporated into the daily routine. Walkers and any necessary assistive devices should be in the home and monitored for safety and maintained in good repair. The amount of time OOB and ambulation distance are increased until normal functions are restored. Efforts to eliminate falls and prevent injury are part of the patient and family teaching. The home should be checked for safety hazards at each visit. (Refer to Chapter 16 for more information.)

Nutrition. A nutritionist should be consulted prior to discharge to assist in the evaluation of nutritional needs and to develop a home nutrition program. Copies of the diet should be available to everyone participating in the patient's dietary activities.

The nurse will be responsible for the assessment of cranial nerves, particularly the lower cranial nerves IX through XII involved in the gag reflex and voluntary muscles for swallowing. The assessment includes evaluation of the patient's ability to chew, swallow, protect the airway from choking and aspiration, and manage different textures and foods; a recording of weight, intake and output, calorie count; condition of the oral cavity and teeth; and a check to determine if the food that is purchased and prepared is adequate.

Patients on steroids or medications that affect fluids and electrolytes, require further evaluation to maintain the integrity of the gastrointestinal tract and also to test for occult bleeding and electrolyte imbalance. For continued healing, patient teaching will focus on the importance of increased metabolic needs during recovery.

The use of supplemental or tube feedings for patients unable to tolerate oral feedings requires additional assessment and teaching to meet the patient's hypermetabolic requirements until adequate oral intake is safe and feasible. Determin-

ing when to switch and what to institute is best done in consultation with the nutritionist/speech therapist. Percutaneous endoscopic gastrostomy (PEG) tubes are widely used to provide long-term nourishment and can be easily managed in the home setting. Protocols provided by the physician or home health organization should be maintained until the PEG tube is discontinued.

The problems of dysphagia, dehydration, and malnutrition should be closely monitored during the home visit in conjunction with the neuroassessment to evaluate any relationship between the neurologic deficits and these potential complications. Creative methods are needed to promote adequate fluid intake and nutrition for the stroke survivor.

In addition, financial considerations may factor into the family's abilities to provide nutrition for the patient. Social services should be notified along with other community agencies as needed.

Bladder elimination. A bladder training program is best initiated during hospitalization and continued at home. Assess the stroke survivor's ability to eliminate by observing toilet routine, degree of continence, use of bladder aids, urinary and dietary intake and output, activity level, skin integrity surrounding the genitalia, and the patient's ability to verbalize toileting needs and/or problems. (Refer to Chapter 15 for more information on elimination problems.)

Bowel elimination. Bowel incontinence may develop from neurologic dysfunction resulting from impaired defecation reflexes and loss of motor control and weakness following a stroke. The nurse will assess:

- Toilet habits
- Bowel evacuation
- Constipation and diarrhea
- Communication skills to verbalize bowel problems
- Balance and strength
- Dietary fluid and fiber
- Stress and anxiety related to bowel evaluation

Every home health care provider is familiar with checking patients for fecal impaction, diarrhea, and skin integrity associated with bowelincontinence and dealing with the patient's embarrassment from loss of bowel control. These same principles are discussed in Chapter 15.

Skin integrity. Thin, dry, flaky skin is vulnerable to prolonged immobility and will quickly break down into pressure ulcers if not well protected. Powders, soaps, and lotions should be used with caution. Mild soap and warm water for remoisturization, gentle toweling to toughen the skin, and meticulous repositioning prevent breakdown. Padding and assistive devices over heels, elbows, and bony prominences are encouraged until the patient is OOB. Strong bleaches and detergents should be avoided in laundering bed linen. Silk sheets are ideal for heavy patients who must be turned frequently. (Refer to Chapter 13 for further guidelines on wound or skin care.)

Stroke prevention. Recovering stroke patients and their family require special teaching to prevent recurrent attacks. The importance of medication compliance, blood pressure control, adherence to diet, smoking cessation, weight control, and other identified controllable risk factors need frequent reinforcement. Teaching the prompt reporting of the earliest warning signs of a "brain attack" for immediate intervention may prevent future death or disability from stroke. The most difficult challenge is motivating the patient to change a lifestyle that precipitated the earlier attack. Wellness promotion and a healthy lifestyle are the most effective therapy we can offer.

Conclusion

Stroke survivors challenge the home health care nurse with many situations during recovery. Patience is needed by everyone during the long period of brain healing and for the edema to subside. Recovery varies from patient to patient. Compensatory coping skills, a high degree of motivation, compliance to a structured regimen, and family support combine for success in overcoming this devastating insult to the brain.

Patient/family/professional resources

Academy of Aphasia (AA)
Boston Veterans Administration
150 South Huntingdon Avenue
Boston, MA 02130
(617)495-4342

Adaptive Environment Center
Massachusetts College of Art
621 Huntingdon Avenue
11th Floor
Boston, MA 02215-5801

National Stroke Association
8480 E. Orchard Road, Suite 1000
Englewood, CO 80111-5015
(303)771-1700
FAX: (303)771-1886

MULTIPLE SCLEROSIS (MS)

Multiple sclerosis is the most common neurologic illness affecting young adults.[3] The disease usually begins in young adulthood with a progressive course characterized by disseminated demyelination of nerve fibers of the brain and spinal cord with remissions and exacerbation that continue throughout life. When myelin is destroyed in multiple areas, the ability of the nerves to conduct electrical impulses to and from the brain is disrupted by the scars, or sclerosis. According to the National Multiple Sclerosis Society, approximately 350,000 people in this country have MS, and each may have a different pattern of demyelination. Symptoms depend on which areas of the central nervous system (CNS) have been attacked and the amount and scatter of lesions. It is one of few diseases that affect women more than men and is more common among Caucasians.

The etiology is unknown; however, most theories suggest an immunogenetic-viral cause where the immune system attacks the body's own myelin. As shown in Table 18-3, symptoms correlate with areas of dysfunction.

Pathophysiology

Multiple plaques in the CNS that consist of demyelinated nerve fibers, sparing of axons, gliosis, and inflammatory cells are the principal pathologic findings in MS. Plaques range in size from 1 mm to 4 cm and are found scattered throughout the white matter, and to a lesser degree in the gray matter. Areas that show a predilection for development of plaques include the optic nerves and chiasm, regions of the brainstem, cerebellum, cerebrum, and cervical spinal cord.[3]

Acute complications

Respiratory failure occurs in patients with MS secondary to aspiration, atelectasis, and pneumonia. Sepsis related to urinary tract infections (UTI) and respiratory infections are not uncommon. Hospitalization is often required during a severe exacerbation for corticosteroid administration, feeding tube placement, insertion of a suprapubic catheter,

Table 18-3 Clinical manifestations of multiple sclerosis

Area of dysfunction	Symptoms
Cranial nerve dysfunction	Blurred central vision; faded colors; blind spots (optic neuritis)
	Diplopia
	Dysphagia
	Facial weakness, numbness, pain
Motor dysfunction	Weakness
	Paralysis
	Spasticity
	Abnormal gait
Sensory dysfunction	Paresthesias
	Lhermitte's sign (electric shock-like sensation radiating down spine into the extremities)
	Decreased proprioception
	Decreased temperature perception
Cerebellar dysfunction	Dysarthria
	Tremor
	Incoordination
	Ataxia
	Vertigo
Bowel and bladder dysfunction	Fecal urgency, constipation, incontinence
	Urinary frequency, urgency, hesitancy, nocturia, retention, incontinence
Cognitive dysfunction	Decreased short-term memory
	Difficulty learning new information
	Word-finding trouble
	Short attention span
	Decreased concentration
	Mood alterations (depression, euphoria)
Sexual dysfunction	Women: decreased libido, decreased orgasmic ability, decreased genital sensation
	Men: erectile, orgasmic, and ejaculatory dysfunction
Fatigue	Overwhelming weakness not overcome with increased physical effort

From Beare P, Myers J: *Principles and practice of adult health nursing,* ed 2, St Louis, 1994, Mosby.

or for spasticity management. As soon as these problems are under control, the patient is discharged for home care.

Treatment

Patients often experience years of frustration until they are finally diagnosed with MS. It has been called "the great imitator" because it can mimic other diseases. After an unexplained remission, patients often dismiss the early signs of MS and disregard the milder symptoms. Magnetic resonance (MR) has emerged as an important neurodiagnostic study to offer earlier supportive evidence; however, diagnosis of MS is one of exclusion

since there is no single test for absolute confirmation. Clinical diagnosis is made when the patient has neurologic dysfunction in more than one area of the nervous system that tends to appear more than once. For some, diagnosis is often a relief when they finally have a name for their illness and can begin treatment. Symptom management (refer to the list in Table 18-3) by a multidisciplinary team is recommended to assist the individual in living a normal life until the onset of an acute attack. Corticosteroids (usually oral prednisone), beginning with a high dose and then tapering will reduce the inflammatory flare-up. Treatment with plasma exchange, immunosuppressive agents, and other modalities have been studied with the best results attributed to a new drug, Betaseron (interferon-beta 1-b). It has been shown to decrease the incidence and severity of exacerbations for patients with relapsing-remitting MS and may actually alter the course of the disease.[4] Other medications may be prescribed for relief of symptoms, e.g., spasticity (baclofen), urinary retention (bethanechol or oxybutynin), or urinary tract infections (antibiotics).

HOME CARE APPLICATION
Assessment

Homebound patients with MS may be wheelchair bound, bedridden or only minimally ambulatory depending on the progression of the disease. A review of the patient's record and a thorough history taken on the initial visit will determine which symptoms are apparent. A complete baseline neuroassessment is needed that will be used for all future comparisons. It is therefore important for the nurse to assess and record findings in a systematic manner. A flowsheet is recommended. Standardized scales may be used, such as the Short Portable Mental Status Questionnaire (SPMSQ) or Mini-Mental State Examination (Figures 18-1 and 18-2), the Bartherl and the Brody Instrumental ADL Scale, the Kurtzke Scale, or the minimal record of disability (MRD). Each patient has unique physiological and psychological requirements that may also include environmental and home modifications.

Nursing interventions

Cognition, behavior, and psychosocial. Changes in cognition, short-term memory, mood swings, and depressive states should be evaluated and given consideration in planning home care. Once family and caregivers understand that changes in behavior are disease-related and not purposeful, it is easier for them to accept and live with these changes.

Strategies such as keeping notes, making a list for daily activities and routines, and reducing stressful episodes are helpful. Fatigue, one of the most common problems experienced by individuals with MS, can interfere in coping with cognition and behavior. The National MS Society describes fatigue in the following ways: (1) normal, due to overactivity, (2) short-circuiting, in which damaged nerves tire with use, (3) lassitude, which is overpowering exhaustion requiring medication, and (4) fatigue of depression, best managed with psychological counseling and/or medication. Fatigue should be evaluated and considered in the overall management of cognitive/behavioral problems.

Euphoria, or loss of control with laughing or crying, can be addressed by the nurse with suggestions (e.g., when you can't stop laughing, think of the saddest thing in your life or pretend that you are in church). Uncontrollable crying or sadness can be countered by visualizing feelings of joy and happy events. Active listening and help with coping skills in an empathetic manner will help the patient learn to manage unwanted behavior and deal with psychosocial concerns.

Mobility. After the amount and safety of ambulation has been planned, the nurse in conjunction with the rehabilitation team can teach or reinforce the following:

- Position changes from a lying or sitting position
- Balance
- Coordination
- Gait
- Toilet, tub, or shower safety
- Strengthening exercises
- Assistive devices that aid in mobility
- Wheelchair/bed/chair transfer techniques
- Application and removal of orthotics, braces, or appliances for improved support for mobility

The nurse will need to use motivational strategies to impress upon patients with MS that they cannot give in to their weakness, ataxia, and fatigue because it will only make them more incapacitated. Pride may interfere in the use of assistive devices such as a cane, wheelchair, or visible tools that bring attention to the illness. Some patients use denial to cope with their disease and do not want to be seen as handicapped. After the nurse explains that energy conservation is more important than pride and will enable the patient to be more mobile, the patient is usually more receptive. Canes, walkers, and wheelchairs can be personalized with artful decorations, paint, and glitter. Safe footwear (usually leather-soled flat tie shoes) is recommended. The nurse should periodically check all equipment to see that it is still appropriate, fits, and is being used.

Sensory. Lhermitte's phenomenon is a sudden, transient, electric-like shock that spreads down the body when the head is flexed forward and is a characteristic finding in MS. Numbness, tingling, loss of joint sensation, and other sensory losses often accompany demyelination from MS. Intolerance of heat from exercising, an overheated environment, a hot bath/shower, or a swimming pool decreases the efficiency of nerve conduction. Keeping the environmental temperature in the cool range helps to avoid discomfort and associated sensory and motor symptoms.

Pain. Pain and discomfort from musculoskeletal dysfunction may result from compensation to maintain balance, from spasticity, or from nerve damage. Correction of the underlying problem or a rehabilitation program may reduce or eliminate the pain. After a complete pain assessment, the physician, nurse, and rehabilitation team can devise remedies to address the patient's pain and discomfort. For the bedridden patient, gentle massage, a warm bath, good body alignment with pillow support to the back and between the legs, a rigid turning schedule with proper protection of the bony prominences, and frequent ROM exercises to decrease spasticity will ease the pain. These interventions will also aid in the prevention of skin breakdown, deep vein thrombosis (DVT) and pulmonary embolism.

Language and communication. Brain lesions that affect speech and swallowing require the nurse to help the patient adapt or seek appropriate communication aids. A speech pathologist referral should be requested to devise a treatment plan to improve speech. Helpful suggestions to the patient include the following:

- Speak slowly
- Use better breath control
- Make a tape recording for feedback of tone, pitch, and inflection
- Use a voice amplifier to generate more volume

Self-care. Enlisting the occupational therapist (OT) to assess the plan interventions for self-care for activities of daily living (ADLs) will help the patient gain independence in bathing, toileting, dressing, eating, cooking, cleaning, and living safely in the home. The use of electronic devices may serve to not only decrease energy use, but also provide more freedom of independence. Depending on the availability of financial resources, there is a wide selection of electronic equipment available. The ability to do housekeeping chores may be minimal or not possible for homebound patients. Every resource should be used to allow for independence until the needs and interventions change during the terminal phase.

Elimination. Bowel problems of constipation and continence plague many patients with MS due to lesions on nerves that control bowel motility. Recommendations made earlier in the chapter are applicable to patients with MS.

The most common problems affecting the bladder are increased frequency, leakage between voidings, storage, incomplete emptying, and difficulty in urinating. Self-catheterization, the use of prescribed medications, and the prevention of UTIs are all important in helping the patient successfully manage MS in the home.

Sexuality. The nurse may find that no one has discussed sexuality with the patient or that the patient has not asked questions regarding changes in sexuality. The neurologic changes may be manifested in the following ways:

- Difficulty in achieving or maintaining an erection for males
- Decreased libido from fatigue, anxiety, embarrassment
- Decreased sensation in the genital area that inhibits arousal for females
- Vaginal dryness for females
- Interference with coitus by the urinary catheter
- Mental, emotional, or psychological concerns

A frank discussion opens the door to dealing with sexual concerns. The nurse may suggest that the couple communicate openly and honestly. Professional help may be needed until the problems can be overcome and the patient can relax and enjoy a satisfying sexual relationship with his/her partner. Attention to dress and appearance, good personal hygiene, and relaxation techniques help set the mood for romance and sexual encounters.

Conclusion

Primary nursing diagnoses and primary themes of patient education are listed in the following boxes. Because patients with MS live a near-normal life

PRIMARY NURSING DIAGNOSES/ PATIENT PROBLEMS

Multiple sclerosis (MS)
- Impaired memory
- Impaired physical mobility
- Sensory/perceptual alterations
- Pain
- Impaired verbal communication
- Self-care deficits
- Alterations in elimination
- Altered sexuality patterns

PRIMARY THEMES OF PATIENT EDUCATION

Multiple sclerosis (MS)
- Information on MS and available resources
- Overcoming physical disadvantages
- Disability prevention/physical fitness
- Coping strategies
- Energy conservation and prevention of fatigue
- Activities of daily living (ADLs)
- Communication

span, they will be faced with a myriad of problems from the remissions and exacerbations that accompany this disease until the nerve fiber degenerates and the symptoms become permanent. Research is promising, but until a prevention or cure is found, nurses will be important in helping the patient attain the best possible quality of life.

Patient/family/professional resources

The National Multiple Sclerosis Society
733 Third Avenue
New York, NY 10017-3288
Phone: (212)986-3240
FAX: (211)986-7981

DEMENTIA: ALZHEIMER'S TYPE

Dementia, Alzheimer's type is a progressive degenerative disease of the brain in which cells die and are not replaced. it results in impaired memory, thinking, and behavior, and is the most common form of dementing illness according to the national Alzheimer's Association (AA), which has developed the following checklist of 10 common symptoms:

- Recent memory loss
- Difficulty performing familiar tasks
- Problems with language
- Disorientation of time and place
- Poor or decreased judgment
- Problems with abstract thinking
- Misplacing things
- Changes in mood or behavior
- Changes in personality
- Loss of initiative

Incidence

With over 4 million Americans afflicted with Alzheimer's disease, it is considered the fourth leading cause of death among adults in the United States. The AA predicts that by the year 2050 over 14 million Americans will have the disease. People are affected regardless of gender, race, ethnicity, or socioeconomic group. The incidence appears to be higher in women. The symptoms usually begin to appear after age 60 with increasing incidence with aging. By the age of 80, up to 40% of the elderly may be affected. Dementia, with impaired intellectual or cognitive function that affects speech, language, memory, and personality is a broad term that often defies diagnosis until autopsy. Terms other than Alzheimer's that nurses may hear associated with dementia include Pick's disease, multiinfarct dementia, organic brain disorder, and organic brain syndrome. In the following sections, dementia, Alzheimer's type will be used to describe the care for patients in the home who suffer from some type of dementia.

Pathophysiology

The cause is unknown; however, there are several theories of causation. The abnormal protein theory suggests that the large concentrations of amyloid-rich plaques, identified on autopsies from patients with Alzheimer's, consist of neurofibrillary tangles most dense in the hippocampus. They are thought to interfere with neural transmission.[2] The brain of patients with the disease becomes atrophic with primary atrophy in the temporoparietal and anterior frontal lobes. The degeneration of neurons in the cerebral cortex allows the ventricles to enlarge, giving a characteristic image on computerized tomography (CT) or magnetic resonance (MR).

It is believed that Alzheimer's is related to a gene on the X chromosome with autosomal dominant inheritance accounting for a small percentage of the disease. Genetic factors, viral agents, and environmental toxins are being studied.

Progression

Alzheimer's dementia may progress in stages that last several years before the onset of the next stage. The Global Deteriorating Scale (GDS) developed by Reisberg et al. is based on the clinical progression of the disease. For example, in stage I for a period of 1 to 3 years there is memory loss and loss of visuospatial skills (e.g., difficulty finding the way around the house, language changes, and personality changes). Changes begin with minor slipups and slight forgetfulness. For the next 2 to 10 years these same symptoms may get worse with the addition of praxis and acalculia. In stage III, intellectual function severely deteriorates; patients are bedridden, mute, incontinent, unable to breathe normally, sleep most of the time, and suffer with rigid limbs or remain in the fetal position. They no longer recognize self or loved ones. A simple way to remember the stages are four words: forgetful, confused, ambulatory, and **dementia.**[6] (See the box titled Signs and Symptoms of Stages of Dementia.) Certain groups of nerve cells no longer function and are destroyed. Death from aspiration, pneumonia, or infection follows the prolonged bed rest.

Treatment

Because there is no treatment or cure to stop the disease progression, care is supportive and symptomatic with the goals of keeping the patient safe from injury (e.g., falling) and from succumbing to complications of immobility. Management is directed at four areas:

- Behavioral
- Cognition
- Slowing the progression of the disease
- Delaying onset of symptoms

The approval of Cognex (tacrine HCL) as a palliative measure during clinical trials was shown to improve scores on the cognitive scale with a tendency for the effect to plateau, and to delay the disease's effects in mild to moderate Alzheimer's. Side effects include liver toxicity, cholinergic effects with nausea, vomiting, and diarrhea. Other medications that may be prescribed during home care are for sleep disturbance, depression, delusions, constipation, and antibiotics for UTIs or respiratory infections.

HOME CARE APPLICATION
Assessment

Patients with Alzheimer's requiring home care are often in the late stage of the disease and present a challenge to the family and to the nurse. When dementia impairs memory and the ability to learn, and is associated with behavior that may not be socially acceptable, caregivers may feel stressed and frustrated in their attempts to help.

After completion of a general physical assessment to evaluate vital signs, weight, nutrition, elimination, hydration, and skin, the nurse should focus on the following neurologic changes:

- Cognition (Mini-Mental State test if appropriate)
- Memory
- Level of consciousness
- Motor—apraxia with impaired ability to perform purposeful activity, ataxia unless bedridden
- Agitation and paranoia
- Combativeness
- Potential for injury

Nursing interventions

Refer to the box titled Primary Nursing Diagnoses/Patient Problems. Stimulation to promote brain activity and reduce agitation and boredom are recommended. A calm, reassuring, and respectful manner is needed to assess and treat the patient. Verbal communications may fail but a demonstration using body language can substitute for teaching the patient appropriate activities such as taking medications, eating, or transferring from bed to commode. Distraction can be used to stop unwanted aggressive behavior. (See the box titled Primary Themes of Patient Education.)

SIGNS AND SYMPTOMS OF STAGES OF DEMENTIA

Early Stage (stage I)
- Memory—forgetfulness, need for notes related to new learning, may appear absentminded
- Disorientation—cannot associate natural cues with time of day, gets easily flustered under stress
- Personality changes—mood swings, changes in affect, may appear depressed, irritable, and develop delusions of persecution, may call 911 to report burglary, may make accusations that people around them are stealing their money and personal items
- Impaired judgment—lack of judgment or unable to make logical decisions (e.g., with finances by taking money out of the bank or giving away personal property), very vulnerable
- Speech and language—inappropriate use of words or unable to name familiar objects
- Concentration—short attention span with impaired ability to concentrate
- Spatial orientation—topographic disorientation
- Activity—may appear careless, nondependable, but otherwise no motor deficits
- Nutrition—within normal limits of premorbid level of nutrition

Late stage (stage II)
- Memory—short-term and long-term memory impaired, may or may not recognize significant others
- Orientation—not oriented
- Personality—apathetic and indifferent to surroundings, socially acceptable behaviors impaired, may say things that offend, verbally abusive, very irritable, sundown syndrome
- Judgment—can not comprehend and make judgments
- Speech and language—aphasia more apparent
- Concentration—lost
- Spatial orientation—disoriented
- Activity—restless, need supervision for ambulation, unsteady, apraxic, difficulty dressing, wandering becomes a safety hazard, may become combative
- Nutrition—may have higher caloric needs related to agitation and restlessness, too restless to sit still long enough for adequate intake of food and fluids unless supervised

Final stage (stage III)
- Memory—lost
- Orientation—lost and impaired, Glasgow Coma Score decreasing
- Personality—intellect so impaired that personality is indefinable, family no longer "knows who this person is"
- Judgment—totally impaired
- Speech and language—may moan and groan to stimuli
- Concentration—totally impaired
- Spatial orientation—totally impaired
- Activity—bedridden, totally dependent, rigid and may assume fetal position, prone to skin breakdown
- Nutrition—difficult to feed, may require tube feeding or PEG tube, weight loss, incontinent of bladder and bowel
- Death—from complications of aspiration, infection, malnutrition, decubitus

The rate of progression from stage to stage varies with the individual and may depend on the quality of care and the prevention of secondary complications. The stages may span a period of 5 to 20 years. Serial EEG, CT, and MR images assist the professional caregiver and families to correlate signs and symptoms of the disease with the neurodiagnostic findings and mental status assessments.

PRIMARY NURSING DIAGNOSES/ PATIENT PROBLEMS

Alzheimer's dementia

- Altered thought processes
- Impaired memory
- Impaired communication skills
- High risk for injury
- Alterations in elimination
- Altered nutrition, less than body requirements
- Constipation/diarrhea
- Sleep pattern disturbance
- Impaired mobility
- Caregiver role strain

PRIMARY THEMES OF PATIENT EDUCATION

Alzheimer's dementia

- Preparation for long-term fatal illness
- Coping skills
- Safety
- Estate planning and/or living will

Simple speech face-to-face, calling the patient's name, and speaking slowly with a single command or statement are more effective than engaging in conversation. Attention span is short and repetition may be required along with a gentle touch.

Dehydration, malnutrition, and weight loss can be prevented by offering small frequent feedings, finger food snacks, feeding the patient, and making sure dentures fit. A large tray of food may provoke confusion whereas one choice at a time that is ground or pureed can be eaten quickly.

Supportive care focuses on a planned schedule of ADLs that begins with awakening the patient at the same hour each day, consistent mealtimes and snacks, toileting the patient every two hours, and preventing long naps that may lead to nocturnal wakefulness. If the patient is ambulatory and wandering is a problem, find a safe place to walk

in a nonstimulating location. Using large muscles for exercise such as walking is a way to decrease agitation. If agitation is related to the need for bladder or bowel evacuation, offer the patient an opportunity to walk to the bathroom or use a bedside commode.

Medications for sleep are appropriate so that the patient is rested and less agitated during the day and also for the family's benefit so that their sleep is uninterrupted during the night; however, a walk before bedtime, a warm bath, and a back massage help relax the patient and may obviate the need for medications. Psychiatric or geriatric clinical nurse specialists can also evaluate the patient and assist in making additional referrals if necessary.

Elder abuse has been recognized in the older patients whose behavior is unpredictable and stressful to the caregivers. When the family's ability to cope is stretched to the limits and the potential for abuse is suspected, the nurse's role is significant in giving the family "permission" to relinquish care to others. Nurses can collect and compile information for community services that offer respite care. The insurance or health care payer may have a program to provide a 1- or 2-week respite program to allow the caregivers a vacation. Moving the patient from the home to a new and strange environment for this short period, while advantageous for the caregiver, may cause the patient to react in negative behavior that could appear as regression. If this happens, families should be warned beforehand and prepared to cope with any temporary regression. The home health care nurse can make arrangements with the respite agency for continuation of the plan of care. The nurse is encouraged to continue seeing the patient during respite care for continuity and to forewarn the family of any behavioral or physical changes to expect on their return.

Protective services must be called if the patient shows evidence of any type of abuse (verbal or physical). The nurse is responsible for detecting abuse and should develop a "high index of suspicion" and confront the patient with questions about the appearance of bruises, fractures, burns, and pinch marks. Check the wrist and feet for evidence of physical restraints or signs of over-medication for chemical restraints. Signs that the patient has not been properly fed or nourished along with poor personal hygiene are important hallmarks of abuse. Ask the patient about family social interaction versus long periods of sensory deprivation and isolation. Reporting of inadequate funds for medical supplies may reveal that the family is reallocating or diverting the patient's finances.

After the diagnosis and recognition of dementia, families are at risk for a strain on relationships that may be expressed with anger, frustration, and resentment. Because dementia affects its victims as they look forward to and approach their retirement years, couples often feel robbed of a lifetime of working hard for the rewards of retirement. Roles must be reversed, plans for the future scrapped, and finances used for treatment and support rather than the pleasures of retirement. A spouse no longer has the mate to turn to for advice and help. On the contrary, the healthy spouse often feels compelled to conceal the stress and strain of the consequences of the illness from the spouse who is ill. The healthy spouse may try to conceal the illness from friends and relatives and go into isolation. Denial may result in frequent doctor visits to find a physician who disagrees with the diagnosis of dementia. Loss of jobs affects income and available funds for everything except necessary expenses.

Children of affected parents may feel embarrassed and refuse to participate in the care or support of the ill parent, causing further hardship for the patient. Fatigue and caregiver burnout are not uncommon. In order to prevent the depletion of lifetime savings or sale of the family home, a divorce may seem to be the only solution. Some couples have chosen this solution to bypass the regulations for health care coverage and support. Medical care and/or home care may not be prescribed during the early phase when these problems are so troublesome.

As the late stage of the illness is reached by the patient, the care and supervision become more intense. The patient may not be safe left alone. Cigarette or pipe smoking becomes particularly dangerous with patients in bed or falling asleep on a sofa or stuffed chair that could catch fire and cause serious burn wounds to the patient. Simple acts like making a cup of coffee may result in leaving a burner turned on that creates a fire, or spilling hot liquid that results in skin burns. Falling in the home when the gait becomes unsteady is problematic as the patient uses poor judgment and no longer understands limitations and safety hazards. The routine of getting up, brushing teeth, dressing, and eating becomes impaired as the disease progresses. It is not only frightening to the patient who has no understanding of the disease process, but it can also be devastating to the family members who must watch and wait with nothing to offer other than help with basic needs.

Physicians may prescribe medications (e.g., haloperidol, thiothixene, loxapine, or thioridazine) to control some of the symptomatic delusions, hallucinations, agitation, depression, or to help the patient sleep.

Eventually the patient will become completely bedridden and totally dependent. Nursing focus is the same as for any bedridden patient with problems of immobility. The family must decide if they can continue home care or if a long-term care facility is in the best interest of the patient. After a family conference, including the physician, caregivers, and social services, the necessary plans for transfer can be completed once the decision is made. Hospice care, long-term skilled care, and even special facilities for Alzheimer's patients are options for the family to consider. The guilt of "giving up" or abandonment should be dealt with during this period to calm the family's emotions. Financial concerns may complicate the decision after the cost of care is considered.

Conclusion

Degenerative disorders pose hardships for everyone concerned. Until further advances are made in pharmacologic therapy to reduce the effects, and until scientific researchers discover the cause of this devastating disease, nurses will play a vital part in helping the patient to function as long as possible until the ravages of the neuronal destruction cause death. The statistics for Alzheimer's in the future are frightening as Americans live longer only to be afflicted with a disease that robs the mind of the ability to think, to learn, to love, and to enjoy the golden years of retirement.

Patient / family / professional resources

Alzheimer's Association
70 E. Lake Street
Chicago, IL 60601-5997
Phone: (800)272-3900

SUMMARY

Three important neurologic diseases commonly seen in the home are stroke, multiple sclerosis, and dementia. Care for other neurologic illnesses has similarities in case management that can be generalized from this information. Reading this chapter, the nurse can see the importance of having a thorough understanding of neuroanatomy and neuroassessment. (For a comprehensive review of neuroscience nursing, the reader is referred to *Neuroscience Nursing* by the author, published in 1994 by Mosby.)

The nurse managing patients in the home may need to plan additional time for patients with neurologic diseases to allow for a detailed history-taking, complete general assessment, and a thorough neuroassessment. Family teaching is more demanding because of a knowledge deficit among the public concerning the cause, treatment, and outcome of neurologic disorders. Recovery may not be an option in some cases with the nursing focus on comfort and palliative care until the disease runs its course. Despair has to be countered with hope; helplessness countered with every possible community resource. Support groups, local chapters for stroke, MS, and Alzheimer's, and related groups (e.g., geriatric services) should be made available to the patient and family. Daycare, eldercare, respite care, and religious organizations can be consulted for possible assistance. The satisfaction of easing the family's burden of care and the joy of managing patients with neurologic dysfunction who can recover in their own environment surrounded by their family is a nursing specialty reserved for the home health nurse.

REFERENCES

1. Barker E: Cranial surgery. In Barker E, editor: *Neuroscience Nursing,* St Louis, 1994, Mosby.
2. Bunting L, Fitzsimmons B: Degenerative disorders. In Barker E, editor: *Neurosci Nurs,* St Louis, 1994, Mosby.
3. Donohoe KM: Autoimmune disorders. In Barker E, editor: *Neurosci Nurs,* St Louis, 1994, Mosby.
4. Kelly CL, Smeltzer SC: Betaseron: the new MS treatment, *J Neurosci Nurs* 26(1):52-56, 1994.
5. National Stroke Association: *Be smart stroke facts,* Englewood, Colo, 1994, The Association.
6. Stolley JM: When your patient has Alzheimer's, *AJN* 94(8): 34-40, 1994.
7. Whitney F: Stroke. In Barker E, editor: *Neuroscience Nursing,* St Louis, 1994, Mosby.

19 The Patient with AIDS

Robyn Rice and **David Ritchie**

The term *acquired immunodeficiency syndrome* (AIDS), a disorder of the immune system, is used to describe only the most severe diseases (e.g., opportunistic infections, neoplasms, wasting, encephalopathy) associated with infection by the human immunodeficiency virus type 1 (HIV-1).[14,16]

AIDS was initially reported in the United States with an outbreak of 25 cases in 1981.[4] Symptomatology was related to an ineffective immune system. We now know that AIDS predisposes individuals to various intermittent and debilitating diseases. These so-called opportunistic infections are rarely seen in people with intact immune systems. For example, *Pneumocystis carinii* pneumonia (PCP) and Kaposi's sarcoma, hallmark diseases of AIDS, normally do not occur in young and middle-aged adults.

HIV infection and *AIDS* are not synonymous terms; primary HIV-1 infection is followed by AIDS. In addition, HIV-1 infection does not usually imply an immediate diagnosis of AIDS. There seems to be some time lag between initial infection and the full-blown manifestation of AIDS.[14] In a study of HIV-1 infected persons, Pantaleo et al.[37] reported that clinical signs and symptoms of AIDS developed after a median time period of 10 years. Of great concern is the fact that HIV-infected carriers may be asymptomatic. Although scientists continue to discover new information about AIDS, at present there is no known cure. The course of the disease has a very wasting effect on the body. Acute infection and co-morbidities eventually result in the patient's death.[18,51]

The social ramifications of AIDS have been tremendous because it appears to be primarily a sexually transmitted disease.[7] In the United States

the homosexual/bisexual population has experienced the majority of reported cases.[11] However, the disease has now moved into the heterosexual population in the United States in increasing numbers.[11]

Sexual taboos, social prejudices, and fears of getting the disease have made case reporting and public education very difficult. In many instances, an almost universal hysteria and phobia have occurred in communities confronted with issues of caring for and living with persons with AIDS (PWAs). For example, it has been very difficult for parents to get children with AIDS enrolled in school and to keep them there.[33] Although community alliances are improving, historically the homosexual population has had problems getting the public involvement and social networking needed to respond to this epidemic. An epidemic it is; surveillance studies indicate that as of 1994, approximately 1 million persons in the United States are infected with HIV-1 with estimates that as of 1995, 250,000 to 350,000 persons will be living with an AIDS diagnosis in the United States.[11]

The revised Centers for Disease Control and Prevention (CDC) case definition of AIDS (used beginning January 1993) has resulted in a substantial increase in numbers of reported AIDS cases.[8] Once changes in the CDC case definition are accounted for, there is expected to be a plateau in overall reported cases of AIDS, although expected trends will continue to show yearly increases.[11]

At present, a person who is HIV positive and has a CD_4 count of less than 200 mm^3 is considered to have AIDS. In addition, the current CDC surveillance case definition of AIDS in the United

---

1993 CDC SURVEILLANCE CASE DEFINITION OF AIDS

CD$_4$ + T-lymphocyte categories
Category I: greater than or equal to 500 cells/µl
Category II: 200-499 cells/µl
Category III: less than 200 cells/µl

Clinical categories
Category A
• Asymptomatic HIV infection (HIV positive with no evidence of illness)
• Persistent generalized lymphadenopathy (chronically swollen glands)
• Acute (primary) HIV infection with accompanying illness or history of acute HIV infections (HIV positive with flulike illness)

Category B
Conditions with symptoms not included in the category C list, but that occur in any HIV positive person and are attributed to HIV infection. Examples of category B illnesses include thrush, early (noninvasive) cervical cancer, fever, or chronic diarrhea.
Category C
HIV positive persons who have or who have had any of the following: Candidiasis of bronchi, trachea, or lungs; Candidiasis, esophageal; Cervical cancer, invasive ('93 revision); Coccidioidomycosis, disseminated or extrapulmonary; Cryptococcosis, extrapulmonary; Cryptosporidiosis, chronic intestinal (>1 month duration); Cytomegalovirus disease (other than liver, spleen, or nodes); Encephalopathy, HIV related; Herpes simplex: chronic ulcers (>1 month duration), or bronchitis pneumonitis, or esophagitis; Histoplasmosis, disseminated or extrapulmonary; Isosporiasis, chronic intestinal (>1 month duration); Kaposi's sarcoma; Lymphoma, Burkitt's (or equivalent term); Lymphoma, immunoblastic (or equivalent term); Lymphoma, primary of brain; *Mycobacterium avium* complex, or *M. kansasii*, disseminated or extrapulmonary; *Mycobacterium tuberculosis,* pulmonary ('93 revision); *Mycobacterium,* other species, any site; *Pneumocystis carinii* pneumonia; Pneumonia, recurrent ('93 revision); Progressive multifocal leukoencephalopathy; *Salmonella* septicemia, recurrent; Toxoplasmosis of brain; Wasting syndrome due to HIV.

Note: The CDC states that HIV-infected persons should be classified using the lowest accurate, but not necessarily the most recent, CD$_4$ count.
Source: Centers for Disease Control and Prevention: 1993 Revised classification system for HIV infection and expanded surveillance case definition for AIDS among adolescents and adults, *MMWR* 41 (RR-17):1-19, 1992.

States cites a number of clinical indicator-diseases associated with AIDS.[8] (See the box above.) In using the CDC case definition for medical management, the lowest, but not necessarily the most recent, documented CD$_4$ + T-lymphocyte count should be used for classification purposes.[8]

Although the new system improves reporting, it has the potential to label HIV-1 positive, asymptomatic persons with the diagnosis of AIDS. This may carry negative psychosocial ramifications for HIV-infected individuals who are otherwise healthy and able to go about their daily routines.[38] Positive benefits of the expanded definition entail increased entitlement benefits that include home

care for eligible individuals. As a result, more PWAs will likely be seen in home care because this is probably the most cost-effective and efficient way to manage many of the health care needs of this population. The likelihood of home management of AIDS is also related to the clinical course of the disease.

Typically, PWAs contract infections and recover, only to contract further infections. Therefore most PWAs go about their normal work routines, receiving only periodic medical attention. Advanced symptomatology of AIDS requires a great deal of nursing care that can be done at home.

The purpose of this chapter is to give a general overview of HIV-1 infection and AIDS in order to assist home health nurses to prepare a plan of care for adult patients.

EPIDEMIOLOGY

More than 70% of persons diagnosed with AIDS since the 1980s have died, with 243,423 reported deaths as of 1994.[7,8] In examining trends of reported cases of AIDS within the heterosexual population, rates are highest among women, ethnic minority groups (Hispanics/African-Americans), and intravenous drug users (IDUs).[11]

Since 1987, with the introduction of zidovudine (ZDV), survival time in individuals diagnosed with AIDS has increased.[27] Although rare, HIV-1 infected people living for more than 15 years with no evidence of symptomatic disease have been reported in the literature.[25] There appears to be shorter survival time among IDUs with AIDS.[50]

The majority of children with HIV-1 infection are born to African-American and Latino women.[9] Maternal-fetal transmission is considered to be the primary mode of infection in children.[8,9]

Although AIDS has been reported in every state, rates are highest in the more heavily populated states.[8,9] The AIDS population primarily resides in metropolitan areas, but the epidemic continues to reach smaller communities.

Laboratory tests to detect HIV-1 infection identify serologic response to the virus.[16] After initial infection, antibodies usually appear within 3 to 6 weeks. Detection of HIV-1 antibodies indicates that the individual has been exposed to HIV-1, initiated an immune response, and is infectious.[14,25]

Initial screening for HIV-1 antibodies is done by the enzyme-linked immunosorbent assay (ELISA). Positive results are confirmed by the Western blot test to establish that the antibody in question is HIV-1 specific.

PATHOPHYSIOLOGY

T-cell lymphocytes (white blood cells) are responsible for cell-mediated immunity, which involves graft rejections, antigen-specific responses to intracellular parasites, and the stimulation of B-cells to make antibodies.[14,25] HIV-1 invades the bloodstream and preferentially infects T-cells.[14,25] After penetrating the T-cell, HIV uses the enzyme reverse transcriptase to copy its own genetic structure into the genome of the infected cell.

The mechanism for activation of the immune system with subsequent viral replication of HIV-1 is still under investigation. Although the infected T-cell appears to remain dormant, an active battle for control of the host may be ongoing. It is known that when stimulated by antigens (for example, by a common cold), the infected CD_4 cell (CD_4 is the receptor for HIV-1 on the T-cell lymphocyte) can reproduce the virus instead of itself.[14,25] The new HIV "buds" out and lyses the infected CD_4 cell, spilling into the bloodstream only to infect other CD_4 lymphocytes. At first, HIV interferes with the function of the CD_4 cell. Eventually, CD_4 cells die or do not reproduce themselves while B-cell function (humoral immunity) remains intact and is often hyperactive.[18] Of note, some HIV-1 strains may be more cytotoxic, destroying CD_4 cells more rapidly than other strains.[25]

Rates of HIV-1 replication may be enhanced by factors such as viral burden, age, gender, coexisting infections, congenital defects, stress, recreational drug use and alcohol use.[14,25] In addition, HIV replication may be minimal if CD_4 cells are not stimulated to reproduce.[18]

The role of HIV-1 in the pathogenesis of AIDS remains a subject for discussion. Current thinking suggests that the presence of HIV-1 along with the existence of other infectious agents may be a major factor driving the pathophysiological manifestations of AIDS.[24,34,52]

The pathophysiology of AIDS is of a progressively destructive nature. Serologically, monocyte-macrophage dysfunction, hypergammaglobulinemia, leukopenia, thrombocytopenia, and anemia can occur. Involvement of alveolar macrophages corresponds to the high incidence of pulmonary infections experienced by PWAs.[36] In addition, the virus enters the central nervous system (CNS) via infected macrophages that cross the blood-brain barrier and cause further damage[26] As a result, the loss of functional CD_4 cells and the infection of macrophages and monocytes appear to correlate with the clinical course of AIDS.[14,16,25]

HIV PRESENTATION AND CLINICAL COURSE OF AIDS

The typical course of HIV-1 infection involves[37] (1) initial infection with HIV-1 virus associated with flulike symptoms, followed by (2) a period of clinical latency (median, 10 years) during which the individual is usually symptom free, followed by (3) physical manifestations of disease, (4) the development of AIDS-indicator disease(s), and (5) eventual death.[35]

Primary infection usually develops within 3 to 6 weeks after exposure.[49] Primary HIV-1 infection can produce clinically symptomatic illness much like mononucleosis, and may require medical treatment. As the infection progresses, almost every body part including the brain is involved.

Although an HIV-infected individual can die from an initial opportunistic infection, it is much more common for a person to suffer episodes of severe illness interspersed with periods of relative wellness. Eventually, recurring infections and related symptoms of AIDS exhaust the body's reserves and ability to respond to therapy, and death results.

MECHANISM OF TRANSMISSION

HIV has been isolated from blood, semen, vaginal secretions, saliva, tears, breast milk, cerebrospinal fluid, amniotic fluid, alveolar fluid, urine, and feces.[7,9,10,11] Blood, semen, vaginal secretions, and breast milk have been implicated in transmission of HIV.[7,9]

AIDS is an insidious disease; it is usually an infected but asymptomatic person who transmits the virus to others. At present, transmission of HIV-1 is believed to occur in three ways:[7,9,11]

1. Through sexual contact
2. Through exposure to infected blood or body fluids
3. From HIV-infected women to their fetus or infant

POPULATIONS AT RISK
Homosexuals and bisexuals

In the United States, homosexual and bisexual males constitute the largest group of the AIDS population.[7,9,11] This is thought to be related to sexual practices and exposure to large numbers of sexual partners. Anal intercourse and practices such as "fisting" (inserting the hand into the anus) cause repeated tearing of mucous membranes and bleeding. Therefore the "receptive partner" is probably at highest risk for HIV infection, al-

though an open sore or lesion on the penis also provides a route of entry for the virus. The risk of oral exposure to HIV-containing semen is unknown and difficult to evaluate, because most homosexuals practice both oral and anal sex.[15] The risk of transmission of HIV via feces is unknown.

Common infections that initially occur in HIV-1 infected homosexuals and bisexuals include genital and perianal warts along with a variety of sexually transmitted diseases. Bowel disease is common in this group.

Intravenous drug users

Cases of HIV-infected IDUs have been reported in increasing numbers since the late 1980s.[9,11] The mechanism of transmission of HIV-1 in IDUs involves sharing used or "dirty" needles.[42] Practices such as "booting," whereby blood is drawn back into the syringe to extract any remaining drug, allow small amounts of HIV-infected blood to be left in the needle. This blood becomes a source of contamination for further infection. The problem of sharing dirty needles/syringes or "works" is magnified by the existence of "shooting galleries" where IDUs meet to share drugs and works.[15]

Offering commercial sex is another primary mechanism of HIV transmission for IDUs. Considering the presence of HIV-1 within the U.S. population, sex without protection may be lethal.[42]

Typical infections reported in HIV-1 infected IDUs included pneumonia, endocarditis with sepsis, tuberculosis, and coinfections with other viruses.[46] Renal disease in HIV-1 infected IDUs is common.[32] Sexually transmitted diseases, especially syphilis, are also common.[42]

Polysubstance abuse among HIV-1 infected IDUs is common and may complicate treatment. For example, mental illnesses associated with drug use include antisocial personality disorders, depression, and anxiety.[43]

Women and children

In addition to the increasing incidence of AIDS among IDUs, HIV has also moved into the heterosexual population, including women.[19] A concentration in the childbearing years raises special concerns regarding the infection of children. Of known pediatric AIDS cases, 80% can be traced to infected mothers.[19] Transmission appears to occur in utero or during labor and delivery when the infant is exposed to HIV-infected blood or other infected body fluids. Although rare, transmission through breast feeding has been reported.[53]

Hemophiliacs

In 1982 the first cases of AIDS among hemophiliacs were reported. The mechanism of transmission was exposure to commercially produced factor VIII concentrate.[31] Since March of 1985, mass screening of donated blood and plasma has almost eliminated this route of transmission. However, at least 70% of the hemophiliacs who received factor VIII from 1979 to 1986 became seropositive for HIV, and about 10% of their spouses also became HIV-infected.[31] What is now different about this risk group as opposed to the others is that fewer new cases of AIDS are being diagnosed.[11]

OCCUPATIONAL AND CASUAL TRANSMISSION

The primary route of exposure for health care workers has been by accidental needlesticks.[20,29] However, surveys of accidental HIV-infected needlesticks among health care workers demonstrat that health care workers are at minimal risk for infection.[20,23,29] McCray et al.[29] studied 124 subjects exposed to HIV-infected needlesticks and defined the rate of risk to exposure as approximately 0.5%.

Case studies have documented other mechanisms of exposure and subsequent HIV infection of home care workers. For example, one woman who provided home health care to a neighbor with AIDS subsequently contracted AIDS.[18] This woman had no known risk factors. The care she provided involved frequent and prolonged contact with the patient's secretions and excretions. The woman did not use gloves and recalled numerous small cuts on her hands and an exacerbation of chronic eczema. Based on an assessment of health care workers exposed to HIV-infected blood, the risk for HIV transmission has been estimated to be less than 0.1% for a single mucous membrane exposure (95% confidence interval = 0.006-0.05).[22]

In studies of family members of AIDS patients, cases of casual transmission are statistically low.[44,53] Activities examined in these studies included kissing, embracing, and sharing common household items (dishes, linens, and toilet facili-

ties) with the HIV-infected family member. However, as of 1995 the CDC has received reports of eight cases of HIV infection that apparently occurred following mucocutaneous exposures to blood or other body substances in persons who received care from or provided care to HIV-infected family members residing in the same household.[10] In the reported cases, exposures occurred after the source patients had developed AIDS; consequently, relatively high HIV titers may have been present in their blood.[10]

HOME CARE APPLICATION

The goals of home care should be directed toward the following:[13]

- Treating disease and ongoing symptoms
- Preventing exacerbations of disease (restoration and maintenance)
- Instructing patients and families regarding self-care management of health care needs at home.
- Anticipating and planning for any assistance the patient may require in performing activities of daily living (ADLs)
- Providing for the psychosocial and spiritual needs of the patient and family

Developing the plan of care

Initial interview. During the first visit, home health nurses should develop a plan of care based on patient and family needs. An ongoing nutritional and physical assessment and an in-depth interview will provide clues to the appropriate interventions for PWAs.

When first interviewing the patient and family, ask them what they think their biggest concerns are and how the home health agency can be of help. Obtaining answers to the questions in the box on p. 328 will help in mutually determining the plan of care. (See also the box titled Primary Nursing Diagnoses/Patient Problems.)

Patient education. Health teaching for patients and their designated caregivers will be very important. (See the box titled Primary Themes of Patient Education.) Patient education strategies should focus on promoting the patient's best level of functioning. Disease process, infection control, diet, equipment, medications, procedural care, bowel/bladder management, and tips for home

INTERVIEWING PATIENTS WITH AIDS AND THEIR FAMILIES FOR ASSESSMENT OF INITIAL NEEDS

What are the patient's living arrangements?

Does the patient's significant other or family know that the patient has AIDS? (It is not uncommon for patients to request that their mother not be told they have AIDS.)

Are there family members or a lover or a significant other who can assist with patient care as needed?

Who cooks and prepares the meals? Would a referral to a registered dietitian be helpful?

What are the patient's finances in terms of getting needed medical supplies? Would a referral to social services be helpful?

Does the patient have transportation to the grocery store or physician, and is there someone who can assist with travel as needed?

Does the patient need help with grooming, cooking, laundry, general housekeeping, etc.? Would a referral to the home health aide or personal chore worker be helpful?

What does the patient and family know about AIDS? Do they have any questions about AIDS or transmission of HIV? What does the patient know about infection control precautions? (For example, how would the patient or family care for an accidental cut on the arm or clean up a blood spill?)

Is the patient sexually active? If so, what means are being used to protect the partner?

Is the patient actively using drugs? Alcohol? (Alcohol and drug abuse can cause serious complications with prescribed therapy and treatment.)

What are the patient's wishes with respect to advanced directives? Does the patient have a living will, durable power of attorney for health care, or health care proxy?

PRIMARY NURSING DIAGNOSES/ PATIENT PROBLEMS

- Fatigue
- Knowledge deficit; home management of AIDS
- High risk for altered body temperature
- Altered nutrition; less than body requirements
- Impaired memory
- Ineffective family coping
- High risk of impaired skin integrity
- Altered oral mucosa
- Incontinence; functional
- Altered sexuality pattern
- Diarrhea; high risk for fluid volume deficit
- Pain

PRIMARY THEMES OF PATIENT EDUCATION

- Disease process; when to call the case manager and physician
- Medications
- Procedural care
- Diet
- Infection control
- Home management of AIDS (infection control, AIDS symptomatology, women's health, procedural care, home safety issues, etc.)
- Postive coping skills
- Energy conservation techniques
- Diet

maintenance should be a part of health teaching. The authors recommend *AIDS Care at Home* by J. Greif and B.A. Golden (published by Wiley in 1994) as a good home reading reference for patients and their caregivers. Instruct the patient/caregiver to immediately call the physician for severe changes in mental status, temperature, pulse, and respirations or with sudden onset of bleeding, diarrhea, vomiting, pain, seizures, or loss of vision or sensation in a body part.

This patient group can be quite challenging to teach. This is due to problems with dementia that affect memory, and to behavioral problems resulting from required lifestyle changes. Any difficulties with noncompliance or nonparticipation with the plan of care must be addressed if treatment is to be effective and safe. (See Chapter 5.)

Medications. During the initial interview, review all medications with the patient including purpose, action, dosage, side effects, and methods of administration. Although experimental studies are ongoing, at present no cure for AIDS exists.

Antiretroviral therapy, vaccines, and immune therapy are principal areas of drug research. See Table 19-1 for medications currently being used to treat HIV and associated infections in the home; be aware of the side effects that should immediately be reported to the physician.

Medication for pain management depends on patient symptoms and stage of the disease. Hydrocodone bitartrate and acetaminophen (Vicodin), oxycodone and acetaminophen (Percocet), and morphine sulfate (Roxanol) are administered for mild, moderate, and severe pain respectively. A continuous infusion of morphine may be required for end-stage disease or for severe, unrelenting pain.

Infection control. During the first visit, assess the patient and family's knowledge of infection control and the management of AIDS. AIDS patients may excrete many other infectious agents (for example, cytomegalovirus) aside from HIV. Infection control precautions, and good personal hygiene should be reinforced on each visit. Therefore instruct patients and family members in universal precautions for blood and body fluids as recommended by the CDC.[5] *Most important, emphasize that gloves must be worn whenever there is the possibility of contact with the patient's blood, vomitus, urine, feces, or other body substances (draining wounds, etc.).*

Instruct patients with AIDS to avoid cleaning the cat box or bird cage (potential source of infections) unless gloves and a mask are worn. They should not clean the fish tank because it may contain mycobacteria, which can cause acute respiratory disease.[17] Keep pets indoors exclusively so they do not pick up any infections to subsequently transmit.[17] Keep pets out of the patient's bed.

When discussing infection control, try to reassure the patient and the family that household transmission of HIV—although possible—is rare. It is important for all household members to follow infection control precautions. However, also make the point that the virus does not just jump off one person and onto another. Reinforce the idea that the *patient* is at greatest risk for infection because AIDS destroys the immune system. Therefore PWAs should avoid situations that would expose them to colds or flus. Family members with a cold or flu should wear a mask when providing care. Sick or ill friends should not visit. Pregnant women should avoid caring for relatives

with AIDS because of the many possible infections that the AIDS patients may have. (See Chapter 5 for patient teaching guidelines.)

Physical assessment and nursing management

AIDS is a disease affecting multiple body systems. In treating existing problems and preventing exacerbation of AIDS, is important for home health nurses to continuously use holistic assessment skills as a basis for practice. In providing physical care, nursing management focuses on symptom control and an understanding of any preexisting health problems, behaviors, or activities that might influence treatment. For example, gay male patients who consume large quantities of alcohol place themselves at risk for developing pancreatitis if on didanosine.[15]

General appearance. Patients typically experience premature aging and graying of hair.[14,26] Hair loss is common. Loss of facial fat, along with profound weight loss, can give these patients a gaunt appearance. Skin and mucosal membranes are typically pale in color. Problems with fatigue, fever, weight loss, and nausea are common.

Fatigue. A common complaint of most PWAs is fatigue. Low flow oxygen therapy and frequent rest periods may be helpful. Promote adequate sleep. Keep needed items at the bedside (e.g., iced water, urinal, and a towel to absorb perspiration). Plan and prioritize activities throughout the patient's day. For example, suggest resting after breakfast and before bathing. (See Chapter 10 for energy conservation tips in the home.) Consider a referral to rehabilitation and home health aide services.

Risk for altered body temperature. Instruct patients to take their temperature the same time each morning. Research suggests that 99.9° F should be the upper limit of the normal body temperature in healthy adults 40 years of age or younger.[21,28] Apply a sheet or loosely woven blanket to the patient's trunk to promote heat loss.[15] If no skin lesions are present and the patient is ambulatory, immerse the patient in a tub bath with a water temperature at 102.2° F.[22] Avoid tepid sponge baths and alcohol sponging; these cause shivering. Use cooling blankets and ice packs when core temperature is rising uncontrollably to prevent seizures.[22] Instruct the caregiver to call an ambulance if the feverish patient has a convulsion, becomes delirious, or is

Tabel 19-1 Medications currently used in the treatment of human immunodeficiency virus (HIV) infection and AIDS

Medication	Dose/route	Side effects	Major use(s)
Antiretrovirals			
Zidovudine (Retrovir)	200 mg PO q8h or 100 mg PO 3-5 times/day	Anemia, leukopenia, myopathy, hepatotoxicity, headache	HIV, $CD_4 > 500/mm^3$
Didanosine (Videx)	125-300 mg PO bid	Pancreatitis, peripheral neuropathy, insomnia	HIV, zidovudine alternative
Zalcitabine (Hivid)	0.75 mg PO tid	Peripheral neuropathy, pancreatitis, oral ulcers	HIV, zidovudine alternative
Stavudine (d4T)	Not yet established	Peripheral neuropathy, anemia, heptotoxicity	HIV, zidovudine alternative
Antifungals			
Amphotericin B (Fungizone)	1 mg IV test dose; 0.25-1 mg/kg/day maintenance dose	Nephrotoxicity, fever, chills, hypokalemia, hypomagnesemia, anemia	Cryptococcal meningitis, histoplasmosis, coccidioidomycosis, candidiasis, blastomycosis
Fluconazole (Diflucan)	50-400 mg PO or IV qd	Gastrointestinal disturbances, hepatotoxicity, rash	Cryptococcal meningitis, candidiasis
Itraconazole (Sporanox)	200-400 mg PO qd	Gastrointestinal disturbances, hepatotoxicity, hypokalemia	Histoplasmosis, blastomycosis, aspergillosis
Ketoconazole (Nizoral)	200-400 mg PO qd	Gastrointestinal disturbances, hepatotoxicity, adrenal insufficiency	Candidiasis, blastomycosis
Clotrimazole (Lotrimin)	10 mg troche dissolved in mouth 5 times/day	Mild local burning, irritation	Oral candidiasis
Flucytosine (Ancobon)	37.5 mg/kg PO q6 (target level: 25-100 mcg/mL)	Anemia, thrombocytopenia, leukopenia, gastrointestinal disturbances	Cryptococcal meningitis (with amphotericin B)
Antivirals			
Ganciclovir (Cytovene)	5 mg/kg IV q12 (treatment); 5 mg/kg IV q24 (maintenance)	Leukopenia, anemia, thrombocytopenia, CNS disturbances	Cytomegalovirus (CMV)
Foscarnet (Foscavir)	60 mg/kg IV q8 (treatment); 90-120 mg/kg/day (maintenance)	Nephrotoxicity, neurotoxicity, electrolyte disturbances, phlebitis	Cytomegalovirus (CMV)
Acyclovir (Zovirax)	200-800 mg PO 5/day or 400 mg PO bid (maintenance); 10 mg/kg IV q8	Nephrotoxicity, neurotoxicity	Herpes simplex virus (HSV), varicella zoster virus (VZV)

Tabel 19-1 Medications currently used in the treatment of human immunodeficiency virus (HIV) infection and AIDS—cont'd

Medication	Dose/route	Side effects	Major use(s)
Antiprotozoals			
Pentamidine (Pentam, IV; Nebupent, aerosol)	3-4 mg/kg IV qd (treatment); 300 mg inhaled q month (prophylaxis)	Nephrotoxicity, hypoglycemia, hyperglycemia, hypotension, hypocalcemia	*Pneumocystis carinii* pneumonia (PCP)
Trimethoprim-sulfamethoxazole (Bactrim, Septra)	15-20 mg/kg/day (TMP) IV qd; 1 DS tablet 3-7 days/week (prophylaxis)	Anemia, leukopenia, thrombocytopenia, nephrotoxicity, rash	PCP
Trimetraxate (Neutrexin)	45 mg/m^2 IV qd x 21 days (plus leucovorin 20-40 mg/m^2 for 24 days)	Neutropenia, anemia, thrombocytopenia, hepatotoxicity, fever	PCP
Atovaquone (Mepron)	750 mg PO tid (with food)	Gastrointestinal disturbances, elevated liver function tests, fever	PCP
Dapsone	100 mg PO qd (treatment); 50 mg PO qd or 100 mg PO 2/week (prophylaxis)	Hemolytic anemia, methemoglobinemia, peripheral neuropathy	PCP
Primaquine	15 mg PO qd (with clindamycin 1200-2400 mg/d)	Hemolytic anemia, methemoglobinemia, gastrointestinal disturbances	PCP
Sulfadizine	1-1.5 grams PO q6 (plus pyrimethamine 50-100 mg PO qd, leucovorin 5-10 mg qd)	Leukopenia, thrombocytopenia, anemia, rash, nephropathy	Toxoplasmosis
Pyrimethamine (Daraprim)	50-100 mg PO qd (treatment); 25-50 mg PO qd (suppressive)	Leukopenia, thrombocytopenia, anemia, glossitis, vomiting	Toxoplasmosis
Paromomycin (Humatin)	500 mg PO qid	Gastrointestinal disturbances	Cryptosporidiosis

Continued

331

Tabel 19-1 Medications currently used in the treatment of human immunodeficiency virus (HIV) infection and AIDS—cont'd

Medication	Dose/route	Side effects	Major use(s)
Antibacterials			
Clarithromycin (Biaxin)	500-1000 mg PO bid	Gastrointestinal and taste disturbances, elevated liver function tests	*Mycobacterium avium* complex (MAC)
Azithromycin (Zithromax)	500 mg PO qd	Gastrointestinal disturbances, elevated liver function tests	MAC
Rifabutin (Mycobutin)	300 mg PO qd	Gastrointestinal disturbances, neutropenia, secretion discoloration	MAC prophylaxis
Growth factors			
Filgrastim (G-CSF; Neupogen)	1-8 mcg/kg subcutaneously qd	Bone pain, fever	For zidovudine- or ganciclovir-induced neutropenia
Sargramostim (GM-CSF; Prokine or Leukine)	1-8 mcg/kg subcutaneously qd	Bone pain, fever, headache	For zidovudine- or ganciclovir-induced neutropenia
Erythropoietin (EPO; Epogen or Procrit)	100 units/kg subcutaneously 3/week	Hypertension, headache, arthralgia, diarrhea	For zidovudine-induced anemia

combative; as the patient will require immediate medical attention.

For chronic recurrent night sweats, instruct the patient to take a prescribed antipyretic before going to bed. Keep an extra set of pajamas and bed sheets on hand at night for profuse diaphoresis. Keep a plastic cover on the pillow.

Be aware that the patient is also at risk for dehydration. Increase caloric and fluid intake as needed (see the gastrointestinal section later in this chapter).

Altered nutrition; less than body requirements. Weight loss and many nutrient deficiencies seen in AIDS patients are a result of the disease. The "wasting" effect of AIDS is related to diarrhea, malabsorption, oral-esophageal problems, fever, and difficulties with swallowing and vomiting. Visually appealing meals, food supplements, and measures to control unpleasant odors may be helpful in promoting appetite.

Malnutrition augments the course of AIDS.[41,48] Therefore a well balanced diet is important to preserve lean body mass and to provide the body with reserves needed to fight infection. Take a dietary history to identify eating habits. Recommend a diet that provides adequate amounts of all nutrients, taking into account particular symptoms or difficulties the patient may be experiencing with eating. Indulge desires for favorite foods. High calorie snacks are recommended. Keep easy to prepare foods such as frozen dinners on hand. The patient should drink liquids a half an hour before eating instead of with meals in order to preserve appetite.[15]

Difficulties with diet may also be related to the patient's ability to chew, swallow, or digest food. For painful sores in the mouth, instruct the patient to avoid acidic foods (such as citrus/pineapple), extremely hot or cold food and beverages; and rough foods (such as raw fruits and vegetables). Encourage patients to eat nonabrasive, easy to eat foods such as ice cream, pudding, noodle dishes, and soft cheeses.[48] Eating popsicles will numb mouth pain. Instruct the patient to use a straw to make swallowing easier.[15] Consider a referral to the registered dietitian and refer the patient to community resources for support services, (e.g., meals-on-wheels).[48]

Knowledge deficit; nausea management. Problems with nausea and vomiting are frequently a side effect of the various medications prescribed to treat the symptoms of AIDS. Discontinuation of the offensive medications is one solution. Administration of antiemetics (Reglan, Compazine) may be useful. Consider the use of cannabinoids such as dronabinol; they may control nausea and stimulate appetite.[40] Nasogastric feedings may be required for patients with severe nausea and vomiting associated with significant weight loss.[48]

Avoid offensive cooking odors by keeping windows open and the home well aerated. Instruct the patient to try cold entrees rather than hot ones because they have less odor and are often better tolerated.[15,48]

Soft foods, liquid meals, or canned supplements may be tolerated better than solids, depending on the type of infection or gastrointestinal disease.[48] The patient may want to avoid greasy, fatty, or spicy foods, because they can aggravate gastrointestinal absorptive disorders.[15,41]

Head, ears, eyes, nose, throat. There are many oral opportunistic disorders associated with HIV (including infections, cancers, and other lesions).[45] Examine the lips for vesicles or pustules indicative of herpes simplex virus (HSV). HSV can be treated with intravenous or oral acyclovir.

Oral cavity disease is common, especially oral thrush and hairy leukoplakia. Oral thrush appears as yellowish-white plaques on the mucosa. These can progress into the esophagus, causing a sore throat and difficulty swallowing. Hairy leukoplakia has a white-ribbed or fibrous appearance and is most commonly found along the sides of the tongue. Fungal infections of the mouth can be treated with clotrimazole troches and lozenges, nystatin, or systemic azole antifungals.[45]

Altered oral mucous membrane. Erosion of the gingiva, associated with painful and bleeding gums, is common in HIV disease. Therefore good dental hygiene should be recommended as a part of the treatment. Patients should routinely brush the teeth using a soft toothbrush and avoid flossing near the gum line. Dental visits should be encouraged.

If an infection or lesion is in the mouth, suggest that patients use Toothettes (small sponge-tipped swabs) when brushing their teeth. This may be followed with a half-strength hydrogen peroxide mouthwash.[17] A Betadine rinse or antibacterial mouthwash (for example, chlorhexidine) may be helpful.

Avoid commercial mouthwashes with alcohol or glycerine that dry out the mouth.[15,17] Suggest commercially prepared artificial saliva for problems with a dry mouth; use lip balms to keep lips moist. Instruct the patient to suck on sugarless hard candies for dryness of the mouth.[15,17]

Acute and painful ulcerations may develop on the soft palate, making eating difficult. Topical applications of viscous lidocaine, triamcinolone acetonide (0.1% in Orabase), or thalidomide may relieve the pain of swallowing. Patients should avoid wearing loose fitting dentures, which may cause a mouth lesion. Consult with the dentist.

Impaired vision. Cytomegalovirus (CMV) retinopathy is the most frequently occurring eye infection in PWAs and essentially destroys the retina. If the infection reaches the optic nerve, a total loss of vision occurs. CMV retinitis is typically treated with ganciclovir. Because PWAs are prone to eye infections, do not allow them to wear contacts overnight.

What is the patient's ability to perform activities of daily living (ADLs)? Check vision and assist patients to cope with any loss. For example, instruct the patient and family to place items required for ADLs in a familiar spot. Talking clocks and watches are available. Patients may enjoy listening to the radio or tapes of books.[6]

Encourage home independence in activities such as feeding. For example, suggest the use of finger foods as snacks and use cups for liquid such as soaps. In addition, describe the location of eating utensils when serving food and identify locations of food on a plate referring to a clock (e.g., the meat is at 6 o'clock and the potatoes are at 2 o'clock).[15,17]

Review general safety measures for the home. Avoid changing or moving furniture in the home and avoid unsecured area rugs.

Cardiopulmonary. Cardiac disorders are common in HIV-infected patients and may include pericardial effusions, mitral valve regurgitation, and dysrhythmias. Kaposi's sarcoma can invade the heart wall, causing valvular dysfunction. Auscultate for abnormal heart sounds and murmurs, and check the patient's heart rate. Report deviations from baseline status and whenever the patient's symptoms to the physician.

Pulmonary infections are also common. Approximately 60% of AIDS patients develop pneumonia.[14] *Pneumocystis carinii* pneumonia (PCP) is the predominant diagnosis. Tuberculosis also occurs in this group. Assess the patient for changes in cough, sputum production, and lung sounds, such changes could indicate a new or recurring lung infection.

Activity intolerance; ineffective breathing pattern. Instruct patients to notify the physician or home health nurse immediately if they experience excessive coughing, shortness of breath, and changes in color or amount of sputum; these are signs and symptoms of pulmonary infection.

If coughing is an ongoing problem, encourage the patient to take cough medications as scheduled. Cough drops and tea with lemon and honey may be helpful.[17] Warm saline gargles may relieve a sore throat. Hydrate the patient with 2 to 3 L of fluid a day if possible to reduce coughing related to viscous pulmonary secretions.[15]

If dyspnea is an ongoing problem, instruct the patient in energy conservation techniques such as pursed-lip breathing and planned rest periods between activities. Have the patient avoid environmental stressors such as cold air, smoke, and air pollution. As appropriate, instruct patients to increase fluid intake to thin their mucus secretions for easier expectoration. Also, room humidification may be helpful. As ordered, encourage use of prn oxygen to help with dyspnea. A referral to rehabilitation services may be appropriate in order to improve activity tolerance.

Neurologic. Depending on central nervous system (CNS) involvement, AIDS patients may experience behavioral changes such as forgetfulness and difficulty with recall. A photophobia may indicate cryptococcal meningitis, which is accompanied by mood swings and headaches. If the spinal cord becomes involved, paralysis may develop. Fluconazole and amphotericin B are being used to treat cryptococcal meningitis.[2,47] The use of fluconazole is promising because this drug does not have the extreme side effects caused by amphotericin B.[2]

Impaired memory. Personality changes and a decline in judgment and comprehension can occur and may be followed by blindness and seizures.[5] The patient may realize that mental functioning is deteriorating and become angry or depressed.

AIDS dementia may result with brain infection. As the disease advances, the patient may lose interest in outside activities and become indifferent and withdrawn. These patients sometimes assume an almost fetal position in bed.

Provide written schedules for patients with mental status changes and encourage everyone involved in the patient's care to adhere to the schedule as much as possible.[15,17] Keep calendars with current dates and pictures of loved ones nearby to help the patient orient to reality. Use clocks with AM and PM indicators. Always address the patient by name and maintain face-to-face contact during interactions. Have the patient dress and groom daily; do not permit patients to go unkempt and unbathed.

Provide for home safety; include the caregiver in all aspects of health teaching. Maintain good lighting. Eliminate throw rugs to decrease the possibility of falls. Remove all loose wires and electrical cords from high-traffic areas.[17] **Never leave household cleansers or other potential poisons in unmarked containers near medications or food.** Instruct patients/caregivers to keep a list of vital telephone numbers within reach at all times (physician, hospital, emergency ambulance service, poison control center, suicide/crisis/substance abuse intervention hotline, police, fire department). Discourage guns in the home.

Dark glasses may help if the patient complains of photophobia. Consider a referral to the psychiatric home health nurse for behavioral problems. (Refer to Chapters 18 and 23.)

Pain. Remember that the patient's self-report of pain is the most reliable indicator of location and intensity. Provide pharmacological interventions to reduce pain and control anxiety. Be aware that opioid analgesic requirements for severe pain are individualized for comfort; physician orders should include "rescue" doses when regularly scheduled doses are insufficient.[15] Nursing care should also focus on patient comfort measures. (See Chapter 25.)

Integumentary. Depressed cellular immunity is responsible for the majority of the viral and fungal infections common with AIDS patients. Skin disorders increase as the number of CD_4 cells declines.[14]

Inspect the skin for lesions, rashes, wounds, or signs of inappropriate needle marks. Examine the axillary and inguinal lymph nodes for swelling or tenderness. Report findings to the physician as appropriate.

Risk for impaired skin integrity. Typically, AIDS patients have very dry, scaly skin. This may be related to malabsorption of fatty acids which causes dryness and premature aging of the skin. Dry skin and problems with immobility and poor nutrition can predispose these patients to pressure sores. If the patient suffers from diarrhea, skin integrity is threatened.

Report reddened areas or signs of skin breakdown to the physician for a wound care protocol. Research suggests that occlusive dressings such as Stomahesive, Op-Site, and Duo-Derm are contraindicated in immunocompromised patients.[15,30]

Bath oils, liquid emollient soaps, and moisturizers can be used to alleviate dry skin. Avoid tub baths if skin lesions are present. As appropriate, instruct the family in wound and skin care. (See Chapter 13.)

Gastrointestinal. AIDS patients are at risk for a variety of gastrointestinal infections and disease. Instruct the patient and caregiver to thoroughly scour all fresh vegetables because AIDS patients are vulnerable to *Salmonella, Shigella,* and other bacteria. Unpasteurized milk products should be avoided, and meats should be thoroughly cooked.

Diarrhea; high risk for fluid volume deficit. Cryptosporidiosis and CMV are frequently the cause of diarrhea with AIDS.[14] Ganciclovir may be useful in treating CMV diarrhea.

A low residue, high protein, high calorie diet is recommended.[12] Potassium-rich foods such as bananas, apricots, or baked potatoes (without butter) will help correct the hypokalemia that is often associated with large fluid losses.[41] It may be necessary to restrict dietary fiber and provide nutrient supplements (Ensure) until diarrhea is resolved.[15,48]

Instruct the patient to avoid raw vegetables and fresh salads. With acute onset of diarrhea, AIDS patients may lose gallons of fluid each day and be at risk for dehydration. Assess the patient for signs and symptoms of dehydration such as hypotension and poor skin turgor. When appropriate, encourage fluids (2 to 3 L a day) and instruct the caregiver to offer fluids to the patient frequently.[15] For severe dehydration, the patient may require normal saline intravenously.[48] It may be necessary to obtain a blood specimen for laboratory evaluation (e.g., SMA6) of electrolyte status. Kaopectate and Immodium, or Lomotil may be useful to treat diarrhea.

Incontinence; functional. Chux, a type of incontinence pad or adult diaper, may be helpful in managing acute episodes of diarrhea. Recommend the use of moisture barrier creams around the anus to prevent excoriation. Instruct the patient and caregiver to cleanse the area with warm, soapy water **and** commercial spray cleansers (e.g., Peri Wash) immediately after episodes of diarrhea; then rinse, pat dry, and apply A and D ointment or skin barrier cream (gloves should be worn during this procedure).[15,17,41] For severe diarrhea, fecal incontinence pouching devices can be worn. Instruct the patient to avoid anal intercourse or oral-anal sexual activities.

Genitourinary. Ask patients if they are having any problems with itching, warts, or sores. Examine areas of concern. HSV often appears around the anus or vulva. These lesions appear as small, red ulcers and are painful. Acyclovir is the treatment of choice for HSV.

Evaluate males for testicular swelling, which could indicate that Kaposi's sarcoma has invaded the inguinal area.[16] A scrotal support or sling may provide comfort.

Ask female patients if they are having any problems with vaginal discomfort or unusual discharge. As appropriate, obtain a specimen for laboratory analysis and institute treatment. *Good personal hygiene should be highly reinforced.*

Altered sexuality pattern; sexual dysfunction. It is advisable to ask the patient about sexual habits. Sexual practice is a very personal and sensitive subject; respect it as such. Encourage safe sex, and discourage multiple sexual partners. Review the proper use of condoms, which have been shown to be helpful in preventing infection (Figure 19-1).[7,17,19] Make sure the patient understands that AIDS is most often transmitted during sex. The patient may wish to refrain from sex or explore other methods of expressing affection.

Incontinence; functional. Urinary incontinence related to neurologic impairment or weakness may become a problem for PWAs. Male patients may benefit from an external or condom catheter in controlling incontinence. A urinary incontinence pouching device can be worn by female patients. Avoid indwelling catheters when possible because of the risk of infection in immunosuppressed patients. Problems with urinary retention can be managed by intermittent or straight catheterization. (See Chapter 15.)

Knowledge deficit; women's health. Women with AIDS may not always continue to menstruate depending on how the physical and emotional stressors of the disease have affected their hormones. It will be important for women with AIDS to keep track of their menstrual period so they can inform their physician of any missed cycles or change in the frequency, flow, or length of their periods. HIV-infected women should be encouraged to use a reliable method of birth control to avoid becoming pregnant because of the risk of transmission of HIV from mother to child.[7,11]

Instruct caregivers to always wear gloves when changing a sanitary napkin or tampon for a female patient. Tampons should be changed every 2 to 4 hours and not worn overnight.[17] Follow local health ordinances regarding disposal of infectious waste.

Instruct women with AIDS to wear cotton underwear in order to avoid vaginitis. In addition, douching is not recommended because it may promote vaginal infections.

When providing care for patients with AIDS, treatment addresses the symptoms of the disease and the infection itself. (Refer to *HIV/AIDS: A Guide to Nursing Care* by J.H. Flaskrud and P. Ungvarski as an additional resource when caring for PWAs.)

Nursing interventions should consider comfort level along with maintenance and restoration of health. Once basic physiological needs are met, it is possible to address the psychosocial and spiritual needs of these patients and their families. Therein may lie the greatest challenge for effective intervention.

Living at home with AIDS

The reality for many PWAs is that they have a horrific disease for which there is no known cure. Psychosocial problems are largely related to loss.[1,15] Perhaps the best insight into what living with AIDS is like comes from considering what patients have lost as a result of the disease:

- General good health, supplanted by a persistent feeling of malaise and weakness
- Independence and mobility, which may create changes in role and identity
- Attractive appearance or body image, as a result of the many infections and skin disorders, cancers, premature aging, and hair and weight loss related to AIDS

How to Use a Condom in Five Easy Steps

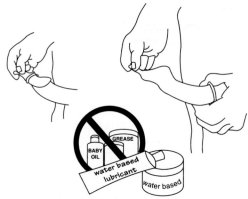

1. Apply the rolled-up condom to the penis when it is erect, leaving space at the tip to act as a reservoir for semen to be collected. If the penis has a foreskin (is not circumcised), pull back the foreskin before putting on the condom.
2. Unroll the condom completely to the base of the penis. (If you decide to lubricate the condom, remember to do so only with water-based lubricants.)

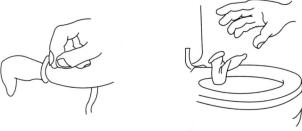

3. Immediately after ejaculation, hold the condom at the base of the penis to secure it in place as you carefully withdraw the penis. Take care not to spill any of the semen inside your partner's body.
4. Dispose of the used condom in the manner in which you dispose of all contaminated waste. (See Chapter 5; Injection Control in the Home.)
5. Wash your penis with soap and water.

Figure 19-1 How to use a latex condom. (From Greif J, Golden BA: *AIDS care at home: a guide for patients, caregivers, and loved ones and people with AIDS,* p. 165. Copyright © 1994 John Wiley & Sons. Reprinted by permission.)

- Appetite and the ability to swallow
- Support systems and networking (possibly family, friends, and lover), as part of the social stigma and fear connected with AIDS
- Financial stability, resulting from job loss and resources drained by medical bills
- The right to a long and happy life

Such losses are not easy for the patient and family to accept. AIDS strikes most patients at a very creative and productive time of life, usually between the ages of 30 and 39.[7] Issues of death and dying are understandably hard for this relatively young population to contemplate, much less accept.

Ineffective family coping. Conflicts among the patient and family/significant others may occur and are exacerbated by the exhaustive nature of the disease. If the patient is gay, the family may still be adjusting to that fact, and feelings of guilt or fear of gossip or social prejudice may incline family members to isolate themselves from relatives, neighbors, or friends who could otherwise be a source of comfort and support.

Considering the losses involved in living with AIDS, the home health nurse should be prepared to witness feelings of anger, guilt, and depression expressed by the patients, families, and significant others.[4] Opening lines of communication is the best intervention when providing care for these patients and their families. Listen to patient and family concerns, and provide reassurance and resources as needed. Maintain confidentiality. Find out what the patient's wishes are with respect to aggressive medical therapy should the patient become unable to make decisions. Make sure the patient's wish is communicated to the family because they may have influence in this decision. If appropriate, do not hesitate to suggest pastoral care or hospice as a way of furthering good communication and support and possibly preparation for death.

Caregivers may become overwhelmed with the patient's multiple health care needs. The key to successful caregiving is to encourage caregivers to attend to their own needs, too. As a result, caregiver respite services or alternate living arrangements for the patient may become necessary. A referral to social services is suggested.

A multidisciplinary team approach is best when providing the many services required by PWAs. Plan visits and coordinate the services of other disciplines on the basis of evolving patient needs and losses during the course of illness. Exploring financial concerns will also give insights into the patient's needs and worries. A community assessment should identify easily accessible grocery stores and transportation for the patient/caregiver.

SUMMARY

It is likely that a larger number of PWAs will be cared for outside the hospital in the next decade. As a result, home health organizations will be providing service for great numbers of these patients.[6,7,11]

In today's society, HIV infection and AIDS are associated with powerful emotional issues and the vast complexities of disease manifestation. Understanding AIDS, its mechanisms of transmission and pathogenesis, along with the psychosocial issues involved with this epidemic equips home health nurses with the scientific knowledge and the sensitivity needed to practice in this special arena of home care.

HIV has no known cure. However, in this world, all things are possible and our patient's hopes for a better tomorrow should never be discouraged. Key interventions are to provide our patients with information that alleviates symptoms of the disease. As professionals, it is important to offer ourselves as caring individuals. For our patients being home, does not necessarily mean being alone. . .

REFERENCES

1. Aranda-Naranjo B: The effect of HIV on the family, *AIDS Patient Care* 7(1):27-29, 1994.
2. Arndt C, Walsh T, McCully L et al: Fluconazole penetration into cerebrospinal fluid: implications for treating fungal infections of the central nervous system, *Infect Dis* 157:178, 1987.
3. Carr G, Gayling G: Aids and AIDS-related conditions: screening for populations at risk, *Nurs Pract* 11(10):25, 1986.
4. Centers for Disease Control and Prevention: Pneumocystis pneumonia—Los Angeles, *MMWR* 30:250, 1981.
5. Centers for Disease Control and Prevention: Recommendations for prevention of HIV transmission in health-care settings, *MMWR* 36:35-185, 1987.
6. Centers for Disease Control and Prevention: Summary of notifiable diseases—United States, *MMWR* 37(54):1-57, 1989.
7. Centers for Disease Control and Prevention: Update: acquired immunodeficiency syndrome—United States 1989, *MMWR* 39(5):81, 1990.
8. Centers for Disease Control and Prevention: 1993 Revised classification system for HIV infection and expanded surveillance case definition for AIDS among adolescents and adults, *MMWR* 41(RR-17):1-19, 1992.
9. Centers for Disease Control and Prevention: Revised guidelines for the performance of CD_4+ T-cell determinations in persons with human immunodeficiency virus (HIV) infection, 1994.
10. Centers for Disease Control and Prevention: Human Immunodeficiency virus transmission in household settings—United States, *MMWR* 43(19):347-356, 1994.
11. Centers for Disease Control and Prevention: Telephone conversation with statistics department in Atlanta, 1995.
12. Culhane B: Diarrhea. In Yasko JM, editor: *Nursing management of symptoms associated with chemotherapy*, Restan, Va, 1984 Restan Publishing.
13. Dhundale K, Hubbard P: Home care for the AIDS patient: safety first, *Nursing 86* 16(9):34, 1986.

14. Fauci A: Immunopathogenic mechanisms of HIV infection: implications for therapeutic strategies, International Conference on AIDS, abstract no PS-01-3, 9(1):9, 1993.

15. Flaskrud JH, Ungvarski P: *HIV/AIDS-a guide to nursing care* Philadelphia, 1995, WB Saunders.

16. Gold JW: HIV-1 infection, diagnosis and management, *Med Clin North Am* 76(1):1-18, 1992.

17. Greif J, Golden BA: *AIDS care at home,* New York, 1994, John Wiley & Sons.

18. Grint P, McEvoy M: Two associated cases of the acquired immunodeficiency syndrome (AIDS), *Communic Dis Rep* 1:42, 1986.

19. Guinan M, Hardy A: Epidemiology of AIDS in women in the states: 1981 through 1986, *JAMA* 257:2039, 1986.

20. Henderson D: HIV infection: risks to health care workers and infection control, *Nurs Clin North Am* 23(4):767, 1988.

21. Holtzclaw BJ: The febrile response in critical care: state of the art science, *Heart and Lung* 21(5):482-501, 1992.

22. Ippolito G, Puro V, De Carli G: Italian study group on occupational risk of HIV infection, the risk of occupational human immunodeficiency virus infection in health care workers: Italian multicenter study, *Arch Intern Med* 153:1451-1458, 1993.

23. Kuhls T, Viker S, Parris N et al: Occupational risk of HIV, HBV, and HSV-2 infections in healthcare personnel caring for AIDS patients, *Am J Public Health* 77:1306, 1987.

24. Lemaitre M, Henin Y, Destousse F et al: Role of mycoplasma infection in the cytopathic effect induced by human immunodeficiency virus type-1 in infected cell lines, *Infection and Immunity* 60(3):742-748.

25. Levy JA: HIV pathogenesis and long-term survival, *AIDS* 7(11):1401-1410, 1993.

26. Libman H: HIV pathogenesis, natural history and classification of HIV infection, *Prim Care* 19(1):1-17, 1993.

27. Lundgren JD et al: Comparision of long-term patients with AIDS treated and not treated with zidovudine, *JAMA* 271(14):1088-1092, 1994.

28. Makowiak PA, Wasserman SS, Levine MM: A critical appraisal of 98.6 degrees F, the upper limit of the normal body temperature, and other legacies of Carel Reinhold August Wunderlick, *JAMA* 268(12):1578-1580, 1993.

29. McCray E et al: Cooperative needlestick surveillance group: occupational risk of the acquired immunodeficiency syndrome among health care workers, *N Engl J Med* 314(17):1127, 1986.

30. McDonnell M, Sevedge K: Acquired immune deficiency syndome (AIDS). In Brown MH et al, editors: *Standards of oncology practice,* New York, 1992, John Wiley & Sons.

31. McGrady G, Janson J, Evatt B: The cause of the epidemic of acquired immunodeficiency syndrome in the United States hemophilia population, *Am J Epidemiol* 126(1):25, 1987.

32. Miller FH, Parikh S, Gore RM et al: Renal manifestations of AIDS, *Radiographics* 13(3):587-596, 1993.

33. Monmaney T: Kids with AIDS, *Newsweek* 9:51, 1987.

34. Montagnier L, Blanchard A: Mycoplasmas as cofactor in infection due to human immunodeficiency virus, *Clin Infect Dis* 17(Suppl 1):S309-S315, 1992.

35. Nahlen BL, Chu SY, Nwanyanwu OC et al: HIV wasting syndome in the United States, *AIDS* 7(2):183-188, 1993.

36. Nash G, Said JW, editors: *Pathology of AIDS and HIV infection,* Philadelphia, 1992, WB Saunders.

37. Pantaleo G, Graziosi C, Fauci AS: The immunopathogenesis of human immunodeficiency virus infection, *N Eng J Med* 328(5):327-335, 1993.

38. Park RA: European AIDS definition (news), *Lancet* 339(8794):671, 1992.

39. Pfeiffer N: Long-term survival and HIV disease-the role of exercise and CD_4 response in HIV disease, *AIDS Patient Care* 6(5):237-239, 1992.

40. Plasse TF, Gorter RW, Krasnow SH et al: Recent clinical experience with dronabinol, *Pharmacol Biochem Behavior* 40(3): 695-700.

41. Resler S: Nutrition care of the AIDS patients, *J Am Dietetic Assoc* 88(7):828, 1988.

42. Rolfs RT, Goldberg M, Sharrar RG: Risk factors for syphilis: cocaine use and prostitution, *Am J Public Health* 80(7): 853-857, 1990.

43. Ross HE, Glaser FB, Germanson T: The prevalence of psychiatric disorders in patients with alcohol and other drug problems, *Arch Gen Psychiatry* 45(11):1023-1031, 1988.

44. Sande M: Transmission of AIDS: the case against casual contagion, *N Engl J Med* 314(6):380, 1986.

45. Sears C: The oral manifestations of AIDS, *AIDS Patient Care* 3(4):8, 1989.

46. Stoneburner RL, DesJarlais DC, Benezra D et al: A larger spectrum of severe HIV-1 related disease in intravenous drug users in New York City, *Science* 242(4880):916-918, 1988.

47. Sugar A, Saunders C: Oral fluconazole as suppressive therapy of disseminated cryptococcus in patients with acquired immunodeficiency syndrome, *Am J Med* 85:481, 1988.

48. The Task Force on Nutrition Support in AIDS: Guidelines for nutrition support in AIDS, *AIDS Patient Care* 3(4):32, 1989.

49. Tindall B, Cooper DA: Primary infection: host responses and intervention strategies, *AIDS* 5(1):1-14, 1991.

50. Tu XM, Meng X, Pagnano M: Survival differences and trends in patients with AIDS in the United States, *J AIDS* 6(10):1150-1156, 1993.

51. Ungvarski P: *Co-morbidities of HIV-1/AIDS in adults.* HIV/AIDS Nursing Care Summit. Washington, DC, Jan 27, 1994.

52. Wang RY, Shih JW, Grandinetti T et al: High frequency of antibodies to mycoplasma penetrans in HIV-infected patients, *Lancet* 340(8831):1312-1316, 1991.

53. Ziegler J, Cooper D, Johnson R et al: Postnatal transmission of AIDS-associated retrovirus from mother to infant, *Lancet* 1:896, 1985.

Special Clinical Issues

20 The Pediatric Patient: Failure to Thrive

Catherine A. White and *Robyn Rice*

The term *failure to thrive* has been used to describe infants and children whose weight and often height fall below expected standards. The term refers to symptoms rather than a specific cause. Although various definitions of this condition have appeared in the literature, there seem to be two distinctive categories: organic failure to thrive and nonorganic failure to thrive. Organic growth failure stems from a variety of physical causes including metabolic diseases, major organ defects, neurologic lesions, and genetic defects. Nonorganic growth retardation, or growth failure for which there is no organic explanation, involves psychosocial factors.

Caring for the failure to thrive child can be complex and frustrating, but also challenging for home health nurses. Both the family and the child are considered the focus for intervention. Interacting within the family environment requires complex and sensitive interventions by home health nurses, and a multidisciplinary team approach is often essential. Family structure, value systems, religious beliefs, educational levels, learning styles, communication patterns, and compliance with recommendations are but a few of the issues relevant to the child's well-being.[2,3,8,18,23] Family participation is elemental to the plan of care.

This chapter reviews family dynamics as related to the psychosocial and physiological manifestations of failure to thrive. There is a strong emphasis in this chapter on the nutritional needs of the failure to thrive patient. This information will assist home health nurses in developing a plan of care for these children and their families.

PATHOPHYSIOLOGY

Both congenital and acquired organic functional disorders can lead to growth retardation. The box on p. 344 lists these disorders and their manifestations. In addition, prenatal events, such as maternal smoking, alcohol or drug abuse (e.g., heroin, cocaine, and crack), therapeutic medication use (e.g., anticonvulsant therapy), and maternal infections can adversely affect the infant's growth rate and development.

A recently published study of preterm and low birth weight infants found failure to thrive to be a common problem. It also found associated "worse" 3-year outcomes in health, growth and development, and cognitive status in this population as compared to normally growing infants.[19] Clinical manifestations of failure to thrive are primarily associated with growth and feeding problems and include the following:[2,14,17]

- Weight below the third percentile
- Sudden or rapid deceleration in the growth rate
- Delay in developmental milestones, especially gross motor and vocalization skills
- Significant environmental and/or psychosocial disruption within the family

Understanding the family and home environment may provide home health nurses with further clues about the lack of growth and development.

PSYCHOSOCIAL ISSUES: UNDERSTANDING THE FAMILY

A *family* may be defined as a group of individuals residing in the same household and sharing significant

---

PATHOPHYSIOLOGICAL MANIFESTATIONS OF FAILURE TO THRIVE[17,33,34]

Cardiac
Congenital heart defects
Acquired congestive heart failure related to bronchopulmonary dysplasia

Respiratory
Bronchopulmonary dysplasia
Cystic fibrosis

Central nervous system
Intracranial hemorrhage
Asphyxia
Meningitis/encephalitis
Other conditions resulting in poor oral motor functioning

Gastrointestinal
Milk or food intolerance
Digestive enzyme deficiency
Malabsorption disease (e.g., Hirschsprung, celiac disease)
Parasite infestation
Infection
Inflammatory or ulcerative conditions
Structural abnormalities (e.g., gastroesophageal reflux, pyloric stenosis)

Renal
Structural abnormalities
Infection
Injury

Endocrine
Cystic fibrosis
Thyroid disorders (hypothyroidism)

Genetic/chromosomal
Idiopathic short stature
Other disorders resulting in poor oral and motor functioning and/or poor growth patterns

---

tion on the plan of care is best accomplished by reviewing family systems theory and dynamics of the family unit.

Family systems theory

The family can be viewed as a social system with shared values and goals. It has a complex communication system and boundaries with variable allowances for movement across the divisions. Relationships within the family are both intimate and purposeful, with an individual member's actions and responses affecting the entire family system.

Viewing the family as a social system gives home health nurses a functional family model useful in developing the plan of care. The following elements are integral parts of this model.

Social system. Predictable responses and behaviors that characterize the lifestyle patterns of the family members are produced by the family's social system. As a component of the system, each member influences the overall living pattern of the family.[5]

Shared goals and values. Goals are developed to satisfy the needs of the family members as a group and to bring the members together. The family goals reflect the members' social status, value system, and fundamental beliefs. By considering the family's goals and values, the home health care nurse gains insight into the decision making capabilities of the family unit and a better understanding of how members assign priorities to their needs. In addition, these goals and values directly determine developmental tasks throughout the life span of the family and can determine nurturance, expectations as social beings, and the release of members into society.[12]

Complex communication system. The communication system governs not only how the members communicate within the family but also how the members communicate within the larger community. Understanding communication lines and barriers is essential in working with the family in the home setting.

Boundaries. Although invisible to the eye, boundaries may provide major obstacles to intervention. Boundaries may prevent members from moving easily within and outside of the family structure and impede the flow of communication. Families of failure to thrive infants tend to set up well defined boundaries that restrict the movement of family members to the point of isolating them

emotional bonds and a commitment to one another.[12,15,27] Significant emotional bonds consist of emotional gratification, affection, care, interdependence, responsibility, loyalty, accountability, and commitment.[13,21] Understanding the impact of illness on the family and the impact of family interaction from the community, neighbors, and sometimes even relatives or friends.

Interrelatedness. As one of the hallmarks of the family system, interrelatedness of the members is an important factor for home health nurses to appraise. The term implies that although each family member responds and reacts as an individual entity, the response affects the entire family structure. As a result, the failure to thrive child sends a ripple that is felt throughout the entire family, and each member responds to the child and illness. Therefore the plan of care for a family must consider each member of the family system.

Dynamics of the family unit

The dynamics of the family unit influence how the family members interact with one another and with the greater community. These dynamics are based on the following elements.

Roles. Family role assignments influence tasks, communication, relationships, and power. Family roles may assume several different patterns:

- Flexible: woman as a mother, wife, and wage earner
- Rigid: woman as homemaker, wife, and mother only
- Reversed: woman as wage earner; man as child care provider
- Changed: woman going back to work after children reach school age; father taking leave from paid work to care for a newborn

Family roles influence the basic functioning of the family unit, and indicate the ability for change.[24]

Rules. Rules reflect the attitudes and values of the family and provide a basis for action and relationships both within and outside of the family unit. Rules may or may not be well delineated and defined, but it is usually expected that they will be followed. When rules are broken, punishment generally ensues regardless of whether or not the rule is known and understood by the family member. Failure to thrive infants may be subjected to rigid rules of behavior that they are not capable of knowing or understanding.

Tasks and functions. Families use tasks or functions to operate effectively and meet responsibilities. These tasks change focus as the family grows and matures. Family functions and individual tasks

are dynamic concepts that change with the family's and members' developmental needs.[8]

Communication. Communication is the basis for interaction, both within the family unit and in the external environment. Communication styles are closely related to roles and rules and provide a basis for decision making. Communication difficulties provide challenges in caring for the family.

Family communication is controlled by a number of influencing variables.[13,32] These variables can include temporary conditions such as illness, fatigue, and stress; or more permanent individual characteristics such as anxious, relaxed, and rigid behaviors. These variables influence family members' interactions and relationships developed and maintained outside of the family structure. Of note, many families of failure to thrive infants have limited communication skills and tend to limit relationships outside the family unit.

Developmental tasks

As a family begins and grows, each additional member adds complexity to the system as a whole.[9] A birth or adoption necessitates changes and restructuring of roles and tasks and affects interaction styles.

During early infancy, the family is faced with the work of identifying the role of parent while maintaining and modifying the established roles of spouse and individual within the system. Studies have indicated that early parenthood is a critical period of adjustment and that marital satisfaction can decrease following the birth of a baby.[10,13,21,27]

Each new addition to the family requires a reorganization. The mother assumes primary caretaking tasks in most situations. Throughout the past three decades, theorists have examined mothering from various aspects, ranging from the concept of an innate mothering instinct[4] to the concept of an acquired mother/infant relationship.[1,7,20] Rubin concludes that mothering is a learned behavior, whereas motherliness is an emotional feeling that develops as the mother has increasing contact with her child.[28] Both Benedek and Rubin view mothering feelings as a reflection of significant relationships in the woman's life. Therefore motherliness does not originate with the birth of a child but evolves from psychic, developmental, and relationship experiences prior to the child's birth.

During early maternal role development the mother usually becomes engrossed with the care and needs of the infant. This early interaction period may be pivotal because the mother's self-esteem is tied closely with her ability to care for her infant. She tends to be very critical of herself; she may view problems related to caretaking tasks as signs of failure. It is important for the mother to feel adequate in these caretaking skills and to be able to assist other family members in caring for the child (as other family members will most likely look to her for caretaking guidance).

It is during psychological maternal role development that the attachment process between mother and infant begins. Rubin discusses the interaction that takes place between the mother and infant in the context of the giving and receiving of food.[29] The mother-infant interaction that months later culminates in attachment is a reciprocal relationship, with signals and responses elicited by both infant and mother.[1,11,29]

The giving and receiving of food is a very visible reciprocal interaction. According to Rubin, "Feeding becomes the criterion of self-esteem for the mother of this child."[3,23,30] Feeding is a continuation of the prenatal nurturing that occurred in the womb. The infant's receiving response adds pressure to the mother's performance. If the feeding goes smoothly, the mother experiences a feeling of satisfaction, which Rubin describes as a "sense of goodness of fit."[16] On the other hand, feeding difficulties may result in frustration and feelings of failure in the mother. The early days and weeks of this mother-infant relationship are spent in attempting to read and interpret cues and make appropriate responses to these cues. According to Rubin,[29] the infant learns about himself or herself through the feeding experience. Feeding and being fed are sensual experiences involving vision, hearing, and touch.

Rubin considers eating a socializing experience. After about 3 to 4 months of receiving gratification through feeding, infants become closely involved with those feeding them. Infants and children generally do not eat alone; thus socialization continues. Even as adults, many pleasurable events center around food and eating in the company of others. Food and eating allow the family and its members to pass on social customs and values.[29]

There is a relationship between giving and feeding.[29] In Rubin's words, "Giving is seen as a major feminine value. To a woman, it is an art, a science, her way of life, her philosophic dialogue with the meaning of life itself. Women assess themselves and other women with respect to their capacity for and effectiveness in giving." This feminine giving reflects a woman's appraisal of herself and her relationships.

Giving is dependent on there being someone willing and ready to receive. Frustration arises when the receiver rejects the gift. For the woman, lack of acceptance of her gift of food serves as a "rejection of her personal self and worth as a human being."[29] Frustration with infant feeding problems may result in the mother feeling rejected and incompetent, which can lead to further discord between the mother and infant.[3,22,23]

HOME CARE APPLICATION

Goals for home care of failure to thrive infants should be based on a thorough assessment of both infant and family. This assessment starts with a medical, family, nutritional, social, and developmental history. Such information should provide an in-depth view of both the infant's progress or lack of progress and the parents' understanding of the medical course and therapy.

Historical database

The historical database provides background information helpful in determining the child's and family's needs related to the plan of care. The box on p. 347 and Figure 20-1 provide guidelines for the database.

Physical assessment

Once the historical database has been obtained, a thorough physical assessment of the infant is necessary. A systematic approach should be used.

General. Observe the general conditions of the infant by assessing: (1) posture and movement, and the child's reaction to being placed on the examining area, and (2) the child's reaction when separated from the mother and the child's interest in the examiner. (Does the child gaze at the examiner or avert the eyes?)

Cardiopulmonary. While the child is quiet, assess the chest for respiratory rate and movement, heart rate and rhythm, and breath sounds.

HISTORICAL DATABASE TO ASSESS FAILURE TO THRIVE[33,34]

Prenatal history

Was the pregnancy planned?

What were the parents' feelings regarding the pregnancy?

When did prenatal care begin?

Did the mother experience any problems during the pregnancy? (Include medical conditions such as high blood pressure, bleeding, infection, and extended nausea and vomiting; and psychosocial problems such as lack of support, loss of a significant person, emotional upset, and extended stress.)

What were the parents' expectations regarding the infant including the sex, appearance, and behavior?

Did the mother use any medications?

Did the mother use alcohol, drugs, or cigarettes?

Birth history

What was the child's gestational age at birth?

What was the birth weight and length?

What was the Apgar score?

What type of delivery occurred (vaginal, forceps, or C-section)?

What anesthetic and/or medications were used during labor?

Were any complications experienced by mother or child?

Did the child have any anomalies?

What was the length of the hospital stay for mother and child?

Were there any problems during the nursery stay, such as elevated bilirubin, feeding difficulties, or breathing difficulties?

What was the parents' initial perception of the infant?

Past medical history

What is the mother's perception of the child's general health?

What illnesses or injuries has the child experienced?

Does the child have any allergies?

Has the child been hospitalized? (Include reason for admission, length of stay, diagnosis, and treatment.)

Do the parents have knowledge of the child's growth progress and/or a copy of the growth record?

Describe the child's stools including frequency and consistency.

Family history

What are the ages and health status of the family members including mother, father, siblings, and other family members living in the home?

Do any specific illnesses run in the family?

What are the heights and weights of the parents, grandparents, siblings, and extended family?

Nutrition history

How is the child fed (bottle—propped or held; solid food—spoon or bottle)?

What is the child fed?

What is the frequency and amount of the feeding? (Ask for a 24-hour recall.)

How is the food prepared and by whom?

Who generally feeds the child?

Continued

HISTORICAL DATABASE TO ASSESS FAILURE TO THRIVE—cont'd

Nutrition history—cont'd

How does the child generally respond to the feeding? (Responses may include crying, spitting up, refusing the bottle after a small amount, enjoying or not enjoying being held, sucking vigorously or poorly, having mild dribbles out of mouth, falling asleep during feeding, or eating well and then falling asleep.)

Does the child cry for long periods of time before eating?

Ask parents to keep a feeding log. This includes all feedings with type, amount, time, and infant's reaction.

Social history

Are the parents employed outside of the home?

Does the family receive any financial assistance such as Medicaid, public aid, child support, WIC, food stamps, or other program assistance?

Who is the consistent child caretaker?

Who lives in the home?

Who makes decisions regarding the child, such as medical care, child care, or discipline?

Does the family and child have a caseworker?

Does the home have a heating/cooling system, refrigerator, running water, and/or working stove?

Where does the child sleep? If in a crib, does it meet safety standards?

What are the child's sleeping patterns?

Are diapers available?

Does the child have adequate clothing?

Are age-appropriate toys and books available?

Does the mother have a support system?

Developmental history

What major developmental milestones have been achieved by the child? (See Appendix 20-1: the Denver II Developmental Screening Test.)

How does the child's development compare with the siblings' development and the parents' expectations?

Skin. Remove the clothing, including the diaper if the temperature allows, to inspect the skin for bruises, abrasions, lacerations, rashes, and skin turgor.

Growth parameters. Weigh the infant using the same scale at each visit. Measure the head-to-rump-to-heel length. Measure the head circumference from the occiput to the frontal area. These data are best plotted on a standard growth grid. It is important to adjust the age for the premature child; for example, a child born at 36 weeks of gestation would have an adjusted age of 4 weeks at 8 weeks postdelivery. The physical assessment should then progress with a head to toe approach. (See Chapter 22 for a complete physical assessment of an infant.)

Evaluate the motor, sensory, coordination, posture, and reflexes relative to the age of the infant. The Denver II (Appendix 20-1) may be useful in evaluating the young child.

Feeding. An important component of the assessment is observing the infant being fed in a natural environment. Feeding is a complex interaction of three important factors:[3,12]

- Oral motor development of the infant
- Availability of nutritionally adequate food
- Behavior of the mother and the infant related to the feeding

Feeding skills are present at birth and develop progressively, as do other motor skills. At birth, the infant's mouth and jaw are strong with well developed neuromuscular functioning, and serve as a mechanism for exploring objects. The innate reflexive action of sucking and swallowing enables the infant to feed. A sucking pattern of feeding in which the tongue and jaw move together predominates during the first 5 to 6 months of life.[13] At about 6 to 8 months of age the sucking pattern

INSTRUCTIONS

1. Record all formula, milk, and food that the baby consumes immediately after each feeding.

2. If your baby is breast fed, record the time of day the baby is fed and how long the baby feeds.

3. If your baby is formula fed, record the time of day the baby eats, the kind of formula the baby is fed, and the amount he/she actually consumes.

    Infant formula preparation:

    Is the formula iron fortified?
    _____ Yes _____ No

    Formula (brand name): _____
    _____ Oz. liquid or
    _____ Tbsp. powder

    Water
    _____ Oz.

    Other (describe): _____
    _____ Oz.
    _____ Tbsp.

    Total prepared formula
    _____ Oz.

4. If the baby spits up or vomits, estimate the amount.

5. Measure the amounts of any other foods carefully in terms of ounces of liquid (e.g., 2 oz. apple juice), level tbsp. (e.g., 2 tbsp. dry rice cereal), or portions of commercially prepared foods (e.g., 1/2 of a 4.7 oz. jar of strained peaches).

6. Does the baby take a vitamin supplement?
    _____ Yes _____ No

    If yes, what kind? _____
    _____ ml. per day

7. Comments: Did baby fall asleep, was he/she restless, etc.

DATE	TIME	FEEDING TYPE AMOUNT	VOMITING	STOOLS	COMMENTS

Figure 20-1 Food diary for infants.

begins to change to more up-and-down movements of the tongue with firmer lip seal and less prominent jaw movement.

Head and trunk control contributes to the infant's ability to feed. The most natural feeding position is a semirecumbent one with flexed posture and the neck protected from any marked extension.

At approximately 6 months of age, chewing behaviors emerge. These movements involve up-and-down jaw movements with unrefined side-to-side movement of the tongue. Lip closure and lateral jaw movement become stronger while tongue action advances so that food is able to be moved around in the mouth.

Spoon feeding is managed effectively at this time as the lips stop moving to prevent leakage during swallowing and help in removing food from the spoon. Tongue movements manage the food bolus and move it to a position to be swallowed. The optimal feeding position for the infant at this age is sitting with the head held upright and the shoulders and hips in alignment. The arms move toward the midline, while the hips and knees are flexed at a 90-degree angle with the feet supported. This position allows coordination of breathing and swallowing, and the opportunity for the infant to explore the environment.

The actual observation of the mother or caretaker feeding the child is a unique opportunity for home health nurses to gather useful information within the family's natural setting. It is best to schedule the home visit around the normal feeding time. The feeding observation allows for the assessment of the following aspects of the child:

Oral motor function. Loss of food from the mouth may reflect poor oral motor function. This loss can affect caloric intake and increase caloric requirements. Oral motor function can be evaluated by observing the previously discussed movements of eating both in and around the mouth, including oral muscle tone, lip and cheek action, jaw movement, sucking movements, tongue activity, and coordination of sucking, swallowing, and breathing. These behaviors should be relatively quiet and smoothly coordinated.

Response to food. Food makes a sensory impact on the oral area, causing the infant to respond with both the mouth and the total body. Abnormal responses may be the result of hyposensitivity or hypersensitivity to the smell, sight, and taste of the food or to the sound of activities surrounding the feeding.

Usual feeding position. Assessment of the feeding position can provide information about oral motor development and the parent-infant relationship. To maintain the natural semireclining, flexed position, the infant is usually held close in the crook of the arm. This position allows the infant and mother/caretaker to gaze at and communicate with each other[21] (Figure 20-2). Distancing of mother and infant from each other may be reflective of interaction difficulties.

Social interaction with the mother/caretaker. Observing the interaction between the mother/caretaker and the infant consists of systematic inspection of the reciprocal behaviors. As discussed earlier, this complex behavioral symphony between the infant and mother provides the basis for early communication of needs and satisfaction. It is influenced by normal developmental growth of each member of the dyad. This communicative behavior is further influenced by the ability of each member to signal, read, and respond to cues. The infant gives signals (fussing, crying) that indicate hunger; the mother picks up the cues and feeds the baby promptly. When this happens, the infant is likely to use the same signals or cues again. The mother, who recognizes her baby's hunger and satisfaction upon being fed, gains a sense of self-confidence from meeting her child's needs. This cycle becomes self-sustaining (Figure 20-3). A similar but less fulfilling cycle can develop when cues are not signaled or read appropriately. This cycle can result in frustration for both parties and poor self-esteem for the mother (Figure 20-4).[3,4,12,23]

The interaction of mother and baby that occurs when the cues are appropriately signaled, read, and responded to is beautiful to observe. Cues that are not read or responded to appropriately can become the focus of feeding difficulties. Infant cues or signals may center around needs such as hunger, burping, positioning, food preference, and satisfaction.

The mother's ability to assess and respond to her infant's cues may be related to her ability to (1) focus attention on the baby during the feeding, (2) read the cues accurately and consistently, and (3) respond to the cues in a timely and appropriate

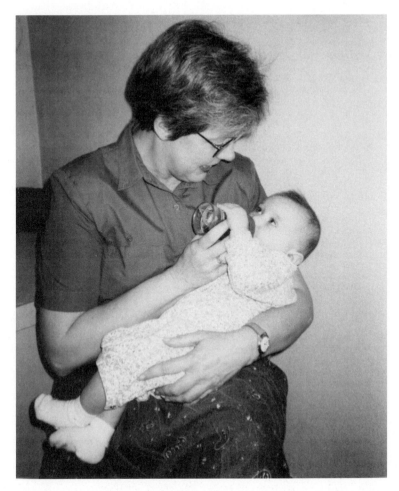

Figure 20-2 Parent-child interaction may be observed during feeding time. (Photo courtesy Robyn Rice.)

manner.[12] These are fundamental mothering behaviors that support positive feeding activities and result in mother/infant satisfaction. Such behaviors can be targeted for nursing interventions through teaching, modeling, and the provision of resources and support.

Nutrition. Nutritional requirements are an essential element of assessment and intervention for infants experiencing failure to thrive. It is known that early feeding practices exert subtle influences on the present and future health of children. During the first year of life—especially the first 6 months—nutritional requirements are greatest.[25]

The energy requirements for healthy infants during the first 6 months of life average 115 kcal/kg and gradually decrease to 105 kcal/kg by the end of the first year. During the second year, 100 kcal/kg will provide sufficient energy for growth.[32] It is necessary to distribute calories appropriately among protein, lipids, and carbohydrates, with the recommended distribution 35% to 65% carbohydrates, 7% to 16% proteins, and 30% to 50% fat. The major sources of calories during the first 6 months are breast milk and formulas, which contain approximately 20 kcal/oz. The daily fluid requirements for an infant are close to 160

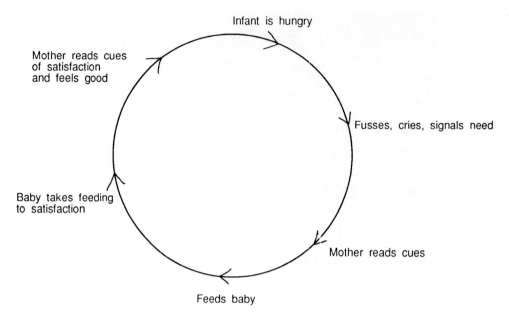

Figure 20-3 Appropriate feeding cues and responses.

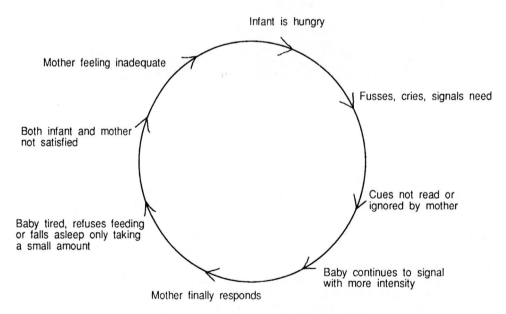

Figure 20-4 Inappropriate feeding cues and responses.

ml/kg and gradually decrease to about 120 to 130 ml/kg by the end of the first year.[26]

In recent years reports have been published regarding increased incidence of diarrhea and/or poor weight gain and growth related to excessive intake of fruit juices. Many parents view fruit juice as healthy and nutritious, and the infant likes the sweetness. Fruit juice consumption can be part of a balanced diet, but should not be substituted for formula or appropriate solid foods.[31]

Developing the plan of care: A multidisciplinary approach

A multidisciplinary approach can be most useful when planning care for failure to thrive infants and their families. Members of the team might include the primary physician, the primary hospital-based nurse, the home health nurse, a registered dietitian, a social worker, and a developmental specialist or rehabilitation therapist. Each member of this team may have a distinctly different perspective for care.[6]

Failure to thrive infants may be hospitalized for confirming diagnosis. Home health nurses, physicians, and consistent health caregivers may share valuable information regarding infant feeding practices, developmental status and progress, and family interaction dynamics.

The registered dietitian can be useful in planning for the nutritional needs of the infant by completing an in-depth assessment and developing an individualized plan to meet the full dietary needs of the child, while ensuring the proper caloric components of the diet.

The social worker's extensive knowledge base of community resources can be used to acquaint the family with resources such as health care and day care facilities, parent education groups, food pantries, and WIC (Women, Infants, and Children) and other agencies providing basic needs such as furniture, appliances, clothing, food, and diapers. Dysfunctional families can benefit from the social worker's skill in counseling.

Developmental specialists or rehabilitation therapists may be able to suggest techniques to improve the infant's oral motor and developmental skills. The role of these therapists may vary from agency to agency, but the assessment and therapeutic interventions they provide may broaden the focus from family interactional problems to infant motor dysfunction.[6]

It is necessary for the team to develop common treatment goals aimed at providing the infant with adequate nutrients for growth and development, providing a positive environment for the infant and family, and promoting positive interaction between the parents and the infant.

Nursing interventions to foster effective parent education

Parent education regarding nutritional needs may include information on formula preparation and bottle hygiene and plans for formula storage if a refrigerator is not available. Additives or concentrated formulas may be needed to increase calories at each feeding. Additives may be used in the form of Polycose or oils. Often the home health nurse may ask the dietitian or physician to direct these interventions.

Human milk or iron-fortified commercial formulas provide the nutritional needs for the infant up to 6 months of age. Solid foods are usually introduced at 5 to 6 months.[25] Eliminate excessive fruit juice consumption.[31] Solid foods during the early months are not compatible with the infant's gastrointestinal abilities and nutritional needs and may contribute to the development of food allergies. (See Appendixes 20-2 and 20-3 for developmental and feeding guidelines for infants.)

If feeding difficulties occur, interventions may center around improving the infant's oral motor abilities while providing the parents with knowledge and skills needed to assist the infant. Attention may need to be given to effective positioning, stimulation of the infant's mouth, or assistance with lip closure, sucking, or chewing. The intervention may be as simple as changing the type of nipple used for feeding.

A consistent feeding plan is important to provide the nutrients necessary for growth; however, consideration of the family's lifestyle is essential for compliance. A complete assessment of the family and feeding practices provides the team with the information necessary to plan and time feedings realistically. The plan should fit the family as much as possible.

Improving the home environment may promote better parent-infant interaction and feeding. This includes providing as many of the basic family needs as possible, thus making the environment less stressful.[6] There are limitations for the home health team, but educating the family about available resources in the community is fundamental to the medical care of the infant. Mothers who are distracted because of stress or conflict may have difficulty feeding and interacting with the child.

Some families are suspicious of helping professionals, including the home health nurse. Overcoming these feelings of mistrust may take time and a caring, nonjudgmental attitude. Home health nurses should remember that many of these parents have poor self-esteem and, in many cases, have been told that they are the source of their infant's problem. Furthermore, families may already be under the care of the state child abuse and neglect agency. It is imperative that home health nurses express interest in the mother as caretaker and her needs. Most of the focus probably has been on the infant, which is appropriate, but when the problem is one of interaction, both members of the dyad must be involved in the therapeutic plan. Interventions used to foster effective parent education include the following:

Address mother/caretaker needs at the beginning of each session. This may take the form of discussing her relationship with family or friends or sharing a nutritious recipe with her. Nurturing behaviors are necessary for both the mother and the infant. Many of these mothers did not experience a nurturing family environment as a child and have difficulty nurturing their own children. "Mothering the mother" is an essential component in the care of both the infant and family.

Listen carefully throughout the visit. Avoid interrupting and lecturing. The use of "should always," "must," or "your problem" can be a source of anxiety for parents with poor self-esteem.

Model interactions that reflect positive parenting techniques. For example, hold the infant while feeding, and talk softly while engaging the infant's gaze. Home health nurses should be careful when modeling care not to make the mother feel inadequate.

Teach normal development and child care. Include the parents in plans for goal attainment. This may be accomplished by providing the parents with information regarding normal development and simple techniques for stimulating the infant.

Foster attachment of the mother and infant. Help the mother identify the infant's cues. Some of these cues might include changes in crying when hungry, increases in body tension when the infant needs burping, or the infant turning to the mother's voice. These may be cues that the mother has not recognized in the past as ways the infant is communicating with her.

Praise parents for desirable parenting efforts. Use this technique for even the smallest positive effort. Praise is nurturing, and many of these mothers are hungry for approval and nurturance. Praise for positive change also opens the door for "teaching moments." Praising the mother for talking softly and positioning herself to face the infant allows the nurse to teach the mother about the importance of cuddling and holding the infant during feeding. Take advantage of every positive reaction from the infant to boost the mother's self-esteem by reinforcing the positive things she does.

Help parents realize that they have options. Allow them to decide their own course of action. Avoid advising the family on what should be done. Rather, point out various options that are available.

When evaluating the progress of the infant and family, all three areas of intervention should be considered: nutritional status of the infant, family environment, and parent-infant interaction. (See the boxes titled Primary Nursing Diagnoses/Patient Problems and Primary Themes of Patient/Family Education.) Professional intervention and evaluation may need to be continued for several weeks or months. In some cases the family may need to be followed for years by professionals. The length of

PRIMARY NURSING DIAGNOSES/ PATIENT PROBLEMS

- Weight below the 3rd percentile
- Sudden or rapid deceleration in the growth rate
- Delay in developmental milestones, especially gross motor and vocalization
- Significant environmental or psychosocial disruption within the family
- Parent-infant interaction dissonance or lack of sensitivity

**PRIMARY THEMES OF
PATIENT/FAMILY EDUCATION**

- Normal infant development and appropriate parental interaction
- Feeding signals, crying, sucking, coughing, spitting, etc.
- Nutrition, diet, and feeding techniques
- Positive parenting skills
- Signs and symptoms of dehydration, when to call the physician

time necessary for effective treatment depends on the individual family. The provision of consistent home health agency personnel usually hastens progress.

SUMMARY

The symptomatology encountered in the failure to thrive child may be indicative of larger problems within the family unit. Home health care of these complex families involves coordinating a multidisciplinary team effort of assessment, planning, teaching, counseling, supporting, and evaluating, with the *family* as the focus of care.

REFERENCES

1. Ainsworth M: Infant-mother attachment, *Am Psychol* 34:932-937, 1979.
2. Barbero G, Shaheen I: Environmental failure to thrive: a clinical review, *J Pediatr* 71:5, 1967.
3. Barnard K, Eyres S: *Child health assessment pt 2: the first year of life,* Public Health Service, HRA, 1979, Bureau of Health Manpower.
4. Benedek T: Psychobiological aspects of mothering, *Am J Orthopsychiatr* 26:272-278, 1956.
5. Bertalanffy LVon: *General system theory,* New York, 1968, George Braziller, Inc.
6. Bithoney W, McJunkin J, Michalek J, Snyder J, Egan H, Epstein D: The effect of a multidisciplinary team approach on weight gain in nonorganic failure to thrive children, *J Dev Behav Pediatr* 12:4, 1991.
7. Bowlby J: *Attachment and loss,* vol 1, New York, 1969, Basic Books.
8. Duvall E: *Marriage and family development,* Philadelphia, 1977, JB Lippincott.
9. Erickson E: *Childhood and society,* New York, 1963, WW Norton.
10. Feldman H, Rogoff M: Correlates of changes in marital satisfaction with the birth of first child. Paper presented at the American Psychological Association Meetings, Sept 3, 1968. Reported in Duvall E: *Marriage and family development,* Philadelphia, 1977, JB Lippincott.
11. Ferholt J: *Clinical assessment of children: a comprehensive approach to primary pediatric care,* Philadelphia, 1980, JB Lippincott.
12. Frappier P, Marino B, Shishmanian E: Nursing assessment of infant feeding problems, *J Pediatr Nurs* 2:1, 1987.
13. Friedman M: *Family nursing: theory & practice,* ed 3, Norwalk, Conn, 1992, Appleton & Lange.
14. Garfunkle J: Failure to thrive in infants and young children, *J Fam Pract* 5. 1977.
15. Goldson E: Neurological aspects of failure to thrive, *Dev Med Child Neurol* 31:816-826, 1989.
16. Gottsacker J: Maternal attachment in relation to failure to thrive. In Brandt PA, Chinn PL, Smith MD, editors: *Current practice in pediatric nursing,* vol 1, St Louis, 1976, Mosby.
17. Harrison L: Nursing intervention with FTT family, *AJNC MCN*1(2):113, 1976.
18. Herman-Staab B: Antecedents to nonorganic failure to thrive, *Pediatr Nurs* 18:6, 1992.
19. Kelleher K, Casey P, Bradley R, Pope S, Whiteside L, Barrett C, Swanson M, Kirby R: Risk factors and outcomes for failure to thrive in low birth weight preterm infants, *Pediatrics* 91:5, 1993.
20. Klaus M, Kennell J: *Parent infant bonding,* ed 2, St Louis, 1982, Mosby.
21. Leavitt M: *Families at risk: primary prevention in nursing practice,* Boston, 1982, Little, Brown.
22. Linscheid R: Feeding disorders during infancy and early childhood, feeding and their medical significance, *Time-savers Publication* 27:3, 1985.
23. Lobo M, Barnard K, Coombs J: Failure to thrive: a parent infant interaction perspective, *J Pediatr Nurs* 7:4, 1992.
24. Miller JR: The family as a system. In Miller J, Janosik E: *Family focused care,* New York, 1980, McGraw-Hill.
25. Pipes PL: *Nutrition in infancy and childhood,* ed 4, St Louis, 1989, Mosby.
26. Rohr FJ, Lothian JA: Feeding throughout the first year of life. In Howard R, Winter H, editors: *Nutrition and feeding of infants and toddlers,* Boston, 1984, Little, Brown, & Co.
27. Rossi AS: Transition to parenthood, *J Mar Fam* 30:26-39, 1968. Reprinted in Reiss IL, editor: *Readings on the family system,* New York, 1972, Holt.
28. Rubin R: Basic maternal behavior, *Nurs Outlook* 9:683-686, 1961.
29. Rubin R: Food and feeding: a matrix of relationship, *Nurs Forum* 6(2):195-205, 1967.
30. Rubin R: *Maternal identity and the maternal experience,* New York, 1984, Springer Publishing.
31. Smith M, Lifshitz F: Excess fruit consumption as a contributing factor in nonorganic failure to thrive, *Pediatrics* 93:3, 1994.
32. Stolz LM: *Influence on parent behavior,* Stanford, Calif, 1967, Stanford University Press.
33. Whaley L, Wong D: *Nursing care of infants and children,* ed 4, St Louis, 1991, Mosby.
34. Wong D, Whaley L: *Clinical manual of pediatric nursing,* ed 3, St Louis, 1990, Mosby.

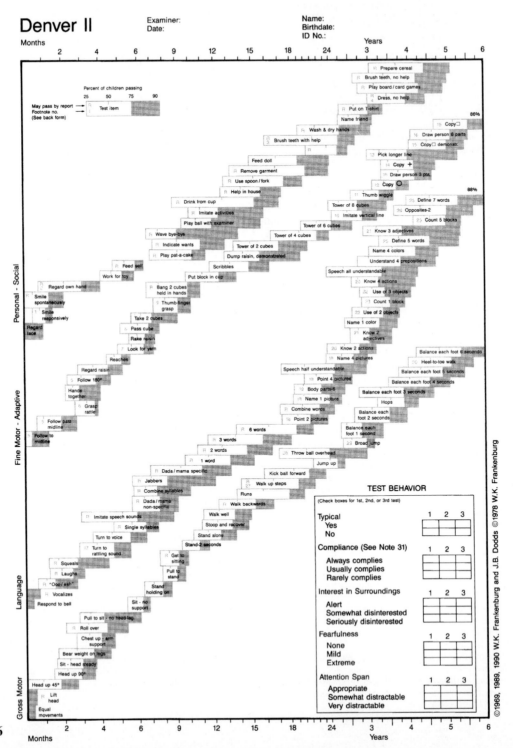

Denver II

DIRECTIONS FOR ADMINISTRATION

1. Try to get child to smile by smiling, talking or waving. Do not touch him/her.
2. Child must stare at hand several seconds.
3. Parent may help guide toothbrush and put toothpaste on brush.
4. Child does not have to be able to tie shoes or button/zip in the back.
5. Move yarn slowly in an arc from one side to the other, about 8" above child's face.
6. Pass if child grasps rattle when it is touched to the backs or tips of fingers.
7. Pass if child tries to see where yarn went. Yarn should be dropped quickly from sight from tester's hand without arm movement.
8. Child must transfer cube from hand to hand without help of body, mouth, or table.
9. Pass if child picks up raisin with any part of thumb and finger.
10. Line can vary only 30 degrees or less from tester's line.|/
11. Make a fist with thumb pointing upward and wiggle only the thumb. Pass if child imitates and does not move any fingers other than the thumb.

12. Pass any enclosed form. Fail continuous round motions.
13. Which line is longer? (Not bigger.) Turn paper upside down and repeat. (pass 3 of 3 or 5 of 6)
14. Pass any lines crossing near midpoint.
15. Have child copy first. If failed, demonstrate.

When giving items 12, 14, and 15, do not name the forms. Do not demonstrate 12 and 14.

16. When scoring, each pair (2 arms, 2 legs, etc.) counts as one part.
17. Place one cube in cup and shake gently near child's ear, but out of sight. Repeat for other ear.
18. Point to picture and have child name it. (No credit is given for sounds only.)
    Fewer than four pictures are named correctly, have child point to picture as each is named by tester.

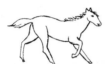

19. Using doll, tell child: Show me the nose, eyes, ears, mouth, hands, feet, tummy, hair. Pass 6 of 8.
20. Using pictures, ask child: Which one flies?... says meow?... talks?... barks?... gallops? Pass 2 of 5, 4 of 5.
21. Ask child: What do you do when you are cold?... tired?... hungry? Pass 2 of 3, 3 of 3.
22. Ask child: What do you do with a cup? What is a chair used for? What is a pencil used for?
    Action words must be included in answers.
23. Pass if child correctly places <u>and</u> says how many blocks are on paper. (1, 5).
24. Tell child: Put block **on** table; **under** table; **in front of** me, **behind** me. Pass 4 of 4.
    (Do not help child by pointing, moving head or eyes.)
25. Ask child: What is a ball?... lake?... desk?... house?... banana?... curtain?... fence?... ceiling? Pass if defined in terms of use, shape, what it is made of, or general category (such as banana is fruit, not just yellow). Pass 5 of 8, 7 of 8.
26. Ask child: If a horse is big, a mouse is __? If fire is hot, ice is __? If the sun shines during the day, the moon shines during the __? Pass 2 of 3.
27. Child may use wall or rail only, not person. May not crawl.
28. Child must throw ball overhand 3 feet to within arm's reach of tester.
29. Child must perform standing broad jump over width of test sheet (8 1/2 inches).
30. Tell child to walk forward, ∞⊂◦∞⊂◦∞⊂◦➤ heel within 1 inch of toe. Tester may demonstrate. Child must walk four consecutive steps.
31. In the second year, half of normal children are noncompliant.

OBSERVATIONS:

Appendix 20-2

Developmental Milestones Associated with Feeding

Age (months)	Development
Birth	Has sucking, rooting, and swallowing reflexes
	Feels hunger and indicates desire for food by crying; expresses satiety by falling asleep
	Has strong extrusion reflex
3-4	Extrusion reflex is fading
	Begins to develop hand-eye coordination
4-5	Can approximate lips to the rim of a cup
5-6	Can use fingers to feed self a cracker
6-7	Chews and bites
	May hold own bottle, but may not drink from it (prefers for it to be held)
7-9	Refuses food by keeping lips closed; has taste preferences
	Holds a spoon and plays with it during feeding
	May drink from a straw
	Drinks from a cup with assistance
9-12	Picks up small morsels of food (finger foods) and feeds self
	Holds own bottle and drinks from it
	Drinks from a household cup without assistance but spills some
	Uses a spoon with much spilling
12-18	Drools less
	Drinks well from a household cup, but may drop it when finished
	Holds cup with both hands
24	Can use a straw
	Chews food with mouth closed and shifts food in mouth
	Distinguishes between finger and spoon foods
	Holds small glass in one hand; replaces glass without dropping
36	Spills small amount from spoon
	Begins to use fork; holds it in fist
	Uses adult pattern of chewing, which involves rotary action of jaw
48	Rarely spills when using spoon
	Serves self finger foods
	Eats with fork held with fingers
54	Uses fork in preference to spoon
72	Spreads with knife
84	Cuts tender food with knife

From Wong DL: *Whaley & Wong's nursing care of infants and children,* ed 5, St Louis, 1995, Mosby.

Appendix 20-3

Guidelines for Feeding during the First Year

Age/type of feeding	Specific recommendations
Birth-6 months	
Breast-feeding	Most desirable complete diet for first half of year
	Requires supplements of fluoride (0.25 mg), regardless of the fluoride content of the local water supply, and iron by 6 months of age
	Requires supplements of vitamin D (400 units) if mother's diet is inadequate or if infant is not exposed to sufficient sunlight
Formula	Iron-fortified commercial formula is a complete food for the first half of the year*
	Requires fluoride supplements (0.25 mg) when the concentration of fluoride in the drinking water is below 0.3 parts per million (ppm)
	Evaporated milk formula requires supplements of vitamin C, iron, and fluoride (in accordance with the fluoride content of the local water supply)
6-12 months	
Solid foods	May begin to add solids by 5 to 6 months of age
	First foods are strained, pureed, or finely mashed
	Finger foods such as teething crackers, raw fruit, or vegetables can be introduced by 6 to 7 months
	Chopped table food or commercially prepared junior foods can be started by 9 to 12 months
	With the exception of cereal, the order of introducing foods is variable; a recommended sequence is weekly introduction of other foods, beginning with fruit, then vegetables, and then meat
	As the quantity of solids increases, the amount of formula should be limited to approximately 900 ml (30 oz) daily
	METHOD OF INTRODUCTION
	Introduce solids when infant is hungry
	Begin spoon feeding by pushing food to back of tongue because of infant's natural tendency to thrust tongue forward
	Use small spoon with straight handle; begin with 1 or 2 teaspoons of food; gradually increase to 2 to 3 tablespoons per feeding
	Introduce one food at a time, usually at intervals of 4 to 7 days, identify food allergies
	As the amount of solid food increases, decrease the quantity of milk to prevent overfeeding
	Never introduce foods by mixing them with the formula in the bottle

*The Academy of Pediatrics recommends breast-feeding or commercial formula feeding for up to 12 months of age. After 1 year whole cow's milk can be given.

From Wong D: *Whaley & Wong's nursing care of infants and children,* ed 5, St Louis, 1995, Mosby.

Continued

Age/type of feeding	Specific recommendations
6-12 months—cont'd	
Cereal	Introduce commercially prepared iron-fortified infant cereals and administer daily until 18 months
	Rice cereal is usually introduced first because of its low allergic potential
	Can discontinue supplemental iron once cereal is given
Fruits and vegetables	Applesauce, bananas, and pears are usually well tolerated
	Avoid fruits and vegetables marked in cans that are not specifically designed for infants because of variable and sometimes high lead content and addition of salt, sugar, and/or preservatives
	Offer fruit juice only from a cup, not a bottle, to reduce the development of "nursing caries"
Meat, fish, and poultry	Avoid fatty meats
	Prepare by baking, broiling, steaming, or poaching
	Include organ meats such as liver, which has a high iron, vitamin A, and vitamin B complex content
	If soup is given, be sure all ingredients are familiar to child's diet
	Avoid commercial meat/vegetable combinations because protein is low
Eggs and cheese	Serve egg yolk hard boiled and mashed, soft cooked, or poached
	Introduce egg white in small quantities (1 tsp) toward the end of first year to detect an allergy
	Use cheese as a substitute for meat and as finger food

21 The Pediatric Patient: Cardiac Anomalies

Jacalyn Wickline Ryberg

He who has health has HOPE and he who has HOPE has everything.

There are approximately 4 million births in the United States each year.* Congenital cardiac anomalies, heart defects that are present at birth, occur in 8 to 14 of every 1,000 live births.[5,10,23] Cardiac anomalies are not always immediately apparent in newborns, and signs and symptoms are often missed during early infancy. Because babies are discharged sooner after delivery than in the past, all babies should be assessed carefully for physiological anomalies. In addition, high-technology health care is increasing the survival rates of these babies, many of whom are discharged into the home environment. Home health nurses need to know about the general incidence, classification, etiology, and pathophysiology of pediatric congenital cardiac anomalies because this patient population will become more prevalent in home care in the years to come.

Reviewing basic pathophysiology will help in understanding characteristic signs and symptoms of congenital cardiac anomalies. Certain congenital cardiac anomalies manifest with specific signs and symptoms after circulatory adjustments have been established (immediately at birth). Other cardiac anomalies may not appear until days, weeks, months, or years later. As one of the major health care providers who see infants and mothers at home for postpartum follow-up, home health nurses need to gather as much information as possible. It is important to obtain complete histories and conduct a thorough physical examination.

The majority of congenital cardiac anomaly deaths are due to heart failure and occur within the first few weeks of life. However, delayed appearances and identifications of congenital cardiac anomalies have been well documented. According to statistics, 46% of congenital cardiac anomalies are diagnosed by 1 week of age, 88% by 1 year of age, and 98% by 4 years of age.[10] The earlier the detection of congenital anomalies, the better an infant's chance of survival.

Advances in cardiac technology have increased the need for home nursing care of fetuses and mothers, newborns, infants, toddlers, and children. Frequently these children and parents have special health care, social, educational, psychological, and parenting needs (Figure 21-1).[4] Often it is the nurse's responsibility to orchestrate and direct the use of available resources to meet these needs.

Before addressing the care of infants and families, a brief review of major congenital cardiac anomalies and symptoms is presented.

PATHOPHYSIOLOGY
Epidemiology

Most fetal cardiac development occurs between the fourth and seventh weeks of fetal life. Multiple factors (environmental, genetic, and intrauterine) account for the majority of congenital cardiac

*For consistency within this chapter, the latest surveillance statistics from the Centers for Disease Control and Prevention's Congenital Malformations Surveillance are used as the reference source.[23]

The author wishes to acknowledge two special colleagues for their assistance in the preparation of this chapter by sharing their expertise: Toni J. Clow, RN, MA, CPNP, Associate Professor, College of Nursing, The University of Iowa; and Robert M. Rice, RPh, MS, Pharmacist, Assistant Director Operations, Department of Pharmacy Services, Medical Center of Central Georgia.

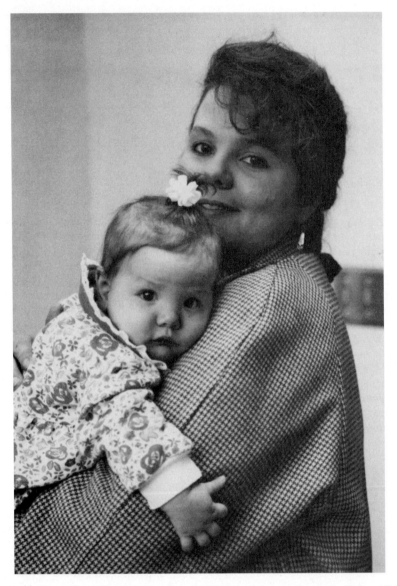

Figure 21-1 A strong bond between parent and child helps to meet the needs of the child with a cardiac anomaly. (Photo courtesy Beverly Teche, Lincoln-Lancaster County Health Department, Lincoln, Neb.)

anomalies. Factors that have been *directly associated* with congenital defects are pharmacologic agents (lithium, thalidomide, trimethadione, hydantoin, and alcohol) and diseases (rubella, maternal insulin-dependent diabetes, and maternal alcoholism). Alcoholic mothers and mothers who

contract rubella during the first 8 weeks of pregnancy have a 50% chance of having a child with a congenital cardiac anomaly, and mothers who have insulin-dependent diabetes mellitus have a 10% chance of having a child with a cardiac anomaly. Babies born of parents with a congenital

Table 21-1 Congenital diseases or syndromes associated with cardiac anomalies

Disease or syndrome	Associated cardiac anomalies
Asplenia syndrome	Ventricular septal defect: single ventricle; common A-V valve; transposition of the great arteries
DiGeorge syndrome	Interrupted aortic arch
Ellis-van Creveld syndrome	Single atrium or large atrial septal defect
Fetal alcohol syndrome	Ventricular septal defect; atrial septal defect; tetralogy of Fallot
Friedreich's ataxia	Cardiomyopathy
Holt-Oram syndrome	Atrial septal defect or single atrium; severe pulmonary vascular disease; total anomalous pulmonary venous return; arrhythmias
Hunter's syndrome	Abnormalities of the mitral or tricuspid valves or coronary artery obstruction
Hurler's syndrome	Abnormalities of the mitral or tricuspid valves or coronary artery obstruction
Laurence-Moon-Bardet-Biedl syndrome	Aortic or pulmonary valvular stenosis, tetralogy of Fallot; ventricular septal defect
Marfan's syndrome	Aortic or mitral valve abnormalities; dissecting aortic aneurysm; myocardial disease
Maternal diabetes (IDDM)	Transposition of the great vessels; ventricular septal defect
Maternal thalidomide ingestion	Tetralogy of Fallot; truncus arteriosus
Neurofibromatosis	Pulmonary valvular stenosis
Rubella syndrome	Patent ductus arteriosus; peripheral pulmonary stenosis
Trisomy 13 (Patau's syndrome)	Patent ductus arteriousus and/or ventricular septal defect with pulmonary hypertension
Trisomy 18 (Edwards' syndrome)	Ventricular septal defect; patent ductus arteriosus
Trisomy 21 (Down's syndrome)	Endocardial cushion defect; ventricular septal defect; patent ductus arteriosus
Turner's syndrome/mosaic (XO/XY)	Pulmonary valvular stenosis
Turner's syndrome	Coarctation of the aorta
William's elfin facies syndrome	Supravalvular aortic stenosis; peripheral pulmonary stenosis

cardiac anomaly have a slightly increased risk of also having a congenital cardiac anomaly. It is important to emphasize that there are few known factors that directly cause congenital cardiac anomalies.[11,16]

Congenital cardiac anomalies may occur as a single anomaly, as one of several congenital cardiac anomalies, or as part of a syndrome. Major congenital cardiac anomalies and associated congenital diseases or syndromes are illustrated in Table 21-1 and are reviewed briefly in the next section.[9,11,17] Signs and symptoms of these anomalies are discussed later in this chapter.

Pediatric cardiac anomalies

Aortic valve stenosis and atresia (incidence 2.1%). With aortic valve stenosis and atresia, a severe aortic narrowing that obstructs blood flow from the left ventricle is present at birth. Hypertrophy of the left ventricle will develop. This defect ranges from mild to severe. Symptoms frequently include irritability, hypotension, tachycardia, and tachypnea. If symptomatic congestive heart failure (CHF) is present at birth, surgery will be needed immediately. In mild cases an infant may be asymptomatic but later display symptoms of a heart murmur in childhood. Symptoms of CHF, angina, ventricular arrhythmias, and syncope occur in severe cases. The child with this condition may appear to be essentially healthy but is at risk for sudden death.

Atrial septal defect (incidence 10.7%). Atrial septal defect (ASD) consists of an opening in the septum separating the left and right atria. Usually it is asymptomatic, but exertional dyspnea and CHF may be present. Repair of the ASD is recommended at 4 or 5 years of age when the defect is thought to be at the optimal size for surgical repair.

Coarctation of the aorta (incidence 2.4%). Coarctation of the aorta is a narrowing in the aortic arch, usually located distal to the origin of the left subclavian artery. It is frequently associated with other cardiac lesions such as ventricular septal defect, patent ductus arteriosus, transposition of the great vessels, atrial septal defect, and aortic stenosis. Coarctation of the aorta may be asymptomatic until adulthood.

Circulation to the lower extremities may be impaired, causing higher blood pressure in vessels rising above the constriction. Coarctation of the aorta is suspected when there are diminished femoral and pedal pulses with upper body hypertension.

Common truncus arteriosus (incidence 0.5%). Inadequate division of the common great vessel—the truncus arteriosus—results in a single large great vessel arising from the ventricles. This vessel gives rise to the systemic, pulmonary, and coronary arteries. Usually a large ventricular septal defect exists. There are four types of truncus arteriosus, each describing the origin of pulmonary arterial circulation from the large trunk. Nearly all infants with truncus arteriosus demonstrate signs of CHF and/or cyanosis within the first months of life. They generally have surgery as infants and again at 4 to 5 years of age.

Endocardial cushion defect (incidence 2.6%). Endocardial cushion defect (ECD) is a congenital heart lesion in the atrial septum, ventricular septum, and atrioventricular valves. There are several forms of ECD, but all are characterized by downward displacement of the atrioventricular valves as a result of ventricular abnormalities. Infants with ECD display severe CHF. Surgical intervention is delayed until as late as 4 or 5 years of age to allow for as much growth as possible because valvular replacement is generally necessary. If growth failure occurs, surgical intervention takes place earlier. Symptoms include increased tachypnea, dyspnea, poor weight gain, diaphoresis, CHF, cardiomegaly, paleness, cyanosis, and frequent respiratory infections.

Hypoplastic left heart syndrome (incidence 2.3%). Hypoplastic left heart syndrome includes a combination of defects consisting of aortic valve atresia, small left ventricles, hypoplastic ascending aorta, and mitral valve atresia. Babies with this condition are cyanotic with grayish skin. Vascular collapse is an imminent reality when their symptoms include hypotension, tachypnea, dyspnea, grunting, nasal flaring, and hypothermia. Prognosis is poor for these babies. Without medical intervention, life beyond 1 month of age is doubtful. Families will need realistic preparation and grief support if they do not opt for a cardiac transplant.[1]

Patent ductus arteriosus (incidence 43.3%). The ductus arteriosus is a blood channel that links the aorta to the pulmonary artery during fetal life. It is believed that blood stops flowing through this channel after respirations begin and that it closes after 3 months of life. If the ductus fails to close, high aortic pressure shunts blood through the ductus into the pulmonary artery, causing left ventricular volume overload, increased left ventricular and diastolic pressure, elevation of the left atrial pressure, and CHF. Increased pulmonary blood flow results in elevated systolic pressure, wide pulse pressure, and bounding peripheral pulse. Clinical symptoms include CHF, fatigue, and growth retardation. Symptoms may be exaggerated by infection, increased environmental temperature, anemia, poor nutrition, and increased activity.

Pulmonary valve stenosis and atresia (incidence 2.7%). With pulmonary valve stenosis and atresia the pulmonic valve cusp that controls the flow of blood from the right ventricle into the pulmonary artery is malformed. The condition varies in degree from mild to severe. In severe cases there may be cyanosis, fatigue, dyspnea, syncope, chest pain, and epigastric pain. The child with this condition is at risk for sudden death.

Tetralogy of Fallot (incidence 2.2%). Tetralogy of Fallot is a set of four congenital cardiac defects consisting of (1) a large ventricular septal defect, (2) pulmonary stenosis, (3) right ventricular hypertrophy, and (4) dextroposition of the aorta. Typically the child with these defects exhibits exertional dyspnea with feeding, crying, and defecating, and may display irritability, pallor, tachypnea, flaccidity, syncope, cyanosis, and digital clubbing. This child usually has a poor growth and development record and is at risk for polycythemia, cerebral vascular accidents, brain abscesses, and sudden death. For compensatory comfort this child may be found in the knee-chest position.

Transposition of the great vessels (incidence 3.3%). Transposition of the great vessels means that the aorta originates from the anatomical right ventricle, and the pulmonary artery originates from the left. The body then has two independent circuits, with pulmonary venous blood returning to the lungs and systemic venous blood flowing from the aorta to the body. To sustain life after birth, either the foramen ovale or the ductus arteriosus, or both, must remain open. Because of the mixing of arterial and pulmonary blood, these infants will have polycythemia and clubbing, which generally appears at about 5 to 6 months of age.[2] If a ventricular septal defect or patent ductus arteriosus is sizable, then pulmonary congestion exhibits as CHF. Symptoms include tachycardia, tachypnea, poor feeding, poor growth, hepatomegaly, cardiomegaly, and labored respirations. Surgical repair is generally done between the ages of 6 months and 3 years.

Tricuspid valve stenosis and atresia (incidence 1.2%). With tricuspid valve stenosis and atresia there is narrowing of the tricuspid valve, which frequently involves a communication between the right atrium and the right ventricle. The condition is identified at birth by the presence of profound cyanosis, tachypnea, and acidosis.

Ventricular septal defect (incidence 12.9%). Ventricular septal defect (VSD) refers to an opening in the septum between the left and right ventricles. As a result of increased volume load on the ventricles and lungs, dyspnea and CHF are symptoms. Children with VSD frequently exhibit CHF, fatigue, failure to thrive, and frequent respiratory infections.

Potential consequences of cardiac anomalies

Cardiac transplant. Cardiac transplant may cause pathophysiological changes as a result of an altered immune system, side effects of the immunosuppressive agents, rejection, and infection. The infant will require close interaction with the primary health care staff.

Signs and symptoms of transplant rejection include low-grade fever, tachycardia, tachypnea, poor feeding, vomiting, diaphoresis, irritability, and hepatomegaly. Since the home health nurse visits the home or talks with the family on the telephone more frequently than any other health professional, it is paramount for the nurse to assess for physiological changes indicating rejection.

Sudden death. The most common reasons for sudden death in children more than 1 year old (excluding sudden infant death syndrome) are infectious diseases and cardiovascular causes. The cardiovascular causes are myocarditis, hypertrophic cardiomyopathy, and congenital coronary artery disease.

Myocarditis accounts for 17% of pediatric cardiac sudden deaths. Children may be asymptomatic or have a mild "viral syndrome" prodrome, subtly exhibited by sinus tachycardia, mild fever, irregular heart rhythm, bradycardia, dyspnea, and tachypnea. More obvious symptoms might include evidence of CHF, galloping heart beat, cardiomegaly, hepatomegaly, tachypnea, and possibly rales.

Hypertrophic cardiomyopathy accounts for 31% of the pediatric cardiac sudden deaths. Historical information may be extremely helpful in identifying at risk children who may need further screening and referral to a pediatric cardiologist. Approximately 60% of the children with hypertrophic cardiomyopathy have a relative with evidence of the disorder. Specific questions should explore family history of sudden death, syncope, accidental death, or "seizures" from arrhythmias.

Children considered at greatest risk are those who have exercise-related syncope, tachyarrhythmias, poorly controlled atrial flutter, dyspnea, weakness, fatigue, chest pain, and acyanosis. A greater risk of sudden death has been linked with family histories of syncope, sudden death, Marfan's syndrome, arrhythmias, mitral valve prolapse, hypertrophic cardiomyopathy, or premature atherosclerotic heart disease.[10,11]

Children with cardiac anomalies are referred to home health agencies from diverse sources. The next section discusses some of the more prominent sources of case identification for referral

REFERRAL NETWORK

Referral networks vary with communities, health care providers, and health care consumers.[8,15] There are at least seven potential referral sources that should be using home health agency services for cardiac follow-up and case identification: (1) obstetric and genetic physicians for prenatal cardiac diagnosis referrals, (2) newborn nurseries for referrals of newborns with congenital cardiac anomalies that are identified at birth, (3) well-child clinics for referrals of infants and children with congenital cardiac anomalies that are identified during well-child exams, (4) tertiary medical centers that provide postsurgical care of congenital cardiac anomalies, (5) tertiary medical centers that care for newborns/infants who are waiting to receive or have received cardiac transplants, (6) newborn nurseries/obstetrical units that provide follow-up of high-risk mothers and infants, and (7) self-referrals by families with children who have identified congenital cardiac defects and are in need of health care. Technological medical advances are continuing to increase survival rates of these children, presenting new challenges for home health nurses as multidisciplinary case managers.

The role of the home health nurse varies and depends on the extent of the problem and the needs of the child and family. Case management referrals save time and money when they include comprehensive nursing process plans of care. Duplication of services and costs can be prevented by using a referral network and implementing the nursing process from assessment through evaluation.[20] Such approaches ensure that families will be spared answering the same questions repeatedly, that referring and receiving services will have comprehensive information, and that the family will receive the benefit of continuous care for the child (Figure 21-2).

DISCHARGE PLANNING

Preparation for discharge and home health care begins upon admission to the hospital or upon diagnosis of the anomaly. During the initial phase of preparation for home health care, several questions should be addressed and discussed. Discharge plans will hinge on answers to the following questions:

- Does the family want the child to go home?
- Is the family able to care for the child at home?
- Does the home environment support any technology that may accompany the child home?
- Are the necessary resources (e.g., monetary, space, hot/cold water, electricity/grounded outlets) available?
- Are the parents able to care for their own needs aside from those of the sick infant?

(Are there signs of abuse, neglect, or substance misuse in the home? *Are there available interagency services that support the well-being of the infant and family?*)
- Is payment for services available?

If the answer to any of these questions is no, the patient is not ready for discharge. Not all patients and families will be ready to begin home care at the same time. The health care system must be sensitive to those who are not ready for discharge and plan accordingly. A nurse case manager may need to become the family's advocate and negotiate with the health care providers and reimbursement agencies to resolve problems. When patients are discharged before they or their families are ready, there is a high incidence of rehospitalization, which in turn is more expensive physically, emotionally, and financially. If families are able to handle home care but insurance carriers will only pay for inpatient care, the nurse case manager may need to be the advocate for the position that home care is more beneficial for the family psychologically, socially, emotionally, physically, and financially.

HOME CARE APPLICATION

The major goal of pediatric home care programs is to normalize the life of the child. Home health nurses come to families with multifaceted backgrounds and expertise. Their roles include advocate, caregiver, case manager, clinician, counselor, problem solver, and teacher.[25]

Assessment

The following discussion of cardiac home care assessment is applicable to all referrals.

Historical database. Background information must be available to all members of the case management team. Historical data collection should include the patient, the family, and the community where the family resides. (See Chapter 20.)

The family, prenatal, pregnancy, delivery, and postpartum histories may have implications for the patient. It is helpful to review birth records, the mother's prenatal records, hospitalization records, and the child's health service records (which would include immunization records, previous histories and physicals with growth grids, and developmental questionnaires and histories). Considerable tact is necessary when collecting personal

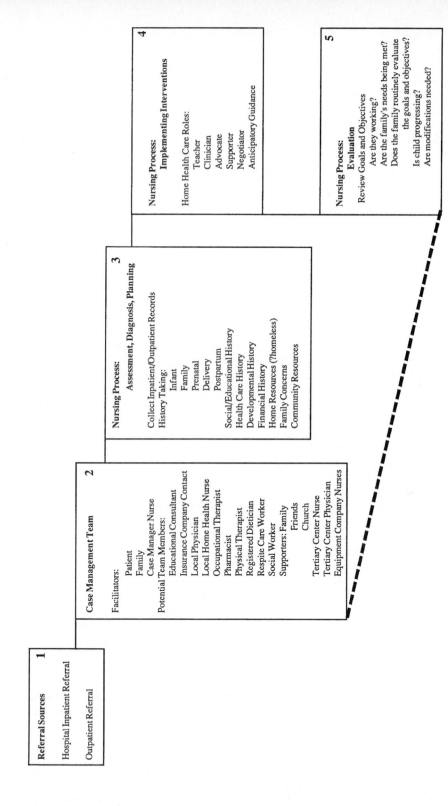

Figure 21-2 The Ryberg model of pediatric referral and case management nursing process. (Courtesy Jacalyn Wickline Ryberg, 1991.)

Referral Sources 1

Hospital Inpatient Referral

Outpatient Referral

Case Management Team 2

Facilitators:
Patient
Family
Case Manager Nurse
Potential Team Members:
Educational Consultant
Insurance Company Contact
Local Physician
Local Home Health Nurse
Occupational Therapist
Pharmacist
Physical Therapist
Registered Dietician
Respite Care Worker
Social Worker
Supporters: Family
Friends
Church
Tertiary Center Nurse
Tertiary Center Physician
Equipment Company Nurses

Nursing Process: 3
Assessment, Diagnosis, Planning

Collect Inpatient/Outpatient Records
History Taking:
Infant
Family
Prenatal
Delivery
Postpartum
Social/Educational History
Health Care History
Developmental History
Financial History
Home Resources (?homeless)
Family Concerns
Community Resources

Nursing Process: 4
Implementing Interventions

Home Health Care Roles:
Teacher
Clinician
Advocate
Supporter
Negotiator
Anticipatory Guidance

Nursing Process: 5
Evaluation
Review Goals and Objectives
Are they working?
Are the family's needs being met?
Does the family routinely evaluate
the goals and objectives?
Is child progressing?
Are modifications needed?

history from the mother. She may be feeling guilty and asking herself, "Why did this happen to my baby?" Because the mother is likely to think that she might have done something during the pregnancy to cause the cardiac anomaly, she needs to be reminded that most cardiac anomalies have multiple causes.[13] Because of sensitive feelings, it is important to gather this historical information only once rather than having each person on the case management team ask the same questions over and over again.[12,15] Along with the historical information, home health nurses should obtain the following information:

1. Knowledge of illness and treatment (parent/child perceptions)
2. Current treatments and medications the child is receiving
3. Current physical, psychological, and developmental effects of the illness and treatments
4. Previous health services the child has received (When? Any particular problems? Were the services before or after diagnosis of the congenital cardiac anomaly?)
5. Past reactions the child has had from immunizations
6. History of prematurity with the baby (Patent ductus arteriosus is more common in preterm infants.)
7. Baby's size compared to gestational age (A significant percentage of babies with congenital heart disease are small for gestational age. The incidence is particularly high for ventricular septal defect, patent ductus arteriosus, atrial septal defect, and tetralogy of Fallot.)
8. Presence of noncardiac congenital anomalies (Congenital malformations tend to clump together. Nearly one fourth of all children with cardiac disease have associated noncardiac anomalies affecting the musculoskeletal system, central nervous system, or gastrointestinal system.)
9. Failure to thrive during infancy. (See Chapter 20.)
10. Recurrent upper respiratory infections, pneumonia, or asthma
11. Specific questions about the family: Have there been changes in the family routines or moods? Have there been changes in financial status? What is the intrafamily support system like and how do the relationship bonds affect the family? What coping strategies are used by the family? (If they are not using effective strategies, the home health nurse should include this in the nursing care plan and teach effective strategies.)
12. *Any* concerns of the parents

Family and home assessment. To minimize confusion, the family and home assessment should be done prior to the baby's discharge. Depending on the needs of the child in terms of equipment, supplies, and health care providers, the home should be appraised, assessed, and reviewed for safety (wiring, carpeting static, wide doorways for equipment), mobility factors (steps, slick floors, electricity, electrical grounding possibilities, backup electricity), accessibility to visitors (dirt roads in rural areas, houses with no house numbers, winter and summer weather conditions), telephone service (with a list of all who are connected with the case conveniently posted), water supply (well water, city water, fire protection), and availability of emergency services (size of nearest hospital and name of the physician who will handle emergencies).

Families often need assistance with finding health care resources and assembling financial resources. Most of the resources needed should be organized while the child is still hospitalized to minimize confusion at homecoming. A social service referral should be considered for assisting families when negotiating with insurance companies, equipment companies, and pharmaceutical vendors. The period immediately after a child requiring intensive acute care arrives at home is a trying and anxious time for the family. They may need the support of several phone calls a day from the nurse during this period. If the family does not have a working telephone, more frequent home visits will be necessary.

Home health agency and community assessment. In planning discharge from the hospital to the home care setting, the home health agency should be assessed for the following:

• Does the agency have a pediatric nurse available to provide consultation, in-service education, and program management?

- Are there written policies on general pediatric care and specialized procedures?
- Is some form of pediatric staff coverage available on a 24-hour basis?
- Is there a mechanism for consultation and record review to improve quality patient care?

Reimbursement for home care costs should be addressed early. Are there alternatives for paying for care other than depletion of the family's financial resources? If there is insurance coverage, it must be explored thoroughly (generally by assertive and creative nurses who do not accept *no* for an answer). Medicaid services differ from state to state, making it necessary to check with state Medicaid offices regarding specific state programs. Social workers are valuable members of the team who generally know Medicaid requirements in detail.

In dealing with the community, parents especially need creative nurse case managers. Nurses can guide families to community resources for backup life support, equipment suppliers, transportation, medications, and educational programs to meet the needs of their children. In addition, they can identify community funds or agency resources available to assist with start-up costs. (See Chapter 3 for more information on community assessment.)

Cardiac physical examination.[7] The examiner should first observe the character of respiration and the contour of the chest, count the respiratory rate,* and then inspect the color of lips, nailbeds, and skin.* Next, the examiner should look for pulsation of neck veins and arteries, palpate pulses in the arms, legs, and neck,* check the precordial impulse and apex beat,* and measure blood pressure.

It is desirable to listen to a quiet child with a stethoscope that is comfortable and familiar, is fitted with a bell and diaphragm, and has tubing measuring no more than 15 inches. It is not necessary to have pediatric chest pieces. The adult-size chest piece works well for infants, and in fact most examiners report that adult-size chest pieces are more effective in transmitting low-intensity and low-frequency sounds.

If the infant is cooperative, it is best to listen to the heart in as many of the following positions as possible: (1) supine, (2) left lateral (or right lateral for transposition of the great vessels), (3) sitting erect, (4) standing, (5) squatting, and (6) standing again immediately after squatting. Generally a murmur is louder after exercise because of the increase in cardiac output. Auscultation after exercise simulates how the heart would sound during a period of fever, infection, or excitement. Valvular areas of the heart to listen to should include the following: (1) primary aortic area (right second intercostal space at the sternal edge), (2) pulmonic area (left second intercostal space at the sternal edge), (3) tricuspid and secondary aortic area (left lower sternal border at the fourth intercostal space), (4) mitral area (the apex of the heart or, in the heart without dilation, at the fourth and fifth intercostal space at the midclavicular line), (5) both infraclavicular areas, (6) over the carotid arteries, (7) in each axilla (at the fourth and fifth intercostal space), and (8) in the posterior aspect of the chest medial and inferior to each scapula. Careful palpation of the carotid, brachial, and femoral pulses is important to exclude associated coarctation of the aorta or interruption of the aortic arch.

Transtelephonic electrocardiography (ECG) has become a valuable tool in the management of children at home. It provides instantaneous information regarding outpatient diagnosis and evaluation of known arrhythmias, pacemaker performance, and drug management. Symptoms of syncope, chest pain, shortness of breath, and palpitations are disconcerting to families, and the presence of ECG transmitters makes it possible to reassure families and children that no serious arrhythmias or conduction disturbances are present. With such a portable, convenient, inexpensive, and instantaneous approach to the assessment of symptomatic cardiac arrhythmias, trips to the emergency department, repeated inconclusive Holter monitorings, or prolonged hospitalizations for ECG monitoring can be decreased.

A single blood pressure norm for children is nonexistent since blood pressure norms change with age and do not reach stable levels until skeletal growth and sexual maturity have occurred. (See Appendix 21-1 for pulse, respiration, temperature, and blood pressure norms.) Measuring height and weight is a means of monitoring growth and development. Development can be monitored with the Denver II, as discussed in Chapter 20.

---

*When an abbreviated examination is necessary, the asterisked items are most sensitive in providing cardiovascular function data.

Respiratory assessment. To accurately evaluate the respiratory rate, place your hand on the chest of a resting infant if the respirations are shallow; otherwise, observe the infant at rest and count the respirations for 1 full minute. Lack of substernal respiratory movement should be noted since normal breathing patterns for infants include chest/abdominal movements in unison. Respiratory rates may be altered by crying, feeding, pain, hypothermia, or hyperthermia. Tachypnea signifies respiratory distress; a rate over 60 breaths per minute for an extended period of time should be considered a warning sign.

Signs and symptoms associated with pediatric congestive heart failure.[11,24] The presence of one of the signs of CHF is not conclusive evidence of cardiac defects, but is serious enough to warrant a thorough medical examination. The following box lists the major signs and symptoms of CHF, and Table 21-2 lists the major medications that are used at home to treat CHF.

CHF is the inability of the heart to pump blood in the quantity that is needed by the body. Common signs of cardiac decompensation in the infant consist of feeding difficulties, failure to thrive, tachypnea, tachycardia, rales, hepatomegaly, and cardiomegaly. Less common symptoms include peripheral edema, ascites, pulsus alternans, gallop heart rhythm, peripheral vasoconstriction with excessive or inappropriate sweating (especially of the face and forehead), and pallor.

Cyanosis is a blue discoloration of the mucous membranes resulting from the presence of circulating reduced hemoglobin. Cyanosis may be minimal in newborns, but intensifies with feedings, crying, or any other activity that requires increased oxygenation. The discoloration may increase around 2 to 3 weeks after birth when the patent ductus arteriosus (PDA) and patent foramen ovale (PFO) close. Severe cyanosis indicates hypoxia and acidosis. (Dark-skinned infants can be evaluated by examining the mucous membranes.)

Diaphoresis is significant perspiration, especially associated with an infant. If the baby has a tense, anxious facial expression, diaphoresis is probably associated with CHF because the infant is unable to get his breath and feels as if he is suffocating.

Dyspnea occurs when engorged pulmonary vessels compromise lung capacity and lung expan-

---

CONGESTIVE HEART FAILURE: SIGNS AND SYMPTOMS IN INFANTS[10,21]

Decreased cardiac output symptoms

Tachycardia
Increased cardiac contractility
Increased vasomotor tone
Peripheral vasoconstriction
Diaphoresis

Decreased renal perfusion symptoms

Sodium and water retention
Poor urine output

Systemic venous engorgement symptoms

Hepatomegaly
Jugular venous distension
Periorbital and facial edema

Pulmonary venous engorgement symptoms

Tachypnea (and decreased tidal volume)
Increased respiratory effort (retractions, nasal flaring)
Grunting (indicates significant distress)
Rales

Less frequent signs and symptoms

Peripheral edema
Ascites
Pulsus alternans
Gallop rhythm
Peripheral vasoconstriction with inappropriate sweating of forehead and face

Behavioral symptoms

Feeding difficulties
Circumoral cyanosis
Failure to thrive
Squatting position
Fatigue

---

sion. Small airways are compressed, causing air hunger. In turn, tachypnea, or faster breathing, occurs. Wheezes are caused by rapid air movement through narrowed airways. Rapid inspiratory air movement through fluid-filled airways causes crackling sounds.

Hepatomegaly, or liver enlargement, is observed with cardiac failure. Because of the engorgement of hepatic veins, the liver can be palpated beneath

Table 21-2 Infant cardiac pharmacology: medications for cardiac therapy[21]

Drug	Age	Dosage
Antiarrhythmics (oral)		
Digoxin (Lanoxin)	Preterm neonate	5-7.5 μ/kg/24 hr*
	Full-term neonate	6-10 μ/kg/24 hr*
	1 month-2 years	10-15 μ/kg/24 hr*
	2 years- 5 years	7.5-10 μ/kg/24 hr*
	5 years-10 years	5-10 μ/kg/24 hr*
Phenytoin (Dilantin)	Children	5-10 mg/kg/24 hr
Propranolol (Inderal)	Children	2-4 mg/kg/24 hr
Quinidine†	Children	15-60 mg/kg/24 hr
Verapamil (Cordilox)	Children	4-8 mg/kg/24 hr
Diuretics (oral)		
Chlorothiazide (Diuril)	Children	20 mg/kg/24 hr
Furosemide (Lasix)	Children	Up to 6 mg/kg/24 hr
Hydrochlorothiazide‡	Children	1-2 mg/kg/dose
Spironolactone (Aldactone)	Children	1.5-3.5 mg/kg/24 hr
Triamterene (Dyrenium)	Children	2-4 mg/kg/24 hr

* Digoxin is calculated in **micrograms**/kg/24 hours while all others are calculated in milligrams.
† May increase serum digoxin levels.
‡ Decrease dose if used with other antihypertensives.
Caution: All medications should be administered cautiously and observed closely since individual patient problems and responses always need to be considered. Each child's response to therapy takes precedence for guiding care.

the right costal margin at the midclavicular. The liver may be 3 to 4 cm beneath the anterior rib cage and should be palpated gently to prevent moving it upward.

Hypoxia occurs when the increase of fluid in the lungs decreases the oxygen transfer across capillary membranes. This decreases the oxygen level in the arterial blood.

Decreased pulses may or may not be exhibited, depending on the cardiac defect. Decreased or absent pulses or variations of blood pressures between the upper and lower extremities are always important and warrant immediate investigation.

Skin that has pallor or is cool and clammy is indicative of arterial blood being shunted away from the skin to vital organs in an effort to conserve oxygen.

Tachycardia is a response to hypoxia in an attempt to maintain cardiac output. To compensate for the decreasing oxygen supply, the sympathetic nervous system increases the heart rate. By boost-

ing cardiac output, this response helps improve the supply of oxygenated blood to tissues. The sympathetic nervous system also triggers vasoconstriction, which increases the blood pressure. Prolonged tachycardia may lead to shock and possibly death.

Planning and intervention

Comprehensive case management. Comprehensive case management not only includes the traditional physical and technical aspects of care, but also includes the anticipatory guidance, advocacy, caring, education, and planning components of patient care.[14] These are the aspects of care that give families the feeling that they are cared for as individuals and are an important factor in the total nursing care process. Most important, the case manager develops a mutually determined plan of care with the family. (See the box titled Primary Nursing Diagnoses/Patient Problems.)

Specific home care plans detail all facets of care provided. They should include documentary logs

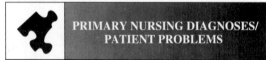

PRIMARY NURSING DIAGNOSES/ PATIENT PROBLEMS

Decreased cardiac output
- Knowledge deficit: disease process and risk complications
- Infant CPR, medications
- Procedural care
- Anticipatory guidance
- Feeding/dietary needs, normal infant growth and development
- Socioenvironmental resources
- Available community services
- Compromised family coping
- Risk for altered parenting

of phone contacts and home visits, designated on-call home health nurses, details of specific visits to provide health care follow-up, developmental evaluations, assessment of parent coping and caretaking skills, education and counseling, confirmation of future follow-up services, and mechanisms to evaluate the delivery of services.[3] (See Chapter 8 for further information on case management.)

Anticipatory guidance. Questions and concerns about the growth and development of all children can be anticipated. For parents of children with congenital heart defects, questions regarding child rearing take on an added significance. For example, letting a child cry and turn blue out of frustration at bedtime would be unwise for parents of children with congenital heart defects. It is important to explore other avenues with these parents. Nurses can help parents establish guidelines for discipline, play, self-feeding, toilet training, and socialization.

Advocacy. Who better to teach families the aspects of accessing the health care system than nurses? The patient needs the services, and the nurse knows how to obtain the services needed. Until nurses actively serve as advocates for patients, patients will not receive the care they need and deserve.

Caring. Caring is an often unidentified component of nursing since it is not a reimbursable commodity. Nyberg[19] identifies several attributes involved in caring: commitment, self-worth, prioritization, openness, and ability to bring about growth. One side of the relationship begins when a person takes an interest that evolves into a commitment to assist another in growing and developing. The other side is receptiveness and willingness on the part of the recipient—the person being cared for. Caring does not imply a short-term relationship and is not always an agreeable or easy path to follow. Caring persons have a strong sense of self-worth and feel cared for in their own lives so that they are able to care for others. Caring relationships have been challenged by a number of factors: infants and children often go home in compromised conditions, they may be technologically dependent, and parents are often expected to assume nursing roles with their children to minimize home health costs. Nurses must never allow the care of the child and family to be compromised; it is the nurse and family who know what is best for patients in their home settings. Assigning priorities is an important part of the caring relationship and means that a person is able to order activities in such a way that there is time and energy for self, patients, family, and professional endeavors.

Parent education.[3,4,22] There are various methods, bridging ethnic and sociocultural diversity, of sharing information with families (see Chapter 6).

Cardiac problems are scary, and they are often synonymous with death to many families. All too often going home with an infant who has a cardiac problem carries overwhelming fears of failure for parents. There are few frightening experiences that quicken the pulse like a baby who stops breathing or whose circulation has stopped. Infant cardiopulmonary resuscitation (CPR) is one thing at the hospital and completely different at home. Cardiac origins rarely are the sole cause of cardiac arrest in infants; more often they are the secondary or tertiary cause. That is why educating parents and child care providers about prevention, recognition of problems, and intervention prior to the need for CPR is essential. (Refer to Appendix 21-2 for a brief review of infant and child CPR.) Along with these fears, parents are consumed with *how* they are going to survive caring for a child with complex needs while maintaining the integrity of an already stressed family, preparing for usual workdays at home or away from home, paying seemingly unending hospital bills, and maintaining a "normal" household. Families deserve the best information and support services to assist them since they do not have the luxury of walking away at the end of the shift.

These families can be best educated through visual methods, auditory-demonstration methods, application methods, and combinations thereof. These methods allow patients and families to control and direct their education in a manner that allows them to absorb what they want *when* they want. The telephone can be a device to clarify and discuss questions, triage client and family needs, evaluate a family's application of information, and direct families to the appropriate resources. The family's level of acceptance and competence can be monitored and evaluated through the use and mastery of information tapes, appointment participation, telephone calls, and home visit requests. Adult learning principles indicate that learning is more effective if learning strategies are begun before discharge and if the family determines what information will be learned in what order and actively participates in setting goals to use the information.

The primary focus of parent education is management of infant illness at home. (See the box titled Primary Themes of Patient/Family Education.) Family instruction regarding diet, feeding, medication, activity levels, safety, signs and symptoms of cardiopulmonary distress, and cardiopulmonary resuscitation is incorporated into the plan of care. In addition, parental use of community resources and support systems should be encouraged by home health nurses. This is accomplished by reviewing available community services when giving instructions to families managing their infant's needs at home. *It is very important to always ask those involved in the infant's care what they want to learn.*

Community resources. Recommendations of child health services should include health services for specific age groups and should be modified to fit the infant's needs.[24] Specific recommendation categories should include activity, anticipatory guidance, child health screening, dental care, development, education, immunizations, nutrition, physical growth, and socialization. Each category should be considered specifically when addressing the needs of the children. Can the standard child health care services be provided or should they be

PRIMARY THEMES OF PATIENT/FAMILY EDUCATION

- Congestive heart failure: recognition and treatment
- Infant CPR and symptoms of distress
- When to call the case manager or physician
- When to call 911
- Medications: purpose, action, dosage, side effects, and methods of administration
- Normal infant growth and development (anticipatory guidance, infant feeding requirements, adequate elimination, sensorimotor stimulation, sleep patterns, and home safety)
- Family dynamics and the chronically ill child (adjustment/positive family coping skills, referral networking, spiritual concerns)
- Parental counseling and positive parenting skills (family-child interaction, providing physical care for the child)
- Socioeconomic resources
- Community services for children with cardiac anomalies

modified, and if so, how? Are there any other needs specific to the infant's health problems that must be addressed? If there is concurrence between the tertiary care and local health care providers for provision of routine child health services and immunizations, it is best for children to receive them locally. By recommending routine well-child care locally, home health nurses ensure that numerous barriers will be removed. Barriers these families frequently encounter include long drives to tertiary care centers, higher health care costs, longer waiting times for appointments, transportation costs, overnight lodging and meal costs, costs associated with time off from work, and family inconvenience.

Evaluation

The final step of the nursing process is evaluation, which assesses patient progress toward meeting the goals and outcomes of care. Evaluation of patient care reflects agency service delivery and appropriate use of resources.[6] Several questions should come to mind when evaluating nursing care of pediatric patients: How is the child doing psychologically, physiologically, socially, and developmentally? Is the child growing as documented by height and weight growth grids? Has there been a rehospitalization? How effectively is the family coping with the stress of home care? Is the child able to stay out of the hospital?

Patient goals and outcomes of care should be reviewed for safety, appropriateness, effectiveness, cost-effectiveness, and legality. General questions one might ask when reviewing patient care include the following: Are the goals and outcomes of care being met? Is the approach working with the child? How is the family doing? Is there a better way to do things? Is the family's/child's health all right? Is there a need for additional information? How is the financial status of the family? Is the family able to manage the child's health care needs in the home setting?

SUMMARY

H. Creighton summarizes today's home care responsibilities in the following excerpt:[7]

"Since early discharges are so common now, there is an increasing incidence of unresolved problems. As a consequence, home care nurses must have superior assessment abilities and be able to make correct decisions to avoid the potential problems accompanying early discharge. Similarly, where home care nurses care for infants with cardiac anomalies, they must thoroughly assess the patient, follow his progress and recognize and be able to effectuate readmission to the hospital when and if necessary. In addition, home care nurses must be cognizant of the community resources and be able to incorporate these in the nursing care plan to meet the patient's needs."

With the development of pediatric home care programs come added responsibilities to be assumed by agencies and home health nurses as they carefully plan and implement programs to improve quality and cost-effective patient care. These specialized pediatric nurses will provide direct patient care in varying settings, engage in independent decision making, collaborate with other health care professionals, and function more autonomously than "traditional" nurses.

If the home health agency does not have a pediatric nurse on its staff, a consultant with expertise in this area is advisable. Furthermore, pediatric in-service training for staff who normally visit adult patients is recommended because weekend and after hour coverage usually involves all patient populations, including infants and children.

As medical technology continues to evolve, the possibilities of health care seem limitless. Children with cardiac anomalies are representative of the types of patients home health agencies will encounter more frequently in the future. The challenge for home health nurses is to balance human need with technology so that these children and their families have long and happy lives.

REFERENCES

1. Bailey NA, Lay P: New horizons: infant cardiac transplantation, *Heart Lung* 18 (2):172, 1989.
2. Blonshine SK: Transposition of the great arteries, *AORN J* 49(4):972, 1989.
3. Brooten D et al: Clinical specialist pre- and post-discharge teaching of parents of very low birth weight infants, *JOGNN* 1:316, 1989.
4. Butler C: High tech tots: technology for mobility, manipulation, communication, and learning in early childhood, *Inf Young Children* 1(2):66, 1988.
5. Callow LB: A new beginning: nursing care of the infant undergoing the arterial switch operation for transposition of the great arteries, *Heart Lung* 18(3):248, 1989.
6. Cragg CA: Nursing ethics: essential component of continuing education, *J Contin Educ Nurs* 19(6):266, 1988.
7. Creighton H: Legal problems of home care nurses, *Nurs Manage* 19 (11):23, 1988.
8. Elsea SJ, Wydeven MS: Low birth weight infants: a system of home health care monitoring, *J Home Health Care Pract* 1(2):37, 1989.
9. Gerraughty AB: Caring for patients with lesions obstructing systemic blood flow, *Crit Care Nurs Clin North Am* 1(2):231, 1989.
10. Gillette PC: Congenital heart disease, *Pediatr Clin North Am* 37(1):27, 1990.
11. Hazinski MG: *Nursing care of the critically ill child,* St Louis, 1991, Mosby.
12. Hutchings SM, Monet ZJ: Caring for the cardiac transplant patient, *Crit Care Nurs Clin North Am* 1(2):245, 1989.
13. Hutti MH: Perinatal loss: assisting parents to cope, *J Emerg Nurs* 14(6):338, 1988.
14. Jaffee MS, Skidmore-Roth L: *Home health: nursing care plans,* St Louis, 1993, Mosby.
15. Kaplan-Sanoff M, Nigro J: The educator in a medical setting: lessons learned from collaboration, *Inf Young Children* 1(2):1, 1988.
16. Moore KL, Persaud TV: *Before we are born: basic embryology and birth defects,* ed 4, Philadelphia, 1993, WB Saunders.
17. Moynihan PJ: Caring for patients with lesions increasing pulmonary blood flow, *Neonatal Pediatr Cardiovasc Nurs* 1(2):195, 1989.
18. Murphy MA: *Decision making in pediatric nursing,* St Louis, 1988, Mosby.

19. Nyberg J: The element of caring in nursing administration, *Nurs Admin Q* 13(3):9, 1989.
20. Pinnell NN, deMeneses M: *The nursing process: theory, application and related processes,* Philadelphia, 1986, Appleton-Century-Crofts.
21. Taketomo CK, Hodding JH, Kraus DM: *Pediatric dosage handbook,* ed 2, Cleveland, 1993-94, Lexi-Comp.
22. Thorne S: *Negotiating health care,* Newberry Park, NY, 1993, Sage.
23. US Department of Health and Human Services: *Congenital malformations surveillance,* Public Health Service/Centers for Disease Control, Atlanta, March 1988.
24. Whaley LB, Wong DL: *Nursing care of infants and children,* ed 4, St Louis, 1991, Mosby.
25. Wolf ZR: Uncovering the hidden work of nursing, *Nurs Health Care* 8(10):463, 1989.
26. Wolf ZR: Pediatric basic life support, *JAMA* 268(16):2251-2261, 1992.

Appendix 21-1

Pulse, Respiration, Temperature, and Blood Pressure Norms for Infants and Children

Normal ranges of heart rates for children (beats/min)

Age	Resting (awake)	Resting (sleeping)	Exercise (fever)
Newborn	100-180	80-160	Up to 220
1 week to 3 months	100-220	80-180	Up to 220
3 months to 2 years	80-150	70-120	Up to 200
2 years to 10 years	70-110	60-100	Up to 180
10 years to adult	55-90	50-90	Up to 180

Modified from Gillette PC: Dysrhythmias. In Adams FH, Emmanouilides GC, Riemenschneider TA, editors: *Moss' heart disease in infants, children, and adolescents,* ed 4, Baltimore, 1989, Williams & Wilkins. In Wong DL: *Whaley and Wong's nursing care of infants and children,* ed 5, St Louis, 1995, Mosby.

Normal temperatures in children

Age	Degrees	Degrees
3 months	99.4	37.5
6 months	99.5	37.5
1 year	99.7	37.7
3 years	99.0	37.2
5 years	98.6	37.0
7 years	98.3	36.8
9 years	98.1	36.7
11 years	98.0	36.7
13 years	97.8	36.6

Modified from Lowrey GH: *Growth and development of children,* ed 8. Copyright © 1986 by Year Book Medical Publishers, Chicago. (Modified and reproduced with permission.)

Normal respiratory rates for children

Age	Rate (breath/min)
Newborn	35
1 to 11 months	30
2 years	25
4 years	23
6 years	21
8 years	20
10 years	19
12 years	19
14 years	18
16 years	17
18 years	16-18

From Wong DL: *Whaley and Wong's nursing care of infants and children,* ed 5, St Louis, 1995, Mosby.

Guidelines for Infant/Child CPR[26]

SEQUENCE OF PERFORMING CPR

1. Determine cause of unresponsiveness or respiratory difficulty.
2. Call for help.
3. Position the victim.
4. Open the airway.
5. Determine whether the victim is breathing.
6. Breathe for the victim.
7. Circulation—check the pulse.
8. Activate emergency medical system—have number available.
9. Perform chest compressions.
10. Coordinate compressions and rescue breathing.

Infant/child CPR variances	Age <1 year	Age 1-8 years
Ventilations per minute	20	20
Compression delivery	Middle and ring finger	Heel of one hand
Compression depth	0.5-1 inch	1-1.5 inches
Compression-ventilation ratio	5:1 (1 rescuer)	5:1 (1 or 2 rescuers)

Source: American Heart Association, 1995.

22 Maternal-Child Nursing: Postpartum Home Care

Annette M. Lynch, Roberta A. Kordish, and Lenore R. Williams

Since birth moved from home to hospital almost a century ago, length of stay (LOS) has steadily declined. The current national debate on health care reform; attention to issues of cost, quality, and access; and emphasis on managed care will continue to drive the length of maternity stay, keeping it as low as possible.

The rapidly decreasing length of hospital stay has directly affected the ability of providers to meet health care needs of mothers, infants, and new families after birth. These needs have been documented in medical, nursing, and sociological research and continue to exist regardless of LOS. Mothers need to recover physically and emotionally. Infants need to make a successful transition to extrauterine existence. Families need to reorganize as they incorporate the infant into the family unit.

Health care needs of childbearing families can be met through implementation of a comprehensive postpartum home care program. Such a program is essential to ensure desired clinical outcomes expected in modern maternity care. It is a proven method to meet the expectations of access, quality, and cost-effectiveness that current health care reform efforts demand.

HISTORICAL PERSPECTIVES

In 1890, 25% of births occurred in a hospital setting; Sloan Memorial Hospital in New York City reported an average LOS of 17.4 days.[25] By 1968, 99.5% of all births occurred in the hospital and the average LOS was 4 to 5 days.[7] From 1970 until the present the LOS has continued to decline because of consumer choice for more homelike, family-centered experiences and payer demand for less costly care (Figure 22-1). The current LOS for all births in the United States is 2.6 days. The LOS for vaginal births ranges from 6 to 48 hours; for cesarean births it ranges from 2 to 4 days.[30,31]

Research has described postpartum home care programs beginning with the Bradford experiment in 1959 in England and spanning the United States and Canada for over 30 years.* In these studies, a shortened hospital stay was combined with follow-up care at home to ensure safe recovery of mothers and infants and to address health care needs of the entire family. Each study demonstrated that a well-planned program resulted in successfully met goals. Common elements of successful short stay maternity programs included (1) guidelines for discharge, (2) preparation of qualified visiting nurses, (3) antepartal contact with the childbearing family, (4) multidisciplinary collaborative program design, (5) timely visits to match the developmental crisis in families, (6) planned mechanisms for referrals when medical or support services were indicated, (7) caregiver accessibility, (8) data on outcomes, and (9) demonstrated cost-effectiveness.

PHILOSOPHY OF CARE

Today the goals of care for childbearing families are a healthy pregnancy, a healthy infant, and parents who are prepared for and confident in their new roles. To achieve these goals, current standards of care advocate early and regular prenatal care and birth in a hospital or birthing center. However, there is no standard that recognizes the needs of mothers, infants, and families following a short LOS. The Association of Women's Health, Obstetric and Neonatal Nurses (AWHONN) recently published a position statement[4] and guidelines for perinatal

---

*References 3, 6, 7, 9, 14, 15, 16, 17, 18, 19, 22, 29, 35, 36, 37.

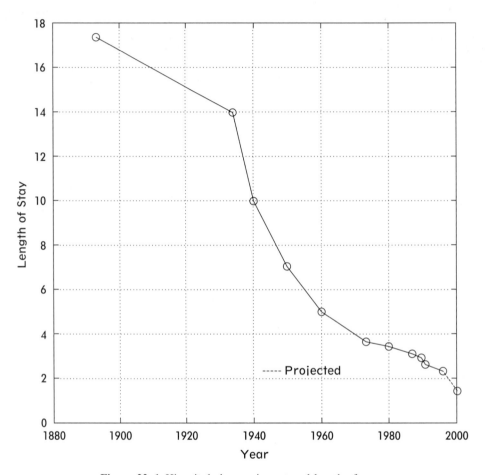

Figure 22-1 Historical changes in maternal length of stay.

home care.[5] In addition, the American Nurses Association (ANA) is developing a similar document[2] to establish skilled postpartum home care as an equally necessary component in meeting national health care goals for childbearing families.

Postpartum nursing has always made a valuable contribution to the recovery of mothers and infants from childbirth, and to the successful launching of new families. Regardless of the environment, such nursing care continues to be necessary to achieve the following goals:

- Monitor and ensure the physical and emotional well-being of family members
- Identify developing complications early, preventing exacerbations and costly rehospitalizations

- Bridge the care gap between discharge and ambulatory follow-up for mothers and infants with primary care providers*

SCOPE OF SERVICES

Differences exist between home care for clients with medically diagnosed conditions and home care for postpartum families. Childbirth is a healthy event. Although services to treat an illness or injury are not indicated, birth does involve a recovery period that must be monitored, and a

---

*Primary care providers exist for both mother and infant. They can include an obstetrician, a certified nurse midwife (CNM), a family practitioner, a pediatrician and/or a pediatric nurse practitioner.

developmental crisis that the new family must resolve to maintain health. A program approach to postpartum home care recognizes these differences and structures services to match this unique population.

A comprehensive and cost-effective skilled postpartum home care program is a hybrid of traditional inpatient postpartum care and traditional home care. It is based on the understanding that when mothers and infants are discharged 6 to 48 hours after vaginal birth or 48 to 72 hours after cesarean birth, only initial stabilization has occurred. Health promotion activities have just been initiated and few learning needs have been identified or met. The intent of such a program is to begin where hospital or birthing center care has ended, neither duplicating nor omitting any essential elements.

These postpartum home care services span the time from late pregnancy to follow-up after birth. They are structured to provide the following:

- Case management from discharge to ambulatory follow-up, usually a 2-week period of time
- Prenatal preparation for both a brief LOS and home nursing care following discharge
- One home visit for two clients (mother and infant) that incorporates intake, initiation, and completion of the plan of care
- Discretionary visits if dictated by nursing or medical needs

Whereas each mother and infant is the focus of a different primary care provider, only the nurse has a whole family perspective. Only the nurse is aware of family dynamics, can assess the health care needs of each family member, and facilitates the initial stages of family reintegration.

The postpartum home care program includes the following services:

- Case management and care by an experienced registered nurse
- Prenatal and previsit contact with the referred family
- Coordination of care with primary care providers, hospital or birthing center nurses, and community agencies
- Visits made 24 to 72 hours following discharge
- Skilled nursing assessment and intervention for mothers, infants, and families

- Use of a risk management documentation tool
- Postvisit phone call(s)
- Availability of a 24-hour help line
- Continuous measurement of quality variables such as health status, complications, readmission rates, client satisfaction, and cost-effectiveness

In addition to the role preparation for the home health nurse outlined in Chapter 3, qualifications for a registered nurse providing skilled postpartum home care include a minimum of 1 year maternal-infant care experience with the theoretical and clinical competencies to assess and care for mothers, infants, and families at home. (See the box below.)

PRACTITIONER COMPETENCIES FOR POSTPARTUM HOME CARE

Didactic content

1. Physiology of lactation
2. Postpartum involution
3. Postpartum missing pieces
4. Postpartum timetable
5. Postpartum depression
6. Physiological transition of infant to extrauterine existence
7. Infant nutrition and feeding
8. Infant growth and development
9. Infant behavior
10. Infant/parent cue/response pattern
11. Infant hyperbilirubinemia
12. Infant metabolic screening
13. Family theory
14. Family developmental tasks
15. Communication theory
16. Teaching/learning theory
17. Crisis theory and intervention

Clinical skills

1. Physical assessment of the postpartum woman
2. Psychosocial assessment of the postpartum woman
3. Physical assessment of the infant
4. Feeding assessment of the infant
5. Specimen collection—maternal (venipuncture or fingerstick, urine and stool, vaginal culture, wound culture)
6. Specimen collection—infant (heelstick, urine)

HOME CARE APPLICATION
Prenatal contact

Case management begins with preparation of clients at 34 to 36 weeks gestation. The nurse can contact the client by phone, in person, or via written communication. The objectives of this contact are as follows:

- Explain the purpose, content, and length of the visit
- Ensure the coordination of care with primary care providers, hospital/birth center nurses, insurers, and community agencies
- Obtain baseline data on the mother and family (health status during pregnancy, preparation for the infant, availability of help at home following hospital discharge, infant feeding method, and pediatric provider)
- Provide anticipatory guidance for identified needs
- Determine address and telephone number of family location following hospital discharge

The nurse gives the client the name, address and phone number of the agency and instructions on how the agency is to be notified of the client's delivery. Documentation of this contact is kept with the client's chart.

Referral process

The home care nurse can be likened to the "next shift." Although some home care agencies have their own coordinators to obtain discharge data, the health care system of the future dictates efficiency. An expedient method for the transfer of information is for the inpatient nurse to "give report" to the home care nurse. This allows the home care nurse to continue or modify the nursing plan of care already established. Since visits should be scheduled within 72 hours of discharge, it is best to obtain the referral information and medical orders for care on the day of discharge. Figure 22-2 shows an example of a comprehensive referral form.

Scheduling visits

The home care nurse determines when the visit should be made based on the prenatal contact, the referral information, and any specific physician order(s). For example, an infant of 37 weeks

gestation who is having feeding difficulty, an inexperienced breast-feeding mother, or a multipara who was discharged on methylergonovine maleate would all warrant visits earlier in the 72-hour time frame.

Mothers should be contacted within 24 hours of discharge to determine recovery status, schedule the visit, verify location, and provide the 24-hour help line number. Considerations for scheduling visits include a mutually convenient time and the presence of support persons. (See the box titled Equipment for Postpartum Home Care.)

Maternal assessment

The nurse determines the mother's progress toward the goal of physical and psychological recovery from childbirth and instructs the mother in self-monitoring techniques. The three major assessment categories are physical, activities of daily living, and psychological. In order to establish a comfort level, it is more appropriate to assess the mother's psychological status, and review activities of daily living prior to doing the physical examination. However, in this section, physical assessment of the mother will be addressed first. Abnormal findings are always reported to the primary care provider.

Physical assessment. Suggest an area of privacy prior to initiating the physical assessment of the mother. The mother needs to assume a supine position on a mattress or sofa. A waterbed is not ideal because of instability. Advise a mother never to feed or sleep with the infant on a waterbed because of the danger of suffocation.

Vital signs. Although the mother's temperature may be elevated during the first 24 hours after delivery and again when the milk comes in, the upper limit of normal elevation is 100.4°F (38°). Tachycardia (>100 beats/min) may indicate a potential for infection, hemorrhage, vaginal hematoma, or other types of cardiovascular compromise. At the time of the home visit, the mother should be normotensive. Elevation may indicate postpartum pregnancy-induced hypertension. Hypotension may indicate excessive bleeding.

Breasts. Identify whether the mother is breast- or bottle-feeding. Inspect and palpate breasts for size, tension, color, heat, and discharge. If the bottle-feeding mother is engorged, assess her understanding of using ice packs, analgesics, a breast

Postpartum Family Referral Form

Date: mo / day / yr

HOLLISTER®
maternal/newborn
RECORD SYSTEM

PATIENT IDENTIFICATION

Patients name
Home address

STREET

CITY   STATE   ZIP

Age _____ Date of birth mo / day / yr Race or ethnicity _____ Religion _____ Marital status _____ Years married _____

	EDUCATION	OCCUPATION
PATIENT		
SPOUSE		

FULL ☐ PART ☐ SELF ☐ UNEMP. ☐ WORK TELE. NO. _____ HOME TELE. NO. _____

	OBSTETRICIAN	PEDIATRICIAN	INSURANCE	HOSPITAL	REFERRING R.N.
NAME					
ADDRESS					DATE / TIME
					mo / day / yr
TELEPHONE _____-_____-_____			_____-_____-_____		___:___ A.M. P.M.

MATERNAL INFORMATION

MATERNAL RECORD # _____

SIGNIFICANT HEALTH HISTORY: _____

_____ BLOOD TYPE Rh _____

PRENATAL INFORMATION

GRAV.	TERM	PRET	ABORT/ ECTOPIC	LIVE	E D C

HISTORICAL RISK FACTORS AND ASSESSMENT

[0] HAD NO KNOWN RISK

[1] WAS "AT RISK"

[2] WAS AT HIGH RISK

PRENATAL HOSPITALIZATION ☐ NO ☐ YES, DATES: _____

INTRAPARTAL DATA

DELIVERY DATE: mo / day / yr TIME OF BIRTH _____:_____ ☐ A.M. ☐ P.M. ☐ VAGINAL ☐ C-SECTION

INCISION: PERINEAL (TYPE) _____ ABDOMINAL (TYPE) _____

ANESTHESIA _____

COMPLICATIONS (INDICATE BOTH MATERNAL AND FETAL / NEONATAL): _____

POSTPARTAL DATA

DATE OF DISCHARGE mo / day / yr TIME _____:_____ ☐ A.M. ☐ P.M.

PHYSICAL STATUS

TEMP	PULSE	RESP.	BP
			/

SIGNIFICANT LAB DATA _____

EMOTIONAL STATUS _____

LEVEL OF MATERNAL / INFANT ATTACHMENT

0 — 1 — 2 — 3 — 4
NONE   HIGH LEVEL

COMPLICATIONS	ACTIVE	RESOLVED
	☐	☐
	☐	☐
	☐	☐

DISCHARGE PLANNING

NEEDS AT DISCHARGE (LEARNING, PHYSICAL, EMOTIONAL): _____

PRESCRIBED MEDS/TREATMENT AT DISCHARGE: _____

REFERRALS: _____

NEWBORN INFORMATION

INFANT'S NAME _____ INFANT'S RECORD NO. _____

☐ FEMALE ☐ MALE APGAR SCORE _____ 1 MIN. _____ 5 MIN.

WEIGHT AT DISCHARGE:

BIRTH WEIGHT _____ LBS _____ GMS. OZS. _____ LBS _____ GMS. OZS.

BIRTH LENGTH _____ CM. IN.

HEAD CIR. _____ CM. IN. THIS INFANT IS CLASSIFIED AS:

CHEST CIR. _____ CM. IN. ☐ PRE-TERM (< 38 WEEKS)

GEST. AGE BY DATE _____ WKS. ☐ TERM (38-42 WEEKS) ☐ POST TERM (> 42 WEEKS)

GEST. AGE BY EXAM _____ WKS. ☐ SGA ☐ AGA ☐ LGA

INFANT BLOOD TYPE / Rh _____

METHOD OF FEEDING

☐ BREAST ☐ BOTTLE TYPE OF FORMULA _____

JAUNDICE

☐ HEAD (3 mg/dl)

☐ HEAD & UPPER CHEST (6 mg/dl)

☐ HEAD & ENTIRE CHEST (9 mg/dl)

☐ HEAD, CHEST & ABDOMEN TO UMBILICUS (12 mg/dl)

☐ HEAD, CHEST & ENTIRE ABDOMEN (15 mg/dl)

☐ HEAD, CHEST, ABDOMEN, LEGS & FEET (18 mg/dl)

LAB DATA	
DATE	BILIRUBIN/HCT

CIRCUMCISION ☐ NO ☐ YES, CONDITION _____

TEMP.	PULSE	RESP.	BP
			/

ABNORMAL FINDING

BEHAVIORAL	PHYSICAL

SPECIAL NEEDS AT DISCHARGE: _____

FAMILY INFORMATION

SUPPORT PERSON(S) NAME _____ RELATIONSHIP _____

LEVEL OF PATERNAL/INFANT ATTACHMENT

0 — 1 — 2 — 3 — 4
NONE   HIGH LEVEL

UNUSUAL FAMILY CIRCUMSTANCE: _____

SIBLINGS: NUMBER: _____ AGES: _____

Hollister
HOLLISTER INCORPORATED, 2000 HOLLISTER DR., LIBERTYVILLE, IL 60048
* TRADEMARK OF HOLLISTER INCORPORATED

VISITING NURSE COPY

POSTPARTUM FAMILY REFERRAL FORM FORM # 5841 392

Figure 22-2 Postpartum family referral form. (Reprinted with permission of Professional Nurse Associates.)

EQUIPMENT FOR POSTPARTUM HOME CARE

1. Record system (Hollister Postpartum Home Care Record System)
2. Foamed alcohol surgical hand scrub
3. Gloves
4. Thermometer and probe covers
5. Sphygmomanometer, regular and large cuffs
6. Stethoscope
7. Penlight
8. Infant scale
9. Tape measure
10. Cord clamp remover
11. Lactation devices (lactaids, shells)
12. Specimen collection supplies (metabolic screening cards; urine specimen containers; lab kit with alcohol swabs, lancets, tenderfoot devices, microtainers, capillary tubes, clay, tourniquet, vacutainer system, gauze sponges, adhesive bandages; specimen labels; specimen bags; sharps container; Clinistix; Dextrostix; culture tubes)
13. Educational materials
14. Community resources information

---

binder, or a tight bra for comfort. There is no antilactogenic medication recommended by the FDA at this time.[20] If the mother is breast-feeding, assess tenderness, nodulation, and milk production; and inspect the nipples for integrity and erectility. If nipple integrity is altered, determine the use and effectiveness of any topical agent. This is an ideal time to teach or reinforce the mother in the technique of breast self-exam (BSE). Inform the breast-feeding mother about changes in breast configuration and in the timing of BSE during lactation. A well-fitting, supportive bra may be worn for comfort. An ill-fitting or underwire bra may cause plugged ducts and ultimately mastitis in the breast-feeding mother.[24]

Abdominal musculature. Following birth, the mother's abdomen is usually soft, distended, and a cause for potential body image alteration. Pregnancy can distend the abdomen and cause an actual separation of the two rectus abdominis muscles (diastasis recti). To assess this phenomenon, have the mother assume a supine position (head flat or elevated with a low pillow, knees bent, feet flat on surface). Instruct the mother to attempt a chin-to-chest maneuver, as if doing a modified sit-up. Measure the width and length of the abdomen in centimeters. Have the mother palpate the diastasis recti to verify the reason for her figure changes and enable her to self-monitor resolution. Instructions in exercise progression can be suggested at this time. If a cesarean or bilateral partial salpingectomy (tubal ligation) incision is present, assess the mother's abdomen for presence of sutures/staples/steri-strips, Redness, Ecchymosis, Edema, Discharge, and Approximation (modified REEDA scale).[10] Physician orders and agency policy should govern the nurse's removing sutures or staples.

Reproductive tract. The puerperium is the period of time from the end of the third stage of labor until the pelvic organs have returned to normal.[23] Usually by 6 weeks postpartum, the uterus returns to its prepregnant state by the process known as involution. During involution the actual number of uterine cells does not change, but each cell decreases in size by approximately 90%.

Approximately 12 hours after delivery, the uterine fundus can be palpated at the level of the umbilicus. It continues to decrease in size by about 1 cm per day.[23] Uterine discharge (lochia) is made up of blood and debris from the necrosis of the decidua (uterine lining). Lochia progression is described in Table 22-1. Lochia should always have a fleshy smell. A strong odor resembling spoiled meat is a sign of infection.

Progression of uterine involution is characterized by the location and consistency of the uterine fundus. When assessing the fundus, first instruct the mother to empty her bladder. The stretched uterine ligaments allow the uterus to move easily in the abdominal cavity. A full bladder can displace the uterus to the right or left of midline. Begin by assessing the perineal pad for the color and amount of lochia, while noting the lochia odor. With the mother in a recumbent position place one hand immediately above the symphysis pubis, and the other on top of the fundus. The fundus should feel firm. If the fundus is relaxed, gently massage it until firm. Assess lochia by noting the type and number of perineal pads and the percentage of pad saturation. Instruct the mother how to monitor normal uterine involution by palpating her fundus, identifying normal involution progression, and rec-

Table 22-1 Lochia progression[10,11,12,23]

Stage	Time postpartum	Characteristics
Rubra	Delivery-3 days	Red, possibly small clots
Serosa	4-10 days	Brownish to pink, serosanguineous
Alba	11-21 days	Yellowish to white

ognizing appropriate lochial flow. Fundal height and lochia can vary slightly due to multiparity, infant size, cesarean birth, or the presence of fibroids. Significant uterine tenderness or foul smelling lochia may indicate the presence of endometritis.

Assess the perineum by having the mother assume a side-lying position with the top leg flexed over the bottom leg. Use a penlight to illuminate the area. Lifting the buttock to visualize the perineum and anal area, note the condition of the perineal body, any laceration/episiotomy (REEDA scale[10]), and the presence/condition of hemorrhoids. Question the mother about perineal hygiene and the use and effectiveness of sitz baths and topical agents.

Elimination pattern. Immediately after delivery, there may be swelling or bruising near the urethra. The bladder has increased capacity following delivery, but the sensation to urinate may not be present as a result of the use of conduction anesthesia. The pregnancy induced ureteral dilatation persists for 2 to 4 weeks after birth. In addition, the body must rapidly rid itself of 2,000 to 3,000 ml of extracellular fluid that accumulates in normal pregnancy. The newly delivered mother experiences diuresis and diaphoresis to accomplish this task. A history of pregnancy-induced hypertension complicates this resolution because of the presence of edema.[23] The bladder should not be palpated above the symphysis pubis. Identify presence of urinary symptoms such as urgency, frequency, dysuria, burning, incontinence, or tenderness. Since any of these signs and symptoms may indicate a urinary tract infection, be prepared to obtain a clean catch urine specimen.

Birth causes decreased intraabdominal pressure. Hormonal alterations may cause decreased intestinal peristalsis. Fear of defecation because of the presence of hemorrhoids and/or laceration/episiotomy may also delay return to normal bowel habits. Assess bowel elimination pattern and identify the use and effectiveness of stool softeners or laxatives.

Lower extremities. Following the delivery of the placenta, there is an increase in clotting factors. This can be exacerbated if the mother has a cesarean delivery, pregnancy-induced hypertension, obesity, or a history of vascular disorders or thromboembolytic disease.[23] Ambulation is recommended to avoid venous stasis. Assess the mother's legs for heat, swelling, redness, or pain. Pain in the calf on dorsiflexion is known as a positive Homans' sign and may indicate thrombophlebitis. To elicit this response, with the leg extended, gently hold the knee flat and dorsiflex the foot. Note the presence of any edema. Measure the extent by depressing the leg surface. Residual edema may not be resolved, especially if the mother has had a prolonged induction of labor, or pregnancy-induced hypertension. Pitting edema of 2+ or more is significant.

Pain. Many mothers experience altered comfort in the postpartum period. Common sites of pain include head, breast, uterus, abdomen, back, perineum, hemorrhoid, and leg. Determine the extent, duration, and cause of the pain. Identify use of analgesics and their effectiveness. Persistent or intractable pain is abnormal.

Activities of daily living. Returning to the realities of household management and infant care may preclude adequate nutrition. If the mother's nutritional needs are not met, recovery may be delayed, and lactation may be inhibited. Decreased appetite may also signify postpartum depression.[23] Obtain a 24-hour diet history (including fluids), assess for nutritional adequacy, and counsel on apparent deficits. Identify intake of iron and vitamin supplements. Most practitioners recommend that lactating mothers continue to take prenatal vitamins.

Fatigue is common. Sleep was interrupted in the last trimester of pregnancy, labor caused energy expenditure, and infant caretaking activities prevent optimal sleep. Identify day and night periods of uninterrupted sleep. Determine maternal activities including infant care, household management, and exercise. The activities of daily living should be correlated with physical and psychological findings in order to determine their appropriateness. Help the family prioritize and reorganize activities to facilitate the mother's recovery.

Psychological assessment. The following factors are important in assessing the mother's psychological well-being.

General comments. Use principles of therapeutic communication such as active listening, maintaining eye contact, reflecting, clarifying, empathizing, encouraging, and the use of touch to elicit information. Ask open-ended questions such as "What has bringing this baby home been like?" to obtain information about feelings, body image, and self-concept.

Integrating the birth experience. The term *missing pieces* refers to a woman's inability to recall her birth events clearly.[1] The labor and birth experience must be resolved before the woman can take on her new role as a mother. Allow the mother time to reflect and determine if missing pieces exist. Reports from the referring institution or information from a support person can clarify details so the mother has a total picture of the birth experience.

Postpartum timetable. Following birth, the mother must progress through tasks of maternal psychological adaptation (Table 22-2). Although the classic stages of "taking in," "taking hold," and "letting go" have been artificially accelerated by the advent of shortened hospital stays, identification of the mother's place on this timetable allows for effective intervention in meeting her needs.

Postpartum depression. The initial exhilaration of delivery is often changed by the time the nurse sees the family in the home. A fluctuation in hormones, fatigue, and feelings of unmet self and societal expectations may precipitate negative feelings during the postpartum period (Table 22-3). Address any negative feelings the mother expresses. Acknowledging that many new mothers feel down (blues), but are not emotionally incapacitated (atypical depression or psychosis) gives families guidelines to do self-monitoring.

Infant assessment

Assess the newborn infant's progress in achieving the goal of healthy adaptation to extrauterine life. The three major assessment categories are physical, nutritional, and behavioral. The presence of parents and other family members allows the nurse to demonstrate infant capabilities and caregiving techniques. Safety of the infant is paramount.

Table 22-2 Maternal psychological adaptation

Phase postpartum	Maternal Characteristics
Taking in (1-2 days)	Passive, dependent, concerned with own needs; verbalizes delivery experience
Taking hold (3-10 days)	Strives for independence; strong anxiety element; maximal stage of learning readiness; mood swings may occur
Letting go (10 days-6 weeks)	Achieves interdependence; realistic regarding role transition; accepts baby as a separate person; new norms established for self

Modified from Rubin R: Puerperal change, *Nurs Outlook* 9:753-755, 1961.

Table 22-3 Postpartum depression[10,11,12,23]

Type	Characteristics	Incidence
Blues	Benign, brief, occurring 2 to 10 days after birth	80%
Atypical	More disabling, physical and psychological symptoms, longer-lasting	10%
Psychosis	Incapacitating, may be long-term, risks of suicide and infanticide	0.5%-3.0%

Never leave the infant unattended. Perform the assessment on a bed, sofa, table with padding, crib, or changing table. To prevent heat loss, only undress the infant for weighing and measuring. Other assessments may be performed with the infant partially clothed. Abnormal findings are always reported to the primary care provider.

In several states, newborn metabolic screening must be repeated if the infant is not at least 48 hours of age at the initial screen. The tests generally include phenylketonuria (PKU), hypothyroidism, and galactosemia. Included in some screening programs are congenital adrenal hypoplasia, homocystinuria, maple syrup urine disease, sickle cell disease and other hemoglobinopathies, tyrosinemia, histidinemia, and various other screening tests.[28,32] Follow the directives of individual state statutes.

Physical assessment.

Descriptive data. Weigh the infant and measure the length from head to heel. Weight loss of greater than 10% of birth weight is reportable. Head circumference (normal range: 33 to 35 cm) may be slightly altered from birth, and molding may initially decrease head circumference. Chest circumference (normal range: 30.5 to 33 cm) should be 2 to 3 cm less than head circumference.

Vital signs. Axillary temperature should register 36.4° to 37.2°C (97.5° to 99°F). Crying or excessive environmental heat will elevate temperature; exposure or environmental cooling may produce hypothermia.

Assess apical pulse (normal range: 120 to 160 beats/min) by auscultation in the fourth to fifth intercostal space, medial to the left midclavicular line. This is the point of maximum intensity (PMI). Displacement of the PMI may indicate cardiac malposition, pneumothorax, or diaphragmatic hernia. Crying can increase the rate to 180 beats/min; sleep can decrease the rate to 100 beats/min. Assessing specific components of heart sounds is difficult because of the rapid pulse and respiratory rate. The first (S_1) and second (S_2) should be clear, with the S_2 being somewhat higher in pitch and sharper. Although murmurs may be heard because of incomplete transition from fetal to newborn circulation, they may also indicate major cardiac anomalies and should always be reported (see Chapter 21). Although irregular rhythm is possible in infants, it is a potential sign of distress/major abnormality and should always be reported.

Respirations (normal range 30 to 60) are irregular and abdominal, with periodic apnea of up to 15 seconds. Breath sounds should be equal and bilateral. Grunting, nasal flaring, and substernal retracting are abnormal findings indicative of respiratory distress.[32] Auscultation of respiratory sounds and cardiac status are best done when the infant is quiet and should be counted for 60 seconds.

Head. The oval contour of the infant's head is usually apparent by the second day of life. Palpate the infant's skull to determine the presence and condition of the **fontanels** and **sutures.** The normal anterior and posterior fontanels feel firm, flat, and are easily demarcated against the skull bones. Depressed fontanels indicate dehydration. A bulging fontanel signifies increased intracranial pressure caused by crying, coughing, or a pathologic occlusion of the flow of cerebrospinal fluid. Residual molding, caput succedaneum, cephalhematoma, or overriding sutures may be present after delivery. Caput succedaneum is identified as a soft swelling caused by fluid in the subcutaneous tissue of the scalp and is not limited by suture lines. A cephalhematoma may be identified by firm swelling that does not cross suture lines. If a vacuum extractor was used during delivery, there may be an area resembling caput succedaneum but appearing slightly cyanotic. Abnormal findings include fused sutures and the presence of a snapping sensation along the lambdoidal suture.

The eyelids may be swollen as a result of the use of prophylactic eye treatment at delivery. Normal **eyes** are symmetrical with pink conjunctiva and white sclera. There may be a subconjunctival hemorrhage caused by capillary rupture at the time of delivery. Pupils should be equal and reactive to light. Infants are able to fixate on an object held 8 to 10 inches away from the eyes, and follow the object to midline. The iris is usually slate grey or dark blue in light-skinned infants and brown in dark-skinned infants.

Normal **ear** position aligns the top third of the pinna with the outer canthus of the eye. Pinnae are flexible with cartilage present. The infant in the alert or light sleep state exhibits the startle reflex when a loud noise is apparent. Some states require parents and hospital staff to complete a screening tool that identifies hearing deficit risk factors.

Infants are obligatory **nose** breathers and are unable to breathe if the nares are occluded. Hold one hand over the infant's mouth and one nostril while noting air passage through the open canal and then repeat on the other side. This is an opportune time for the nurse to instruct the family on nasal suctioning with a bulb syringe.

Assess the **mouth** for a high-arched, intact palate and the uvula at midline. Assess tongue mobility. A shortened frenulum may cause immobility and impair breast-feeding. Check for the sucking, rooting, and gag reflexes. Mucous membranes should be pink. Thrush (a white, patchy coating on the tongue or buccal membranes) is an abnormal condition requiring treatment. If a mother has vaginal moniliasis at the time of birth, transmission to the infant's oral mucosa is almost ensured. Thrush interferes with infant feeding, may cause candidal diaper dermatitis, and can be transmitted to the nipples and breasts of the nursing mother.[32]

Neck. The infant's neck is usually short, thick, and surrounded by skin folds. There is complete range of motion. Identify movement, shape, and the ability of the infant to exhibit some degree of head control. Palpate clavicles for the presence of crepitus, which indicates fracture. This may or may not be accompanied by brachial plexus palsy.[32]

Chest. The chest appears almost circular with symmetrical expansion. The xiphoid process is prominent. Due to the influence of maternal hormones, breasts of infants of either sex may be enlarged and exude a milky white discharge ("witches' milk") around the third day of life.

Cardiovascular. In addition to heart sounds (see the section on vital signs), assess brachial and femoral pulses for strength and equality. Color changes in the skin may indicate cardiac compromise (see the section on skin). For a detailed assessment of cardiovascular anomalies see Chapter 21.

Abdomen. The abdomen is almost cylindrical in nature. Bowel sounds are audible with a stethoscope. The liver can be palpated approximately 1 to 3 cm below the right costal margin. A liver that is larger may indicate hepatomegaly, especially in the presence of jaundice. Occasionally the tip of the spleen can be palpated approximately 1 cm below the right costal margin, and a skilled prac-

titioner can palpate the kidneys soon after birth. Abdominal masses are abnormal.

The **umbilical cord** is white, gelatinous, and moist at birth. The cord may still be clamped from birth. Inspect the cord for drying and if not moist, remove the clamp. Instruct in cord care and placement of the infant's diaper below the level of the cord to promote continued drying and prevent infection. Tub baths are not recommended until the cord stump falls off, usually 7 to 14 days after birth. Although some serosanguineous drainage may occur, there should be no active bleeding. The presence of erythema, purulent drainage, and foul odor indicate an infection.

Genitalia. The **female** infant at term may exhibit swelling of the clitoris and labia majora, especially with a breech presentation. A hymenal tag may be present at the posterior end of the vagina, gradually disappearing by a few weeks of age. Due to the influence of maternal hormones, vaginal discharge is usually white, mucousy, and may be blood tinged (pseudomenstruation). Explain to parents that this is normal and usually disappears by 4 weeks of age.

Inspect the **male** infant for urethral opening at the tip of the penis. The uncircumcised male has a foreskin covering the glans. Forcibly retracting the foreskin is not necessary for hygiene and may cause adhesions. Smegma, a thick white substance, may be present. If the infant is circumcised a yellow exudate may be present on the glans. This granulation is part of the normal healing process and should never be removed. Petrolatum may be applied to prevent adherence of the circumcised penis to the diaper. Bleeding or swelling are abnormal. If a Hollister Plastibell is used for circumcision, the residual plastic ring usually falls off in 5 to 8 days. No petrolatum should be used with the Plastibell because it may cause deterioration of the plastic.

The scrotum in the term male infant is usually large and pendulous, with greater edema in the breech infant. Testes are normally palpated in the scrotal sac. Undescended testes in the inguinal canal, inguinal hernia, scrotal masses, or hydrocele are abnormal.

Skeletal. Place the infant on the abdomen. Inspect the back for any curves, masses, or openings along the spinal column. Any degree of spina bifida or pilonidal cyst or sinus is abnormal.

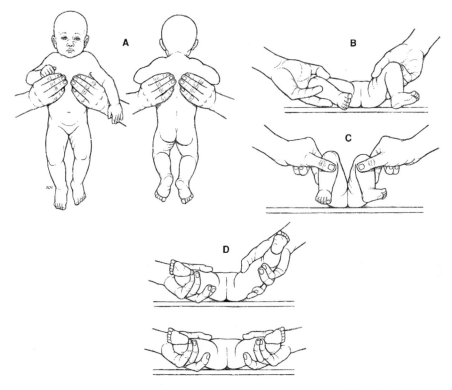

Figure 22-3 Signs of congenital dislocation of the hip. **A,** Asymmetry of gluteal and thigh folds. **B,** Limited hip abduction with flexion. **C,** Apparent shortening of femur, indicated by knee height when knees are flexed. **D,** Ortolani click (under 4 weeks of age). (From Wong DL: *Whaley and Wong's nursing care of infants and children,* ed 5, St Louis, 1995, Mosby.)

Extend the legs to examine for symmetry and equality of gluteal and thigh folds. Inspect the anus at this time for fissures or fistulas.

Examine the extremities with the infant in a supine position. Asymmetry, limited range of motion, malformations, polydactyly, and syndactyly are abnormal. Check for congenital dislocation of the hip by techniques shown in Figure 22-3. The Ortolani test should be reserved for experienced practitioners.

Elimination. Infants void 3 to 4 times per day in the first few days of life. By the end of the first week, the infant who is adequately hydrated will void 6 to 10 times per day. Urine is almost colorless although there may be some orange-red urine crystals present. Stool frequency can vary widely from one per feeding to one every few days.[23] (See Table 22-4 for descriptions of stool patterns.)

Neuromuscular. The term infant is in a flexed posture, and exhibits neither hypotonia nor hypertonia. Occasionally the infant may demonstrate trembling activity. Several reflexes are present at birth and are bilaterally equal, indicating central nervous system integrity. (See Table 22-5 for assessment of representative newborn reflexes.) Diminished or unequal responses are abnormal. Expect the infant's cry to be strong and lusty. Cries that are high-pitched, shrill, weak, groaning, absent, or exceeding 4 hours per day are abnormal.

Skin. The skin is smooth and pink. By the second day, there may be some dry and peeling areas, especially in the postmature infant. Acrocyanosis or transient mottling may occur when the

Table 22-4 Infant stool patterns[23,37]

Type	Characteristics	Time frame
Meconium	Thick, tarry, dark green	Birth-2 days
Transitional	Loose, green-brown to yellow-brown, seedy	2-5 days
Breast-fed	Mushy, golden yellow, often after each feeding, odor similar to sour milk	posttransitional
Formula-fed	Firm, pasty, yellow-brown, strong odor	posttransitional

Table 22-5 Selected infant reflexes[23,32]

Reflex	Assessment technique	Expected response
Moro	Stimulate by sudden noise, movement, or change in position/equilibrium.	Extends and abducts all extremities. Forms "C" shape with thumbs and forefingers. Adducts, then flexes extremities.
Palmar grasp	Place finger in palms.	Grasps examiner's finger.
Babinski	Stroke outer sole of foot upward from the heel across the ball of the foot.	Hyperextends toes, dorsiflexes great toe, fans toes outward.

infant becomes chilled. Pallor or generalized cyanosis may indicate cardiovascular compromise and are considered abnormal. Normal variations include telangiectatic nevi, mongolian spots (especially seen in infants of African, Asian, and Hispanic descent), milia, miliaria, erythema toxicum, and birthmarks. Petechiae or ecchymoses may be present if birth was traumatic. A scalp lesion may result if an internal electrode was used for fetal monitoring.

Jaundice. Jaundice is one of the most common conditions present in infants, with incidence of 50% to 80% reported.[10,21,28,33,34] Physiologic jaundice is caused by an accumulation of bilirubin, a product of red blood cell (RBC) breakdown. A high volume of fetal RBCs is needed to circulate oxygen in utero. At birth, natural destruction of excess RBCs occurs. The infant's immature liver is unable to remove the bilirubin as rapidly as the demand is made. This physiologic process is compared with other types of jaundice in Table 22-6. Physiologic jaundice can be exacerbated by ethnic predisposition (Asians, Native Americans, Eskimos), maternal medical complications (diabetes or infection), birth injury, or hypoxia. Assess the jaundice level by visual inspection. Jaundice appears in a cephalocaudal progression and usually resolves in the opposite direction. Use the "rules

of three"[27] to estimate the approximate serum bilirubin level as follows:

- Head (3 mg/dl)
- Head and upper chest (6 mg/dl)
- Head and entire chest (9 mg/dl)
- Head, chest and abdomen to umbilicus (12 mg/dl)
- Head, chest and entire abdomen (15 mg/dl)
- Head, chest, abdomen, legs and feet (18 mg/dl)

A serum bilirubin verifies the estimated level of significant jaundice. A serum bilirubin level of greater than 20 mg/dl in the term infant is associated with kernicterus, cerebral encephalopathy from the deposit of unconjugated and highly toxic bilirubin, which can result in brain damage. Draw a serum bilirubin by heelstick per agency protocol and medical order. Warm the heel prior to site preparation. Puncture the outer aspect of the heel no deeper than 2.4 mm (Figure 22-4). A free flow of blood is necessary. Squeezing the heel or scraping it on the collection tube may cause excessive hemolysis, giving a false high bilirubin level. Apply pressure to the site with gauze until bleeding has stopped, and then apply an adhesive bandage. Use universal precautions when obtaining and transporting specimens. (See Chapter 5.) Protect the specimen from light during transport to

Table 22-6 Types and characteristics of neonatal jaundice*

Type	Etiology (incidence)	Onset	Progression	Prevention treatment
Physiologic jaundice	RBC hemolysis and immature liver function (5%-80% of all infants)	After 24 hours, usually 2nd or 3rd day	Peaks 3rd to 5th day, declines 5th to 7th day	Sufficient caloric/fluid intake resulting in increased stooling. Possible phototherapy.
Breast-feeding associated jaundice	Decreased caloric and fluid intake associated with insufficient milk production in early breast-feeding (10%-25% of breast-fed infants)	Usually 2nd to 3rd day	Peaks 2nd to 4th day	Early initiation of breast-feeding. Breast-feeding 8-12 times per 24 hours. Temporary formula supplement may be required if infant exhibits significant dehydration, poor feeding behavior, lethargy, and infrequent stooling. Possible phototherapy.
Breast milk jaundice	Beta-glucuronidase in some mothers' milk inhibiting conjugation and fecal excretion of bilirubin (1%-4% of breast-fed infants)	After 7 days	Peaks 10-15 days	Diagnosis may be confirmed by temporary cessation (24-48 hours) of breast-feeding with formula replacement. Monitor levels. Requires no intervention in most cases.
Pathologic jaundice	Excessive RBC hemolysis caused by RH/ABO maternal-fetal incompatibility	Within first 24 hours	Variable	Requires medical management. Treatment related to etiology. May include phototherapy and/or exchange transfusion.
	Deficient carrier protein or binding sites caused by prematuring, sepsis, hypoxia, or certain drugs	After first week of life		
	Liver/metabolic disease or malformation	Within first 24 hours		

*References 10,21,23,28,32,33,34

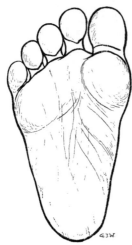

Figure 22-4 Puncture sites for infant heelstick specimens. (From Wong DL: *Whaley and Wong's nursing care of infants and children,* ed 5, St Louis, 1991, Mosby.)

prevent bilirubin breakdown (which could result in a false low reading).

Nutrition assessment. In the first few days of life, the infant may lose up to 10% of birth weight.[23] Therefore an infant nutritional assessment is an important aspect of home visits. This is particularly true when evaluating for failure to thrive. (See Chapter 20.)

Breast-feeding. Due to its immunologic, nutritional, and psychological advantages, breast milk is the optimal food for infants. There are three stages of milk production in the lactating mother: colostrum (thick, yellow), transitional milk (2 to 4 days after birth), and mature milk (approximately 2 weeks postpartum). Mature breast milk has a high fluid component, resembles skim milk, and provides 20 calories/oz. Although breast-feeding is more economical, it does require adequate nutrition, hydration, and rest for the mother.

Breast-feeding is a learned behavior. To promote an adequate milk supply, the breast-feeding infant should feed on demand, 8 to 12 times per day during the first few weeks of life. Encourage the mother to alternate the breast she offers first and to offer both breasts at each feeding without time restriction to stimulate milk production. Alternate feeding positions (cradle, side-lying, football) to prevent nipple trauma. Position the infant "tummy-to-tummy." Ensure the infant's mouth is wide open with tongue down. Check that the mother's nipple and as much of the areola as possible is grasped before latch and sucking begin. Improper latch may cause painful, cracked, and bleeding nipples (see the section on maternal assessment). Assess for nutritive sucking (characterized by coordinated suck-swallow and audible swallowing). Discourage use of supplemental bottle feedings and pacifiers in the first 2 weeks to prevent nipple confusion and refusal of the breast. Parents can gauge adequate nutrition and hydration by infant satisfaction between feedings, and 6 to 8 wet diapers per day. Assure parents that it takes 2 to 3 weeks for breast-feeding to be established. Weight gain of 0.5 oz per day in the first 6 months of life is appropriate for the infant who is breast-fed.[23]

Bottle-feeding. Bottle-fed infants are fed with a commercially prepared formula, usually recommended by the primary care provider. These formulas are available in ready-to-feed, concentrate, and powder. Assess the parents' knowledge of formula preparation and storage. Instruct parents to feed the infant cradled in the en face position, and never to prop bottles. Infants need about 2 hours of sucking time each day.[32] Allowing the infant approximately 20 minutes to take a feeding every 3 to 4 hours will ensure sucking needs are met. Calculate the nutritional needs for each infant, based on 50 calories/16/day and 20 calories/oz of formula. Infants who receive formula gain 1 oz per day in the first 6 months.[23] Instructing families about infant nutritional needs can prevent underfeeding or overfeeding. An infant who is overfed can be irritable, may frequently regurgitate, and exceeds recommended weight gain. Suggest burping the infant at the middle and end of each feeding. The infant who cries prior to being fed or feeds too rapidly may need to be burped prior to feeding and more frequently to prevent gastric distentions, excessive gas, and regurgitation.

Whether the infant is breast- or bottle-feeding, the nurse should observe and assess the following:

- Method of feeding
- Frequency of feeding
- Length of time or amount at each feeding
- Feeding reflexes (root, suck, swallow, gag)
- Environment during feeding

- Infant and maternal care-response patterns before, during, and after feeding (See Chapter 20, Social Interaction with the Mother/Caretaker.)
- Amount, frequency, and character of regurgitation
- Type and pattern of use of a pacifier

Behavioral assessment. Assess the infant's sleep/activity pattern for the preceding 24 hours by identifying the amount of time in the sleep, awake-alert, and awake-crying states. Often parental expectations, do not coincide with the reality of an infant who is "always crying." Although the duration of crying is highly variable, 1 to 4 hours per day is considered normal. Infants under 3 months of age may have colic, a condition manifested by long periods of intense crying, drawing the legs up to the abdomen, and inability to be comforted.[38]

Consolability is the ability of the infant to self-quiet or be quieted with assistance. The level of consolability can be measured after an infant has been crying for at least 15 seconds. The infant who is difficult to console may evoke intense feelings of helplessness in parents. Identifying individual differences in consolability will help parents cope with infant crying. Does the infant continue to cry regardless of consoling maneuvers such as movement, enfolding, sounds, or sucking? Does the infant respond to minimal consoling maneuvers by caregivers? Does the infant make an effort to self-console by sucking on fist, fingers or tongue?

Family assessment

Incorporation of a new family member is a developmental crisis, the resolution of which is facilitated by the presence of supportive others. The nurse is part of this support network. Identify family members living in the home, others whom the family can mobilize for support (parents, grandparents, neighbor, friend), and family dynamics. (See Chapter 20.)

Environmental safety. Determine safety in the home. (See Chapter 21.) Accidents are the highest cause of death for children under 2 years of age. Identify any potential for injury and counsel parents.

Knowledge of infant capabilities. Knowledge of physical, sensory, and behavioral capabilities of the infant enhances family interaction and parental

development. Physical capabilities include reflexes and developmental milestones of the first month of life. Informing parents that infants interact with all senses helps them understand the need for appropriate sensory stimulation. Identify behavioral capabilities by assessing the infant's response to and interaction with the environment.

Family-infant interaction. Most parents develop an expectation of their infant during pregnancy. When the reality of their infant's sex, appearance, and/or temperament does not correlate with this "fantasy" infant, bonding is delayed and interaction may be compromised. Assess both expectations and current perceptions of parents about their infant.

Communication, a reciprocal process involving a sender and a receiver, is an integral part of parent-infant interaction. Assess the parents' awareness of, interpretation of, and response to infant cue patterns. Determine the level of both verbal and tactile response to infant cues. Some factors influencing diminished parental response may include lack of knowledge, anxiety, or cultural variations. Absence of or negative parental response (demonstrated by neglecting, scolding, shaking, or striking the infant) necessitates referral to social services.

Response patterns may also be influenced by parental attitudes toward discipline and spoiling. Attitudes may be shaped by the parents' own childhood experiences, experience with other children, or by extended family participation in care. A belief that infants require discipline may predict abusive behavior. Assess discipline by observing interactions with other children in the home, and/or through questions such as:

- Are you concerned about spoiling your infant?
- When and how do you think you will start disciplining your infant?
- What do you remember about your parents disciplining you?

Assure parents that the newborn infant cannot be "spoiled" by responding to cues.

Infant care abilities of the family. Assess family members' ability to bathe, diaper, clothe, and feed the infant, to provide appropriate skin, cord, and circumcision care, and to offer sensory stimulation.

In addition, determine the family awareness of health promotion and illness prevention activities. Increased infant irritability, lethargy, hypothermia, or hyperthermia, signs of dehydration, recurrent and/or forceful vomiting, diarrhea, and poor feeding are signs of illness that require medical evaluation.

Adjustment to parental roles. A change in factors such as division of labor, financial status, and communication between partners can add stress to the lives of new parents. Help identify strengths and potential problems, and support parents in developing effective coping mechanisms. Families experiencing financial difficulties may be eligible for federal programs (such as WIC) or for state/county programs (such as family assistance, housing assistance, or utilities financing). Be aware of available programs and refer families where appropriate.

Family violence occurs at some time in 50% of all homes in the United States. It is not limited by socioeconomic status or race. The addition of a new family member may exacerbate an existing abuse cycle. Assess for adult domestic violence, especially toward women, through such questions as:

- Are you in a safe relationship?
- Do arguments ever involve slapping, pushing, shoving, or threats with a weapon?

Be aware of community resources and refer to domestic violence hot lines or shelters where appropriate. A business card format with hot line/shelter phone numbers and a safety plan for escape (see the following box) is a safe, convenient way to relay this information.

Sexuality. The usual medical advice to mothers is to avoid sexual intercourse until the postpartum checkup. Partners may desire to engage in sexual activity prior to that time. Intercourse is safe when lochia has ceased and the perineum is healed. Inform the couple that the breasts of a nursing mother may leak during orgasm, and that vaginal dryness can cause discomfort. Fatigue in one or both partners can interfere with sexual expression. Failure to identify these factors can cause concern and adversely affect the couple's sexual relationship at a time when mutual support is vital. Partners need to be informed that conception is possible prior to the return of menses. Address

---

SAFETY PLAN FOR VICTIM SURVIVORS OF DOMESTIC VIOLENCE

Have the following items hidden in one central place:
- About $50 in cash
- Extra keys for car and house
- A small bag with extra clothing for you and children
- These important documents:
  - Bank accounts
  - Insurance policies
  - Marriage license
  - His date of birth
  - Social security numbers (his, yours, and children's)
  - Birth certificates (yours and children's)
  - List of important phone numbers (family, friends)
  - Sentimental valuables
  - Children's school records

Source: Ohio Department of Human Services, Domestic Violence Network.

---

family planning preferences. If contraception is desired, suggest options. Over-the-counter measures (e.g., foam and condoms) can be used prior to the woman's visit to her health care provider for the postpartum checkup. Although some oral contraceptives are safe to take during breast-feeding, they are transmitted in breast milk. Newer hormonal contraceptives (Depo-Provera or Norplant) have the advantage of being longer acting, but significant side effects have been reported. Since the inner pelvic structure changes following birth, a diaphragm must be refitted. Uterine healing and cervical closure occurs over a 4-week period, precluding placement of an IUD prior to this time. Due to irregularities incurred in the menstrual cycle during lactation, natural family planning may not be effective.

Adjustment of siblings. Parents bringing home a second or subsequent child may have concerns about the impact the new infant will have on the family constellation. Determine reactions of the sibling(s) through observation and interview. Identify developmental stages of older children that could positively or negatively influence their adjustment. Encourage parental reinforcement of positive behaviors and appropriate limit setting when indicated.

Coping abilities. A family copes through identifying their needs, seeking information, reorganizing their lifestyle, mobilizing their resources, and adapting to the changes in their lives. Most families exhibit strength and growth potential with the addition of a new family member. When ineffective coping exists, facilitate appropriate intervention and counseling.

Planning and intervention

Postpartum home care programs usually include one visit. Based on maternal and infant nursing diagnoses,[35] patient teaching is a major intervention. (See the boxes titled Primary Nursing Diagnoses and Primary Themes of Patient/Family Education.) Mothers have difficulty learning and retaining in the first 2 days postpartum.[8,13,26] Learning occurs in incremental steps. Reinforce teaching with written materials. Select brochures or pamphlets that are culturally sensitive, appropriate to language and reading level, and specific to the needs identified. Pay careful attention to brochures written by product manufacturers. Although educational, they are also marketing tools. In addition, brief written recommendations for self and infant care ("nursing prescriptions") can help the mother recall key interventions to meet identified needs. (Refer to Chapter 6.)

Families may have ongoing needs for support and/or social services beyond the scope of the postpartum home visit. In these circumstances, do not hesitate to refer to appropriate organizations or agencies (e.g., support groups for parenting or postpartum depression, LaLeche League, county health departments).

Evaluation

Evaluation is the final step of the nursing process. In a postpartum home care program, this is done by a follow-up phone call 7 to 10 days after the final visit. Individual needs may require calls being made sooner or more frequently. During the phone call, ask questions to determine physical and emotional status of the mother. Areas for maternal assessment include breasts, nutrition, elimination, lochia, incision/laceration, sleep/activity pattern, and emotional needs. Areas for

PRIMARY NURSING DIAGNOSES/ PATIENT PROBLEMS

Maternal

- Pain, related to episiotomy/perineal laceration, cesarean incision, breast engorgement, backache, uterine cramping.
- Altered nutrition: less than body requirements
- Constipation
- Risk for infection (cesarean/BPS incision, urinary tract, episiotomy, uterine, breast)
- Risk for injury (elevated blood pressure, anemia, postpartum hemorrhage, postpartum PIH, thrombophlebitis, domestic violence)
- Ineffective individual coping
- Anxiety
- Risk for caregiver role strain
- Fatigue
- Hyperthermia

Infant

- Ineffective breast-feeding
- Altered nutrition: less than body requirements
- Risk for injury (hyperbilirubinemia, heart murmur, anemia)
- Risk for infection (cord, eye, circumcision)
- Risk for altered body temperature
- Effective breast-feeding

Family

- Knowledge deficit (infant care, feeding, growth and development)
- Family coping: potential for growth
- Altered sexuality patterns

infant assessment include feeding, elimination, condition of cord and circumcision, and sleep/activity pattern. Assess family support and adjustment. If problems identified during the visit have not been resolved or new problems are detected, suggest additional interventions or make referrals. Ascertain that the mother and infant are scheduled to receive follow-up care via primary care providers. Terminate the relationship and document findings.

SUMMARY

The challenge is before us: refine the model of maternity care to meet the needs of mothers,

PRIMARY THEMES OF PATIENT/FAMILY EDUCATION

- Maternal pain management
- Maternal nutrition
- Signs and symptoms of postpartum complications
- Modification of activities of daily living to promote rest and recovery from childbirth
- Health maintenance
- Infant care
- Infant feeding (general)
- Breast-feeding
- Normal infant growth and development
- Signs and symptoms of infant illness
- Family planning
- Community resources: socioeconomic, breast-feeding support, domestic violence, postpartum depression, infant CPR classes
- Identification and management of emergencies

infants, and families while containing costs; yet maintain professional standards of practice. This challenge presents an opportunity for nurses to control the quality of health care and define the scope of professional practice.

Postpartum home care is a natural progression in the redesign of maternity care. It is a common-sense application to the overwhelming needs for public access to health care that exist in our society today. As hospital stays shorten, concepts of providing prenatal care for all women should certainly be applied to the postpartum recovery period.

The majority of women have a healthy pregnancy and birth. Yet it is a national standard that all women receive prenatal care in order to identify complications early and to provide health promotional activities. The majority of women and newborns will have a healthy recovery after birth. However, no one can predict which baby will have problems feeding or be septic, or which mother will develop an infection or postpartum depression. In addition, women and families need access to information to oversee their own recovery. Therefore in order to manage associated risks and health educational needs, postpartum recovery, as a national standard, should be monitored in the home by skilled maternity nurses.

The necessity, safety, quality, and cost-effectiveness of comprehensive short stay maternity programs have been established. Promulgating a national standard, which includes postpartum home care as a component of maternity care, is a priority for nurses if we are to ensure the safety and well-being of infants, mothers, families, and—in the long run—society itself.

REFERENCES

1. Affonso D: Assessment of maternal postpartum adaptation, *Public Health Nurs* 4(1):9-20, 1987.
2. American Nurses Association: Position statement. *Postpartum and infant home care as a national standard of care* (In progress).
3. Arnold L, Bakewell-Sachs S: Models of perinatal home follow-up. *J Perina Neonatal Nurs* 5(1):18-26, 1991.
4. Association of Women's Health, Obstetric, and Neonatal Nurses (AWHONN): Position statement. Issues: shortened maternity and newborn hospital stays, *Voice* 2(5):20, 1994.
5. Association of Women's Health, Obstetric, and Neonatal Nurses (AWHONN): *Didactic content and clinical skills verification for professional nurse providers of perinatal home care,* 1994.
6. Avery M: An early discharge program: Implementation and evaluation, *J Obstet Gynecol Neonatal Nurs* 11(4):233-235, 1982.
7. Bennett MD: Influence of health insurance on patterns of care: maternity hospitalization, *Inquiry* 12: 59-63, March 1975.
8. Brooten D et al: A randomized trial of early hospital discharge and home follow-up of women having cesarean birth, *Obstet Gynecol* 84(5):832-838, 1994.
9. Carty E, Bradley C: A randomized, controlled evaluation of early postpartum hospital discharge, *Birth* 17(4):199-204, 1990.
10. Cohen S et al: *Maternal, neonatal and women's health nursing,* Springhouse, Pa, 1991, Springhouse Publishing.
11. Cunningham F et al: *Williams obstetrics,* ed 19, Norwalk, Conn, 1993, Appleton & Lange.
12. DeCherney A, Pernoll M, editors: *Current obstetric and gynecologic diagnosis and treatment,* ed 8, Norwalk, Conn, 1994, Appleton & Lange.
13. Eidelman A et al: Cognitive deficits in women after childbirth, *Obstet Gynecol* 81(5, part 1):764-767, 1993.
14. Evans C: Description of a home follow-up program for childbearing families, *J Obstet Gynecol Neonatal Nurs* 20(2):113-118, 1991.
15. Gillerman H, Beckham M: The postpartum early discharge dilemma: an innovative solution, *J Perinat Neonatal Nurs* 5(1):9-17, 1991.
16. Haupt BJ: Deliveries in short stay hospitals: United States, 1980, *NCHS Advancedata 83* 12:1,82-96, Oct 8, 1982.
17. Hellman I et al: Early hospital discharge in obstetrics, *Lancet* 1:227-232, 1962.
18. Jansen P: Early postpartum discharge, *Am J Nurs* 85(5):547-550, 1985.
19. Lemmer C: Early discharge: outcomes of primiparas and their infants, *J Obstet Gynecol Neonatal Nurs* 16(4):230-236, 1987.

20. Miller-Slade D: Ask the experts (Parlodel), *Voice* 2(11):11, 1994.
21. Newman T, Maisels M: Evaluation and treatment of jaundice in the newborn: a kinder, gentler approach, *Pediatrics* 89:809-818, 1992.
22. Norr K, Nacion K: Outcomes of postpartum early discharge 1960-1986. A comparative review, *Birth* 14(3):135-141, 1987.
23. Olds S et al: *Maternal-newborn nursing: a family centered approach,* ed 4, Redwood City, Calif, 1992, Addison-Wesley.
24. Riordan J, Auerbach K: *Breastfeeding and human lactation,* Boston, 1993, Jones & Bartlett.
25. Ropp A, Thorn K: Historical perspectives. In *Short stay postpartum programs.* Presented at a course conducted by the Nurses' Association of the American College of Obstetricians and Gynecologists, Pittsburgh, June 1986.
26. Rubin R: Puerperal change, *Nurs Outlook* 9:753-755, 1961.
27. Scanlon J: *A system of newborn physical examination,* Baltimore, 1979, University Park Press.
28. Seidel H et al: *Primary care of the newborn,* St Louis, 1993, Mosby.
29. Theobald G: Home on the second day: the Bradford experiment: the combined maternity scheme, *Br Med J* 2:1364-1367, 1959.
30. US Department of Health and Human Services: *Health United States and prevention profile,* DHHS Pub No 90-1232 189-190, Hyattsville, Md, 1990.
31. US Department of Health and Human Services: *Health United States 1993,* DHHS Pub No 93-1232, Hyattsville, Md, 1994.
32. Whaley L, Wong D: *Nursing care of infants and children,* ed 5, St Louis, 1995, Mosby.
33. Wilkerson N: A comprehensive look at hyperbilirubinemia, *MCN* 13(5):360-364, 1988.
34. Wilkerson N: Treating hyperbilirubinemia, *MCN* 14(1):32-36, 1989.
35. Williams L, Cooper M: Nurse-managed postpartum home care, *J Obstet Gynecol Neonatal Nurs* 22(1):25-31, 1993.
36. Williams L, Cooper M: A new paradigm for postpartum care, *J Obstet Gynecol Neonatal Nurs* (resubmitted for publication November, 1994).
37. Yanover M et al: Perinatal care of low risk mothers and infants: early discharge with home care, *N Engl J Med* 294(13):702-705, 1976.
38. *Your baby and crying,* Columbus, Ohio, 1993, Ross Laboratories.

23 The Mental Health Patient

Dorothy O. Hauk

Psychiatric home care prevents or shortens psychiatric hospitalization for the acutely depressed individual and the schizophrenic patient.[33,40,46] Patients with both acute and chronic mental disorders benefit from services that stabilize and maintain them in their home environment.[38,45] The focus topics for this chapter have been limited to depression and schizophrenia, but home health patients come with as much diversity as do patients in any other mental health care setting. The services that psychiatric home care can provide include the following:

- Assessment and evaluation of mental status
- Assessment of medication effectiveness and side effects, administration of medications, and management of medication compliance
- Assessment of family and community support systems and their effectiveness
- Instruction in basic information concerning the diagnosed mental illness
- Instruction in actions and side effects of all medications
- Instruction in ways to develop and implement problem solving strategies, coping skills, and skills of daily living
- Individual and family psychotherapy
- Crisis intervention
- Assistance and support to families and caregivers
- Community resource information and referrals
- Reporting to the attending psychiatrist and other physicians concerning the response to medication, the mental status of the patient, and any change in medical condition

- Encouraging regular follow-up with physician and clinic appointments
- Evaluation of the entire process

Assessment is always the first step for the professional nurse. Along with the usual vital signs, additional factors such as weight, nutrition, elimination, history, support systems, activities, and sleep patterns are considered. The home health nurse also assesses the patient's mental status with an appropriate tool.

Following assessment, a care plan is developed to meet the multiple needs of the mental health patient. Patients are included in this phase insofar as they are capable and willing to participate in developing the care plan. The principal care provider is included in mutual planning and realistic goal setting whenever possible. Interventions frequently include individual and family therapy, instruction in medication actions and side effects, crisis intervention, assistance in the development of problem solving skills, coping mechanisms, and assistance in the activities of daily living. Injections of neuroleptic medications and venipuncture for the monitoring of drug levels are frequently a part of the services rendered by home health nurses.[17]

Ideally, home health agencies employ a mental health nurse experienced in working with the mentally ill to care for patients with mental disorders. However, this is not always the case, and home health nurses may be called upon to attend to the complex needs of the mentally ill.[51] Medicare now reimburses for psychiatric home nursing for patients who have a primary diagnosis of mental illness and whose care is supervised by a

399

psychiatrist. Home health nurses who care for these patients require preparation in one of the following ways:

- RN with a master's degree in psychiatric or mental health nursing
- RN with a BSN degree and 1 year of related work experience in an active treatment program for adult or geriatric patients in a psychiatric health care setting
- RN with a diploma or AD degree and 2 years of related work experience in an active treatment program for adult or geriatric patients in a psychiatric health care setting
- ANA certification in psychiatric or community health nursing

Other qualifications may be considered on an individual basis.[13,35]

Home health nurses encounter patients with mental illness for the simple reason that many patients have multiple diagnoses (e.g., the newly diagnosed diabetic patient with an acute depressive disorder). Planning care for the physiological and psychological needs of patients with mental health disorders represents a challenge for the home health nurse. This chapter reviews the two most common mental disorders treated in the home: depression (both acute and chronic) and schizophrenia. The information presented will assist home health nurses in developing a care plan for these patients. (The reader is referred to Chapter 18 for clinical guidelines for patients who experience dementia.)

As home health nurses review nursing care of the mentally ill, a definition of mental illness is necessary. "Mental illness cannot be observed any more than mental health can be seen—both are categories. What can be observed are various behavioral manifestations that may or may not be labeled as deviant."[18]

Depression

ETIOLOGY AND PATHOPHYSIOLOGY

The etiology of depression is presently unknown. Theories range from psychoanalytic to cognitive to biologic to sociocultural. At present there is no overriding evidence to support any one theory. An integrated causation theory is most favored.[37] Depression occurs at all ages, occurs more frequently in women than in men, and occurs more frequently in persons who live alone. A history of depression predisposes the individual to another episode, especially if loss or stress has been part of the patient's recent experience. Medications can also be a causative factor in the development of depression.[14,16] Research has suggested that those receptor sites to which neurotransmitters (such as serotonin and norepinephrine) attach in the brain become disregulated, leading to poor transmission of impulses and, consequently, depression. Drug therapies and electroconvulsive therapy (ECT) are often effective in "resetting" these receptors to restore normal mental activity.[10]

Many drugs may cause signs of depression. These include antihypertensives, cardiovascular preparations, antiparkinsonian medications, hypoglycemics (oral), psychotropic medications, antimicrobials, steroids, analgesics, and others.[10] (See the box titled Drugs Causing Signs of Depression.)

Treatment modalities vary according to the individual patient, diagnostic classification, and treatment methods and results of past hospitalizations. Antidepressant medications and ECT are the most common physiological treatments used today. A wide variety of psychotherapeutic approaches assist recovery of the depressed individual.

Studies indicate that combining antidepressant drug therapy and psychotherapy is more effective than using either modality alone.[36]

HOME CARE APPLICATION
Assessment

Depression is a mental disorder that nurses will encounter frequently in home care. Depression is categorized, according to the *Diagnostic and Statistical Manual of the American Psychiatric Association (DSM IV)*, as one of the major depressive disorders, a disturbance of mood not caused by any other physical or mental disorder.

A major depressive episode includes five or more of the following symptoms having been present during the same 2-week period. It represents a change from the person's previous functioning. At least one of the symptoms must be depressed mood or loss of interest or pleasure.

DRUGS CAUSING SIGNS OF DEPRESSION

Antihypertensives
Reserpine
Methyldopa
Propranolol
Clonidine
Hydralazine
Guanethidine

Cardiovascular
Diuretics
Digitalis
Lidocaine
Procaine

Antiparkinsonians
Levodopa

Hypoglycemics (oral)

Psychotropics
Sedatives
Barbiturates
Benzodiazepines
Meprobamate

Antipsychotics
Chlorpromazine
Haloperidol
Thiothixene

Hypnotics
Chloral hydrate

Antidepressants
Amitriptyline
Doxepin

Antimicrobials
Sulfonamides
Isoniazid

Steroids
Corticosteroids
Estrogens

Analgesics
Narcotic
Morphine
Codeine
Meperidine
Pentazocine
Propoxyphene

Nonnarcotic
Indomethacin

Others
Cimetidine
Cancer
    chemotherapeutics
Alcohol

From Marianne Smith, RN, Elderly Services Coordinator, Abbe Center for Community Mental Health, Iowa City.[10]

1. Depressed mood most of the day, nearly every day
2. Diminished interest or pleasure in activities
3. Significant weight loss when not dieting, or weight gain
4. Insomnia or hypersomnia nearly every day
5. Psychomotor agitation or retardation nearly every day
6. Fatigue or loss of energy nearly every day
7. Feelings of worthlessness or excessive or inappropriate guilt nearly every day
8. Diminished ability to think or concentrate, or indecisiveness, nearly every day
9. Recurrent thoughts of death, recurrent suicidal ideation without specific plan, or a suicide attempt or a specific plan for committing suicide[2,3]

The presenting symptoms may endure for a few weeks or for long periods of time. They may be quite intense or mild. They may be confined to a one-episode experience or occur over and over in the life of an individual.[2,3]

Primary nursing diagnoses and patient problems for depression are listed in the following box. In

PRIMARY NURSING DIAGNOSES/ PATIENT PROBLEMS

Depression
• Social isolation
• Suicidal ideations
• Medication compliance
• Nutrition, hydration, weight loss, or weight gain
• Loss of interest, lack of enjoyment in usual interests
• Altered sleep patterns
• Diminished physical activity, fatigue
• Irritability, anxiety
• Feelings of guilt, worthlessness
• Poor concentration, indecisiveness

developing a plan of care, a complete physical assessment and history is taken. This should include information regarding previous episodes of depression or other mental illness. Suicide potential should be evaluated. A depression assessment

Zung Depression Scale

	A little of the time	Some of the time	Good part of the time	Most of the time
1. I feel downhearted and blue	1	2	3	4
2. Morning is when I feel the best	4	3	2	1
3. I have crying spells or feel like it	1	2	3	4
4. I have trouble sleeping at night	1	2	3	4
5. I eat as much as I used to	4	3	2	1
6. I still enjoy sex	4	3	2	1
7. I notice that I am losing weight	1	2	3	4
8. I have trouble with constipation	1	2	3	4
9. My heart beats faster than usual	1	2	3	4
10. I get tired for no reason	1	2	3	4
11. My mind is as clear as it used to be	4	3	2	1
12. I find it easy to do the things I used to	4	3	2	1
13. I am restless and can't keep still	1	2	3	4
14. I feel hopeful about the future	4	3	2	1
15. I am more irritable than usual	1	2	3	4
16. I find it easy to make decisions	4	3	2	1
17. I feel useful and needed	4	3	2	1
18. My life is pretty full	4	3	2	1
19. I feel that others would be better off if I were dead	1	2	3	4
20. I still enjoy the things I used to do	4	3	2	1

Figure 23-1 The Zung Depression Scale. (From Zung WWK: A self-rating depression scale, *Arch Gen Psychiatry* 12:63, 1965.)

scale may be used for this evaluation. The Zung Self-Rating Depression Scale (Figure 23-1)[57,58] provides information for measuring the intensity of the patient's depression when the test is administered. It is easily used in the home setting and easily tabulated later. For the geriatric patient, the Yesavage Geriatric Depression Scale (Figure 23-2)[9] may be more appropriate. It can be administered quickly and involves only "yes" and "no" answers, which are easier for the elderly patients to follow. Because the depressed individual may exhibit signs of paranoia or cognitive impairment, the Folstein Mini-Mental State assessment tool is frequently useful for determining the presence of dementia (Figure 23-3).[21]

The possibility of abuse of the elderly patient must always be considered by the home health nurse during the course of home visits. Laws defining elder abuse are not the same from state to state, but most states now have elder abuse reporting laws. Five types of abuse have been identified and can be helpful to the home health nurse in assessing abuse.

Physical abuse. Bodily harm or mental distress may be active (assault) or passive (negligence). The Select Committee on Aging defines negligence to be an act of carelessness, a violation of right, or a breach of duty resulting in injury (such as the lack of food, drink, medication, or allowing the development of pressure sores).

Zung Depression Scale Conversion Table

A table for the conversion of raw scores to the SDS index

Raw score	SDS index	Raw score	SDS index	Raw score	SDS index
20	25	40	50	60	75
21	26	41	51	61	76
22	28	42	53	62	78
23	29	43	54	63	79
24	30	44	55	64	80
25	31	45	56	65	81
26	33	46	58	66	83
27	34	47	59	67	84
28	35	48	60	68	85
29	36	49	61	69	86
30	38	50	63	70	88
31	39	51	64	71	89
32	40	52	65	72	90
33	41	53	66	73	91
34	43	54	68	74	92
35	44	55	69	75	93
36	45	56	70	76	95
37	46	57	71	77	96
38	48	58	73	78	98
39	49	59	74	79	99
				80	100

To obtain the patient's depression rating, the completed scale is scored with the indicated value for each item, and totaled; this raw score is then converted to an index based on 100 (see above). The scale is so constructed that a low index indicates little or no depression and a high index indicates depression of clinical significance. The table below shows SDS depression rating obtained in normal controls and in patients with diagnoses of depression, anxiety reaction, personality disorders, and transient situational adjustment reaction.

Diagnosis of validating groups	Mean SDS index	Range
Normal controls	33	25-43
Depressed hospitalized	74	63-90
Depressed out-patient	64	50-78
Anxiety reactions	53	40-68
Personality disorders	53	42-68
Transient situational adjustment reaction	53	38-68

Figure 23-1, cont'd. For legend see opposite page.

Choose the best answer for how you felt over the past week

1. Are you basically satisfied with your life?	yes/**no**
2. Have you dropped many of your activities and interests?	**yes**/no
3. Do you feel that your life is empty?	**yes**/no
4. Do you often get bored?	**yes**/no
5. Are you hopeful about the future?	yes/**no**
6. Are you bothered by thoughts you can't get out of your head?	**yes**/no
7. Are you good in spirits most of the time?	yes/**no**
8. Are you afraid that something bad is going to happen to you?	**yes**/no
9. Do you feel happy most of the time?	yes/**no**
10. Do you often feel helpless?	**yes**/no
11. Do you often get restless and fidgety?	**yes**/no
12. Do you prefer to stay at home, rather than going out and doing new things?	**yes**/no
13. Do you frequently worry about the future?	**yes**/no
14. Do you feel you have more problems with memory than most?	**yes**/no
15. Do you think it is wonderful to be alive now?	yes/**no**
16. Do you often feel downhearted and blue?	**yes**/no
17. Do you feel pretty worthless the way you are now?	**yes**/no
18. Do you worry a lot about the past?	**yes**/no
19. Do you find life very exciting?	yes/**no**
20. Is it hard for you to get started on new projects?	**yes**/no
21. Do you feel full of energy?	yes/**no**
22. Do you feel that your situation is hopeless?	**yes**/no
23. Do you think that most people are better off than you are?	**yes**/no
24. Do you frequently get upset over little things?	**yes**/no
25. Do you frequently feel like crying?	**yes**/no
26. Do you have trouble concentrating?	**yes**/no
27. Do you enjoy getting up in the morning?	yes/**no**
28. Do you prefer to avoid social gatherings?	**yes**/no
29. Is it easy for you to make decisions?	yes/**no**
30. Is your mind as clear as it used to be?	yes/**no**

Scoring instructions: Score bold answers as 1 point
Rating: 0-9 = normal; 10-19 = mild depressive; 20-30 = severe depressive

Figure 23-2 The Yesavage Geriatric Depression Scale. (From Brown JH: The role of the home health care nurse in mental health assessment of the elderly, *J Home Health Care Pract* 2:1, 1989.)

Financial abuse. Money may be stolen from an elder outright or property may be transferred to another by force, deceit, fraud, or misrepresentation.

Psychological abuse. Name calling, verbal assaults, protracted and systematic efforts to dehumanize, or threats to instill fear can be as harmful as physical violence.

Sexual abuse. Most often perpetrated by a grandson or son-in-law, sexual abuse may be covered up by other children.

Self-abuse or self-neglect. A range of behaviors is possible from simple physical neglect to suicide. This abuse is often precipitated by actions and attitudes of loved ones that lead to feelings of loneliness and rejection in the elder.[30]

Typical patients referred to a home health agency have recently been hospitalized with either some manifestation of depression or, less common, a bipolar disorder. Depressive and manic episodes have usually alternated over weeks or months. Reactive depression resulting from some loss, real or perceived, is frequently seen. Its management calls for the listening skills learned early in nursing education.[26]

Physical appearance provides significant information in determining the presence of depression.[37] Is

Mini-Mental State Exam

Instructions: Ask all questions in the order listed and score immediately.
Record total number of points.

Maximum score	Score	
5	( )	1. Ask the patient to name the year, season, date, day, and month. (1 point each)
5	( )	2. Ask the patient to give his/her whereabouts: state, county, town, street, address. (1 point each)
3	( )	3. Ask the patient to repeat three unrelated objects that you name. Repeat them and continue to repeat them until all three are learned. (1 point each)
5	( )	4. Ask the patient to subtract 7 from 100, stopping after five subtractions, or to spell the word "world" backwards. (1point for each correct calculation or letter)
3	( )	5. Ask the patient to repeat the three objects previously named. (1 point each)
2	( )	6. Display a wristwatch and ask the patient to name it. Repeat this for a pencil. (1 point each)
1	( )	7. Ask the patient to repeat this phrase: "No ifs, ands, or buts!" (1 point)
3	( )	8. Have the patient follow a three-point command such as, "Take a paper in your right hand, fold it in half, and put it on the floor!" (1 point each)
1	( )	9. On a blank piece of paper write, "Close your eyes!" Ask the patient to read it and do what it says. (1 point)
1	( )	10. Ask the patient to write a sentence on a blank piece of paper. It must be written spontaneously. Score correctly if it contains a subject and a verb and is sensible. (Correct grammar and punctuation are not necessary.) (1 point)
1	( )	11. Ask the patient to copy a design you have drawn on a piece of paper (two intersecting pentagons with sides about one inch). (1 point)

Total score _____   Maximum score = 30

Scoring: Scores of 23 or less: a high likelihood of dementia
            Scores of 25-30: normal aging or borderline

Figure 23-3 The Mini-Mental State Exam. (From Folstein MF, Folstein SE, McHugh PR: "Mini-Mental State": a practical method for grading the cognitive state of patients for the clinician, *J Psychiatric Res* 12:189-198, 1975.

BEHAVIORAL SIGNS OF DEPRESSION

- Sadness, crying, discouragement, brooding
- Anxiety, panic attacks, irritability, paranoia
- Talking of feeling sad, blue, depressed, that nothing is fun, down in the dumps
- Withdrawal from usual activities
- Loss of libido
- Inability to express pleasure
- Feelings of worthlessness
- Unreasonable fears
- Self-reproach for minor failings
- Delusions of poverty
- Critical attitude toward self and others
- Passivity
- Increased or decreased body movements
- Pacing, wringing hands, pulling or rubbing hair, body, or clothing
- Sleep disturbances
- Weight and appetite changes
- Fatigue
- Preoccupation with physical health, somatic complaints
- Difficulty concentrating, thinking, making decisions
- Slowed speech, flat affect
- Thoughts of death and/or suicide; suicide or suicide attempts
- Constipation
- Tachycardia

Adapted from Buckwalter K, Stolley J: Managing mentally ill elders at home, *Geriatr Nurs* May/June 1991.

PRIMARY THEMES OF PATIENT EDUCATION

Depression
- Medication effects and side effects, reasons for taking medications
- Missed-dose management of medication
- Information about electroconvulsive therapy
- Information about mental illness; when to call the doctor
- Coping strategies
- Grief resolution
- Suicide prevention
- Community alliances

the patient well groomed or unkempt? Does the patient have obvious injuries or deformities? Does the patient appear generally healthy or generally ill? In recognizing depression, the nurse must look for known symptoms and behaviors, as identified in the box titled Behavioral Signs of Depression.[11,32]

Medication response

As part of the assessment, home health nurses must carefully monitor the effectiveness and side effects of any antidepressant or other medication the patient is receiving. Many drugs used to treat illnesses common to the elderly are associated with depression.

In addition, determining whether patients are taking their medication is important. If a significant other is present and willing to assume the responsibility for medication compliance, the problem of compliance may be solved. However, patients often live alone and are potentially unreliable, forgetful, or easily confused by the medication regimen set up for them.

If this is the case, home health nurses must find an alternative way to help these patients comply with their medication regimen. Methods of promoting compliance include making out a schedule in graphic form, filling small envelopes with the appropriate medication for each time period and clearly marking the envelope with the date and time of day the medication is to be taken, or suggesting that patients obtain a commercially produced medication box with compartments. Without medication compliance, psychiatric patients will almost invariably deteriorate and end up in the hospital.

Because some medications take weeks before reaching peak activity levels, it is extremely important to monitor for effectiveness with changes in behavior and symptomatology. In addition, blood levels should be monitored and the patient observed for possible side effects and interactions of all medications being administered.[44]

Patient education

Primary themes of patient education for depression are listed in the box above.

Medications. Many depressed patients are at risk for discontinuing medication of their own volition because they may not like the side effects they have noticed. They also may not believe the drug is having any effect on them at all, or they may believe they are cured and no longer need the medication. When patients are informed of the slow onset of therapeutic response from many drugs, they are much more likely to accept the prescribed regimen and follow instructions. These instructions often require frequent repetition because many patients have difficulty concentrating or may have memory problems that make learning difficult or impossible.

Patients also must be taught how to manage those inevitable times when they will forget or when they are unable to take their medication on the normal schedule set up for them. The following are general instructions for missed-dose management:

- Take the missed dose as soon as possible.
- If the missed dose is remembered when the next regularly scheduled dose is due, take only the regularly scheduled dose.
- Take any remaining doses for the day as prescribed.
- Do not take double doses.[56]

Drug specific missed-dose management instructions are even more valuable to the patient, and are available in a medication teaching manual published by the American Society of Hospital Pharmacists. This information can be even more helpful in maintaining a drug's action, in returning the patient to regular dosing intervals, and in preventing additional side effects from excessive dosing.[56]

If patients can be taught to associate medication taking times with some routine daily activities (such as mealtimes, early morning awakening, or bedtime), habits can be formed that make medication taking as routine as other habits of daily life. Patients must be made aware of the reasons they are taking each medication, the effects and side effects of each medication, and the consequences if the regimen is not followed. The only way medication compliance can become truly effective is when patients understand the medication program they have been given, and then take responsibility for following through with the program.[49,53]

Mental illness. Within the patient community, and particularly within the aging population of the community, there is a widespread ignorance about mental illness. Occasionally a patient will be resistant to the very idea of any form of mental illness and will not permit a mental health nurse or a psychiatrist to assess or treat problems that have emerged. This patient, and perhaps this patient's family, may require considerable education about mental illness before any treatment can even be considered.

Families are helped considerably by learning of organizations such as Alliance for the Mentally Ill, an organization made up of persons who are mentally ill, families and friends of mentally ill persons, and professionals who work with such individuals. Families may also benefit from reading books such as *Surviving Schizophrenia: A Family Manual* by E. Fuller Torrey (published by Harper & Row, New York, 1978) and *Caring Family: Living with Chronic Mental Illness* by Kayla Bernheim, Richard Lewine, and Caroline Beale (published by Contemporary Books, Inc, Chicago, 1982).

Electroconvulsive therapy. Another area in which depressed patients may require instruction involves electroconvulsive therapy (ECT). Patients may have received a series of ECT in the hospital, or they may be receiving such treatment on an outpatient basis. One of the primary problems of ECT is temporary loss of memory. Some patients cannot even remember having been instructed that memory loss is usually only temporary. These patients may be very bewildered and frightened by the memory loss and need to be reminded repeatedly that it is usually of a temporary nature.

Patients and families may also fear ECT because they have heard horror stories about this treatment. They need to know that ECT has shown effective and safe results in the treatment of depression. ECT acts by altering neurotransmitters in certain areas of the brain, such as the hypothalamus and the pituitary. Through the use of muscle relaxants and anesthesia, the likelihood of physical damage during the seizure is minimal. An electrical current is sent through the brain by electrodes placed at the temples. ECT works rapidly and improvement is evident more quickly than many other methods, such as psychotherapy. The patient will be lethargic for a time following the treatment, and will need someone to provide transportation to and from the treatment setting.

Interventions

Establishment of a nurse-patient relationship. Mentally ill patients often do not request home care services, and sometimes they refuse to allow nurses to enter their home. Because they are often ambivalent about receiving home care services, the establishment of a nurse-patient relationship must begin immediately. Without such a relationship, future visits may not be allowed, and the many needs of these patients will not be met. Home health nurses must accept that occasionally such relationships are not possible because of personality factors or because of the illness of the patient (e.g., paranoia, obsessive-compulsiveness, or depression). Sometimes patients are too ill to be at home, but for whatever reason they are unable or unwilling to be hospitalized. Home health nurses, preferably in consultation with a mental health nurse or a mental health clinical specialist, are often successful in establishing this essential nurse-patient relationship.[22,23]

After a relationship is established, work can begin toward mutual exploration of problems and maladaptive behaviors.[37] The ability of patients to participate in such exploration may depend on the effectiveness of the medication in lifting the patient's mood and providing the energy level necessary to participate actively in problem solving. Because depressed patients tend to make progress slowly, any progress—however slow and tenuous—is significant. Problems such as anxiety, powerlessness, suspicion, low self-esteem, anger, negative thinking, impulse control, or egocentricity can be addressed and dealt with until success is achieved in some area. Success with one area can serve to increase self-esteem and enhance the possibility of success in other areas. Depressed patients often have deficiencies in social skills and interpersonal relationships. Social skills training may be of major benefit to assist patients out of a cycle of failure and depression.

Brief psychotherapy. A brief model of psychotherapy described by Aguilera,[1] using the crisis theory introduced by Caplan,[12] may be useful to home health nurses working with depressed patients.[55] According to the model, when a stressful event occurs certain balancing factors assist a person toward equilibrium or resolution of the problem. If one or more of these factors are inoperative or weak, a crisis will be experienced. These factors include the following:

- The patient's perception of the event
- Persons available to provide the patient with support
- Coping mechanisms the patient has used effectively in the past

By using this model, home health nurses determine what the precipitating event means to the patient and how this event affects the future (i.e., whether the patient views the matter realistically or in a distorted fashion).

Next a determination must be made about persons who are available to provide support to help solve the problems. A lack of support may easily lead to development of a full-blown crisis, with patients experiencing feelings of being overwhelmed and completely alone.

Last an assessment is made of the patient's usual mode of coping with similar situations of stress (i.e., what is usually done when there is a problem). Coping mechanisms may be conscious or unconscious and may be exhibited in behaviors such as aggression, regression, withdrawal, or repression.[1]

Interventions are established in conjunction with information derived from assessment. This information includes the extent to which the situation has disrupted the patient's life and ability to function. Questions about work or school may give information about the patient's past accomplishments, ability to handle stress, activities of interest, etc. The degree of disruption of patients' lives and the degree to which their problems are affecting significant others is of supreme importance. The home health nurse routinely attempts to spend time with a patient's significant other to obtain another perspective of the events. This is often more easily accomplished in the home environment than in formal counseling settings because support persons are frequently present during the initial visits, even if they do not live with the patients.

Consideration is then given to cause-effect relationships. Tentative clarification of problems is reflected back to the patient. Clarification continues until the home health nurse and the patient agree on what the problems are, and both are able to focus on possible solutions to reduce the anxiety generated by the crisis. Specific ideas and direction of actions are mutually agreed upon by patient and nurse. An agreement is reached whereby the patient will test identified solutions to determine their feasibility and effectiveness in addressing the problems identified.

The agreed on solutions are evaluated during the next visit for their effectiveness. If they proved ineffective, new solutions are identified and agreed upon. It is imperative that patients be active participants in this negotiating-problem solving process. If they are not, and the home health nurse does all the "work," the patient has very little commitment to implement the designated solutions.

Before the visits are discontinued, plans for establishing realistic goals for the future are mutually negotiated between the patient and nurse. Evaluation of the entire process must be made at the end of the therapeutic experience, with the fundamental question being, Has this individual returned to his or her usual level or a higher level of equilibrium in functioning?

Crisis intervention theory works well with many patients and situations specific to home care. Because the patients themselves do not usually seek the counseling, and because the idea of home care for psychiatric disorders is usually conceived by physicians, social workers, hospital nurses, or family members, the patient's initial commitment to therapy is often minimal or nonexistent. A part of the home health nurse's role becomes that of salesperson. The idea of working toward a solution must be sold to patients in such a way that they agree to the process and commit themselves to working on mutually agreed upon solutions. Usually the nurse's listening skills and interest in patients' problems quickly dispel any resistance that patients might have toward such visits. However, the fact remains that some patients do not want to work on their problems regardless of the therapist's skill. Some cannot remember what solutions were set forth for testing, and some are too ill to focus on any problem solving. In some cases the home health nurse may choose to negotiate a transfer of a patient to another nurse or seek consultation with the mental health clinical nurse specialist. Hopefully another

person can find the key that will unlock resistance to treatment.

Home health nurses may begin therapy during the initial visit by focusing attention on short-term, here and now problems that can be worked on immediately. This is done by assisting patients to achieve some small success, thereby planting in their mind the experience of feeling successful and having hope for the future. Later when depression has lifted and the nurse-patient relationship has solidified, work can begin on the more difficult problems that must be addressed if patients are to achieve a lasting sense of control over their lives.[19,24,25,37,43,52]

A sample patient care plan for depression problems is presented in Table 23-1.

Grief resolution. Perhaps the most frequent problem causing depression in the elderly population is the inability of the patient to resolve the grief experienced with the death of a spouse, special friend, or child. There may also be grief associated with loss of health, diagnosis of terminal illness, loss of home or familiar environment, or any other experience that is a major loss for the individual.

Encouraging reminiscence helps the patient to work through the grief. Exploring how the patient has solved similar problems in the past gives insight for solving problems in the present and future. By listening to others who have gone through much the same experiences, the patient will have a sense of not being alone. To learn that others have survived such losses means that the patient can survive too. The homebound patient may not be able to go to support groups during the interval of time the home health nurse is visiting, but encouragement and information can be given about such groups so that later, when health improves, the patient can follow through. If a support group is medically prescribed or directed, the patient may sometimes attend and still be considered homebound.[7,31,39]

Nursing care of the suicidal patient

Assessment of suicide potential. Suicide potential is evaluated by direct and specific questions. The fear that bringing up the subject of suicide with depressed patients instills in them the idea of killing themselves is unfounded; giving patients permission to discuss the subject openly and honestly may reduce the tension within them at that moment. Predicting suicide potential is an inexact

Table 23-1 Patient care plan: Depression

Nursing problem	Interventions	Outcomes	Evaluation
			Date/Initial
Alteration in mental status r/t depressed feelings, loneliness, preoccupation with physical problems, poor ego strength, unresolved problems of childhood, poor body image Date: _____	Assess mental status for increased depression: Downhearted feelings Tearfulness Insomnia Altered eating patterns Anxiety Loss of interest Irritability Difficulty making decisions Lack of enjoyment in usual interests Suicidal ideations	Pt. will verbalize that depression has lifted by: _____ by: _____ Pt. will have no more than 2 signs and symptoms of depression by: _____ by: _____ Pt. will identify ways to deal more effectively with social isolation by: _____ by: _____	U/R _____ U/R _____ U/R _____ U/R _____ U/R _____ U/R _____
	Counsel pt. in ways to increase activities, ways to deal with health losses, ways to decrease social isolation, ways to assert self effectively, ways to become less sensitive to the remarks of others	Pt. will begin to use identified patterns of dealing with social isolation by: _____ by: _____	U/R _____ U/R _____
		Pt. will acknowledge sad feelings, and will begin to deal with them positively by: _____ by: _____	U/R _____ U/R _____
		Pt. will make contract not to harm self and contact MD/RN when having these feelings by: _____ by: _____	U/R _____ U/R _____
	Instruct pt. in actions and side effects of medications: 1 2. 3.	Pt. will verbalize knowledge of actions and side effects of medications by: _____ by: _____	U/R _____ U/R _____
	Assess effectiveness and side effects of medications	Pt. will demonstrate compliance with medication regimen by: _____ by: _____	U/R _____ U/R _____

science, but the following questions provide useful guidance:

- Are you thinking about killing yourself right now?
- Do you have a plan?
- Do you have what you need to carry out this plan right here with you?
- Do you trust yourself to keep your thoughts and feelings under control?

If the patient answers yes to the first question, it is imperative to continue. Having a plan is much more serious than simply having thoughts of suicide. If the plan is vague and there is no convenient way to carry it out, the threat is probably not immediate. However, if the plan is in place, the necessary means are available, and the patient does not feel under control, the danger is critical for this patient and must be taken seriously.

To assess these three critical elements in more detail and gain insight into a patient's suicide potential, consider the following:

- Is the method chosen relatively lethal?
- Does the patient have the means available?
- Is the suicide plan specific? Can this patient tell exactly when he or she plans to do it?

Some behavioral clues the patient may exhibit while at risk for suicide are as follows:

- Verbal threats about committing the act
- Planning the act in detail
- Alcohol or drug abuse
- Giving away personal items, especially those that have been cherished for the patient's entire life
- Hallucinations
- Marked restlessness, anxiety, or agitation
- Delusions about severity of real or imagined physical illness, such as cancer[16]

Beyond evaluation of the patient's suicide plan, the home health nurse should note several other factors: (1) the age and sex of the patient (elderly men present the greatest threat of actual suicide), (2) any stressful event that may have precipitated the suicidal behavior (any significant loss, real or imagined), (3) any sudden change in the patient's life situation, (4) symptoms of severe depression, (5) the support system available to help the patient through this stressful situation, (6) the patient's past lifestyle (stable or unstable, chronic suicidal behavior or acute episode), (7) the communication style that exists between the patient and significant others, and (8) the reaction of significant others to the suicidal behavior (helpful or nonhelpful, supportive or unbelieving, hopeful or hopeless in response).[1]

Home health nurses must observe carefully those patients who are known to be depressed and suicidal. During extreme depression the patient will not have the energy to attempt suicide, and will also feel numb emotionally. After treatment has progressed, energy returns and with it those feelings of grief and sadness that made suicide a possibility. The patient may again be at risk for suicide.[16]

Interventions. Home health nurses are not able to place suicidal patients in isolation or provide constant supervision, as might be done in the hospital setting. If patients are actively suicidal (such as holding a knife to the chest or holding a handful of pills), the decision is easy: the emergency unit is called and the patient is hospitalized. If the suicide plan is chosen, the means are available, and the patient is alone and vulnerable, the nurse's plan of action is more difficult. Physicians must certainly be notified of unstable situations. If a supportive person is available, that person must be informed of the patient's suicidal state of mind. Removal of lethal amounts of medication from the home may be all that is necessary to prevent a medication overdose. A 1-week supply of medication is rarely lethal to the average patient.

Probably the most critical aspect of nursing care is the nurse's communication of care and concern to the patient. Counseling can assist patients to cope with immediate problems by finding ways to reduce the anxiety and stress of the moment and by identifying coping strategies that were helpful in the past and can be applied to the immediate future. The therapy of touch (such as holding the patient's hand or giving a hug) often provides the strength these patients need to live and work on the problems that plague their existence. Beyond this, home health nurses must accept human limitations. Nurses cannot remain in the home forever and they cannot be certain the patient is safe once they have left the patient's home.

Ideally the patient would be sent immediately to the hospital when suicide thoughts become known to the nurse or the physician. This is no longer always possible when the suicidal thoughts remain in spite of careful and repeated medication changes and hospitalizations, because of the constraints of medical insurance or Medicare and Medicaid coverage. However, care and concern can be verbalized and communicated. The promise of specific follow-up visits gives the suicidal patient a reliable thread of strength for the immediate future.

Schizophrenia

ETIOLOGY AND PATHOPHYSIOLOGY

Schizophrenia is the most common and disabling of the mental health disorders. It is thought to stem from some malfunction of the brain and is known as a thought disorder. There is no unique symptomatology for schizophrenia at this time, and American categories are not accepted in other countries. Clinically no two individuals are alike.[36]

The pathology of schizophrenia is unknown but it may result from excessive activity of the neurotransmitter dopamine in the brain. Weinberger and Kleinman[50] call attention to brain-imaging techniques that reveal structural and functional abnormalities in certain brain regions. Genetics plays a role in the disorder. A sibling of a person with schizophrenia has a 1 in 10 chance of developing the disease, whereas the general population has only a 1 in 100 chance. The usual onset of the disorder occurs in late adolescence or early adulthood; it generally develops before age 30. The disorder is found in all races and is more common in men than in women.

There is no cure for schizophrenia although 25% of this population recover spontaneously. The majority become chronically ill with symptoms usually lasting throughout the life span.

Treatment consists of administering antipsychotic medications, which act on chemicals in the brain to reduce hallucinations and delusions. About 5% to 20% of schizophrenic patients do not respond to medication. These individuals spend their lives in and out of hospitals, uncontrolled, often homeless, sometimes permanently institutionalized in state hospitals. Most live in the community, either in their own apartments (with the support of case managers), or with parents, siblings, or other family configurations. These individuals increasingly need care from psychiatric home care nurses.

HOME CARE APPLICATION
Assessment

Characteristic symptoms. Characteristic symptoms of schizophrenia include two or more of the following, with each present for a significant portion of time during a 1-month period:

1. Delusions
2. Hallucinations
3. Disorganized speech
4. Grossly disorganized or catatonic behavior
5. Negative symptoms, e.g., affective flattening, alogia (inability to express oneself through speech), or avolition (inability to make decisions, or decide what to do)

Social/occupational dysfunction. For a significant portion of the time since the onset of the disturbance, one or more major areas of functioning (such as work, interpersonal relations, or self-care) have been markedly below the level achieved prior to the onset.

Duration. Continuous signs of the disturbance persist for at least 6 months. This must include at least 1 month of the characteristic symptoms and may include periods of prodromal or residual symptoms.

Schizoaffective and mood disorder exclusion. Schizoaffective disorder and mood disorder with psychotic features have been ruled out because either (1) no major depressive, manic, or mixed episodes have occurred concurrently with the active-phase symptoms; or (2) if mood episodes have occurred during active-phase symptoms, their total duration has been brief relative to the duration of the active and residual periods.

Substance/general medical condition exclusion. The disturbance is not due to the direct physiological effects of a substance (e.g., a drug of abuse or a medication) or a general medical condition.

Relationship to pervasive developmental disorder. If there is a history of autistic disorder or another pervasive developmental disorder, the ad-

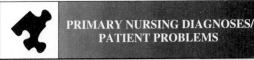

**PRIMARY NURSING DIAGNOSES/
PATIENT PROBLEMS**

Schizophrenia
- Delusions and hallucinations
- Social dysfunction, isolation, withdrawal
- Medication compliance/noncompliance
- Medication side effects
- Paranoia
- Low motivation, apathy, feelings of failure
- Denial of illness

ditional diagnosis of schizophrenia is made only if prominent delusions or hallucinations are also present for at least a month (or less if successfully treated).[2,3]

Narrow classifications of schizophrenia seldom stand up in clinical experience, but the disorder is recognizable through observation of behavior. Behavior emerges in aloofness, suspiciousness, episodes of impulsive destructiveness, immature emotional responses, exaggerations, ambivalence, and inappropriateness. Severe states include withdrawal into a fantasy life in which usual social customs and personal care are disregarded.[34] Primary nursing diagnoses and patient problems for schizophrenia are listed in the box above.

Medication response

Assessment of the effectiveness and side effects of drugs is particularly important for schizophrenic patients, who sometimes forget or disregard appointments with their physicians. Home health nurses may be the only link these patients have with their physician for months at a time.

One of the most frequent reasons for seeing schizophrenic patients in the home is to administer injections of fluphenazine decanoate (Prolixin) or haloperidol decanoate (Haldol) on an intermittent schedule, usually every 2 to 4 weeks. The rationale for these visits may be that these patients are noncompliant in going to the mental health center for regular injections or that they have no one who can or will assume the responsibility for getting them to the center.

Although injections are the primary purpose for these visits, nurses must assess the effectiveness

and side effects of the medications. It is necessary to make certain that no problems are emerging and that the medication dosages remain adequate for the patients' needs. Some particularly troublesome problems must be guarded against. Home health nurses are frequently in the unique position of being the only health care professional seeing these patients on a regular basis. It is therefore imperative that home health nurses be aware of neurological impairments common to antipsychotic drugs, such as extrapyramidal symptoms (EPS), tardive dyskinesia, and neuroleptic malignant syndrome. They should report these conditions promptly when symptoms emerge.[8] Some physicians will choose not to treat EPS, especially if the symptoms seem minor. A safe course is to lower the dose at the first sign of EPS. A third approach is to add an anti-EPS agent to the medication regimen, or to give it prn when EPS appears.

Extrapyramidal symptoms (EPS). EPS can appear in several forms, which are usually not difficult to assess and are usually easy to treat.[8]

Dyskinesia is a defect in voluntary movement. It may consist of sustained or intermittent muscle spasms that produce abnormal postures and contortions of the eyes, face, neck, or throat. Slower dystonic movements and postures occur when the trunk or extremities are involved. An oculogyric crisis, when the eyes roll back and up, can be a serious problem. Further developments can include life-threatening events when the tongue, neck, or pharyngeal areas become distorted, blocking the airway. The physician must be notified, and an anti-EPS agent must be given at the first sign of acute dyskinesia.

Parkinsonism (drug-induced) consists of signs and symptoms identical to idiopathic Parkinson's disease: rigidity, postural abnormalities, slowed movements, blunted spontaneity, and tremor (especially of the hands and fingers). "Pill rolling" movements of the fingers and "cogwheel" rigidity of the arms are rather easily assessed. Such symptoms are controlled by antiparkinsonian agents, such as trihexyphenidyl, amantadine, or benztropine.

Akinesia consists of a fixed and flat facial expression, a dulled speech, an apathetic manner, and lethargy or excessive sleeping. It can be confused with psychosis, organic brain syndrome, or depression. One in three patients taking long-term antipsychotics develops akinesia. It is reversed by lowering the dose of the antipsychotic and adding anticholinergics.

Akathisia is noted for restlessness and motor agitation. Shuffling, tapping, shifting of weight from foot to foot, or rocking may be part of the agitated picture. A more severe manifestation might be running or pacing constantly, or being unable to stand or sit for any length of time. The patient reports feeling "nervous inside," "jumpy," "wired," or "wound-up." Delusions or psychotic thoughts may be present. A single dose of an antipsychotic can trigger this EPS. Sometimes self-destructive behaviors such as suicide or homicide may result from severe akathisia. Confusing these behaviors with anxiety and increasing the dosage of antipsychotic medication, or giving antianxiety medication, only worsens the problem. Anticholinergics can be given routinely or prn to effectively control the problem.

Tardive dyskinesia. To identify tardive dyskinesia as early as possible, home health nurses should be alert to chewing movements, licking and smacking of the lips, sucking, repetitive protrusion of the tongue or tongue movements within the oral cavity, tongue tremor or wormlike myokynic (twitching) movements on the tongue surface, grotesque grimaces, and facial spasms. Early signs after initiating neuroleptic drug therapy consist of facial tics, ill-defined oral or ocular movements, chewing, rocking, or swaying. Frequently, tardive (meaning late or delayed) dyskinesia appears late in treatment, often after 3 to 6 months of taking antipsychotic medications.

These chronic, involuntary movements may also be observed in the extremities and trunk, with restless, agitated movement of the hands, feet, fingers, and toes. The physician must be informed as early as possible of such developments so that the offending neuroleptic drug can be discontinued while the condition is still reversible. The longer tardive dyskinesia goes on, the more likely it is to become irreversible.[34]

Neuroleptic malignant syndrome (NMS). Approximately 1% of all patients treated with neuroleptic medications develop neuroleptic malignant syndrome, the most serious form of EPS. Schizophrenic patients must be assessed by home health nurses for signs and symptoms of the syndrome.

NMS has been described as an exaggerated form of neuroleptic-induced parkinsonism.[20] Hyperthermia (a sudden and rapidly rising temperature) is the main signal indicating neuroleptic malignant syndrome, along with central nervous system symptoms such as confusion, seizures, and autonomic instability (widely fluctuating blood pressure, tachycardia, and diaphoresis). Creatine phosphokinase (CPK) is elevated. Diffuse tremor, dystonic posturing, and changes in mental status that may lead to stupor or coma may also be present. Rapid and severe muscle rigidity with difficulty moving or breathing is the final indicator of this potentially fatal syndrome. NMS often goes unrecognized by health care professionals. Treatment consists of immediate discontinuance of the antipsychotic medication, and appropriate support of cardiovascular, respiratory, and renal functions.[2,8,29]

Problems frequently arise when the patient is taking other drugs with the neuroleptics. A knowledge of drug interactions will assist the home health nurse in assessing such problems. The following list provides information on how other drugs interact with neuroleptics:[49]

- **Alcohol** can augment the effects that neuroleptics have on the central nervous system, increasing the likelihood of oversedation and dizziness.
- **Antacids** can inhibit the absorption of the phenothiazine neuroleptics, reducing their effectiveness.
- **Anticholinergic drugs** intensify the anticholinergic effects of neuroleptic drugs, causing more dry mouth, blurred vision, constipation, and ejaculatory problems.
- **Anticoagulants** can become more active when taken with phenothiazines, increasing the risk of bleeding. When given with haloperidol, anticoagulants may be less effective.
- **Antidepressants** in the tricyclic family—e.g., imipramine (Tofranil) and nortriptyline (Pamelor)—can raise neuroleptic blood levels, increasing the likelihood of adverse effects.
- **Antihypertensives** become more potent when taken with neuroleptics. Propranolol (Inderal) and other beta blockers may exacerbate neuroleptics' cardiotoxic effects.
- **Bromocriptine (Parlodel)** may need to be given in larger doses to control parkinsonism-like symptoms when the patient is taking

antipsychotics. By raising dopamine levels in the brain, bromocriptine—like other antiparkinsonian agents—can intensify the symptoms of schizophrenia.

- **Carbamazepine (Tegretol)** can lower neuroleptic blood levels, reducing the effectiveness of the drug.
- **Corticosteroids** are more efficiently absorbed when taken with neuroleptics, making them more potent.
- **Digoxin (Lanoxin)** is more likely to reach toxic levels when taken with antipsychotic agents.
- **Levodopa (Larodopa)** is less effective when taken with neuroleptics, which also are less effective.
- **Methyldopa (Aldomet),** when taken with haloperidol, may cause dementia.
- **Monoamine oxidase inhibitors** such as isocarboxazid (Marplan) and phenelzine (Nardil) can intensify the hypotensive effects of neuroleptics.
- **Morphine** and other narcotic analgesics can make patients taking neuroleptics more drowsy and increase the risk of respiratory side effects (e.g., bronchospasm, laryngeal edema, and suppression of the gag and cough reflexes).
- **Phenytoin (Dilantin)** and neuroleptics can reduce each other's effectiveness.
- **Quinidine (Duraquin)** affects the myocardium more powerfully when taken with neuroleptics, increasing the risk of hypotension, bradycardia, and heart block.[49]

Patient and care provider education

Primary themes of patient education for schizophrenia are listed in the following box.

The typical schizophrenic patient seen by home health nurses lives alone in a subsidized apartment or lives with an aging parent in the family home. Frequently these patients have social workers assigned to them through the department of mental health for case management. Their relationships may range from frequent visits to remote, sporadic contact. Patients usually know who their case manager is but frequently they are unable to make judgments about whether their needs are being met because they know no other system and have nothing with which to compare their experience. Case managers nearly always have overwhelming caseloads to contend with.[28]

The effects that recently discharged schizophrenic individuals have on primary care providers must be noted by home health nurses. Threats to personal safety—including actual or threatened physical, social, or emotional abuse—constitute the single greatest concern of primary care providers. The older the provider is, the greater the potential negative impact on the care provider's quality of life when the patient is discharged to the home. The negative impact on the quality of life of care providers is related to the number of years that the schizophrenic person has been ill.[42]

Care providers, if present, are an integral part of home health nurses' care and concern. The needs of these individuals must be addressed. They need instruction regarding medication regimens and side effects. An understanding that schizophrenia is a devastating brain disorder, and not the result of poor parenting, relieves the guilt often found in families. Time must be spent educating families about the disease and about ways to cope with delusions, hallucinations, and "acting out" behavior. Nursing care of schizophrenic patients includes attending to their physical and medical needs. Doing this may require monitoring vital signs, weight, and blood sugar levels for diabetic patients; urine screening; venipuncture for any needed blood specimens; and assessment and instruction concerning any bowel problems.

The detached patient. Nursing care of schizophrenic patients also involves establishing an

PRIMARY THEMES OF PATIENT EDUCATION

Schizophrenia
- Information about pathology, progression, symptomatology; when to call the physician
- Medication effects and side effects; reasons for taking medications
- Extrapyramidal symptoms; tardive dyskinesia; neuroleptic malignant syndrome
- Drug interactions with neuroleptics
- Care provider education on dealing with specific patient symptoms
- Development of interpersonal relationships
- Skills development
- Community alliances

emotional bond with patients who are often detached, withdrawn, or hallucinating. Communication is often difficult and patience on the part of the home health nurse is essential. Patients frequently view efforts to establish a relationship with them as an attempt to deprive them of the protective facade they have built around themselves. Home health nurses must allow patients time to become familiar with them and to test their reliability. Home health agencies should take this into account and consistently send the same nurse to the same patient as often as possible.

In assisting patients who remain detached in establishing a relationship, home health nurses must identify the behaviors patients use to avoid relating. Home health nurses can then help patients relinquish these behaviors by helping them to see that there is no need for avoidance.

Home health nurses also must rely heavily on any healthy aspects of behavior presented by the patients. They must learn never to take rejection seriously or personally. Nurses can discover clues about what raises anxiety levels by carefully watching patients' behavior and noting what is being discussed when avoidance begins. They can then assist patients in overcoming anxiety and developing some success in relating to other human beings. No one approach works for all patients, so nurses must be resourceful and willing to attempt innovations when original strategies fail. The belief that all patients are potentially reachable is an essential attitude for nurses who work with the mentally ill.[18]

The elusive patient. Patients who do not keep appointments, either by running away when they know their nurse is coming or by refusing to answer the door, pose another problem for home health nurses. Later the patient may or may not offer an excuse such as "I forgot," "I had to go to my doctor," or "I didn't hear your knock." The nurse should wait for a few minutes and then leave a note clearly stating when the visit was scheduled to occur, when the next visit will be, and that the patient is expected to be present and available at that time. Patients often test their nurses to see if they mean what they say and will care enough to come back.

If the behavior persists, family or friends may have to intervene and assist in making sure that patients are available for visits. Home health agencies can seldom afford to allow nurses to go repeatedly to homes only to find no one at home or no one to answer the door. Once such patients and nurses meet again home health nurses must confront patients with the behavior, conveying an attitude of concern and interest in understanding what actually happened.

Home health nurses need to be honest in stating their feelings of worry and annoyance at being "stood up," presenting their own reality to the patients, and letting patients know that their behavior has affected someone else. A contract or some understanding must be established between patients and nurses, or the visits will have to be terminated and the physician notified that home visits are not working with the patient.[18]

The suspicious patient. Suspicious patients present special problems to home health nurses because they frequently do not allow the nurses into their homes, or they do not allow nurses to give injections or make assessments. They also are very difficult to engage in any kind of problem solving activities. Their suspicion is grounded in a persistent tendency to mistrust or doubt the sincerity or honesty of others. They are unable to consider any viewpoint valid except their own. They cannot admit that they might ever be wrong about anything.

Home health nurses must approach suspicious patients with a goal of helping them learn to trust. They must very carefully define their own role in working with these individuals because such patients tend to misinterpret words and behaviors. Home health nurses must also be very honest and extremely consistent to build trust. Any trust that does develop is fragile and can be destroyed by even a casual remark or action. Suspicious patients tend to avoid interpersonal relationships because they cannot believe another person could ever be reliable.[18]

A sample patient care plan for the suspicious or paranoid patient is presented in Table 23-2.

Rehabilitation: A model for home care. Psychiatric disorders, particularly schizophrenia, are associated with severe and persistent disability. A psychiatric rehabilitation model has been developed with an overall goal of ensuring that patients with a psychiatric disability acquire those physical, emotional, social, and intellectual skills needed to live, learn, and work in the community, with the least possible amount of support from nurses and other helping professionals.[4]

Table 23-2 Patient care plan: Paranoia

Nursing problem	Interventions	Outcomes	Evaluation
			Date/Initial
Alteration in mental status r/t suspicion and fear of interpersonal relationships	Assess mental status for S/S of paranoia, violence, physical assault of others, verbal abuse of others	Pt. will have no episodes of violent or verbally abusive behavior by: _____ by: _____	U/R _____ U/R _____
Date: _____	Counsel pt. on working through fears of relating to other people, on developing an increased ability to trust other people	Pt. will verbalize/admit to having suspicions and fears of other people by: _____ by: _____	U/R _____ U/R _____
		Pt. will verbalize feelings of anxiety, inadequacy, and helplessness by: _____ by: _____	U/R _____ U/R _____
		Pt. will verbalize learning of the ability to clarify doubts, suspicions, and possible misinterpretations of other people's motives by: _____ by: _____	U/R _____ U/R _____
		Pt. will identify coping behaviors that have been effective in the past by: _____ by: _____	U/R _____ U/R _____
	Assess medication regimen for effectiveness and side effects	Pt./S.O. will demonstrate compliance with medication regimen by: _____ by: _____	U/R _____ U/R _____
	Instruct Pt./S.O. in actions and side effects of medications: 1. 2. 3.	Pt./S.O. will verbalize actions and side effects of medications by: _____ by: _____	U/R _____ U/R _____

This model involves (1) teaching patients specific skills necessary to function effectively, and/or (2) developing community and environmental resources that support and strengthen present levels of functioning. Home health nurses provide care in an ideal setting for such skill training because the home environment usually is less threatening to schizophrenic patients than anywhere else.

Social withdrawal, apathy, slovenliness, and anhedonia (lacking in interest of pleasure) do not respond well to neuroleptic drugs. Sometimes such negative symptoms respond well to clozapine

(Clozaril). Drugs do not teach life and coping skills. Most schizophrenic patients need to learn or relearn social and personal skills to survive in the community. By meeting patients in the home environment, home health nurses can help individuals and families select appropriate goals and then assist these patients in developing skills. The main disadvantage faced by the home health nurse is the infrequency of visits (usually 1 to 2 times per week, or even less frequently if the identified reason for services is to provide an injection every 2 to 4 weeks). Self-care, medication and symptom management, establishment of relationships, money management and consumerism, residential living, recreational activities, food preparation, and choice and use of public agencies are areas in which the skills of schizophrenic patients either have been lost or were never developed. It is important to remember that persons with a psychiatric disability can learn useful skills.[4,5,41,42]

If such skill training is not possible because the deficits are too great, the strategies of home health nurses may be directed toward helping patients compensate for their disabilities by (1) locating environments that accommodate the deficits and symptoms and (2) adjusting patients' and families' expectations to a level that is realistically attainable.[4,5,27,48] An ongoing support person can significantly reduce the disability by simply being available. Home health nurses can provide support as long as the case remains open.

Inherent to a rehabilitation model for schizophrenia are three guiding attitudes that nurses must maintain:

1. Optimism that change is possible
2. Belief that motivation for change can come from within the patient and the environment if carefully implemented
3. Confidence that even small changes can improve the patient's quality of life[4,5,47]

SUMMARY

Schizophrenia and depression are two of the many mental health disorders that a nurse encounters in the home setting. No two patients will manifest identical symptoms. As inpatient hospitalization stays are reduced (because of DRG criteria, insurance limitations, or reduced federal, state, and local funding), more and more mentally ill persons are discharged to their homes in states of disequilibrium and instability.

Home health nurses have a unique opportunity to assist these individuals toward optimal health through (1) careful assessment of medical and psychological needs, (2) medication management, (3) short-term case management, (4) crisis intervention, (5) skills training, (6) family and personal counseling, (7) support and problem solving, (8) assistance in securing community resources and alliances by a social service referral, (9) assistance with personal hygiene by a home health aide when necessary, (10) instruction in nutritional concerns by the nurse and/or a registered dietitian, and (11) referral to a physical therapist or occupational therapist if the need arises.[6,12,54] Knowledge about mental health resources that are available in the community, the state, and the country are invaluable to this population of patients because they are so often unable to obtain this information for themselves.[15,28]

No other area of nursing provides nurses with so much information about the environment in which such patients live and the people with whom they share their lives. For an hour or so, with each visit, nurses share that life with their patients and have the opportunity to assist in the process of implementing change so that patients' lives may be fuller and their trips to the hospital less frequent.

REFERENCES

1. Aguilera DC: *Crisis intervention: theory and methodology,* ed 6, St Louis, 1989, Mosby.
2. American Psychiatric Association: *Diagnostic criteria from DSM-IV,* Washington, DC, 1994, The Association.
3. American Psychiatric Association: *Diagnostic and statistical manual of mental disorders,* ed 4, Washington, DC, 1994, The Association.
4. Anthony WA, Liberman RP: The practice of psychiatric rehabilitation; historical, conceptual, and research base, *Schizophr Bull* 12:540, 1986.
5. Anthony WA, Margules A: Toward improving the efficacy of psychiatric rehabilitation: a skills training approach, *Rehabil Psychiatry* 21:101, 1974.
6. Baier M: Case management with the chronically mentally ill, *J Psychosoc Nurs Ment Health Serv* 25:17, 1987.
7. Bateman A et al: Dysfunctional grieving, *J Psychosoc Nurs Ment Health Serv* 30:5, 1992.
8. Blair DT: Sorting through EPS, *Geriatr Nurs* 244-246, Sept/Oct 1991.
9. Brown JH: The role of the home health care nurse in mental health assessment of the elderly, *J Home Health Care Pract* 2(1): 1989.
10. Buckwalter KC: How to unmask depression, *Geriatr Nurs* 7/8:179, 1990.

11. Buckwalter KC, Stolley J: Managing mentally ill elders at home, *Geriatr Nurs* 136-139, May/June 1991.

12. Caplan G: *Principles of preventive psychiatry,* New York, 1964, Basic Books.

13. Carson VB: Doing psych but talking med-surg language. . . . *Caring* 32-41, June 1994.

14. Cosgray RE, Hanna V: Physiological causes of depression in the elderly, *Perspec Psychiatr Care* 29(1):26-28, 1993.

15. Crosby RL: Community care of the chronically mentally ill, *J Psychosoc Nurs Ment Health Serv* 25:33, 1987.

16. D'Arrigo T: Depression and recovery in home care patients, *Caring* 42-46, June 1994.

17. Dittbrenner H: Psychiatric home care: an overview, *Caring* 26-30, June 1994.

18. Doona ME: *Travelbee's intervention in psychiatric nursing,* ed 2, Philadelphia, 1979, FA Davis.

19. Duffey J, Miller MP, Parlocha P: Psychiatric home care: a framework for assessment and intervention, *Home Health Care Nurs* 11(2):22-28, 1993.

20. Fogel BS, Goldberg RJ: Neuroleptic malignant syndrome (letter), *N Engl J Med* 313:1292, 1985.

21. Folstein MF, Folstein SE, McHugh PR: "Mini-Mental State": a practical method for grading the cognitive state of patients for the clinician, *J Psychiatric Res* 12:189-198, 1975.

22. Forchuk C et al: Incorporating Peplau's theory and case management, *J Psychosoc Nurs Ment Health Serv* 27:35, 1989.

23. Forchuk C, Brown B: Establishing a nurse-client relationship, *J Psychosoc Nurs Ment Health Serv* 27:30, 1989.

24. Frisch N: Home care nursing and psychosocial-emotional needs of clients, *Home Health Care Nurs* 11(2):64-65, 1993.

25. Gomez GE, Gomez EA: Depression in the elderly, *J Psychosoc Nurs Ment Health Serv* 31:28, 1993.

26. Harris MD: Psychiatric evaluation and therapy, *Home Health Care Nurs* 11(2):66-67, 1993.

27. Hellwig K: Managing patients in the community setting, *J Psychosoc Nurs Ment Health Serv* 31 (12):21-24, 1993.

28. Hoffmann NE: Mental health resources in the United States, *Caring* 48-52, June 1994.

29. Hooper JF, Herren CK, Goldwasser H: Neuroleptic malignant syndrome: recognizing an unrecognized killer, *J Psychosoc Nurs Ment Health Serv* 27:13, 1989.

30. Janz M: Clues to elder abuse, *Geriatr Nurs* 220-222, Sept/Oct 1990.

31. Joffrion LP, Douglas D: Grief resolution: facilitating self-transcendence in the bereaved, *J Psychosoc Nurs Ment Health Serv* 32(3):13, 1994.

32. Kelley JH, Lehman L: Assessment of anxiety, depression, and suspiciousness in the home care setting, *Home Health Care Nurs* 11(2):16-20, 1993.

33. Klebanoff JA, Casler CB: The psychosocial clinical nurse specialist: an untapped resource for home care, *Home Health Care Nurs* 4:36, 1986.

34. Kolb LC, Brodie HK: *Modern clinical psychiatry,* ed 10, Philadelphia, 1982, WB Saunders.

35. Kozlak J, Thobaben M: Treating the elderly mentally ill at home, *Perspec Psychiatr Care* 28 (2):31-35, 1992.

36. Malone J: Schizophrenia research update: implications for nursing, *J Psychosoc Nurs Ment Health Serv* 28:4, 1990.

37. Maurer FA: Acute depression: treatment and nursing strategies for this affective disorder, *Nurs Clin North Am* 21:413, 1986.

38. Miller MP, Duffey J: Planning and program development for psychiatric home care, *J Nurs Adm* 23(11):35-41, 1993.

39. Peachey NH: Helping the elderly person resolve integrity versus despair, *Perspec Psychiatr Care* 28(2):29-30, 1992.

40. Pelletier LR: Psychiatric home care, *J Psychosoc Nurs Ment Health Serv* 26:22, 1988.

41. Plante TG: Social skills training: a program to help schizophrenic clients cope, *J Psychosoc Nurs Ment Health Serv* 27:7, 1989.

42. Seymour RJ, Dawson NJ: The schizophrenic at home, *J Psychosoc Nurs Ment Health Serv* 24:28, 1986.

43. Shires B, Tappan T: The clinical nurse specialist as brief psychotherapist, *Perspec Psychiatr Care* 28(4):15-18, 1992.

44. Smith M, Buckwalter KC: Medication management, antidepressant drugs and the elderly: an overview, *J Psychosoc Nurs Ment Health Serv* 30(10):30, 1992.

45. Soreff S: Indications for home treatment, *Psych Clin North Am* 8:563, 1985.

46. Talbot J: Community care for the chronically mentally ill, *Psych Clin North Am* 8:437, 1985.

47. Thompson J, Strand K: Psychiatric nursing in a psychosocial setting, *J Psychosoc Nurs Ment Health Serv* 32(2):25, 1994.

48. Torrey EF: *Surviving schizophrenia, a family manual,* rev ed, New York, 1988, Harper & Row.

49. Vallone DC, Stephanos MJ: Minimizing adverse drug reactions, *RN* 36-40, Nov 1990.

50. Weinberger DR, Kleinman JE: Observations on the brain in schizophrenia. In Frances AJ, Hales RE, editors: *Psychiatry update, the American Psychiatric Association annual review,* Washington, DC, 1986, American Psychiatric Association Press.

51. Wernert P, Runyon E: Healing mind and body, *Caring* 22-25, Dec 1992.

52. Whall AL: What is the nursing treatment for depression? *J Psychosoc Nurs Ment Health Serv* 31(12):37-38, 1993.

53. Wilkinson L: A collaborative model: ambulatory pharmacotherapy for chronic psychiatric patients, *J Psychosoc Nurs Ment Health Serv* 29:12-26, 1992.

54. Worley NK, Albanese N: Independent living for the chronically mentally ill, *J Psychosoc Nurs Ment Health Serv* 27:18, 1989.

55. Yoest MA: The clinical nurse specialist on the psychiatric team, *J Psychosoc Nurs Ment Health Serv* 27:27, 1989.

56. Zind R et al: Educating patients about missed medication doses, *J Psychosoc Nurs Ment Health Serv* 30(7):10-14, 1992.

57. Zung WWK: A self-rating depression scale, *Arch Gen Psychiatry* 12:63, 1965.

58. Zung WWK, Richards CB, Short MJ: Self-rating depression scale in an outpatient clinic, *Arch Gen Psychiatry* 13:508, 1965.

24 The Geriatric Patient

Nancy Van Fleet Wilens

One clinical issue consistently challenging our society is the provision of quality home care for elderly persons. The increasing number of older adults requiring diverse health care services necessitates the development of cost-effective, quality care.[27] More and more older adults are deciding to live at home even though many of them have chronic health problems that they cannot handle alone. Four out of 10 persons 65 years of age or older require assistance, and the need for home health assistance increases with age.[19]

The high cost of health care and a desire for independence are two primary factors that influence the older adult's decision to remain at home as long as possible. Additionally, the demands for home health care are growing in response to the diagnostic-related groups (DRGs) and managed care groups, which encourage shorter hospital stays and provide limited reimbursement for acute care services.

The purpose of this chapter is to provide information that will assist home health nurses in developing a plan of care for older adults. Included in the chapter are a profile of the elderly population, a review of the normal physiology of aging, a description of the characteristics of elderly patients receiving home health care services, and an examination of patient care issues relevant to the needs of older adults.

DEMOGRAPHICS
Age

Persons 65 years of age or older represent 12.7% of the U.S. population.[12] Their numbers will continue to increase, although it is predicted that this growth will be slow during the 1990s because of the relatively small number of babies born during the Great Depression of the 1930s.[30] The most rapid increase can be expected between the years 2010 and 2030 when the baby boom generation reaches age 65.[12] By the year 2000, it is expected that 13% of the population will be 65 years of age or older; this percentage may climb to 20% by 2030.[12]

In addition, during this century the average life span for Americans has risen from 47 years to 75 years.[7] In other words, a child born in 1991 can expect to live 75.5 years, about 28 years longer than a child born in 1900.[12]

Living arrangements

The majority (67%) of noninstitutionalized older persons live with family members[12]; only 31% live alone. The percentage of older persons living in nursing homes dramatically increases with age. At present, approximately 5% of persons 65 years of age or older, 6% of persons from 75 to 84 years of age, and 24% of persons 85 years of age or older are living in nursing homes.[12]

The elderly population is less likely to change residence than other age groups. 29% of older persons live in inner cities whereas 44% live in suburbs.[12]

Income

The median income of older persons is $14,548 for men and $8,189 for women.[12] Approximately 23% of family households with a person 65 years of age or older have incomes of less than $15,000; 40% of these households have incomes of $30,000 or more.[1] The incomes of 12.9% of the elderly population are at or below the poverty level.[12]

Housing

Seventy-seven percent of the elderly population own their own homes and 23% are renters.[12] The housing of elderly Americans is generally older and less adequate than that of younger age groups, and structural problems are common.

Employment

Employment status does not often change for individuals after the age of 65. 12% of older Americans (3.6 million) are in the labor force; this constitutes 2.8% of the U.S. labor force.[12]

Education

Among older individuals, the median number of years of education completed varies by race and ethnic origin: 12.2 years for whites, 8.5 years for blacks, and 8.0 years for Hispanics.[7] However, the educational level of the older population is gradually rising.

PHYSIOLOGY OF AGING

Many physiological functions decline at a rate of approximately 1% per year after age 30.[3] A decline in any one major organ system such as the cardiovascular, respiratory, or genitourinary system is not always significant. It is the gradual deterioration of several organ systems that typically affects the functional ability of the older individual.

Goldstein[16] defines aging as "a progressive unfavorable loss of adaptation and a decreasing expectation of life with the passage of time that is expressed in measurement as decreased viability and increased vulnerability to the normal forces of mortality." Age-related functional loss follows several patterns. A function can be totally lost, as is the female reproductive ability, or a function can be retained with an altered level, as occurs with musculoskeletal disease or kidney changes. As age-related changes occur, some people develop chronic problems and therefore become more vulnerable to illness.

For home health nurses to accurately assess an older person, it is important that they have a clear understanding of how the human body ages.

Cardiovascular

With age the heart loses elasticity; therefore decreased contractility and cardiac output occur in response to increased metabolic demands. In-creased systolic and diastolic blood pressure result from increased peripheral resistance and pulse pressure. These changes in cardiac output and peripheral resistance cause a decrease in organ perfusion. By age 80 renal blood flow is reduced by half and cerebral blood flow by 20%.[3] Electrical changes produce a decrease in the heart rate and an increase in premature beats. The heart rate during rest changes little with age. Pedal pulses may be weaker as a result of arteriosclerotic changes. Lower extremities may be cool to the touch and appear mottled on inspection.

Respiratory

A decrease in pulmonary blood flow and diffusion is found in older adults. Respiratory accessory muscles undergo degeneration that results in decreased muscle strength. The maximum breathing capacity, vital capacity, residual volume, and functional capacity all diminish with age.[3] Airway closure occurs at higher tidal volumes in an older adult. Ventilation is less than adequate in dependent lung regions where perfusion is greatest. As a result a decrease in PAO_2, the amount of oxygen in the blood, would be associated with a significant decrease in oxygen delivery in someone over age 60.[29] Respiratory disorders such as chronic obstructive pulmonary disease (COPD) or emphysema put an elderly patient at greater risk for hypoxemia than a younger patient. (See Chapter 10.)

Integumentary

The amount of subcutaneous adipose tissue decreases with age, resulting in poor thermal insulation. Extremities are cooler and perspiration decreases. There is less fat distributed on the extremities and more on the trunk. Epidermal sweat glands and hair follicles atrophy, pigmentation increases unevenly, and the supporting collagen and elastin degenerate. These changes cause discolored, thin, dry, and wrinkled skin.[42] Senile purpura and senile keratosis are common. Such changes in the integument, along with poor peripheral circulation, predispose the elderly population to tissue breakdown and the formation of dermal wounds. (See Chapter 13.)

Hair color may be dull gray, white, yellow, or yellow-green. Hair distribution thins on the scalp, axillae, pubic area, and all extremities. Nail growth slows with age; nails become hard, thick, and brittle and are difficult to keep groomed. Insufficient calcium may make fingernails and toenails turn yellow. Older adults often need to be referred to a podiatrist because they are unable to reach their feet, see their feet, or manipulate clippers to cut the nails.

Genitourinary

The glomerular filtration rate (GFR) and kidney mass decrease with age. By age 80 the GFR declines by 50% and creatinine clearance declines by 33% compared with age 50.[21] Men may have increased micturition as a result of prostatic enlargement. Women have a decrease in perineal tone and therefore have urgency and stress incontinence. (See Chapter 15.)

Reproductive

In older males, testosterone production decreases, the phases of intercourse are slower, and there is a lengthened refractory time. No changes are seen in libido and sexual satisfaction. Testes decrease in size, sperm count decreases, and seminal fluid has a diminished viscosity.

Female estrogen production decreases with menopause, and breast tissue diminishes. The uterus decreases in size, and mucous secretions cease. Uterine prolapse may occur as a result of muscle weakness.

Gastrointestinal

Chewing is impaired because of partial or total loss of teeth, malocclusion, or ill-fitting dentures. Swallowing is made more difficult by diminished salivary secretions. A decrease in esophageal peristalsis causes an increased incidence of hiatal hernia with gaseous distension. Digestive enzyme production is decreased and fat absorption is delayed, affecting the absorption rate of fat-soluble vitamins A, D, E, and K. Intestinal peristalsis is reduced, causing a decrease in motility and, as a result, constipation. Gastric emptying is markedly slower in older persons. Some studies report that transit time for a liquid meal in elderly persons is more than double that for young adults.[14]

Musculoskeletal

Muscle strength and function decrease with loss of muscle mass. Bone structure is more porous but maintains normal demineralization. Connective tissue increases in density and contains less water as a person becomes older. Joints are less mobile, and tightening and fixation occur.[17] Physical activity will delay loss of function. Posture changes with age, and kyphosis is often seen. A decrease in total size occurs. (For example, normal height decreases 1 to 3 inches from that in young adulthood.) This decrease in size occurs as the body loses protein and water. These losses occur in proportion to a decrease in basal metabolic rate.

Neurologic

The majority of the elderly population have normal cognitive function in learning, memory, and abstract thinking.[20] A common concern of the aged is forgetfulness, which becomes a problem when it interferes with the performance of activities of daily living. It has been found that an elderly person may take longer to learn and remember new information but is capable of doing so.[1,20]

Slowing is one of the most significant nervous system changes.[20] This affects learning new information, motor tasks, and reaction to multiple stimuli. Activities that show a functional decline include getting up from a chair, writing rapidly, and buttoning or zipping clothing.[20]

Proprioception in the lower extremities is less efficient with age. As a result the elderly person often demonstrates a gait change, such as a Parkinson-like gait. Gait changes, combined with reduced position sense, complicate the older person's ability to maintain balance.

Elderly persons often experience a change in sleep patterns. They get a normal amount of sleep but awaken frequently during the night and therefore stay in bed longer. Frequent complaints of the older person are insomnia and disrupted sleep.

Sensory

All senses gradually decline with advanced age. Sight, hearing, and taste all diminish because of anatomic changes. Tactile sensitivity and perception of vibration decrease.

As the eye ages, structural and functional changes take place. The eyelids atrophy and become wrinkled. The lenses lose elasticity and frequently become opaque and cloudy, causing cataracts and a sensitivity to glare.[4] Changes in the iris and pupil slow down the ability to adapt to darkness. Sclerosis of the iris causes the pupils to become smaller, which limits the amount of light reaching the retina.[3] Many older adults find it difficult to drive at night because of a visual inability to adapt to darkness and bright lights. A decrease in lacrimation (tearing) causes many older people to complain of dry eyes.

The four most common diseases that affect vision are cataracts (opacity of lens), macular degeneration (retina), glaucoma (increased intraocular pressure), and diabetic retinopathy.[3] Conditions that should be reported to the physician are blurred vision, double vision, changes in pupil color, a film over the eye that does not go away with blinking, and frequent changes in the prescription for corrective lenses.

Hearing and vestibular function normally decrease with aging. Significant hearing impairments are found in 90% of nursing home residents and 30% of the ambulatory noninstitutionalized elderly population.[3]

Gustatory sensation has a diminished acuity because the tongue papillae and taste buds decrease in number with aging. These changes can result in a loss of appetite and inadequate nutrition.

Tactile sensitivity for touch and pain decreases with age, and the ability to detect vibration is reduced, especially in the feet. These changes are thought to be a result of slowed peripheral nerve conduction and central conduction of peripheral impulses associated with aging.

Understanding the normal aging process and how it may interfere with activities of daily living will improve home health nurses' abilities to identify significant changes in the condition of their patients. Knowledgeable nurses will readily recognize changes in the patient's status that should be communicated to the physician and incorporated into the plan of care.

THE ELDERLY HOME HEALTH PATIENT

To develop a realistic and meaningful plan of care, home health nurses need to be familiar with the health characteristics of elderly patients admitted to home health services.

Van Ort and Woodthi[45] studied 66 elderly patients admitted to home care to determine the home care patient and caregiver characteristics and to identify the nursing needs of these patients. In their study 70% of the home care patients were

women from 70 to 89 years of age, 50% of whom were married. A majority (80%) of the patients were living with a caregiver; only a small number (14%) were living alone. Patients received home care an average of 19 days, having approximately three health-related visits a week.

This study also identified the most frequent medical and nursing diagnoses for elderly home health patients; 75% of the primary medical diagnoses fell into four categories—orthopedic, cardiovascular, diabetes, and pulmonary-related. This corresponds with Fowles' list of the most common ailments found in the noninstitutionalized elderly population. The box on page 430 lists nursing diagnoses related to the geriatric patient.[12]

This study is significant because it reflects the health care problems found most frequently among the elderly—problems related to dementia, nutrition, immobility, polypharmacy, and safety. These problems represent the patient care issues that home health nurses should consider in designing and implementing plans of care that promote symptom management and enhance patients' return to optimal health.

PATIENT CARE ISSUES IN THE HOME SETTING
Dementia

Elderly patients often complain about memory problems and seek professional advice. As many as 10% to 15% of persons over the age of 65 may have cognitive impairment.[2] Once a dementia is recognized the cause or type should be determined.

Dementia is a clinical syndrome characterized by a decline from a previous level of intellectual function.[6] It has many different causes. True cognitive impairment or dementia takes place when there is deterioration in at least three of the following: cognition, memory, language, recognition, visual spatial skills, and personality.[2] Some illnesses that cause dementia can be stopped or reversed, but the illnesses most frequently associated with dementia are not reversible.[26]

Four common treatable causes of dementia in the elderly are drugs, hypothyroidism and other metabolic conditions, destructive or mass lesions of the central nervous system, and depression.[25,30] The most common untreatable type is dementia of the Alzheimer's type (DAT), which is present in

65% to 75% of the patients seen in dementia clinics.[26] A diagnosis of DAT is based on four criteria:[3] (1) global cognitive dysfunction that interferes with daily activities, (2) gradual onset, with symptoms lasting for 6 months or longer, (3) progressive deterioration over time, and (4) lack of strong evidence for another illness causing the dementia.

Nurses caring for elderly patients need to recognize the difference between dementia and delirium, both of which occur frequently in the elderly. Delirium is characterized by a sudden change in the level of consciousness and is therefore a cognitive change. It is usually associated with an acute illness. Fever, hypoxemia, and other metabolic dysfunctions associated with acute illness can affect consciousness or mental state, thereby producing delirium.

Frequently, dementia and depression are both present in elderly people at the same time.[38] It is difficult to distinguish between depressed elderly individuals and those with a true dementia, but there are some differences. Depressed patients are dysphoric, with mild or no cognitive impairment. The onset of depression is often abrupt and the patients frequently have a history of affective problems. Patients with dementia are less aware of cognitive problems, have a more gradual onset of symptoms, and have serious deficits in memory, thinking, judgment, and problem solving abilities.[47] Such deficits eventually lead to these patients being totally dependent on others for care.

The care of a patient with an illness causing dementia is complex and requires a multidisciplinary approach that considers the needs of both the family and the patient. Few people with chronic illnesses such as Alzheimer's disease receive in-home nursing care.[4] Therefore home health nurses assist these patients intermittently when acute health problems occur. See the box titled Developing a Plan of Care for the Dementia Patient and Caregiver at Home. (For further information about Alzheimer's disease and depression refer to Chapters 18 and 23.)

Nutrition

Since aging is associated with a decline in body function, nutrition is also affected. People age at different rates and to different extents, but the effects on body functions appear similar. The

---

DEVELOPING A PLAN OF CARE FOR THE DEMENTIA PATIENT AND CAREGIVER AT HOME

1. Provide ongoing education about the disease process.
2. Identify effective techniques that assist patients and caregivers with day-to-day tasks.
3. Assist patients and families with behavioral management strategies that facilitate appropriate behavior.
4. Locate community resources that assist with respite care and long-term care decisions, especially for the patient living alone.
5. Provide ongoing emotional support for patients and caregivers.
6. Identify safety issues, such as environmental modifications.
7. Assume a case management role as the patient advocate.

---

ability to digest food and use nutrients depends on the range of age-related changes in the body. Morley and Silver[33] list five factors that affect the nutritional status of the older adult: social factors, psychological factors, physical factors, anorexia of aging, and disease.

Social factors that affect eating behaviors include poverty, problems with food shopping and preparation, and lack of socialization at mealtime. It sometimes is assumed that the reason older adults eat inadequately is lack of knowledge about nutrition, but often the reason is poverty.[39] Older persons may skip meals, eat pet food, and exist on snack foods because they have limited financial resources. Lack of transportation and physical impairment may also interfere with their ability to buy and prepare food. Since 30% of the elderly population live alone, there is often a decreased interest in preparing nutritious meals. Socialization at meals enhances the intake of a well balanced diet.

Bereavement and depression are psychological factors that may affect nutrition in the elderly person. It is estimated that one third of people over age 60 have a depressed mood.[15] When people are sad, blue, or depressed, they often lose interest in eating and may lose weight without trying. Decreased appetite is a very common symptom of depression.[47]

Physical conditions that affect eating behavior are immobility, inability to feed oneself, and difficulty chewing. It has been found that nutritional intake is related to dentition and self-perceived chewing problems.[18] Persons who believe they have a chewing problem will eat less and therefore have a decreased intake of protein and calories and an increased carbohydrate intake. Some carbohydrates are softer and more tolerable than proteins.

Factors that contribute to anorexia or weight loss with aging are decreased basal metabolic rate, hunger, and feeding drive. Not only do older people have a decreased metabolic rate but also they become physically less active. Deterioration of taste, smell, and visual acuity may cause older adults to lose pleasure in eating. There is a natural decline in gastric secretions with age, and as a result digestion is less efficient. A change in gastric hormones affects the drive to eat.[33] The gastrointestinal tract sends messages to the central nervous system that cause a feeling of fullness when food passes through the intestines.

The most extreme changes in nutritional status in older adults are caused by diseases. For example, with dementia, memory deficits affect the amount of food eaten, and therefore weight loss is common.[11] Patients with dementia are at increased risk for malnutrition because of indifference (they do not care about eating), memory loss (they cannot remember if they have eaten), and impaired judgment (they do not recognize the need to eat). Many elderly patients are dependent on others for providing adequate nutrition, and their needs are not always met.

Meeting the nutritional needs of the elderly is complicated by individual differences in aging and by the roles played by social, psychological, and physical factors in each patient's lifestyle. A thorough assessment of a patient's food intake is necessary to determine caloric and nutritional status. This assessment should include medical, social, nursing, and dietary histories, and a physical examination. Home health nurses must be aware of normal aging changes that may mask themselves as a nutrient deficiency. Patients are at nutritional risk when they have three or more of the warning signs listed in the following box.[37]

WARNING SIGNS OF POOR NUTRITIONAL HEALTH

- Disease
- Eating poorly
- Tooth loss/mouth pain
- Economic hardship
- Reduced social contact
- Multiple medicines
- Involuntary weight loss/gain
- Needs assistance in self-care
- Elder years above age 80

Immobility

Impaired physical mobility is a state in which the individual experiences a limitation of the ability for independent physical movement.[23] Most diseases and rehabilitative states involve some degree of immobility. Approximately 30% of those 85 years of age or older have extreme limitations in the activities of daily living.[28] These limitations are of major significance to the health care system.

Alteration in mobility may be short-lived or chronic. A patient who is hospitalized because of an acute medical problem is at risk for developing a chronic problem as a result of the hazards of immobility. Observable signs and symptoms of immobility are associated with many different acute health conditions. (See Chapter 15.)

The hazards of immobility affect all people with impaired physical mobility, but older adults are at increased risk. Age and disease affect functional reserves, and more energy is needed to maintain functional status as capabilities and resources decline.[5] Many organ systems are affected by decreased mobility.[32] These systems and the effects of immobility are listed in Table 24-1. The hazards of immobility make it important for home health nurses to maximize mobility within the limits of the patient's condition.

Mobility is potentially the most important factor in assessing the independence of the elderly and their needs for health care.[5] Restricted ability to move affects the performance of all other tasks. The ultimate nursing goals are maintenance of mobility and prevention of impairment.

Table 24-1 Hazards of immobility

Organ system	Hazard
Skin	Skin breakdown
Musculoskeletal	Muscle weakness
	Increased immobilization
	Backache
	Joint stiffness
	Disuse osteoporosis
Cardiovascular	Increased workload of heart
	Orthostatic hypotension
	Thrombus formation
	Peripheral edema
Respiratory	Decreased chest expansion
	Stasis of secretions
	Pneumonia
	CO_2 narcosis
	Respiratory acidosis
Renal	Difficult urination
	Urinary stasis
	Renal calculi
Gastrointestinal	Constipation
	Fecal impaction
Psychological	Depression
	Boredom

When selecting interventions for a patient who has limited mobility, the nurse needs to consider three things: the condition that caused the disability, the medical restrictions on activity, and the individual's abilities and limitations.[38] Risk factors also should be taken into consideration when instituting a plan of care. Risk factors associated with immobility in the elderly population include contractures, severe dementia, poor vision, hip or leg fractures, and environmental safety.[41,43]

Polypharmacy in a shoe box

Of all prescription drugs ordered, 25% are for the elderly.[9] Because many elderly people have at least one chronic health condition, they are more likely than other age groups to be taking multiple medications. This makes them highly susceptible to adverse drug reactions caused by multiple drug use, which is the most common reason for such reactions. Adults over the age of 65 are twice as likely as other age groups to have an abnormal response to medication.[24]

The problem of adverse reactions is often compounded by improper management and administration of medications at home. Self-medication errors and subsequent adverse reactions may be related to (1) methods of storage or organization in which both current and out-of-date medications are stockpiled in shoe boxes, bowls, paper bags, or dresser drawers, (2) impaired visual acuity and memory associated with aging, (3) a knowledge deficit regarding the action of medication and need for adherence to medication, and (4) multiple physicians ordering multiple medications.

Numerous age-related physiological changes affect the absorption, distribution, and metabolism of medications. These changes may alter the reaction to medication and influence the type and dosage of medication prescribed by physicians.

A decline in gastric acid secretions and motility affects the rate at which drugs are absorbed. Medications that rely on acid in the stomach for dissolving often do not produce the expected therapeutic response in older adults.

Distribution to tissues is less effective because of changes in cardiac output that affect circulation. An increase in body fat compared with total body mass causes drugs to build up in the adipose tissue. Therefore drugs are active longer as a result of slower distribution throughout the body.[9]

Metabolism, detoxification, and excretion of medications are altered by age-related changes in the kidney and liver. Decreased glomerular filtration rate, tubular reabsorption, and cardiac function lead to a less efficient kidney. Medications are not filtered as rapidly and are present in the body longer. The time it takes for drugs to be excreted is almost doubled with advanced age.[9] Decreases in the size and function of the liver alter the enzyme system. The detoxification of drugs declines, causing medications to remain in the bloodstream longer.

To avoid adverse reactions and yet achieve therapeutic levels, elderly patients usually require lower doses of medication. Since no two individuals are alike, drug response will vary. All home health nurses should keep current on the use and side effects of medications. There are many risks associated with drug therapy in older adults, and the benefit from drug therapy should outweigh any problems a drug may induce.

The initial home health visit should include a thorough nursing assessment of drug usage in the elderly patient. (See the home care application section later in this chapter.) From this assessment the nurse can develop a plan of care that promotes safety and prevents noncompliance in medication use. This plan should include ongoing patient education and assessment of medication administration, tolerance, and effectiveness.

Safety

Risk for injury is a nursing diagnosis that should routinely be considered with an elderly individual requiring home care assistance. This is defined as "interactive conditions between individual and environment which impose a risk to the defensive and adaptive resources of the individual."[23]

Elderly people are more susceptible to accidents, falls, and elder abuse as their capabilities diminish.[41] Internal and external factors work together to influence this susceptibility. Among these are biological factors such as sensory dysfunction, physiological factors such as immobility, and increased demands on caregivers related to growing older. Deficits of sight, hearing, equilibrium, and reaction time[10] (all of which predispose older adults to accidents) may be a result of aging, a result of disease, or a side effect of medication. Specific accidents common among the elderly are related to fire, carbon monoxide poisoning (from a faulty heating system), medication reactions, drowning, and auto use.[10] The elderly have a high rate of hospital admission and death as a result of trauma.[10] Prevention of accidents can be enhanced by a comprehensive assessment of the home situation. Escher, O'Dell, and Gambert[10] describe a mnemonic, "ACCIDENTS," to help home health nurses assess the older adult's risk for an accident in the home (see the following box). This assessment may lead to interventions that range from simple oral or written reminders to suggestions for changing a person's lifestyle. The family and/or caregiver should be included in the plan of care to prevent accidents in the home.

Falls are the leading cause of death from injury in persons older than 65.[44] Although the majority of falls do not cause sufficient injury to require medical attention, serious injury from falls is significant. Approximately 250,000 hip fractures per year occur among persons 65 years of age or

---

ASSESSMENT OF POTENTIAL RISKS FOR ACCIDENTS IN THE HOME

- Activities of daily living (level of function)
- Cognition, emotional state (memory, depression)
- Clinical findings (health history)
- Incontinence
- Drugs (complete inventory)
- Eyes, ears, environment (sensory deficits)
- Neurologic deficits (gait, balance)
- Travel history (driving ability)
- Social history (alcohol, drug)

From Escher JE, O'Dell C, Gambert SR: Typical geriatric accidents and how to prevent them, *Geriatrics* 44:54, 1989. Reprinted with permission.

---

older, with an annual cost of $7 billion.[22] The people who fall most often are those who have multiple medical impairments or functional disabilities. These individuals should be identified in the plan of care as being at risk for falls.[28] The risk of falling is greater among older adults who have decreased abilities and are taking a number of medications. Other factors that may indicate a risk of falling are confusion, corrective lenses, nocturia with urgency, weakened or impaired gait, the use of assistive devices, and a history of falls.[34] The patient who uses furniture or railings for support, has poor balance, or requires assistance when rising from a chair is assessed by the nurse as having impaired gait. By thoroughly and accurately assessing the patient's status on the initial home visit and pursuing the appropriate safety measures, home health nurses can identify characteristics and physiological changes that place a patient at risk of falling and implement measures to prevent falls.[44] The mnemonic ACCIDENTS may assist home health nurses in assessing functional ability and safety in the home.

Elder abuse represents a shocking and still largely hidden phenomenon affecting hundreds of thousands of our nation's most helpless and vulnerable citizens.[13] It crosses all classes of society and occurs in large urban areas and small towns.[36] Estimates suggest that between 500,000 and 2.5 million elderly people in the United States are victims of abuse, neglect, exploitation, or abandonment each year.[31] Because the abused elderly

---
CLINICAL INDICATORS OF NEGLECT

- Poor hygiene
- Decubiti
- Dehydration
- Poor skin integrity
- Impaction
- Contractures
- Malnutrition
- Urine burns/excoriation
---

are reluctant to admit that their children, their loved ones, or those entrusted with their care have mistreated them, only one out of every six cases is ever reported.[31] Home health nurses who are knowledgeable of signs and symptoms of elder abuse can assist in providing a safe, clean environment and protection from those who are not genuinely concerned about the health and best interests of the older adult.

Neglect is a situation in which a caregiver intentionally or unintentionally fails to some degree in providing care for an individual. Signs that could be suggestive of neglect are alterations in nutrition evidenced by weight loss or dehydration, impaired skin integrity evidenced by pressure sores, or alterations in elimination evidenced by a decrease in bowel movements. Neglected patients may appear dirty and ill-clothed, with hair and nails that show no signs of personal grooming. Their environment may display features such as poor ventilation or heating, bug-infested or filthy surroundings, and isolation from the rest of the household. (See the box titled Clinical Indicators of Neglect.) Careful evaluation is needed when neglect is suspected. It is important for the nurse to remember that every caregiving situation is different and to consider the intent of the caregiver. In assessing older adults, it is also important to differentiate the effects of age-related changes or disease from the effects of neglect. Even conscientious caregivers can experience great difficulty with the nutrition, skin care, and elimination needs of the impaired older adult.

Characteristics of those susceptible to abuse include the following: over the age of 65, living with a spouse or another person, poor health, and significant dependence on caregivers for basic needs, love, and social interaction. This dependency may lead to abuse or neglect when caregivers lack the resources to meet the demands made on them.[7] Potential abusers may be members of families that have high levels of stress (e.g., alcoholism, marital problems, financial difficulties)[13] or a pattern of violence within the family,[35] pathologic individuals who inflict harm for unknown reasons, or individuals who are unable to meet the physical and emotional needs of an elderly patient.

The presenting symptoms of abused individuals often fall into two categories: physical and behavioral. Physical abuse may result in unexplained fractures of the skull, nose, or facial structures. Other physical signs of abuse include abrasions, bleeding, bone fractures, bruises, burns, and drug toxicity. Because physical evidence of abuse does not always exist, home health nurses also need to be sensitive to behavioral signs that may indicate abuse. Behavioral signs of abuse include cowering, and guarded, indifferent, or passive behavior.

The health condition and home environment of geriatric patients should be assessed by home health nurses in determining the potential for injury. Accidents, falls, and mistreatment are only a few of the many outcomes that may result from the physical decline that accompanies increasing age.

HOME CARE APPLICATION

When assessing the geriatric patient, attention should be directed toward the following goals of home care:[46]

- Treating the symptoms of disease
- Maintaining functional ability
- Preventing impairment of physical ability
- Providing patient/family instruction regarding care management in the home
- Identifying or anticipating assistance the patient/family may require in performing activities of daily living (ADLs)
- Identifying physical and environmental safety issues
- Providing for the psychosocial and cultural needs of the patient/family
- Locating community resources to meet short-term and long-term needs of the patient and family

During the first visit, home health nurses should develop a plan of care based on the special needs of the elderly patient and family as related to health problems. (See the boxes titled Primary Nursing Diagnoses/Patient Problems and Primary Themes of Patient Education.) Because many different nonfatal, chronic health conditions interfere with the independent functioning of older adults, home health nurses must consider many factors when evaluating the elderly patient in the home. The assessment should be structured to identify patient problems and the appropriate interventions to be initiated. When planning care for these patients, there may be a need for multidisciplinary referrals and various state and community resources.

PRIMARY NURSING DIAGNOSES/ PATIENT PROBLEMS

- Knowledge deficit
- Altered thought processes
- Impaired physical mobility
- Activity intolerance
- Impaired skin integrity
- Altered comfort
- Self-care deficit
- Ineffective respiratory function
- Potential for noncompliance with the therapeutic regimen

PRIMARY THEMES OF PATIENT EDUCATION

- The normal physiology of aging
- Medications: purpose, action, dosage, side effects, and methods of administration
- Safety issues: recognition and treatment
- Dementia: recognition and treatment
- Hazards of immobility and treatment (skin care, exercise programs, proper body positioning, range of motion exercises, pressure reduction/relief devices, bowel and bladder management)
- Diet: food selection, dentition, appetite, weight

When first interviewing the patient and/or family, consider issues and questions that influence the plan of care (for example, the patient's primary concerns, health history, recent life changes, daily activities, cognitive patterns, and support systems).[40]

Primary concerns

Determine the reasons the patient or caregiver sought home health care. Ask why the patient requires skilled nursing care. Investigate the patient's stated problems. The information may be obtained from the patient or the family by asking the following specific questions:

- What changes in health status have taken place?
- When did these changes begin?
- How have they affected lifestyle?
- How can the home health agency be of help?

The patient's and family's perceptions of changes will help focus the assessment.

Health history

Patterns of recurrent injury or illness disclose situations involving physical or psychological abuse, financial limitations, and the effectiveness of past treatment. Questions to ask include the following:

- When and where did the patient last receive health care?
- What was the outcome?
- How often has the patient been hospitalized and for what reasons?
- For what reason was the patient referred to home care services?

Medication use

Patients should be asked to *show* the home health nurse all medications they have in the home, including over-the-counter medications. Asking the patient how, when, and why each drug is taken is very important. This information should be checked against prescription bottles and physician orders. The following questions may assist home health nurses in reviewing patients' medication history, their habits, and their knowledge:

History:

- What medicines are you taking? Please show them to me.
- How long have you been taking each medication?
- How and when do you take your medication?
- Do you ever forget to take your medicines? If you do forget them, what do you do?
- Where do you purchase medications? Is cost a problem?
- How often are your medicines reviewed by your physician?
- Have you ever had an unpleasant reaction to medication?

Storage:

- What medications do you have at home that you are not currently using?
- Where do you keep medications?
- How long do you keep a medication before discarding it?

Problems:

- Do you have any problems taking medications such as tablets, eye drops, or insulin?

A thorough medication history may prevent adverse reactions to medications. If the history reveals problems with reading medication labels or remembering when to take medications, systems such as the following may be helpful:

1. Medication placed into envelopes marked in large black letters that are easily read
2. Pills placed in an egg carton or plastic organizer
3. Prefilled insulin syringes stored in the refrigerator
4. Cross-off-the-pill chart, devised by home health nurses, on which patients "X" out time and dosage box or square after the medication is taken
5. A talking medication dispenser (there are several brands now out on the market)
6. Medication boxes or "punch cards" dispensed by the pharmacist
7. Use of a magnifying glass to read labels
8. Color coding the tops of medication bottles for easy reference
9. Assistance of caregivers to administer and monitor the patient's medication regimen

Patient education in regard to purpose, side effects, route of administration, and *when* to take the medication, should be a routine component of the plan of care. Medications should be reviewed on *every visit* with emphasis upon both compliance and patient response.

It may be necessary for the home health nurse to do a pill count to verify medication compliance for certain elderly adults who may be confusional at times. Home health nurses should always do pill counts in front of the patient in order to avoid possible problems with paranoia.

Recent life changes

The impact of recent changes in a patient's life is frequently overlooked. Elderly people are very likely to experience stressful changes such as the death of a spouse, the loss of close friends, a decrease in financial resources, or separation from family.

Physical problems such as weight loss or malnutrition may be a result of serious life changes. As indicated earlier, a person who is sad, blue, or depressed may lose interest in eating, preparing meals, or socializing. Often a referral to the registered dietitian, mental health nurse, or social worker is helpful to resolve some of these problems.

Daily activities

Factors to assess are the activities of daily living: ambulating, bathing, dressing, toileting, and eating. The level of function in these areas indicates the amount of assistance needed in the home. Referrals are made for assistance according to the needs of each individual patient. The home health aide can assist the patient with personal care such as bathing and grooming. Rehabilitation services can assist the elderly patient to improve mobility and independence by providing a therapeutic exercise regimen that increases strength and endurance along with patient education regarding use of assistive devices for safe ambulation and transfer activities.

Cognitive patterns

Assessment of cognition includes a review of recent stressful life changes and current medication routine. Focus on a patient's reasoning ability, memory, behavior, mood, and activities to determine intellectual function. Changes in cognitive ability should be investigated when they interfere with a patient's functional capacity and safety in the home.

Support systems

The last step in doing a thorough assessment of an elderly patient is an evaluation of available support systems. Answers to the following questions will influence the plan of care:

- What are the patient's living arrangements?
- Are there family members or a significant other who can assist the patient as needed?
- Who cooks and prepares the meals?
- What is the home environment like? (Consider safety issues such as handrails, steps, lighting, rugs, and clutter.)
- Is there evidence of patient abuse or neglect?

Investigating the patient's support system will guide the selection of interventions. Intraagency referrals and external referrals to other health care professionals are made according to the individual needs of the patient.

If patient abuse, neglect, or inadequate living arrangements are believed to exist, home health nurses must share their concerns with their managers and the patient's physician. Issues of neglect should be addressed with the family. A phone call to the local elderly abuse hot line or State Division on Aging is certainly an option.

SUMMARY

As a result of a gradual decline of physiological function, older adults may experience deterioration of several organ systems that affect functional ability. Common health concerns or problems among the elderly include knowledge deficits, impaired mobility, impaired skin integrity, altered comfort, and self-care deficits.

Nursing care of older adults requires special skill and sensitivity. The goal of a successful plan of care for older adults is to maintain their maximum potential. Regardless of the specific disease process or treatment that serves as the basis for the home health referral, decisions for nursing intervention must be based on the unique behavior of the individual. A comprehensive assessment by the home health nurse is the key to developing an effective plan of care. This is facilitated by having knowledge about the physiology of aging, the specific issues relevant to the elderly population, and resources available. This not only will promote symptom management but will enhance the geriatric patient's return to optimal health and an independent lifestyle.

REFERENCES

1. Albert ML: *Clinical neurology of aging,* New York, 1984, Oxford University Press.
2. Beck JC, Benson DR, Scheibel AB et al: Dementia in the elderly: the silent epidemic, *Ann Intern Med* 97:231, 1982.
3. Berman R, Haxby J, Pomerantz R: Physiology of aging, part I, normal changes, *Patient Care* 1:20, 1988.
4. Braun K, Rose C: Geriatric patient outcomes and costs in three settings: nursing home, foster family, and own home, *J Am Geriatr Soc* 35:387, 1987.
5. Brown MD: Functional assessment of the elderly, *J Gerontol Nurs* 14:13, 1988.
6. Consensus Conference: Differential diagnosis of dementing diseases, *JAMA* 258:3411, 1987.
7. Darney AJ: *Life expectancy at birth and age 65, Statistical record of older Americans,* Detroit, 1994, Gale Research, Inc.
8. Davis D: Elderly abuse: a national disease, *Caring* 1:5, 1986.
9. Eliopoulous C: *Gerontol nurs,* ed 3, Philadelphia, 1992, JB Lippincott.
10. Escher JE, O'Dell C, Gambert SR: Typical geriatric accidents and how to prevent them, *Geriatrics* 44:54, 1989.
11. Fairburn CG, Hope RA: Changes in eating in dementia, *Neurobiol Aging* 9:28, 1988.
12. Fowles D: *A profile of older Americans,* Washington, DC, 1993, Program Resources Department, American Association of Retired Persons and Administration on Aging, US Department of Health and Human Services.
13. Fulmer T, Street S: Abuse of the elderly: screening and detection, *J Emerg Nurs* 10:131, 1984.
14. Geokas MC, Conteas CN, Majirmdar APN: The aging gastrointestinal tract, liver and pancreas, *Clin Geriatr Med* 1:177, 1985.
15. Gianturco D, Busse E: Psychiatric problems encountered during a long-term study of normal aging volunteers. In Isaacs A, Post F, editors: *Studies of geriatric psychiatry,* New York, 1978, John Wiley & Sons.
16. Goldstein S: The biology of aging, *N Engl J Med* 285:1120, 1971.
17. Gordon GS, Genant HK: The aging skeleton, *Clin Geriatr Med* 1:95, 1985.
18. Gordon SR et al: Relationship in very elderly veterans of nutritional status, self-perceived chewing ability, dental status and social isolation, *J Am Geriatr Soc* 33:334, 1985.
19. Johnson K: Exploring home health care opportunities as a result of the prospective payment system, *Caring* 4:54, 1985.
20. Katzman R, Terry R: *The neurology of aging,* Philadelphia, 1984, FA Davis.
21. Kaysen GA, Meyers BD: The aging kidney, *Clin Geriatr Med* 1:207, 1985.
22. Kelsey JL, Hoffman S: Risk factors for hip fracture, *N Engl J Med* 316:404, 1987.

23. Kim MJ, McFarland GK, McLane AM: *Pocket guide to nursing diagnoses,* ed 4, St Louis, 1991, Mosby.

24. Lamy PP: Adverse drug effects, *Clin Geriatr Med* 6:293, 1990.

25. Larsen EB, Bernard LO, Williams ME: Evaluation and care of elderly patients with dementia, *J Gen Intern Med* 1:116, 1986.

26. Larsen EB, Reifler BV, Featherstone HJ, English DR: Dementia in elderly outpatients: a prospective study, *Ann Intern Med* 100:417, 1984.

27. Lowenstein S, Schrier R: Social and political aspects of aging. In Schrier R, editor: *Clinical internal medicine in the aged,* Philadelphia, 1982, WB Saunders.

28. Lund C, Sheafor M: Is your patient about to fall? *J Geriatr Nurs* 11:37, 1985.

29. Mahler PA, Rosiella RA, Loke J: The aging lung, *Clin Geriatr Med* 2:215, 1986.

30. Marsden CD, Harrison MJG: Outcome of investigations in patients with presenile dementia, *Br Med J* 2:249, 1972.

31. Matlaw J: Elder abuse: ethical and practical dilemma for social work, *Health Social Work* 6:85, 1986.

32. Miceli DG: Evaluating the older patient's ability to function, *J Am Acad Nurs Pract* 5:167, 1993.

33. Morley JE, Silver AJ: Anorexia in the elderly, *Neurobiol Aging* 9:9, 1988.

34. Morse JM, Tylko SJ, Dixon HA: Characteristics of the fall prone patient, *Gerontologist* 27:516, 1987.

35. Patwell T: Familial abuse of the elderly: a look at caregiver potential and prevention, *Home Health Care Nurs* 4:10, 1985.

36. Pillemer K, Finkelhor D: The prevalence of elder abuse: a random sample survey, *Gerontologist* 28:51, 1988.

37. Posner BM, Jette AM, Smith KW, Miller DR: Nutrition and health risks in the elderly: the nutrition screening initiative, *Am J Public Health* 83:944, 1993.

38. Reifer BV, Larsen EB, Hanley R: Coexistence of cognitive impairment and depression in geriatric outpatients, *Am J Psychiatr* 139:623, 1982.

39. Roe DA: Geriatric nutrition, *Clin Geriatr Med* 6:319, 1990.

40. Santo-Noval DA: Seven keys to assessing the elderly, *Nursing* 8:60, 1988.

41. Selikson S, Damus K, Hamerman D: Risk factors associated with immobility, *J Am Geriatr Soc* 36:707, 1988.

42. Shenefelt PD, Fenske NA: Aging and the skin: recognizing and managing common disorders, *Geriatr* 45:57, 1990.

43. Tinetti ME, Speechley M, Ginter SF: Risk factors for falls among the elderly persons living in the community, *N Engl J Med* 319:1701, 1980.

44. Tinetti ME, Williams F, Mayewoski R: Fall index for elderly patients based on number of chronic disabilities, *Am J Med* 80:429, 1986.

45. Van Ort S, Woodthi A: Home health care providing a missing link, *J Geriatr Nurs* 15:4, 1989.

46. Yurick AG, Spier BE, Robb SS, Ebert NJ: *The aged person and the nursing process,* ed 3, Norwalk, Conn, 1989, Appleton & Lange.

47. Zung WW: Depression in the normal aged, *Psychosomatics* 8:287, 1967.

25 The Hospice Patient

Diane Huntley and *Robyn Rice*

Hospice is both a service and a philosophy. It is also a term that is unfamiliar to some, misunderstood by others, and mispronounced by many. (The word is correctly pronounced 'hahs-pis.')[2,8,16,19] The origin of the word *hospice* dates back to the Middle Ages when the expression was used to describe a shelter or haven for the weary traveler.[3,6] From that beginning, the term has come to be associated with support and care. In hospice, dying is looked upon as a normal part of living. Consequently, hospice programs assist patients and families to prepare for death in a positive manner. Shelter from discomfort is provided to enable dying patients to approach death in a peaceful way while living the remainder of their lives to the fullest. Therefore hospice is not a place but is instead a philosophy of comfort and caring. Hospice embraces the philosophy that quality of life is much more important than quantity and emphasizes caring rather than curing.[18]

The modern hospice concept began in 1967 with the founding of St. Christopher's Hospice in southern London by Dame Cicly Saunders, a nurse, physician, and social worker.[2,3,6] She believed that cancer pain could be better controlled by administering regular doses of pain medicine rather than giving the medicine on an as-needed basis. She also stressed the importance of listening to patients, really hearing and paying attention to what they have to say. Sometimes, just the listening itself produces a dramatic decrease in patients' pain.[19]

Contemporary hospice care began in the United States and Canada with groups in Connecticut, New York, and Montreal. Today approximately 2,000 programs exist in the United States.[2] Ideally, each program includes an inpatient unit and a home care service. Home is where most patients want to be, and their wish is usually supported by the family.[3,16,17] The home is viewed as a familiar, comfortable, and realistic place for patient care. Inpatient services are used when problems arise that cannot be handled at home.[3,6,17]

Hospice programs are frequently a division of home health services. This is particularly true for Medicare-certified hospice programs affiliated with Medicare-certified home health agencies. Ideally a specially trained hospice nurse provides and coordinates care for terminally ill patients. However, changes in staffing and flexibility of services often bring home health nurses into contact with hospice patients. The purpose of this chapter is to review the hospice philosophy and to provide guidelines for the care of terminally ill patients. This information will help all home health staff gain insights into caring for these patients and their families.

MEDICARE GUIDELINES

Hospice care is reimbursed under Medicare Part A. Coverage can be 100% for persons with Medicare or Medicaid; private insurance plans have varying degrees of coverage. For terminally ill patients, hospice benefits have advantages not available with standard Medicare coverage (Table 25-1).[17]

Patients must meet certain criteria to qualify for hospice benefits. They must have a life expectancy of 6 months or less according to the physician's best estimate, they must not be undergoing or contemplating any active treatment for their disease, and they should have decided to forgo resuscitative measures (e.g., CPR) at the time of their death. In other words, there are no blood transfusions, no radiation, no chemotherapy or experimental drug

Table 25-1 Comparison of standard Medicare and hospice benefits

Standard Medicare benefits	Medicare hospice benefits
Patient must be homebound to qualify for home care	Homebound status not required
Prescription drugs not covered	Drugs related to terminal illness fully covered, small co-payment required
No custodial home care allowed	Custodial home care may be provided by home-makers and home health aides
Medical equipment and supplies: pays 80% of allowed charge after deductible	Medical equipment and supplies fully covered if related to terminal illness
No respite care allowed	Inpatient respite care allowed for limited days during each benefit period
No more than 8 hours of home care a day allowed	Continuous care available, up to 24 hours a day if needed
Inpatient hospital care is subject to a deductible and co-payment after 60 days per benefit period	Short-term inpatient care, fully covered, no deductible or co-payment ever required

From Nassif JZ: *The home health care solution,* New York, 1985, Perennial Library, p. 284. Reprinted with permission.

administration (as a cure), usually no intravenous fluid administration, and no CPR or respirators for these patients. Gray areas include feeding tubes, surgery, and parenteral measures for pain control. The use of these measures is evaluated by individual hospice programs. Comfort measures such as the administration of oxygen and antibiotics are a part of the hospice philosophy.

ADMISSION TO A HOSPICE PROGRAM

Admission into a hospice program follows certain guidelines. After a physician has stated on a medical assessment form the opinion that the illness is terminal, an evaluation of the patient's physical and psychological problems must be documented by a nurse or social worker. If the patient meets agency admissions criteria, the patient is notified and necessary consent forms are signed.

An important criterion for admission to a hospice program is that the patient and family should be able to discuss the patient's diagnosis and prognosis openly.[8] Otherwise intervention by the hospice team will be less effective. Open discussion of death and dying does not mean that all hope has been removed; rather, it reduces the stress that is involved when caregivers and patients have to watch what they say to one another. At the time of assessment and after admission to the hospice program, home health nurses should answer patients' questions honestly. However, it is not necessary to force a discussion of topics about which no one is ready to speak. In time, patients will usually tell the nurse what they want to know and are ready to hear. Many patients would like to plan their own funeral services but find this a scary topic of discussion. Sometimes anxiety can be relieved if patients update their wills or make amends with an estranged friend or relative. Facilitating these kinds of discussions can assist both patient and family to realize that death is actually going to occur.[2,3] Consequently, admission into a hospice program can help terminally ill patients and their families say their last good-byes.

PATIENT PROFILES

Approximately 90% of hospice patients are suffering from cancer, the most common types being lung and breast cancers.[3] Other patients may have terminal heart and lung conditions such as severe valvular disease or end-stage chronic obstructive pulmonary disease (COPD), neurologic conditions such as amyotrophic lateral sclerosis, or acquired immunodeficiency syndrome (AIDS). In adult hospice programs, many patients are in their 70s, although ages will range from late teens to 100 years of age or older.[12] There are hospices for children, but these specialized programs are not covered in this chapter.

THE HOSPICE TEAM: A MULTIDISCIPLINARY APPROACH

Each member of the hospice team has a special role. However, roles will sometimes intermingle.

Home health nurses' duties include checking vital signs and medications, assessing skin and appetite, evaluating elimination and pain control, providing emotional support, checking and determining general strength, and assessing sleep pattern and mental status. More specifically, home health nurses may change a catheter, dress a wound, irrigate a central venous catheter, or give an enema. Home health aides are responsible for personal care such as nail, mouth, skin, and hair care, linen changes, and bathing. Physical therapists evaluate strength and provide an exercise program and assistance with ambulation as indicated. Occupational therapists assist with activities of daily living and the use of energy saving techniques. The registered dietitian assesses the patient's appetite and gives suggestions regarding dietary supplementation. Chaplains are available for counseling and prayer regardless of the religious preference or lack of faith involved.[18] Social workers assist with financial concerns and family problems. A speech/language pathologist may be needed to improve communication or to aid with swallowing difficulties.[3,6]

Throughout the patient's time at home a very important part of the hospice team—the volunteer—can make a caregiver's life less stressful.[8,18] Each volunteer, working without compensation, tries to do what will help the family the most. This may include shopping for the family (or staying with the patient while the family shops), feeding the patient, or doing laundry. It is up to those involved to decide what is most helpful. If possible, it is best to introduce the volunteer early, before the family has a real need. In the beginning the volunteer can do small chores; then if the time comes when the family has a crisis, they will be less likely to feel shy about asking their volunteer for help.

Burnout among hospice team members happens but does not have to become an insurmountable problem.[2,8] Difficult circumstances or highly emotional family situations can be stressful for team members. The work can be very intense. Every case is seen to its logical conclusion—and beyond. It is not unusual for a hospice team member to remain in contact with caregivers for many years. There is much interpersonal giving. Regular support sessions or staff conferences help to alleviate work-related stress. Talking with other members of the hospice team and getting feedback (and perhaps

a hug) can do a lot to raise lagging spirits. It cannot be overemphasized that team members, like the caregivers, must first take care of themselves.[8]

HOME CARE APPLICATION
Hospice goals of care and fundamentals of patient education

Goals to strive for under the hospice philosophy include general and palliative measures. The focus of care is pain control, a peaceful death, assistance for the caregiver, and an understanding of the meaning of life.[3,12] (These goals are incorporated into the plan of care. See the box below and on p. 438.) Providing care and comfort includes simple acts such as smoothing sheets, rubbing backs, and drying bottoms. Wrinkled sheets, aching backs, and wet bedclothes become major worries when a person is ill, and counseling will not be effective until these problems are handled. Competent counseling helps both patients and families see death as inevitable and as a positive event. Looking at life and death in this manner strips away feelings of isolation and makes it easier to view death as a natural part of life. Discussing the patient's terminal condition openly and honestly is the best way to help patients and families cope. It is not a question of taking hope away but instead one of redirecting the patient's goals toward immediate needs such as pain control.[4] This search for meaning in life can provide insightful answers and an acceptance of what has happened.[19]

Symptom control: Physical problems

Symptom control is of primary importance for hospice patients. Symptoms can be few and easily

PRIMARY NURSING DIAGNOSES/ PATIENT PROBLEMS

- Alteration in comfort: pain
- Alteration in nutrition, less than required
- Knowledge deficit re: disease process, dying process, diet, medications, hospice services
- Self-care deficit
- Grieving (anticipatory/patient and family)
- Alteration in elimination: bowel and/or bladder
- Alteration in coping: individual, family
- Alteration in skin integrity

PRIMARY THEMES OF PATIENT EDUCATION

- Signs and symptoms of dying; when to call the case manager and physician
- Comfort measures: mouth care, skin care, positioning
- Medications: purpose, action, dosage, side effects, route
- Equipment use
- Symptom management: nausea, vomiting, bowels, pain
- Emotional support for caregivers
- Hospice team services
- Concept of palliative care
- Bereavement services

GUIDE FOR PAIN ASSESSMENT

1. Location (anatomical site)
2. Description (aching, sharp, knifelike)
3. Intensity (mild, moderate, severe)
4. Duration (constant, intermittent)
5. Response to pain (crying, immobility, withdrawal)
6. Current relief measures (What helps? What makes pain worse?)

handled, or may be many, varied, and complex. Home situations range from calm and well organized to hectic and chaotic. When home health nurses arrive at the home for the first time, they assess the immediate needs and priorities of the patient and family. This may involve setting up a medication schedule or giving instruction on positioning and transfers. Nurses should try to do what is most helpful for patients and their caregivers. The nurse must include the patient and family in establishing the plan of care. Trying to impose the nurse's priorities on the family can lead to frustration for everyone.[4]

Symptom control is important not only for patient comfort but also for caregiver peace of mind. Some of the most common physical symptoms are pain, loss of appetite, weakness, constipation, urinary incontinence, dyspnea, skin problems, insomnia, difficulty swallowing, cough and mucus production, edema, nausea, and confusion.[6,11]

Pain. When the word *cancer* is mentioned, people often think immediately of excruciating pain. If patients do not have pain at hospice admission, many families assume that it is just a matter of time before the pain will start. Patients and families should be reassured that up to one half of all cancer patients do not experience pain.[6,15,17]

When pain is a problem, many think only of the physical component. However, pain actually has many facets and is not necessarily related to the terminal diagnosis. For example, a terminal cancer patient may still have pain from arthritis, or a terminal heart patient may suffer from the discomfort of constipation. The pain experience can be difficult to describe and define. If patients are confused or lethargic, the source of the pain and the fact that pain is occurring can be missed. The interaction between the physical and psychological components of pain will determine what patients experience and how they express their experience.

Acute physical pain can make patients anxious and restless, whereas chronic pain is exhausting and depressing. Only patients can describe the character, onset, duration, amount, and location of their pain. (See the box titled Guide for Pain Assessment.) Some patients will say "my arm hurts." Others will describe their pain in much more detail. A full description may be helpful but is not always necessary for effective treatment.

Psychological pain includes the affective, cognitive, and behavioral components. Affective states such as depression, anger, or fear will profoundly influence patients' perceptions of pain and may also impinge upon successful treatment. Cognitively, patients' awareness of pain may be influenced by what they know about pain and what meaning this knowledge has for them. In regard to the behavioral aspect, patients will express pain differently—from restlessness to moaning, or from a simple "ouch" to loud screams. Some patients deny pain even when it is there. Perhaps they have never taken much medication and refuse to start now; others feel it is important to suffer to some degree before dying. As a result, pain control can be a complicated process and oversimplification can interfere with effective pain management.[15]

There are many effective interventions for pain control. Regular doses of narcotics in conjunction with medications such as antidepressants may be used. Morphine can be given by tablet, liquid, or suppository—administration methods that are appropriate in the home. The usual dose of pain medication may not be sufficient to control the pain of terminally ill patients. Consistent assessment is necessary to determine whether the present dose is effective. Variables such as age and tumor site should be considered when implementing pain control.[21] Fortunately, most physicians and patients no longer worry about the patient becoming addicted. It is one thing to take a drug for its "high," another to take the drug for the control of pain. Sometimes families need to be reassured about this. Flexibility and thorough assessment are the keys to effective pain control.

Generally, less invasive analgesic approaches are preferable to invasive palliative approaches.[21] Oral administration is preferred because it is convenient and usually cost-effective.[1,21] If patients cannot take oral preparations, transdermal or rectal routes should be offered.

Many caregivers prefer not to administer suppositories, and this route is contraindicated for patients who have diarrhea, anal/rectal lesions, or mucositis. Suppositories must be used every 2 to 6 hours to maintain pain control; this schedule may be exhausting for caregivers.[21] The transdermal route is convenient but more costly. This route is not suitable for rapid dose titration, but is very effective for stable pain. The transdermal route also allows caregivers to be relieved of a potentially demanding medication schedule because the patch is changed every 2 to 3 days. Long-acting medications, administered every 8 to 12 hours, can also be very effective. Long-acting medications prevent the problem of the patient waking in the middle of the night in severe pain. The continuous pain control can help both the patient and caregiver to sleep at night.[6] Parenteral routes are generally the last route chosen. The intramuscular route is avoided because of unreliable absorption, pain, and inconvenience to both patients and caregivers.[21] Continuous infusions of narcotics can provide excellent pain relief. However, caregivers must be able to manage the equipment, and home health nurses need to be available 24 hours a day for teaching, support, and problems. Both intravenous and subcutaneous routes are acceptable. Often a combination of routes is used to treat pain.

Radiation therapy may be used for control of cancer pain, primarily for bone metastasis. Localized radiation therapy can provide enough pain relief to substantially (although often temporarily) improve the patient's quality of life.[2,21]

In conjunction with medication, instruction on positioning and use of relaxation or distraction techniques will assist with pain control. Pain medication should be given in a consistent amount on a regular schedule, not when a patient asks for it. After an adjustment in pain medication, sometimes the patient may seem overly sedated. Before reducing the dose it is important to assess whether the patient is sleeping because of previous sleep deprivation related to unrelieved pain or because of the new dosage. If the sedation does not decrease in 48 to 72 hours, the narcotic dose can be lowered. Adding a nonsteroidal antiinflammatory drug will boost analgesia without sedation. Central nervous system stimulants such as caffeine or dextroamphetamine can decrease sedation if reducing the dose and increasing the frequency do not work.[21] If pain control is still not sufficient, a new narcotic may need to be tried.[15] Tables 25-2 and 25-3 list drugs commonly used for pain relief and those not recommended for treatment of cancer pain.

Anorexia. Anorexia is very prevalent among terminally ill patients. Delayed digestion, a constant feeling similar to seasickness, and decreased or increased olfactory and gustatory sensations all contribute to this symptom. A new narcotic regimen can influence appetite, as can hypercalcemia, copious sputum, uncontrolled pain, or medication taken for problems other than pain. Nausea and vomiting can have a multitude of causes.[8] Antiemetics may be given as needed but are probably more effective for nausea or vomiting if administered on a regular schedule. Delayed digestion can be helped by small, frequent meals that are easy to digest. Good oral hygiene can help with intake.[11]

Accommodating patients' food desires can be important. Even if a meal of hot, spicy food seems out of line, if patients ask for it, it may be just right for them that day.[16] Many cancer patients cannot tolerate meat, and some cannot bear the taste of anything sweet. Frequently, nutritious meals must be abandoned. Liquid supplements can add vitamins and calories and are easy to consume. Giving patients very small mouthfuls of food and pureeing the food will make eating easier and reduce the

Table 25-2 Analgesic dosage and comparative efficacy to standards

Drug	Proprietary names (not all-inclusive)	Average analgesic dose (mg)	Dose interval (hours)	Maximal daily dose (mg)	Pediatric dose (mg/kg)	Analgesic efficacy compared to standards	Plasma half-life (hours)	Comments
Acetaminophen	Numerous	500-1000 PO	4-6	4000	10-15 PO q4-6h	Comparable to aspirin 650 mg	2-3	Rectal suppository available for children and adults
Salicylates								
Aspirin	Numerous	500-1000 PO	4-6	4000	10-15 PO q4-6h	—	0.25	Because of risk of Reye's syndrome, do not use in children under 12 with possible viral illness; rectal suppository available for children and adults
Diflunisal	Dolobid	1000 PO initial, 500 PO subsequent	8-12	1500	—	500 mg superior to aspirin 650 mg, with slower onset and longer duration; an initial dose of 1000 mg significantly shortens time to onset	8-12	
Choline magnesium trisalicylate	Trilisate	1000-1500 PO	12	2000-3000	25 PO bid	Longer duration of action than aspirin 650 mg	9-17	
Propionic acids								
Ibuprofen	Motrin, Rufen, Nuprin, Advil, Medipren	200-400 PO	4-6	2400	10 PO q6-8h	Superior at 200 mg to aspirin 650 mg	2-2.5	
Naproxen	Naprosyn	500 PO initial, 250 PO subsequent	6-8	1250	5 PO bid	—	12-15	

440

Naproxen sodium	Anaprox	550 PO initial, 275 PO subsequent	6-8	1375	5 PO bid	275 mg comparable to aspirin 650 mg, with slower onset and longer duration; 550 mg superior to aspirin 650 mg	—	
Fenoprofen	Nalfon	200 PO	4-6	800	—	Comparable to aspirin 650 mg	2-3	
Ketoprofen	Orudis	25-50 PO	6-8	300	—	Superior at 25 mg to aspirin 650 mg	1.5	
Indoleacetic acids								
Indomethacin	Indocin	25 PO	8-12	100	—	Comparable to aspirin 650 mg	2	Not routinely used because of high incidence of side effects; rectal, IV forms available for adults
Pyrrolacetic acids								
Ketorolac	Toradol	30 or 60 mg IM initial, 15 or 30 mg IM subsequent	6	150 first day, 120 thereafter	—	In the range of 6-12 mg of morphine	6	IV route is investigational only
Anthranilic acids								
Mefenamic acid	Ponstel	500 PO initial, 250 PO subsequent	6	1500	—	Comparable to aspirin 650 mg	2	In U.S., use is restricted to intervals of 1 week

From American Pain Society: *Principles of analgesic use in the treatment of acute pain and cancer pain*, Skokie, Ill, 1992, American Pain Society.

Table 25-3 Drugs and routes of administration not recommended for treatment of cancer pain

Class	Drug	Rationale for not recommending
Opioids	Meperidine	Short (2-3 hour) duration. Repeated administration may lead to CNS toxicity (tremor, confusion, or seizures) (Cleeland, 1985; Kaiko, Foley, Grabinski, et al., 1983; Szeto, Inturrisi, Houde, et al., 1977). High oral doses required to relieve severe pain, and these increase the risk of CNS toxicity (American Pain Society, 1992; Weissman, Burchman, Dinndorf, et al., 1992).
Miscellaneous	Cannabinoids	Side effects of dysphoria, drowsiness, hypotension, and bradycardia preclude its routine use as an analgesic (American Pain Society, 1992).
	Cocaine	Has demonstrated no efficacy as an analgesic or coanalgesic in combination with opioids (American Pain Society, 1992).
Opioid agonist-antagonists	Pentazocine Butorphanol Nalbuphine	Risk of precipitating withdrawal in opioid-dependent patients. Analgesic ceiling (Kallos and Caruso, 1979; Nagashima, Karamanian, Malovany, et al., 1976). Possible production of unpleasant psychomimetic effects (e.g., dysphoria, hallucinations) (American Pain Society, 1992; Martin, 1984; Weissman, Burchman, Dinndorf, et al., 1992).
Partial agonist	Buprenorphine	Analgesic ceiling. Can precipitate withdrawal (American Pain Society, 1992; Weissman, Burchman, Dinndorf, et al., 1992).
Antagonist	Naloxone Naltrexone	May precipitate withdrawal. Limit use to treatment of life-threatening respiratory depression (Ellison, 1993).
Combination preparations	Brompton's cocktail	No evidence of analgesic benefit to using Brompton's cocktail over single opioid analgesics (Twycross, 1977; Walsh, 1984; Weissman, Burchman, Dinndorf, et al., 1992; Wisconsin Cancer Pain Initiative, 1988).
	DPT (meperidine, promethazine, and chlorpromazine)	Efficacy is poor compared with that of other analgesics. High incidence of adverse effects (Nahata, Clotz, and Krogg, 1985).
Anxiolytics alone	Benzodiazepine (e.g., alprazolam)	Analgesic properties not demonstrated except for some instances of neuropathic pain. Added sedation from anxiolytics may limit opioid dosing (American Pain Society, 1992; Weissman, Burchman, Dinndorf, et al., 1992).
Sedative/hypnotic drugs alone	Barbiturates Benzodiazepine	Analgesic properties not demonstrated. Added sedation from sedative/hypnotic drugs limits opioid dosing (American Pain Society, 1992).

Routes of administration	Rationale for not recommending
Intramuscular (IM)	Painful. Absorption unreliable (American Pain Society, 1992). Should not be used for children or patients prone to develop dependent edema or in patients with thrombocytopenia (Weissman, Burchman, Dinndorf, et al., 1992).
Transnasal	The only drug approved by the FDA for transnasal administration at this time is butorphanol, an agonist-antagonist drug, which generally is not recommended. (See opioid agonist-antagonists above.)

From US Department of Health and Human Services, Public Health Service, Agency for Health Care Policy and Research: *Management of cancer pain, clinical practice guidelines,* No 9, Pub No 94-0592, March 1994, Rockville, Md.

energy required for chewing. Small plates of food are also more appetizing and less overwhelming. Encouraging fluid intake by offering frequent sips of liquids will do much to maintain comfort.[10,15] Medication such as steroids, megestrol acetate, and metoclopramide can enhance appetite and intake.[21] For the most part, caregivers should approach meals in a matter-of-fact way, serving food and removing the leftovers without comment. Too much urging to eat on the part of caregivers can soon make mealtime a battleground where no one wins.[10,11] Patients may then find food a convenient way to control their lives and the lives of their caregivers.

Weakness. Decreased food and fluid intake, decreased activity, fever, and shortness of breath all contribute to a lack of energy and drive. As a result, strength and vitality decline. Sometimes a mild exercise program can be physically and psychologically beneficial. Energy conservation techniques can help patients perform activities more efficiently. A referral to rehabilitation services may prove helpful. Providing instruction on cane, walker, or wheelchair use may improve mobility and patient outlook. Being able to move from bedroom to kitchen or even outdoors can lift spirits immeasurably. Adding rails to the bathtub or toilet or raising the height of the toilet in small increments to facilitate use can contribute to feelings of well-being and accomplishment.

Many patients say they have no drive to do anything and no ability to concentrate on a task. Instead, they spend hours each day thinking about the past and future. Some lament the fact that now that they have time to read or do needlework, they no longer have any desire to do these things. One patient remarked, "I never got to see the redwoods. How I wish I could see them." He was strong enough to take the trip and his family urged him, "We'll take you." But he said, "No, it's really not that important." What he may have meant was that the thought of the trip was too overwhelming, and it was easier to sit in his chair and imagine.[11]

Constipation. A problem frequently encountered in the terminally ill patient is constipation. An assessment of bowel function should be done on the initial visit and a bowel program established. Sometimes the problem is not actually constipation but is instead related to a poor intake

and/or narcotic use. In this circumstance, a large daily bowel movement is an unrealistic expectation. It is important to know the patient's past bowel habits. Many older people believe that a daily bowel movement is essential for good health and may have used laxatives for many years to produce this result. In contrast, other patients may have had a bowel movement only every 3 or 4 days. Even with decreased food and fluids, decreased activity, and the addition of pain medication to the patient's regimen, the goal still should be to have a bowel movement at least every 3 days.[13] If this does not occur, the patient should be checked for a fecal impaction. If present, enemas should be used to remove or soften the impaction. If enemas are unsuccessful, the impaction should be removed manually.

The proper and consistent use of stool softeners, laxatives, suppositories, and/or enemas should then be instituted to try to prevent recurring impactions and to promote more regular bowel movements.[13,15,21] A suppository followed if necessary by an enema will usually produce the desired results.[5] One teaspoon of lactulose three times a day will help prevent a high impaction. Patients may have difficulty increasing fiber and fluids in their diet. Liquid supplements that include fiber in their ingredients may prove helpful. In some patients the problem is diarrhea, not constipation. This can often be controlled with medication and a change in diet.[11,16]

Edema. Another common problem is edema, usually occurring in the lower extremities. Edema can be due to a simple cause such as immobility or to more complex causes such as blockage by a tumor, cardiovascular conditions, or liver disease. Treatment may involve the administration of diuretics or digitalis preparations, elevation of the affected part above the level of the heart, the application of elastic hose, or the removal of restricting garments.

Urinary problems. Both urinary incontinence and retention can be controlled with the insertion of a Foley catheter.[3,11,16] However, the families of many patients with incontinence prefer to forgo the indwelling catheter and use pads, diapers, or an external catheter. (See Chapter 15.)

Dyspnea. Dyspnea can result from a patient's weakened condition or may be due to actual lung pathology. Home oxygen therapy administered by nasal cannula can provide relief and comfort. Many lung cancer and terminal COPD patients continue to smoke and must be warned about combining oxygen and cigarettes. Occasionally there is a singed nose or mustache when patients "forget" that they must turn off the oxygen before smoking, but usually patients and families are overly cautious. Patients who continue to smoke may say that smoking is the only pleasure left in their lives. (See Chapter 10.)

Skin problems. Dry and/or itchy skin can be another persistent problem. This may be due to poor diet, decreased fluids, medications, the disease process itself, or just the patient's natural propensity for dry and flaky skin. Increasing fluids, using oils in the bathwater, reducing the number of baths, and applying moisturizing lotions are helpful interventions. Fingernails should be kept short and without rough edges. Patients say that itching is more uncomfortable than pain, and an amazing amount of damage can be done when a patient begins scratching. Oral medications can be beneficial in the control of itching.[15]

The more immobile, lethargic, incontinent, and anorexic the patient, the higher the risk for pressure ulcers. Regular repositioning of a bedfast patient is essential to prevent skin breakdown.[11] Sometimes terminally ill patients have particular positions they prefer, and families are reluctant to move the person out of that position. Caregivers need to know that even a few minutes off a preferred side or back can reduce the likelihood of developing pressure areas. (See Chapter 13.)

Insomnia. Insomnia is a problem that often requires attention in the terminally ill patient. The causes are many and varied. For example, some patients begin sleeping more and more during the day and thus have difficulty sleeping at night. These patients are more relaxed during daytime hours and find that sleep comes easily. They are reassured by the daylight and by their awareness that people are moving around and checking on them. In contrast, the nighttime is quiet. Patients may fear that if they call for help they will not be heard, or they may fear the darkness, perhaps even associating it with death. Consequently, sleep patterns may become reversed and be exhausting for the family. Caregivers find themselves being up both day and night. Solutions include using sleeping medications to try to restore the normal sleep pattern and counseling patients in an effort to relieve some of their fears of dying. In addition, daytime naps by caregivers when patients are sleeping may help reduce fatigue.

Sometimes patients have a problem simply with going to bed too early. It is not unusual for patients to complain of waking up at 2:00 AM and then admit that they go to bed at 6:00 PM. They often go to bed early out of boredom or just as a way to make the time pass. Patients should be encouraged to try to alter their sleep time or they must learn to lie quietly at 2:00 AM so that the rest of the family can sleep.

Dry mouth and dysphagia. Dry mouth and difficulty swallowing are very prevalent problems. The latter condition is frightening for both patients and caregivers. Causes include decreased fluid intake, incoordination of the swallowing mechanism, medications, and the disease process itself. Saliva substitutes can help ease dry mouth and improve the health of mouth tissue. If patients are able to increase fluids, this is the most helpful course. Sometimes hard candies and chewing gum can be of temporary benefit. Perhaps a medication that is drying to the mouth can be discontinued. Small sips from medicine cups can be used to allow easier swallowing. Straws are not always helpful because patients may have trouble drawing up the liquid and have difficulty stopping the flow once it is started. Offering fluids by eyedropper or syringe can make it possible for patients who have difficulty swallowing to take in at least small amounts. These devices can make it easier to control the amount of fluid being administered. Popsicles, ice chips, sherbet, soft foods, or thick liquids may be tolerated better than plain water or other thin liquids. Nevertheless, it is imperative that patients be aware that fluids are being administered. To prevent choking, caregivers must watch patients swallow before giving the next sip. The lips may also be dry and parched when the mouth is dry. Frequent application of petroleum jelly to the lips provides some comfort.[10,11]

Coughing. Another problem frequently encountered is coughing. Sometimes the cough sounds productive, but the patient is too weak to bring up the sputum. The administration of expectorants, bronchodilators, and perhaps percussion or postural drainage can assist in the expectoration of the mucus. Only occasionally are cough suppressants prescribed, primarily to suppress a dry cough that is exhausting or keeping the patient awake at night.[22] If sputum shows infection, patients may be treated with antibiotics, especially if the infection is interfering with their comfort. Caregivers are encouraged to keep track of sputum's color, consistency, and amount and to report these characteristics to the home health nurse. Some patients produce abnormal amounts of mucus not related to a cough or sputum. These patients will be constantly expectorating saliva because they feel their mouths being flooded with this fluid. Keeping an emesis basin or two at hand and emptying the basin frequently will promote comfort.[11]

Confusion. Confusion is one of the hardest symptoms for families to handle. Family members may find themselves in a constant state of stress because of the patient's unpredictable behavior. Reorienting patients is sometimes impossible. Even when approached gently and matter-of-factly, confused patients may become very angry when told they are in one place while they insist they are in another. Patients can also exhibit extraordinary strength. It is not unusual for patients considered bedridden to suddenly get up and walk. For example, one patient (a very large man) had been able to be transferred only by a Hoyer lift. One night he got out of bed without anyone's knowledge, walked to his favorite recliner, sat down, and slept. He was not able to get up from that recliner except by the Hoyer lift and, in fact, never walked again.

In some circumstances, behaviors can be controlled with tranquilizers. Sometimes, however, caregivers feel so much stress from the unpredictability of patients' conduct that they become exhausted and are fearful of sleeping at night lest patients harm themselves. In these cases the family may feel better with extra help during the nighttime hours, either from hospice staff, a volunteer, or by rotating family members. Sometimes the patient may have to be placed in a nursing home for respite or an extended stay.[3]

Symptom control: Psychological problems

Having touched first on the most frequently seen physical problems does not mean the psychological problems are less important. Both patients and families may exhibit Kubler-Ross's stages of death and dying, which include denial, anger, bargaining, depression, and acceptance.[7,12,15,20]

Denial. Some patients will deny to the end that their disease is really terminal, and families may have to help them with their denial. Poor relationships among family members are usually not improved or resolved when someone is terminally ill. In fact, it is more likely that relationships will deteriorate even further as family members try to fix the blame for an intolerable situation. On occasion, rifts are healed as family members try to make amends for past disputes, but often longstanding feuds continue and counseling will be needed before and after the patient dies.[20] Hospice care can help the family work together, getting family members to talk and opening up lines of communication between parents and children. Emotional support from the team helps the family to cope.[6] A cooperative effort seems to decrease turmoil. Families find that having an outside person such as the home health nurse who can be called on for advice and counsel makes them feel more confident in their care and more able to share in caregiving chores.

It is also important to explore patients' needs for spiritual guidance. Home health nurses should encourage visits by the patient's own minister or by the chaplain who is part of the hospice team. Whatever the patient's faith, the nurse must support that faith if it seems helpful and meaningful to the patient.[18] Volunteers can be enlisted to read spiritual writings aloud if the patient so desires. Team members need not worry about saying the "wrong thing" about religion but instead should show care and concern and the ability to listen.[14] Organizing patients' care can provide caregivers with common goals. Hospice personnel can promote stability and give direction or guidance by acting as moderators or supervisors. The disorganization so often seen during the first few visits decreases as family members begin to make lists and diaries and take turns with different chores. If one caregiver is repelled by mucus and another by stool, they may soon learn to laugh at this, and one may take over the area repulsive to the other. Often by the time patients are close to dying, family members who at first were arguing over whether the patient needed one blanket or three are able to gather around the bedside hugging and holding one another.

Providing the encouragement that families may need involves the whole hospice team. Whether the family requests minimal or maximal assistance in the home depends on the family's support systems and personal life experiences. For example, a man in his 80s who has not had much experience with tasks such as changing diapers and cleaning up emesis may feel overwhelmed by these chores. Women without the experience of raising children may feel the same way. Some caregivers feel very insecure but ask for direction and then do what needs to be done. Others take one look at the situation and call for the home health nurse or aide to remedy it. Frequently, all a family needs is for someone to simply listen.[6]

One of the barriers to good communication between patients and caregivers is the mutual use of certain defenses and reactions.[7] Denial of the disease and especially its terminality is common among both patients and their loved ones. Often it is patients who are more realistic about the future, probably because they are the only ones who actually know the extent of their own pain, weakness, or anorexia. There is nothing wrong with hope, but unrealistic hope can be destructive and stand in the way of patient comfort.

Anger. Anger by either the patient or caregivers can also prevent honesty and forthrightness among those involved in the care. Sometimes patients are the angry ones, distressed because they are sick instead of someone else. Caregivers may feel the same way. Family members or patients may be angry with the physicians, hospital, or others in the health care field about procedures done or not done. One source of irritation may be the person's decision about treatment. Terminally ill persons may have decided from the start that they do not want chemotherapy or radiation. Patients who have seen someone with a severe adverse reaction to such therapies may feel that they do not want to take that chance themselves. Caregivers may not agree with the decision and may bring the subject up now and then, in subtle and hurtful ways. Other sources of irritation and anger may be expressed among caregivers who do not get along, or when caregivers want patients to do tasks that the patients do not want to do. For example, caregivers may show their displeasure when patients do not eat, leading patients to exercise control by not eating. Situations can become quite tense and may require counseling.

Families can be just as angry when a patient does not die as when he does. In some cases, caregivers will take the physician's prognosis very literally, almost counting down the days. If the time passes and the patient does not die, both the patient and family may become confused. "What is going on?" they demand. In other words, they may be asking if the physician was wrong, if maybe the patient is actually getting better. This is the time to reemphasize taking each day as it comes, that life is uncertain and that, at best, predictions are guesses. Usually as emotional responses subside and more rational thinking takes over, patients and their families are able to proceed with more stability and in a more realistic fashion.

Bargaining. Bargaining seems to take several different forms. It may be overt, as when a patient says, "I just have to make it until my first great-grandchild is born," or patients may simply think, "After my sister comes to visit me, then I will be ready." At times the family will urge the patient to hold on ("we have had this trip planned a long time and we know John will take good care of you while we are gone"). Amazingly the patient often will stay strong enough to make it to and through the event but may deteriorate quickly afterward. If the patient's and family's attachment to a date or event are the same, everyone seems to work toward that goal. However, anger or silence can result if the patient is not interested in reaching the milestone that the family wants. Communication may be impaired, with the goal becoming more important than the patient. Recognizing that bargaining is taking place can lead to resolution.

Depression. Depression is also a barrier to communication. If the patient and/or the caregiver is depressed, withdrawal leads to silence or to negative talk that can be difficult for everyone. Soon the nondepressed people will start to avoid the depressed one to protect their own outlook. Counseling and the use of antidepressants can be helpful. Certainly there is reason for terminally ill patients to be depressed and for those who love them to feel sad also. True clinical depression is rare, but if the depression seems unreasonably deep or long, or suicide is mentioned, home health nurses should be concerned and take appropriate action.[7] Alerting the physician and discussing the patient's feelings with the patient and the family are ways to offer support. A referral to the psychiatric home health nurse may be helpful because suicides occasionally do occur.[7]

Acceptance. Some patients may never accept the fact that they are going to die, especially if deterioration is rapid. Patients may be fearful and anxious regarding what will happen to them or to their family after they die. Encouraging patients to talk about their fears, grief, and concerns may resolve feelings of anger and depression as the end nears. If medication for anxiety and depression is considered, benzodiazepines (Xanax and Valium) are helpful and do not significantly interfere with the patient's level of consciousness. With such interventions, most hospice patients approach their last hours in a calm and peaceful manner surrounded by their loved ones and frequently their nurse.

Caregivers' concerns and need for support

Taking care of a dying person is stressful, exhausting, and traumatic for caregivers. Caregivers frequently lack confidence, saying, "I am not a nurse (i.e., social worker) so I am probably doing everything wrong." It is important to reassure them that if they go by their instincts, they will usually do the right thing. Caregivers are actually more experienced than they realize with tasks such as feeding or bathing. Telling caregivers that knowing the patient gives them an advantage may boost self-confidence. Instilling confidence in caregivers is important so that they feel they are doing a competent job, and later feel that they did all they could to make the dying person's last days or weeks comfortable.

"What should I expect—I mean in regard to dying?" is a question often asked by caregivers. Many caregivers fear that the death will be sudden or agonizing because of things they have seen in movies and on television. To learn that patients' conditions usually worsen gradually until they are finally bedridden and that their death will be expected and peaceful relieves caregivers from a lot of anxiety. Another frequent query is, "What will we do when the pain gets excruciating?" Reassuring families that there is usually a medication with a dosage and frequency to take care of problems with patient pain is comforting. "I felt so bad last night when I lost my temper" is another often heard statement. For some reason, caregivers feel that they should be able to have unending patience with their sick loved ones. However, it is not unusual for patients to awaken their caregivers and then forget what they wanted the caregiver to do. After several nights of this occurring numerous times, tempers get short. In other instances, patients may insist on a treat such as strawberry shortcake at 3:00 AM. When their caregiver finally gets the treat all prepared, the patient may decide that it does not look as good as was imagined and refuse to eat it. The caregiver feels exasperated and then guilty for any outburst. It is important to reassure caregivers that they cannot be expected to be calm every moment. Stress and fatigue make these predicaments look much more serious than they are. They should apologize, explain the reason for the outburst, and then move on.

"How can I get more rest?" is another question commonly asked. Sleeping when the patient sleeps, enlisting the help of friends and neighbors, letting the housework go, and relying more on volunteers are all possible solutions. Caregiving is a full-time job, and even though there may be several people involved, usually there is one main caregiver who accepts responsibility for the majority of the patient's care. If phone calls are interrupting rest periods, caregivers must firmly state that this is rest time, especially if the call will raise the caregiver's anxiety level. If the caregiver is unable to pleasantly ask the person to call back, it might be helpful to have a volunteer stay by the phone during the rest period so that the caregiver can at least relax. Finally, a concern that caregivers often raise is, "I want to go out, but I am afraid to leave the house for fear something will happen while I am gone." Of course this is a worry; however, cabin fever can be depressing. Enlisting the help of a friend, relative, or volunteer to stay with the patient while the caregiver shops, has lunch, or gets a haircut will give a surprising lift to the spirits.

Caregivers often need as much tender loving care as patients. One of the kindest questions a home health nurse can ask of the caregiver is, "How are you doing?" Caregivers often feel that all the emphasis is on the patient, and this simple question lets them know that they, too, are valuable and appreciated. They must be reassured that they are doing the best they can for the patient and that is all anyone can do.

The time of death and after

During the active dying process, families are instructed to call the nurse and not to call any emergency service. As the patient gets close to dying, some caregivers will ask the nurse or other hospice team member to stay with them; others want private time with their loved one. Most families appreciate support during this time and also at the time of death.

At this time patients need to feel that they are not alone. Family members should be reassured that holding the dying person's hand and providing small comforts and caring words are meaningful and natural and will be remembered in a positive way. Also families need to know that hearing is the last sense to leave the patient and that they should not speak at the bedside as though the patient has already died. Often families provide strength and encouragement to patients as they are dying. Touching the person who has just died is encouraging and confirms the reality of the situation. It is important to reassure family members that not being able to close the dead person's eyes or mouth is not unusual. Just after the patient dies, the nurse calls the physician, the funeral home, and others who need to be contacted so that the family is free of these concerns. The nurse bathes the patient and stays in the home until the body is removed. Medication is disposed of and equipment is organized for pickup. Saying, "He certainly died peacefully," or relating a touching moment can be comforting to the family. The nurse should use the word *died* rather than a euphemism and should be kind and caring but not overly sentimental. If the home health nurse shares a few tears with the family, this is nothing to be embarrassed about. The nurse should offer to call the minister, priest, rabbi, or other spiritual counselor. The nurse should stay with the family until they seem calm and arrangements have been made. The family is told that the hospice team will stay in touch and is informed that sadness, anger, guilt, and depression are all normal responses. The grieving process may take a long time, and its length will vary for each individual. Family members may need to be told that there is no feeling that they "should" or "should not" have after a certain number of months have passed.

As part of the bereavement follow-up, a letter of condolence is sent out from the agency.[9,19] Phone calls may be made to the family members to check on how they are doing and to inquire whether they need assistance of any sort, or have any questions that need answering. Formal follow-up by phone or letter is made at 1 month, 3 months, 6 months, and 1 year.[3,9] Home visits may be made at those intervals. In addition, invitations to a monthly bereavement group typically are sent during that period. If more intensive counseling is needed, that also is provided. The monthly bereavement meetings may be a mixture of serious and frivolous topics. There is always the opportunity to "vent your spleen," but there are also meetings that are purely social and fun.[9] Most hospice programs also sponsor a yearly memorial service to honor and remember those who have died during the year. This is beneficial for families and staff.

SUMMARY

Working with patients who are dying provides many insights into living and the wonders of life. It is essential that those working in hospice look at their own lives and at their own feelings about death before they try to help others. Although very few people want to die tomorrow, for the hospice patient, the family at home, and the hospice team, living each day to its fullest makes death less frightening.

Care and comfort for terminally ill patients are very important. Therefore home health nursing interventions are primarily palliative and supportive. To die peacefully at home in a familiar spot with those they love gathered around is the way many would prefer their lives to end. With hospice care, that wish is within the patient's and family's reach. For in moments of darkness and despair, to touch and be touched signifies our very real and human need for one another.

REFERENCES

1. American Pain Society: *Principles of analgesic use in the treatment of acute pain and cancer pain,* Skokie, Ill, 1992, American Pain Society.
2. Baer K: Dying with dignity: a guide to hospice care, *Harvard Health Letter,* special suppl, April 1993.
3. Beresford L: *The hospice handbook: a complete guide,* Boston, 1993, Little, Brown.
4. Buncher P: Hospice nursing: daily challenges, daily rewards, *Caring,* p. 67, Nov 1993.
5. Colburn L: Preventing pressure ulcers, *Nursing 90* 12:63, 1990.

6. Cundiff D: *Euthanasia is not the answer: a hospice physician's view,* Totowa, NJ, 1992, Humana Press.
7. Ferszt G, Barg FK: Psychosocial support. In Baird SB: *A cancer source-book for nurses,* Atlanta, 1991, The American Cancer Society.
8. Gentile M, Fello M: Hospice care for the 1990's, *J Home Health Care Pract* 3:1, 1990.
9. Gianino PM: Providing hospice bereavement follow-up services: practicing the art of doing more with less, *J Home Health Care Pract* 3:1, 1990.
10. Holdeen CM: *Nutrition and hydration in the terminally ill patient: the nurse's role in helping patients and families.*
11. Kaiser C: *Home hospice: a caregivers guide,* Wilton, Conn, 1990, Home Health Care.
12. Kubler-Ross E: *On death and dying,* New York, 1972, Macmillan.
13. Levy MH: Pharmacologic management of cancer pain. Lecture at Cancer Pain Symposium, Augusta, Me, June 24, 1994.
14. Lutheran Medical Center: *Hospice,* St Louis, 1986, National Medical Enterprises.
15. McPherson ML: Pharmacologic management of pain and symptoms in terminally ill cancer patients, *J Home Health Care Pract* 3:1, 1990.
16. Murkland S: Nutritional management of the home hospice patient, *J Home Health Care Pract* 3:1, 1990.
17. Nassif JZ: *The home health care solution,* New York, 1985, Perennial Library.
18. Pierce JL: Spiritual care: the soul of hospice, *J Home Health Care Pract* 3:1, 1990.
19. Storey P: Goals of hospice care, *Tex Med* 86:50, 1990.
20. Ufema J: Insights on death and dying, *Nursing 90* 12:22, 1990.
21. US Department of Health and Human Services, Agency for Health Care Policy and Research: *Management of cancer pain,* Rockville, Md, 1994, HCFA.
22. West TS: *Hospice medicine distressing symptoms,* Essex, Conn, 1987, Hospice Education Institute.

IV Future Trends

26 Paradoxes of Progress: Implications for Home Health Care

Jacquelyn M. Clement, Elizabeth A. Buck,
Carol A. Keene, and Jacalyn Wickline Ryberg

In many ways, the home care challenges that face nursing are stimuli to return to age-old efforts and standards. It is said that history repeats itself, and there seems to be some truth in the notion that society does turn back to basics when new eras emerge and progress moves too swiftly. This fundamental paradox lays the foundation for exploration of home health care trends in America, which are examined in this chapter.

What does the future of home health care hold? Given the present issues confronting the nation from this perspective, two overriding concerns surface: the needs of the individual versus the needs of society, and quality of life versus quantity of life. Questions related to these concerns are: Who is the consumer of the future? How does emerging technology fit into tomorrow's health care? What ethical issues will we face as health care changes? What impact will the responses to such issues have on the practice of home health care nursing?

WHO IS THE CONSUMER OF THE FUTURE?

The most dramatic factor in the United States that will influence the sociopolitical context of health care is the growing diversity of the American population. The complexity of our society is reflected in varying age groups, work settings, economic classes, family structures, educational levels, and ethnic origins. Understanding the nature of this diversity is a prerequisite to considering reforms in health care, since individual needs will necessarily be addressed within a socioeconomic framework imposing limits upon the response to these needs.

CHARACTERISTICS OF DIVERSITY
The aging society

Never before in the United States have four distinct phenomena occurred in the manner and dimensions that we now face: (1) people are living longer, healthier, and more vigorously than ever before, (2) the birth rate has declined, creating a large population of older adults that is not offset by a high birthrate, (3) the "oldest old" (85 years of age or older) is the fastest growing segment of our population,[6] and (4) a large segment of the baby boom population, now middle-aged, will soon be part of the "elder boom." These phenomena of aging in America largely reflect the changes and growth in society that have coincidentally accompanied the prominence of the baby boomers and the resulting attention given to this large group as it approaches the geriatric stages of life.[11] Cumulatively the effect of all these factors adds up to a distinctively different older citizenry. This has created some shifting of national priorities and some intergenerational tensions as attempts are made to address newly identified needs.

From 1960 to 1990, the number of individuals 85 years of age or older increased by 232%, while the total population grew by just 39%.[6] The majority of these oldest old individuals are without disability and live within the community. However, they are also subject to functional impairment and chronic disease. Since approximately 50% of those living in the community will need some assistance with everyday activities, this growing segment of the population clearly presents service opportunities for home health nurses.[6] At the same time, this growth presents challenges to health care reform. For example, patients with recognized physical therapy needs should have direct access to rehabilitative services without the mediation of acute care.

The elder boom

The dramatic increase in the population of persons 65 years of age or older—the elder boom—has made it a powerful sociopolitical group. Their needs, issues, problems, and interests have moved to the forefront as driving forces of change. Since health care is a major concern of this population, health care delivery is taking on new dimensions and dynamics, which promise continuing intensification of such emerging challenges as increasing costs, consumerism, and changing availability of high-technology care.[11]

The world in which we live is already changing to accommodate the needs of the elder boomers and, more specifically, the older old. Simple things such as larger typeface in newspapers, books, and greeting cards are increasingly available. Television, radio, and print media will continue to launch new efforts to be responsive to the interests of elderly Americans. The emergence of computers as tools of recreation, entertainment, conversation, education, and communication is already having a major impact on the hobbies and habits of the elderly and will continue to be a key factor in the day-to-day life of this group. Safety and comfort issues require additional attention as more elderly people drive cars, exercise, participate in sports, and continue to be active in jobs. Science and technology must continue to respond not only to these challenges, but to the challenges of supporting the altered sensory needs and the intellectual needs of a productive elderly population.[11]

The overall message that is important as preparation is made for the future in nursing and home health is to erase today's image of the elderly population and see in its place a transformed aging population that has new dimensions of health care needs. The health care industry as a whole will experience new challenges and unimagined opportunities in the future. As facilitators of patient care, home health nurses will play pivotal roles in meeting these challenges and in making possibilities a reality.

Baby boomers

Baby boomers, those individuals who were born between 1946 and 1964, number 76 million—one third of the U.S. population.[11] Because the baby boomers are such a large proportion of the population, society has focused heavily on the needs and issues of this group. In the 1960s, the hippie movement was very visible; the 1970s continued to focus on Vietnam issues and on the fashion, music, and political statements of the baby boomers. The 1980s brought a health conscious consumerism, exercise, dieting, materialism, and emphasis on the preservation of youth; the 1990s seem to be bringing a fresh awareness and appreciation of the environment, natural resources, and education, along with a new sensitivity to the issue of aging. In evidence of this sensitivity, one needs only to note the plethora of articles and television programs on subjects such as menopause and arthritis.

The first of the baby boomers will become elder boomers in 2011. Their concerns are already shaping the concerns of society as a whole and plans for the future. For example, boomer entrepreneurs are already inventing devices and health care aids, and developing new models for long-term care facilities to meet the multiple and varied needs of elderly groups. American society is being subtly reshaped, not only by contemporary elder boomers, but also by these soon-to-be elder boomers whose needs, by their sheer quantity, are anticipated to be different from those of the elderly population as we now know it.

Diverse work settings

It is anticipated that individuals will change career paths several times during their lives. We will rarely see the person who retires at age 65 after 45 years in the same job. People will not only change jobs, but they will also be more apt to redirect their talents in entirely new areas of interest several times during their lives. The incidence of a "middle-age career hiatus" may increase with people returning to the work environment after "dropping out" for a few years to attend school, experience travel and leisure, or start a second or third family. The locale of the workplace is already changing, with more people conducting work out of their homes, using computer networks, teleconferencing equipment, fax machines, and telephones as means of communicating. These varying characteristics of the contemporary workforce have contributed to insecurity about the provision of health care which, in turn, has been an impetus to the call for universal health care.

Restructuring of the family

Personal and family relationships as we have known them are also changing dramatically. A recent study by the U.S. Census Bureau revealed that half of American children live in something other than the traditional nuclear family (a married couple living with their biological children and no one else). The phenomena of "blended" and "blended multigenerational" families will continue to increase. Based on 1991 data only 56% of white children, 26% of African-American children, and 38% of Hispanic children live in a traditional nuclear family.[25] Even the nuclear family is different from what it was several decades ago, given the number of women now employed outside the home. In addition, the incidence of single parent families continues to rise.

Longevity has also influenced family structure. Longer lives may result in multiple marriages in one lifetime and the incidence of individual relationships that span 70-plus years becoming more common. Other potential changes include multigenerational housing consisting not only of the typical "sandwich generation," but of four generations living under one roof as young adults now return to their parents' homes (Figure 26-1). The incidence of cohabitation among the elderly may increase due to economic conditions. These structural changes will necessarily affect the ways in which health care is delivered in the future.

Educational levels

Consumers of the future will be more mature, more sophisticated, and more health conscious than ever, despite the current trend of young people receiving less formal education than their baby boomer parents. In addition, consumers will increasingly participate in decisions about their own health care and be involved in, and knowledgeable about, quality care issues. Individuals are already becoming aware that they determine their own health. They are absorbing reams of health care information that in the past was not made available to laypersons. In fact, one of the greatest challenges that the health care consumer faces today is sifting through the vast amount of information that is available in an effort to make knowledgeable decisions. For the first time in the history of the United States, this nation will have a population in which many individuals will be informed health care consumers from a relatively early age and will make conscious decisions about long-term health issues during their youth. Among today's consumers, some already are becoming the watchdogs of health care providers; this tendency will increase considerably as expanding varieties of providers participate in the delivery of health care. As a result the composition of review boards for health care evaluation will evolve to include a larger proportion of members representing the public. Ethics committees, consisting in part of laypeople, already are being mandated by accrediting bodies for health care facilities, including home health care agencies. Public accountability for health care decisions and issues of quality will continue to grow as individual citizens are required to take more responsibility for their health care.

Cultural sensitivity

All health care providers, and particularly nurses, are facing the challenge of providing culturally competent care. This imperative, that care be not only available and accessible, but also appropriate, is driven by the health care data indicating differentials of disease incidence among ethnically diverse groups. The need for cultural sensitivity extends beyond disease analysis to understanding cultural variations and diverse value systems, as well as developing skills prerequisite to working with ethnically diverse populations.[7]

SOCIOPOLITICAL CHALLENGES

In light of the demographic changes, there are multiple sociopolitical challenges, paradoxical in nature, to which health care must respond. For example, although the U.S. health care system is well supported on a national basis, limitations must be placed on the use and availability of technological resources because of the need for cost containment of services. In addition, U.S.

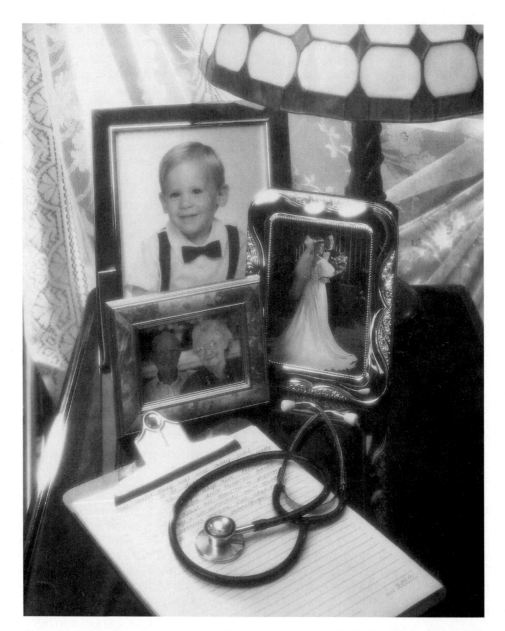

Figure 26-1 It has become more common for several generations of a family to live together under one roof. (Photo courtesy Nebraska Methodist Home Health.)

health care is also the most advanced technologically. The consequences of our fascination with technology, coupled with the consequences of our denial of death, are leading us to reexamine our values and to question whether the quantity of life is worth more or even as much as the quality of life. Americans are beginning to place a greater value on quality of life (although unfortunately without a commitment to the health promotion activities required to reach it). This dissonance is a prime example of the paradox of progress in health care. The desire for quality of life afforded by the technological revolution has been the key impetus for the social revolution seeking the transformation of health care. We must continually question whether technology is serving our goal, and whether our goal is spurring technology to the desired end. We must ensure that future technological advances improve the quality of life, not merely its quantity. Efforts to increase the quantity of life may need to be curbed so as not to jeopardize the quality of life.

When we place this problem within the sociopolitical framework, the good of the many versus the good of the few becomes a pivotal issue. It is this dilemma that created the controversy in a recent attempt to form a universal health care policy. The prizing of autonomy, it appears, must be tempered with social responsibility. This is not merely an economic or sociopolitical issue, but more importantly a moral issue for each and every citizen. A key example of the tension between self-determination and social responsibility is the growing moral debate over the question of medical futility.

It is paradoxical that this country is experiencing an increase in culturally diverse populations while health care legislation is calling for more standardization in health care delivery. This call for standardization presumes a common set of values among the citizenry. Until we can agree upon a set of values that can serve as a basis for our health care policy, efforts at standardization will be futile.

The most immediate and pressing incongruity for the health care worker in day-to-day practice is the call for holistic and caring (not mechanized or fragmented) treatment in an age of ever-increasing advancement in technology. The dehumanization of the patient in the biomedical model, with its focus on disease and its ignoring of illness, has generated a dehumanization within the health care profession itself. It is crucial that the caring aspects of health care reemerge as the central force directing the development of a national health care policy, together with reform of the curricula of all health care professionals.

COST OF HOME HEALTH CARE: A NATIONAL PERSPECTIVE

None of the tremendous efforts to decrease the escalating rate of health care costs has been effective. The cost of health care in the United States continues to grow out of proportion to any other part of the federal budget. The United States is currently spending over 16% of its gross national product on health care, and this percentage is expected to continue to rise. One of the attempts to curb the costs of health care was the prospective payment system introduced by the federal government in 1983. Due to the financial incentives associated with this system, hospital lengths of stay decreased, resulting in an increased need for services outside of the hospital. Consequently, since 1983 the home health care industry has been the fastest growing segment of the health care delivery system. The Bureau of Labor Statistics indicates that home care employment has increased by 19.2%, and the U.S. Department of Health and Human Services predicts that 8,000 more registered nurses will be needed in home health care by the year 2000.[16,17]

Other factors continue to contribute to the increased need for and diversity of home health services. These include (1) the growing number of older adults, as discussed earlier in this chapter, (2) the increased consumer interest in self-care, which has generated a preference for receiving care at home rather than in institutions, and (3) the increase in the number of individuals receiving long-term chronic care, such as patients with AIDS, individuals with Alzheimer's disease, crack babies, and persons on ventilatory support and/or total parenteral nutrition (TPN). Major health problems like these, previously seen primarily in institutional care settings, are now being managed in the home by the families and professional home care nurses. Nurses have had to develop more sophisticated skills in the areas of high technology, care of the terminally ill, and care for and support of whole families.

Because of the fragmentation of the current health care delivery system and an historical inability of the federal government to decrease health care costs, health care is moving into the free market by a managed care system with federal subsidies of services changing in the foreseeable future. Though home health care has been a major provision in most of the proposed federal legislation and should be included in future bills, federal policy is moving the locus of action to the state level. Hence, home health nurses *must* take the initiative in policy making efforts at the state level to ensure that provisions for adequate service to patients in their homes are included in any legislation passed. This legislation should support mechanisms to guarantee continuity of care for all aspects and levels of individuals' health care needs.

In addition, home health nurses must be willing to educate the public on the clear need for federal and state health care legislation that includes home health care as an integral part. To do this, home health nurses must remain informed about proposed legislation and must maintain close contact with their federal and state legislators to keep them apprised of the unique health care experiences of patients and their families in the home setting. No one envisioned the difficulties that the prospective payment system would cause for consumers, families, and health care providers. This point is highlighted by the fact that there is a national call for capitation in home care. Capitation certainly offers the promise of economic efficiency but may well represent the paradox of increased limitations in home care service to the public. Therefore it is essential that all those who are involved in the transformation of health care policy and delivery remain attuned to the needs of patients and their families.

However, doing these things is not sufficient to make these efforts successful. The failure of this nation to provide all its citizens with a basic health care package is, at least in part, traceable to different interest groups eschewing a common effort in the name of consumer advocacy to protect their own insular interests. Home health nurses must not fall prey to the paradoxical view that health care legislation can occur only through the diverse, if not divisive, efforts of splinter groups. Home health nurses must take the initiative to collaborate with other nurses, physicians, and other health care professionals to ensure that the educative effort of health care professionals is a concerted one. This implies that home health nurses will become politically and professionally active.

THE HOME HEALTH NURSE'S ROLE IN THE CHANGING HEALTH CARE SYSTEM

Collaboration with others in educating the general public and policy makers is but one of the educational roles of home health nurses. We must also ensure that all nursing school graduates are educationally prepared for a health care system that is vastly different from the current system. The health care system will continue to experience accelerated change as the needs of the health care consumer become more diversified; this only serves to accentuate the need for reform of the nursing curriculum at all levels.[12]

Education of the home health care nurse must begin at the associate degree level. Home health experiences previously limited to baccalaureate programs must also be included as part of the essential framework in associate degree nursing curricula. These experiences should provide associate degree students with a wide variety of opportunities to apply basic patient care concepts to the home setting. Because nursing is in a transition from a predominantly hospital-based or acute care setting to a heavily focused community-based care setting, all new nursing graduates must be prepared to assume community-based roles consistent with their levels of education. The baccalaureate nurse will need to be educationally prepared to assume expanded roles as new independent nursing care models develop, roles that will require increased independence, authority, and responsibility in settings very different from the traditional hospital setting. Moreover, the continuing development and proliferation of diverse patient care models commensurate with the expansion of nursing roles will demand further clarification of differentiated levels of practice between associate degree graduates and baccalaureate graduates of nursing. Furthermore, because the preparation of the baccalaureate graduate will soon be equivalent to that of the current master's graduate in this area, master's degree programs in community-based care must change. To provide leadership requisite for future nursing practice, these programs must evolve with new curricula central to both community health and home health care. The new curricula must be supportive of case management, advanced nursing practice, interdisciplinary collaboration and research, national and international networking, and entrepreneurial skills.

Since the focus of practice in such a new program would be responsive to developing health care needs, an important characteristic of master's prepared nurses will be their ability to conduct research that will lead to quality care in community-based settings. For example, research might explore such basic issues as how care is delivered in the home, how the family copes with increased responsibility, how the frail elderly manage self-care, the cost benefits of home care, and outcome analysis. Although much is known about the pathophysiology of disease, little is known about the sociopolitical context in which home health care is delivered. Moreover, research must not be limited only to disease (the biomedical phenomenon as defined by the medical community), but must also embrace illness (the experience as articulated by the patient).[14,23] If research does not reflect this holistic context of home care, policy considerations will be mired in unrealistic definitions, views, and expectations.

Successful health restorative, rehabilitative, and palliative interventions by nurses—supported by methodologically sound research studies—will increasingly direct major funds into home health as an economically preferred alternative to hospitalization. The implementation of these interventions will be spearheaded by home health nurses as the concept of managed care continues to become a reality. Home health nurses, being in the best position to detect real and potential health problems, are able to direct patient care toward early interventions that reduce the need for more intensive and expensive care.

A recent growth in the area of community-based nursing practice is encouraging a model of case management in the home health agency in which professional nurses plan and provide hands-on physical care and provide health teaching, while also participating in the supervision of home health aides who provide less skilled areas of care for the patients. Since the home setting has become more acute, and the acute care setting is continuing to downsize, the risk exists that more professional nurses will enter home care with relatively minimal acute care skills. Consequently, professional nurses need to develop expertise previously associated with acute care experience, in the home care setting. Learning many of these skills in the home is different from learning them in the hospital because of the lack of on-site collegial, multidisciplinary support in the home setting. The challenges for nurse educators will be to prepare novice nurses with working skills in the home care setting.

Because of the expanding education and role of home health nurses, third-party reimbursement for nursing services is a natural expectation. However, efforts to get third-party reimbursement for nurses at some state levels will continue to be an uphill battle because of the powerful medical lobby's resistance to expanded roles for nurses. The need to provide affordable access to quality care particularly in rural communities, will be the driving force supporting reimbursement legislation. Direct reimbursement for nurses practicing in more autonomous roles will need to be negotiated so as not to contribute to an increase in overall health care costs.

DIRECTIONS FOR EMERGING TECHNOLOGY

With the projected demographics, the continuing emergence of new technology in health care, and rising health care costs, the future use of technology in home care will take distinct paths. Several clear directions for technology in home health nursing will be in information systems, in patient assessment devices used to predict and sustain patients' physiological needs, and in palliative care and safety needs. Although life-promoting technologies will continue to be used for patients who have an optimal chance for recovery, there will be more informed decision making by patients and their families regarding the appropriateness of choosing such technology in the home setting. Families will face such decision making with new challenges in the areas of personal societal cost-effectiveness, accessibility of options as a result of rationing, and quality versus quantity of life. Elderly patients, many of whom currently spend a large proportion of health care dollars during the last months of their lives in acute care settings, will instead make the choice to live their last days at home under the care of family and home health care nurses. These predictions are made with consideration of increasing sensitivity to quality of life issues, the future demographics of our society compounded by the aging of the baby boom generation, the increased recognition of the individual's power of self-determination, the effects of health care rationing, and the impact of continually rising health care costs.

Information systems of the future will be the "cognitive prostheses" for nurses and health care providers.[21] It is predicted that scientific information affecting nursing practice is proliferating so rapidly that home health nurses, in particular, will rely heavily upon information systems for identification of patient health patterns and direction for nursing care needs. At the 1990 American Nurses' Association Convention, June Abbey, Associate Dean for Research and Evaluation and Director of the Center for Nursing Research at Vanderbilt University School of Nursing, described computers as "memory extenders" and physiological monitoring devices as "sensor extenders."[21] These "extenders" will be the tools with which nurses in the future collect patient information and from which phenomena are identified and nursing interventions developed. These same computer systems will provide nurse researchers with opportunities to access and organize health data for the development of research to predict patient needs and patient responses to interventions. As health care conglomerates develop through mergers among numerous health care facilities, computer networks containing individual and aggregate patient data will emerge and expand to provide not only documentation of individual health records, but also the basis of monitoring health care trends and identifying patterns of health needs. Laptop computers and computer systems are already being used in some home health care agencies, and their usage will continue to increase as additional technologies are developed.

Palliative care and safety issues will take high priority in technological developments for home health care in the future. Increased focus will be given to providing comfort measures to chronically ill elderly persons rather than to prolonging life as an end in itself. For example, the use of electronic devices to measure physiological status (blood pressure, pulse and cardiac output, etc.) and to deliver an appropriate dose of analgesia may be available in the home for personal use by the patient. The development of safety mechanisms and communication devices will continue to expand as more older adults are alone in their homes. Patients will have the ability to communicate via computers, television sets, phone systems, and safety alarm systems at an increasingly sophisticated level. Families will have access to new technology in the home that will increase the possibility of providing care for chronically ill members of the family. Devices such as electronic lifts and easily accessible bathtubs will be installed

for long-term home care. Health care services such as physical therapy (already available in the home) will become increasingly common in home care as more portable equipment is developed. A variety of other services will be provided more and more in the home setting; these may include professional hair care, foot and nail care, income tax assistance, pet care, shopping assistance, and clothing repair and tailoring. Homes themselves will be designed and constructed with features to accommodate the potential needs of the aged and chronically ill. Home planners will be more sensitive to the need for single floors, main floor laundry areas, limited stairways, widened doorways and hallways for wheelchairs and other equipment, and adequate communication and security systems.

ETHICAL ISSUES IN HOME HEALTH CARE

Ethical issues occur on a day-to-day basis at the micro-level, in the delivery of health care in the noninstitutionalized home setting. The micro-level, however, is intrinsically interwoven with the macro-level, the highly institutionalized health care delivery system, enmeshed in sociopolitical and economic dimensions also reflects issues of justice regarding the distribution of resources both to and within the health care industry. This intersection of the micro- and macro-levels in patient care provides a further reason for home health nurses to play a key role in the development of public policy regarding health care. Once developed, public policy will specify guidelines concerning the nature and extent of health care services to be delivered in the home.

Micro-level ethical issues

The impetus for home health care to become a major player in the health care system can be traced to several factors including (1) the elder boom and the concomitant increase in the need for care of chronic illness, (2) the high cost and predicted shortage of nursing homes, (3) the current hospital-based prospective payment system with its economic incentive to discharge patients as soon as possible, (4) the general preference of older adults and their families for home health care rather than institutional care, and (5) the goal to decrease fragmentation and inefficiencies of service while promoting increased continuity and quality of patient care. Although considerations of demographics and of cost containment generate several ethical issues at the macro-level, it is the preference of individuals for home health care that is telling at the micro-level. This preference signals a choice that bestows a special value on home care as a means of meeting the health needs of individuals while preserving their control over day-to-day activities as long as possible. Home health care is prized so highly because it is seen as the avenue of health care delivery that best preserves the autonomy of the individual.

The fact that home health care is so viewed by the general public underscores the importance of nursing's holistic approach to patient care. Such an approach is particularly conducive to meeting patient expectations in the home, since the holistic focus necessarily includes efforts to maximize the autonomy of patients (i.e., their capacity to be self-determining and to make choices in accord with their own goals and values) and to treat their illness, not merely their disease. But as recent discussions have pointed out, concern about autonomy in home health, which at present chiefly involves the chronically ill patient, is to be distinguished from the autonomy paradigm of acute care in institutionalized settings, a paradigm that has dominated bioethics since its inception.[8,13] In acute care, a key goal of both the health care professional and the patient is to restore, where possible, the patient's autonomy by curative treatment. In chronic care, the correlative goal is to preserve the autonomy of the patient as long as possible, recognizing that chronic illness impairs restoration of autonomy to the level possessed prior to the onset of the illness. Home health nursing thus involves assisting patients to integrate exacerbations of chronic illness into their daily lives in such a way as to maximize their decision making capacity and feelings of self-worth, and to retain sufficient independence to ward off institutionalized care. Given the nature of chronic illness and the increasing life span of the elderly, patients will most likely undergo several reintegrations of changes in health status as independence decreases. The home health nurse will face the continuing challenge of responding to evolving patient needs as chronic illnesses progress and become more debilitating.

The ethical issues that home health nurses will confront at the micro-level will come primarily from the human relationships they will encounter in home settings. Issues prevalent in nursing practice, such as honesty, confidentiality, and beneficence, are not merely the preserve of the acute setting but remain the moral cornerstone of the relationship between the patient and the nurse whatever the setting. Thus conflicts that arise in regard to these values in acute care can also emerge in home care. Beyond such commonality, however, there are certain factors peculiar to the home setting that require consideration.

First, patients at home are in a familiar setting where they have been accustomed to exercising some measure of control. In contrast to the institutional setting, in the home it is not the patient who is a stranger in a strange land, it is the nurse. This situation not only may create less compliance on the part of patients, but also may mask whether they have sufficient autonomy (i.e., knowledge and freedom) to make decisions relative to their health care needs. Home health nurses must bear in mind that competence (to use the legal terminology) and autonomy are not all-or-nothing concepts. The fact that a patient is competent to perform a particular task does not thereby imply competence to make a particular health care decision. As Buchanan and Brock have shown, competence is decision-relative and decision-specific.[2]

Family members residing with the patient add another dimension to the complexity of respecting and nurturing the patient's autonomy while managing health care needs in the home setting. Given the increase in multigenerational families living under one roof, the home may be the family members' home. Because of the impact of care decisions upon family members, some of whom may be caregivers, the question of "who decides" cannot automatically be resolved by an appeal to the primacy of patient autonomy. On the other hand, family caregivers may themselves find their autonomy diminished, their independence curtailed, and their emotional and economic resources dissipating. Such circumstances only serve to highlight how complex the determination of "who decides" is. There are no general answers to this question; determinations must be made on a decision-by-decision basis. The complexity of family relationships within the home setting and the attendant attenuation of the primacy of patient autonomy is but a microcosm of the limits that are imposed on individual desires and needs when considered within any social or communal framework.[20]

The "who decides" issue that home health nurses presently face will change because of the projected dramatic changes in the family. Furthermore, by the year 2030, it is expected that 30 million elderly persons will have no caregiver, compared with 8.4 million in 1984.[22] Thus the question will arise, Who will be there to decide on behalf of patients who cannot decide for themselves? This issue emphatically demonstrates the limits of the autonomy paradigm and the need to search for additional models to guide decision making when the autonomy model falters or fails.

Still another cluster of issues that will arise in the home setting concerns the role and nature of technology in home health care. As mentioned previously in this chapter, technology is not good in itself. Since it may be used for good or ill, health care professionals must consider its use judiciously, whatever the setting. That individuals tend to prefer the home setting over the institutionalized setting signals not only their desire to be in familiar surroundings, but also their felt need to be in surroundings that bear their personal stamp. Though the home setting should not be unduly romanticized (given the possibility of dysfunctional families and/or of high stress with high tech in the home), it has traditionally been perceived as the individual's ultimate refuge. Hence, as advanced technology in health care enters the home, home health nurses must be ever mindful that the home is considered to be the patient's sanctum from abstract and barren institutionalized settings. Moreover, as chronically ill patients "take a turn for the worse," there is a need to acknowledge that the lines of life support can readily become the chains of an existence burdensome to the patient, and a mere prolongation of dying.[1] The use of advanced technology in home health care thus requires special consideration, so that no harm is done to the patient's sense of integrity or to the concept of the home as a refuge. Perhaps, to assist in keeping a balanced perspective on the role of technology in health care, all home health nurses should be required to have training in hospice care. Such training might also serve them well as

they confront moral concerns within the health care profession itself about the concept of medical futility. The hospice concept is often posed as an alternative in current discussions about the morality of assisted death (whether the latter takes the form of euthanasia or of assisted suicide), an issue that is not insulated from the home setting.

Because of ethical challenges such as these, it is imperative for nurses to work closely with other disciplines in creating new approaches to dealing with complex situations. The recent movement toward the development of ethics committees by home health agencies is a welcome step in this direction. But collaborative research projects are requisite as well if nurses are to be at the forefront of multidisciplinary teams moving toward the development of paradigms to address the new frontier in home health care suggested by the projected demographics.

Macro-level ethical issues

It is not only at the micro-level that challenges to the autonomy paradigm are and will continue to emerge. Home health care faces issues of an ethical nature at the macro-level that beset the health care industry as a whole, issues of justice in the distribution of resources both to and within the health care system. As Veatch predicted in 1972, the success of the biotechnology revolution, in effecting both increased longevity and a certain improvement in the quality of life, has generated a social demand that health care coverage be made accessible to all citizens of the United States.[24]

Approximately 37 million Americans presently fall outside the system of coverage. This is generally conceded to be scandalous, given the professed values and global stature of the United States. Consequently, as suggested earlier in this chapter, there are ever-increasing cries for change in the health care system, for provision of some national plan to rectify current injustices. Although federal legislative efforts in this cause have recently been deferred, the forces of justice at the grassroots will not allow political gridlock to thwart provision of a basic health care package for all citizens of this country. The United States is now the only country of the developed nations to be lacking in a national health care plan. Public discussion will continue to focus on the means for this provision. Whatever the means ultimately determine, certain issues must still be resolved.

To date the United States has taken an irrational, patchwork approach to health care policy, which has produced a "nonsystem" that is spawned by attending to special interest groups.[19] One sign of the chaos in the present health care system is that $145 billion was spent on health care for the elderly in 1988, with less than 0.5% invested in research for improving the quality of life of the elderly.[22] To try to dissect issues as they relate to specific population groups or specific care settings would be a meaningless exercise. The only way that these issues can be addressed effectively is within the context of health care as a whole. As noted previously, the nursing profession must speak in one voice in the development of a comprehensive plan, not in differing voices of nursing groups representing special interests.

All health care professionals must contribute to the resolution of macro-level ethical issues. What does the claim that there is a right to health care mean? How does the right to health care interact with other rights of individuals, groups, and society as a whole? What constitutes a decent standard of health care? It is not merely the social demand for coverage and access for all citizens that prompts this last question, but also the demand for cost containment. If limits are to be acknowledged, their content must be established. What should be the role of quality measures in the issue of health care allocation? What constitutes a just allocation of limited resources?

Given the demographics of American society, the question of justice is pushed still further.[10] What constitutes a just distribution of resources across generations? Clearly, rationing of resources must be a necessary accompaniment of future reforms and health care policies, as Callahan has argued.[4] Unless the general public accepts this, there will never be a universal health care plan in this country.

It has been argued that age-based rationing of resources, for example, is ethically justifiable. Callahan has described his view of a natural life span, at the end of which death comes as an inevitable part of the life cycle. He basically eschews using high-technology lifesaving treatments on individuals beyond their late 70s to early 80s, suggesting that such individuals have realized virtually all of

their goals by that time of life. Callahan cautions, however, that such individuals should not be abandoned by the health care system, but should receive increased support for chronic illness through measures such as palliative care.[5]

Another argument for age-based rationing has been advanced by Daniels,[9] who seeks to overcome the perception of the resource issue as an intergenerational conflict. What he proposes is that individuals budget their own benefit package, making selections of health care resources to meet their considered needs at each stage of life. If they are prudent deliberators, such individuals would be more likely to give emphasis to lifesaving treatments early in life and low-technology services in their later years. By proposing that this budgeting process be left in the hands of the individual, Daniels offers a view in which generations do not compete for health care resources. There are, however, several legitimate concerns about age-based rationing. First, the elderly are not a homogeneous group. Any attempt to implement a strict age-based criterion for allocation of health resources presents incongruencies that apparently contributed to Callahan's initial waffling on setting a specific age limit for providing high-technology interventions to the elderly and his subsequent retreat from such specification in favor of a life cycle framework devoid of a strict age-based criterion.[3] Secondly, arguments for age-based rationing appear to assume that, given the costs of high-technology, a greater proportion of resources is now being used for dying persons than in the past. However, a recent study on Medicare payments in the last year of life from 1976 to 1988 calls this assumption into question, concluding that such payments for persons 65 years of age or older have changed very slightly and that expenditures for care during the last 60 days of life considered as a percentage of payments for the last year of life have held steady at 52%. Not only did this study conclude that increased costs for persons in the final year of life do not differ in magnitude from the overall growth of Medicare expenditures, but it also showed a pattern of lower Medicare payments for older decedents as compared with younger decedents.[18] Thirdly, and most importantly from an ethical standpoint, attempts at categorization by age specification undercut the one-to-one relationship between the care provider and the individual patient that is the very foundation of health care as a moral enterprise. To focus on age as a basis for rationing and cost containment is dangerous because it is so simplistic. Such a focus ignores the many other variables (medical condition, likelihood of success, etc.) worthy of serious consideration in individual life-sustaining decisions.

Another controversial arena that must be faced is that the existence and acceptance of technology in health care does not make its use moral. As Hippocrates reminds us, acting in the patient's best interests requires that we recognize that there are times when the disease so overpowers the patient that medicine is impotent. The use of medicine in such cases may be immoral. This does not mean, however, that the patient is abandoned by the health care system. To the contrary, this is precisely the point at which home health care becomes the cornerstone of efforts to provide palliative care when curative measures are not an option. Ever-emerging technology is already reshaping the locus of issues regarding treatment refusal, advance directives, rationing, and medical futility. They will no longer be the preserve merely of the acute, institutionalized setting, but will enter the home setting as well.

These matters which have to date largely been debated by the judiciary are now being considered as critical ingredients of a national health care plan. Home health care nurses and their patients are already confronting these issues daily. The micro-level cannot await decisions at the macro-level. This places a tremendous burden on the health care delivery system, the educational system, and ultimately—and most importantly—on each individual nurse to collaborate with other concerned sectors in seeking resolution of these most perplexing questions about living and dying.

SUMMARY

The direction for the future of home health care without a doubt will require careful reflection and thoughtful decisions in the integration of demographic, economic, educational, technologic, and ethical issues. It is imperative that we as a nation recognize that the future holds unprecedented challenges in all these arenas. To reap the benefits of understanding from the past and apply them to projections for future decision making in an informed and responsible manner is a critical task

for all health care providers. Home health nurses, recognizing that their role in the future of our nation's health will be pivotal, must play a major part in providing quality and cost-effective patient care. Consequently, nurses must speak in one voice to be responsive to the trust that the public imparts to the profession. Only by doing so can we ensure that the needs of individuals, and the needs of our nation, will be met in humane and caring ways.

REFERENCES

1. Arras J et al: The technological tether: an introduction to ethical and social issues in high-tech home care, *Hastings Center Report* 24(5): special suppl, 1994.
2. Buchanan A, Brock D: Deciding for others, *Milbank Q* 64: suppl 2, 1986.
3. Callahan D: Aging and the goals of medicine, *Hastings Center Report* 24(5):39-41, 1994.
4. Callahan D: Symbols, rationality, and justice: rationing health care, *Amer J Law Med* 18(1&2):1-15, 1992.
5. Callahan D: *Setting limits,* New York, 1987, Simon & Schuster.
6. Campion EW: The oldest old, *N Engl J Med* 330(25):1819-1820, 1994.
7. Cassetta RA: Cultural competency: essential to HIV/AIDS care and prevention, *Am Nurs* 15, July/Aug 1994.
8. Collopy D, Dubler N, Tuckerman C: The ethics of home care, *Hastings Center Report* 20(2): special suppl, 1990.
9. Daniels N: *Am I my parents' keeper?* New York, 1988, Oxford University Press.
10. Daniels N et al: Meeting the challenges of justice & rationing, *Hastings Center Report* 24(4):27-42, 1994.
11. Dychtwald K, Flower J: *Age wave, the challenges and opportunities of an aging America,* Los Angeles, 1989, Jeremy P Tarcher.
12. Hills MD, Lindsey E: Health promotion: a viable curriculum framework for nursing education, *Nurs Outlook* 42(4):158-162, 1994.
13. Jennings B, Callahan D, Caplan A: Ethical challenges of chronic illness, *Hastings Center Report* 18(1): special suppl, 1988.
14. Jennings D: The confusion between disease and illness in clinical medicine, *Can Med Assoc J* 135:865-870, 1986.
15. Joint International Research Group of the Institute for Bioethics, Maastricht, the Netherlands, and The Hastings Center, Briarcliff Manor, NY, USA: What do we owe the elderly? *Hastings Center Report* 24(2): special suppl, 1994.
16. Jones K: Evolution of the prospective payment system: implications for nursing, *Nurs Econ* 7:299, 1989.
17. Kent V, Hanley B: Home health care, *Nurs Health Care* 11:234, 1990.
18. Lubitz JD, Riley GF: Trends in Medicare payments in the last year of life, *New Engl J Med* 328(15):1092-1096, 1993.
19. Mitchell PH, Krueger JC, Moody LE: The crisis of the health care nonsystem, *Nurs Outlook* 38:214, 1990.

20. Murray T et al: Individualism & community: the contested terrain of autonomy, *Hastings Center Report* 24(3):32-35, 1994.
21. Sigma Theta Tau International: Focusing on information technologies, *Reflections* 16(3):1, 1990.
22. Three times more elderly to be alone in 2030, *St. Louis Post Dispatch,* p. 18A, Aug 24, 1989.
23. Toombs SK: The temporality of illness: four levels of experience, *Theor Med* 11:227-241, 1990.
24. Veatch R: Models for medicine in a revolutionary age, *Hastings Center Report* 2(3):5-7, 1972.
25. What Americans think, *Washington Post National Weekly Edition,* p. 37, Sept 5-11, 1994.

Epilogue: Dealing with Change

Robyn Rice

> *Even if you are on the right track, if you just sit there*
> *you will get run over.*
> *—Will Rogers*

Home health nurses are hearing a lot of new words at work these days, words such as *bundling, co-payments, capitation,* and *"encounters"* rather than *"home visits."* These words reflect the tremendous amount of change going on in home care and the health care industry as a whole, change that is driven by a public demand for easily accessible yet cost-efficient health care.

In the midst of such change, home health nurses will see large regional and vertically integrated health care networks emerge as managed care systems. As a result, home health nurses will likely witness a decline in the number of freestanding community-based home health agencies.

Once the patient enters these managed care networks, all health care services will be provided. The patient will essentially write one check for all services delivered in the system. The money will be taken and divided up among services used based on capitation. Hopefully, bureaucratic paperwork will diminish.

In these managed care systems, there will be a shift from hospital care to home care; some patients will never see the hospital. Productivity for health care professionals will likely be forced up as a way to lower overall cost. Yet there will be an increasing emphasis upon total quality management (TQM) as a means to address issues such as cost-effectiveness of service delivery, clinical outcomes, and patient satisfaction with care.

As part of change, new ways of caring for patients will emerge, again resulting from a public demand for cost containment of services. For example, as a future trend, home health nurses will very likely see government reimbursement for home custodial care (which is, at present, not a covered service under the Medicare home health benefit). This would be a means to keep patients with chronic disability at home and prevent repeated, expensive rehospitalizations for exacerbations of disease process. Health promotion and rehabilitation nursing would certainly be emphasized with home custodial care.

In the midst of all this change, what are home health nurses to do? home health nurses must be willing to adapt to the times. *More important, they must survive the change.* It is important to recognize that Change presents great opportunities to move forward. If nurses who work in home care were asked to compare what they are doing today as opposed to what they were doing 10 years ago, many would say "unbelievably exciting things." Such are the opportunities for people who actively work to create their future.

How do home health nurses deal with change? They meet it head-on and begin to work together to shape change for a better tomorrow. In implementing clinical policy, it is important for home health nurses to have a voice that drives policy making. Therefore nurses should actively support state and national organizations in home care and in nursing. In terms of working with regulatory agencies, it will be important for home health nurses to monitor the *effectiveness* and *appropriateness* of future government recommendations for infection control, waste management, employee safety, and quality improvement. In preserving professional standards of practice, it will be important for home health nurses to understand the purpose of home care and, as circumstances arise, to be able to articulate their role and the role of the patient and service delivery. Likewise it will be important for home health nurses to be a player in their own communities, becoming involved in what goes on at town hall. At work, home health nurses should become active in promoting quality patient care and professional standards of practice through the auspices of case management and clinical leadership strategies. On a professional development level, home health nurses must continue to advance their level of expertise through professional certifications, workshops, and further schooling. On a personal level, home health nurses *must* make a commitment to professional unity as a platform for political processes.

No one has a crystal ball to say exactly how the future is going to be for home health nursing. The times ahead will be exciting ones. They certainly promise change, change, and more change. The best way for home health nurses to deal with change is to get *involved.*

Index

Page numbers in *italic type* refer to figures. Tables are indicated by *t* following the page number.